Zoonoses

Infectious Diseases Transmissible Between Animals and Humans

Zoonoses

Infectious Diseases Transmissible Between Animals and Humans

Rolf Bauerfeind

Institute for Hygiene and Infectious
Diseases of Animals
Justus Liebig University Giessen
Giessen, Germany

Alexander von Graevenitz

Department of Medical Microbiology
University of Zurich
Zurich, Switzerland

Peter Kimmig

Department of Parasitology
University of Hohenheim
Stuttgart, Germany

Hans Gerd Schiefer

Medical Microbiology
Justus Liebig University Giessen
Giessen, Germany

Tino Schwarz

Central Laboratory and
Vaccination Center
Stiftung Juliusspital,
University of Wuerzburg,
Wuerzburg, Germany

Werner Slenczka

Institute for Virology
University Hospital of Marburg
and Giessen
Marburg/Lahn, Germany

Horst Zahner

Institute for Parasitology
Justus Liebig University Giessen
Giessen, Germany

Library of Congress Cataloging-in-Publication Data

Names: Bauerfeind, R. (Rolf), editor. | Von Graevenitz, Alexander, editor. | Kimmig, Peter, editor. | Schiefer, H. G. (Hans Gerd), 1935-editor. | Schwarz, Tino F., editor. | Slenczka, Werner, editor. | Zahner, Horst, editor.
Title: Zoonoses: infectious diseases transmissible between animals and humans/editors, Rolf Bauerfeind, Justus Liebig University Giessen, Giessen, Germany; Alexander von Graevenitz, University of Zurich, Zurich, Switzerland; Peter Kimmig, University of Hohenheim, Stuttgart, Germany; Hans Gerd Schiefer, Justus Liebig University Giessen, Giessen, Germany; Tino Schwarz, University of Wuerzburg, Wuerzburg, Germany; Werner Slenczka, University Hospital Giessen and Margurg, Marburg/Lahn, Germany; Horst Zahner, Justus Liebig University Giessen, Giessen, Germany.
Other titles: Zoonosen. English
Description: Fourth edition. | Washington, DC: ASM Press, [2016] | ?2016 | Includes bibliographical references and index.
Identifiers: LCCN 2015037193 | ISBN 9781555819255 (alk. paper)
Subjects: LCSH: Zoonoses.
Classification: LCC RC113.5.Z6813 2016 | DDC 616.95/9–dc23 LC record available at http://lccn.loc.gov/2015037193

ISBN 978-1-55581-925-5
e-ISBN 978-1-55581-926-2
doi:10.1128/9781555819262

Printed in Canada

10 9 8 7 6 5 4 3 2 1

Address editorial correspondence to: ASM Press, 1752 N St., N.W., Washington, DC 20036-2904, USA.
Send orders to: ASM Press, P.O. Box 605, Herndon, VA 20172, USA.
Phone: 800-546-2416; 703-661-1593. Fax: 703-661-1501.
E-mail: books@asmusa.org
Online: http://estore.asm.org

Contents

Preface   xiii

Introduction   xv

Abbreviations   xvii

---

1   Viral Zoonoses   1

1.1   **Introduction   1**
  1.1.1   Classification Principles   1
  1.1.2   Zoonotic viruses   1
    1.1.2.1   Bat-borne viruses   3
    1.1.2.2   Zoonotic viruses as B-weapons   4
    1.1.2.3   Global distribution of zoonotic agents   4
  1.1.3   Cycles of Arbovirus Infections   5

1.2   **Zoonoses Caused by Alphaviruses   8**
  1.2.1   Agents   8
  1.2.2   Alphaviral Zoonoses   8
  1.2.3   Eastern Equine Encephalitis   10
  1.2.4   Western Equine Encephalitis   12
  1.2.5   Venezuelan Equine Encephalitis   14
  1.2.6   Semliki Forest Fever   16
  1.2.7   Sindbis Fever   17
  1.2.8   Epidemic Polyarthritis (Ross River Fever) and Barmah Forest Fever   18
  1.2.9   Chikungunya Fever   21
  1.2.10   O'Nyong-Nyong Fever   24
  1.2.11   Mayaro Fever   25

1.3   **Zoonoses Caused by Flaviviruses   26**
  1.3.1   Agents   26
  1.3.2   Complexes of the *Flaviviridae* with Clinical Importance   27
    1.3.2.1   Virus Complex Transmitted by Ticks   27

         1.3.2.2   *Virus Complex Transmitted by Mosquitoes: Japanese Encephalitis Virus and Related Encephalitis Viruses* *27*

         1.3.2.3   *Agents Causing Yellow Fever and Dengue, Forming Two Closely Related Virus Complexes* *27*

    1.3.3   Zoonoses Caused by Tick-Borne Flaviviruses 32

         1.3.3.1   *Tick-Borne Encephalitis (TBE) European Subtype (Central European Encephalitis) and TBE Eastern Subtype (Russian Spring-Summer Meningoencephalitis)* *32*

         1.3.3.2   *Louping Ill* *37*

         1.3.3.3   *Powassan Virus Encephalitis* *38*

         1.3.3.4   *Kyasanur Forest Disease and Alkhurma Virus Hemorrhagic Fever* *39*

         1.3.3.5   *Omsk Hemorrhagic Fever* *40*

    1.3.4   Zoonoses Caused by Mosquito-Borne Flaviviruses 41

         1.3.4.1   *Japanese Encephalitis* *41*

         1.3.4.2   *Murray Valley Encephalitis and Kunjin Virus Disease* *44*

         1.3.4.3   *St. Louis Encephalitis* *46*

         1.3.4.4   *Rocio Encephalitis* *48*

         1.3.4.5   *West Nile Fever* *49*

         1.3.4.6   *Usutu Virus* *52*

         1.3.4.7   *Wesselsbron Fever* *52*

         1.3.4.8   *Yellow Fever* *53*

         1.3.4.9   *Dengue Fever (Dengue Hemorrhagic Fever and Dengue Shock Syndrome)* *58*

1.4   Zoonoses Caused by Bunyaviruses 65

    1.4.1   La Crosse (California Encephalitis) Virus, Snowshoe Hare Virus, and Tahyna Virus 68

    1.4.2   Oropouche Fever 70

    1.4.3   Crimean-Congo Hemorrhagic Fever 71

    1.4.4   Rift Valley Fever 73

    1.4.5   Sandfly Fever 76

    1.4.6   Zoonoses Caused by Hantaviruses 78

         1.4.6.1   *Hemorrhagic Fever with Renal Syndrome (Old World Hantaviruses) and Hantavirus Pulmonary Syndrome (New World Hantaviruses)* *78*

1.5   Zoonoses Caused by Reoviruses (*Coltiviridae* and *Orbiviridae*) 83

    1.5.1   Genus *Coltivirus* 83

         1.5.1.1   *Colorado Tick Fever* *83*

    1.5.2   Genus *Orbivirus* (Kemerovo Complex) 85

    1.5.3   Genus Rotavirus 85

1.6   Zoonoses Caused by Arenaviruses 88

    1.6.1   Lymphocytic Choriomeningitis 89

    1.6.2   Lassa Fever 92

    1.6.3   Zoonoses Caused by New World Arenaviruses (Agents of Hemorrhagic Fever) 95

1.7   Zoonoses Caused by Filoviruses 97

    1.7.1   Marburg Virus Hemorrhagic Fever 99

    1.7.2   Ebola Virus Hemorrhagic Fever 104

1.8 Zoonoses Caused by Rhabdoviruses 109
  1.8.1   Rabies 110
  1.8.2   Vesicular Stomatitis 117

1.9 Zoonoses Caused by Paramyxoviruses 119
  1.9.1   Newcastle Disease 120
  1.9.2   Zoonoses Caused by Hendra Virus 122
  1.9.3   Nipah Virus Encephalitis 124

1.10 Zoonoses Caused by Orthomyxoviruses 127
  1.10.1   Influenza-Viruses 127
       1.10.1.1 Swine Influenza Virus H1N1 129
       1.10.1.2 Avian Influenza Viruses H5N1, H7N7, H7N9, and H9N2 131
  1.10.2   Thogotoviruses 133

1.11 Zoonoses Caused by Picornaviruses 134
  1.11.1   Swine Vesicular Disease 134
  1.11.2   Foot-and-Mouth Disease 135
  1.11.3   Encephalomyocarditis 138

1.12 Hepatitis E 139

1.13 Coronaviruses 140
  1.13.1   SARS: Severe Acute Respiratory Syndrome 141
  1.13.2   Middle East Respiratory Syndrome Coronavirus
            (MERS-CoV) 144

1.14 Retroviruses 147
  1.14.1   Primate T-cell-Lymphotropic Viruses: PTLV 1 and PTLV 2
            (HTLV 1 and 2) 147
  1.14.2   Lentiviruses: HIV 1 and HIV 2 149
  1.14.3   Endogenous Retroviruses 152

1.15 Zoonoses Caused by Herpesviruses 153
  1.15.1   Herpes B Virus: Simian Herpes Infection 153

1.16 Zoonoses Caused by Poxviruses 156
  1.16.1   Zoonoses Caused by Orthopoxviruses 158
  1.16.2   Individual Orthopoxvirus Infections 159
       1.16.2.1 Monkeypox 159
       1.16.2.2 Vaccinia Virus 160
       1.16.2.3 Buffalopox 163
       1.16.2.4 Camelpox 163
       1.16.2.5 Cowpox 164
       1.16.2.6 Elephantpox 164
  1.16.3   Parapoxvirus Infections 165
       1.16.3.1 Contagious Ecthyma of Sheep (Orf) 165
       1.16.3.2 Milker's Nodules (Pseudocowpox) 166
       1.16.3.3 Papular Stomatitis 166
  1.16.4   Zoonoses Caused by Yabapoxviruses 167
       1.16.4.1 Tanapox Virus 167
       1.16.4.2 Yaba Monkey Tumor Virus 167

1.17 Zoonoses Associated with Prions 167
  1.17.1 Bovine Spongiform Encephalopathy and the New Variant of
          Creutzfeldt - Jakob disease 169

2   Bacterial Zoonoses 175

2.1   Introduction 175

2.2   Anthrax 175

2.3   Bartonelloses 179
  2.3.1   Cat Scratch Disease 180
  2.3.2   Endocarditis due to *Bartonella* Species 182
  2.3.3   *Bartonella* Infections in Immunocompromised Patients 182

2.4   Borrelioses 183
  2.4.1   Lyme Borreliosis 183
  2.4.2   Relapsing Fever 189

2.5   Brucelloses 191

2.6   Campylobacterioses 195

2.7   Chlamydioses 198
  2.7.1   Psittacosis/Ornithosis 199
  2.7.2   Chlamydioses Transmitted from Mammals 201

2.8   Ehrlichioses/Anaplasmosis 202

2.9   Enterohemorrhagic *Escherichia coli* (EHEC) Infections 206

2.10 Erysipeloid 211

2.11 Glanders 214

2.12 Leptospiroses 216

2.13 Listeriosis 219

2.14 Mycobacterioses 223
  2.14.1 Infections with the *Mycobacterium tuberculosis*
          Complex 223
  2.14.2 Infections with *Mycobacterium marinum* 228
  2.14.3 Possible Zoonotic Mycobacterioses 229
          2.14.3.1 Infections with M. avium *subsp.* avium *230*
          2.14.3.2 Infections with M. avium *subsp.* hominissuis *230*
          2.14.3.3 Infections with M. avium *subsp.* paratuberculosis *231*
          2.14.3.4 Infections with M. genavense *232*

2.15 Pasteurelloses 232

2.16 Plague 234

2.17 Q Fever 238

2.18 Rat Bite Fever 242

2.19 Rickettsioses 244
 2.19.1 General Features 244
 2.19.2 Rocky Mountain Spotted Fever 248
 2.19.3 Mediterranean Spotted Fever 249
 2.19.4 African Tick Bite Fever and Other Spotted Fever Diseases 251
 2.19.5 Rickettsioses in Central Europe 252
 2.19.6 Rickettsialpox 252
 2.19.7 Epidemic Typhus 253
 2.19.8 Murine Typhus 254
 2.19.9 Tsutsugamushi Fever (Scrub Typhus) 256

2.20 Salmonelloses 257

2.21 Staphylococcal Infections 262

2.22 Streptococcal Infections 264
 2.22.1 General Features 264
 2.22.2 *Streptococcus equi* infections (Group C) 264
 2.22.3 *Streptococcus suis* Infections (groups R, S, and T) 266
 2.22.4 *Streptococcus pyogenes* (serogroup A) Infections 267
 2.22.5 *Streptococcus agalactiae* (serogroup B) Infections 267
 2.22.6 Infections with other *Streptococcus* spp 267

2.23 Tularemia 269

2.24 Vibrioses 272
 2.24.1 Cholera 273
 2.24.2 Disease due to other *Vibrio* spp. and closely related species 275

2.25 Yersinioses (Enteric Infections due to *Yersinia enterocolitica* and *Y. pseudotuberculosis*) 276

2.26 Rare and Potential Agents of Bacterial Zoonoses 280
 2.26.1 *Actinobacillus* Infections 280
 2.26.2 *Aeromonas* Infections 280
 2.26.3 *Arcobacter* Infections 281
 2.26.4 *Bordetella* Infections 282
 2.26.5 *Capnocytophaga* Infections 283
 2.26.6 *Corynebacterium pseudotuberculosis* Infections 284
 2.26.7 *Corynebacterium ulcerans* Infections 285
 2.26.8 *Dermatophilus congolensis* Infections 286
 2.26.9 *Helicobacter* Infections 287
 2.26.10 Melioidosis (*Burkholderia pseudomallei* Infections) 288
 2.26.11 *Rhodococcus equi* Infections 290
 2.26.12 *Trueperella pyogenes* Infections 291

3 Fungal Zoonoses 293

3.1 Introduction 293

3.2 Dermatophytoses Caused by *Microsporum* spp 293

3.3 Dermatophytoses Caused by *Trichophyton* spp 296

3.4 Sporotrichosis 298

3.5 Pneumocystosis (*Pneumocystis* Pneumonia) as a
Potential Zoonotic Mycosis 300

4 Parasitic Zoonoses 303

4.1 Introduction 303

4.2 Zoonoses Caused by Protozoa 306
4.2.1 Amebiasis 307
4.2.2 Babesiosis 312
4.2.3 Balantidiasis 315
4.2.4 Chagas' Disease (American Trypanosomiasis) 317
4.2.5 Cryptosporidiosis 324
4.2.6 Giardiasis (Lambliasis) 328
4.2.7 Leishmaniasis 330
4.2.7.1 *Visceral Leishmaniasis (Kala-Azar)* 332
4.2.7.2 *Old World Cutaneous Leishmaniasis* 337
4.2.7.3 *American Cutaneous and Mucocutaneous Leishmaniases
(Espundia and Related Forms)* 339
4.2.8 Microsporoses 341
4.2.9 Monkey Malaria (Simian Malaria) 345
4.2.10 Sarcosporidiosis 348
4.2.11 Sleeping Sickness (African Trypanosomiasis) 351
4.2.12 Toxoplasmosis 355
4.2.13 Other Zoonotic Protozoal Infections 362

4.3 Zoonoses Caused by Trematodes 363
4.3.1 Cercarial Dermatitis 363
4.3.2 Clonorchiasis 366
4.3.3 Dicrocoeliais (Distomatosis) 368
4.3.4 Dwarf Fluke Infections (Intestinal Dwarf Fluke Infections) 369
4.3.5 Fascioliasis 370
4.3.6 Fasciolopsiasis 374
4.3.7 Opisthorchiasis 375
4.3.8 Paragonimiasis (Pulmonary Distomatosis) 376
4.3.9 Schistosomiasis (Bilharziosis) 378
4.3.10 Other Zoonotic Trematode Infections 383

4.4 Zoonoses Caused by Cestodes 384
4.4.1 Coenurosis 385
4.4.2 Diphyllobothriasis (Broad Tapeworm infection) 386
4.4.3 Dipylidiosis 389
4.4.4 Echinococcosis 390
4.4.4.1 *Alveolar echinococcosis* 390
4.4.4.2 *Cystic Echinococcosis (Hydatidosis)* 395
4.4.5 Hymenolepiasis (Dwarf Tapeworm Infection) 399
4.4.6 Sparganosis 401

4.4.7   Taeniasis saginata (including Taeniasis asiatica)   402

4.4.8   Taeniasis solium and Cysticercosis   405

4.4.9   Other Zoonotic Cestode Infections   408

     4.4.9.1   *Intestinal Infestation: Etiology, Occurrence, and Transmission   408*

     4.4.9.2   *Extraintestinal Infestation: Infection with* Taenia crassiceps   *409*

4.5   Zoonoses Caused by Nematodes   409

    4.5.1   Angiostrongyliasis   410

        4.5.1.1   *Cerebral Angiostrongyliasis (Eosinophilic Meningoencephalitis or Eosinophilic Meningitis)   410*

        4.5.1.2   *Intestinal Angiostrongyliasis   411*

    4.5.2   Anisakiasis (Herring Worm Disease)   412

    4.5.3   Capillariases   415

        4.5.3.1   *Hepatic Capillariasis   415*

        4.5.3.2   *Intestinal Capillariasis   416*

        4.5.3.3   *Pulmonary Capillariasis   417*

    4.5.4   Dioctophymiasis   418

    4.5.5   Dracunculiasis (Guinea Worm Infection)   418

    4.5.6   Eosinophilic Enteritis   420

    4.5.7   Filariases   421

        4.5.7.1   *Brugia Filariasis (Lymphatic Filariasis)   422*

        4.5.7.2   *Dirofilariasis   425*

    4.5.8   Gnathostomiasis   426

    4.5.9   Gongylonemiasis   427

    4.5.10   Hookworm Infection (Infection with *Ancylostoma ceylanicum*)   428

    4.5.11   Lagochilascariasis   429

    4.5.12   Larva Migrans Cutanea (Creeping Eruption)   430

    4.5.13   Larva Migrans Visceralis   432

    4.5.14   Oesophagostomiasis   434

    4.5.15   Strongyloidiasis   435

    4.5.16   Syngamiasis   438

    4.5.17   Thelaziasis   439

    4.5.18   Trichinellosis (Trichinosis)   440

    4.5.19   Trichostrongylidiasis   445

    4.5.20   Other Zoonotic Infections by Nematodes   446

4.6   Zoonoses Caused by Acanthocephala   447

    4.6.1   Acanthocephaliosis   447

4.7   Zoonoses Caused by Arthropods   449

    4.7.1   Zoonoses Caused by Ticks   449

        4.7.1.1   *Tick Bites   449*

        4.7.1.2   *Tick Toxicoses (Tick Paralyses)   454*

    4.7.2   Zoonoses Caused by Mites   455

    4.7.3   Zoonoses Caused by Diptera   459

        4.7.3.1   *Dipteran Bites   460*

        4.7.3.2   *Myiasis   464*

    4.7.4   Zoonoses Caused by Fleas (Siphonaptera)   467

        4.7.4.1   *Flea bites   467*

        4.7.4.2   *Tungiasis (Chigoe Flea infestation)   469*

    4.7.5   Infestations by Heteroptera (Bed Bugs and Triatomine Bugs)   471

4.8 Zoonoses Caused by Pentastomids   473
    4.8.1   Pentastomidosis, Linguatulosis (Halzoun, Marrara Syndrome)   473

Appendix A   477

A.1   Animal Bite Infections   477
    A.1.1   Dog Bites and Bites by Foxes, Skunks, and Raccoons   477
    A.1.2   Cat Bites   478
    A.1.3   Simian Bites   478
    A.1.4   Alligator Bites   479
    A.1.5   Squirrel Bites   479
    A.1.6   Lizard Bites   479
    A.1.7   Fish Bites   479
    A.1.8   Bat Bites   479
    A.1.9   Shark Bites   479
    A.1.10   Hamster/Guinea Pig/Ferret Bites   479
    A.1.11   Camel Bites   479
    A.1.12   Opossum Bites   480
    A.1.13   Horse Bites   480
    A.1.14   Rat and Mouse Bites   480
    A.1.15   Sheep Bites   480
    A.1.16   Snake Bites   480
    A.1.17   Pig Bites   480
    A.1.18   Seal Bites   480
    A.1.19   Bird Bites   480
    A.1.20   Bear Bites   480

Appendix B: Infections and Intoxications Transmissible by Foodstuffs of Animal Origin   483

B.1   Viruses   483

B.2   Bacteria   484

B.3   Fungi (Mycotoxins)   486

B.4   Parasites   486

B.5   Fish Poisoning   488

B.6   Shellfish Poisoning   488

B.7   Phytotoxins Transmitted by Bats   496

Appendix C: Iatrogenic Transmission of Zoonotic Agents   499

Appendix D: Zoonotic Diseases Notifiable at the National Level   503

Index   505

Preface

Zoonoses are infectious diseases transmissible from vertebrate animals to humans and vice versa under natural conditions. They comprise a complex spectrum of diseases due to the diversity of pathogenic agents involved. They may confront veterinarians as well as general practitioners, pediatricians, infectious disease specialists, and microbiologists with special diagnostic and therapeutic problems. While we did not intend to write a handbook of zoonoses, we wanted to cover not only well-known diseases but also rare ones that may be of importance to physicians active in developing countries and to travelers going to distant or rarely visited areas.

Our book is based on the 4th German edition of *Zoonosen: Zwischen Tier und Mensch übertragbare Infektionskrankheiten* which was published in 2013 by Deutscher Ärzte-Verlag, Cologne, Germany. It has been thoroughly revised, updated, and amended.

We have tried to present the most significant aspects of the great variety of zoonotic diseases in a concise manner. However, in some cases readers may even need more detailed information.

We express our appreciation to Christine Charlip, Director, and Larry Klein, Production Manager of ASM Press for their constant encouragement, assistance and advice. We are indebted to Professor Gaby Pfyffer von Altishofen, Lucerne, for helpful suggestions and constructive criticism of the chapter on mycobacterioses, and Dr Tanja Matt, Zürich, for technical help with the figures on transmission chains. We also want to thank Prof. Peter Mayser, Giessen, for valuable advice on the chapter on fungal zoonoses and Prof. Brigitte Frank, Hohenheim, for her support in the translation. And all of us, particularly those involved in translating the German text into English, are deeply grateful to our families for their patience, tolerance, and support.

Finally it is the particular concern of the authors to commemorate our co-author Hans Gerd Schiefer who unfortunately died shortly before completion of this edition. His work and participation had been extremely important for this book.

Introduction

Numerous human infectious diseases are caused by agents that are directly or indirectly transmissible from various animal species to humans. Today, more than 200 diseases occurring in humans and animals are known to be mutually transmitted. They are caused by prions, viruses, bacteria (including rickettsiae and chlamydiae), fungi, protozoa, and helminths, as well as arthropods. An Expert Committee of the World Health Organization defined zoonoses in 1958 as "diseases and infections which are naturally transmitted between vertebrates and humans." This definition is still valid.

Originally, zoonoses were regarded as animal diseases (in Greek *zoon* means "animal"). In the 19th century, the meaning of the word changed. Thus, in 1855, R. Virchow included in his book, *Handbuch der Speciellen Pathologie und Therapie*, the chapter "Infectionen durch contagiöse Thiergifte" ("Infections Caused by Animal Contagious Poisons") with the subtitle "Zoonosen" ("Zoonoses"). Shortly after this, the word "zoonoses" received a double meaning for the first time. W. Probstmayer (1863) stated in the *Etymologisches Wörterbuch der Veterinärmedizin und ihrer Hilfswissenschaften* (Etymological Dictionary of Veterinary Medicine and its Auxilliary Sciences) "zoonoses are (i) animal diseases and (ii) diseases of humans transmitted from animals by means of a vector or contact." Today, no difference is made with regard to the direction of transmission, that is, animal to human or human to animal, although attempts exist to describe precisely the direction of transmission. The term "zooanthroponoses" referred to diseases transmitted from animals to humans, and the term "anthropozoonoses" referred to diseases transmitted from humans to animals. However, the latter play only a minor role in the epidemiology of zoonoses. The term "zoonosis" still underlies conceptual changes. For instance, increasing epidemiological knowledge has put into doubt the traditional associations of some infectious diseases with zoonoses. Diseases that do not require a vertebrate reservoir because of their occurrence in water, in soil, on plants, or in food or fodder, whence they are transmitted to vertebrates (including humans), are also called sapronoses, saprozoonoses, or geonoses.

Zoonoses are a persisting threat to the human society. Classical infectious diseases, such as rabies, plague, and yellow fever, well known for centuries, are zoonoses that have not been eradicated despite major efforts. And the importance of zoonoses still increases. In recent years, new zoonotic entities, for example, Lyme borreliosis, ehrlichiosis, infections with enterohemorrhagic *Escherichia coli*, cryptosporidiosis, and hantavirus pulmonary syndrome, have been detected.

The steadily increasing threat that zoonoses pose to humans have many causes that differ from country to country. Overpopulation, wars, and progressive deterioration of living conditions may cause migration of countless people into slums of large cities, with a subsequent breakdown of hygiene and public health care. The proximity of their dwellings to huge garbage dumping grounds and their dependence on water contaminated with sewage facilitate contact with rodents, stray animals, and their parasites.

Scarcity of food forces millions of humans to clear woodlands for cultivation and to produce new settlements in areas where animal populations and their pathogenic agents were formerly separated from humans. Humans may participate unwittingly in unknown parasite-host cycles and become a new link in an infectious chain. In many of these cases, humans, as accidental hosts, are in no way adapted to the new pathogenic species, which may result in high mortality.

Artificial irrigation changes the ecology of whole countries. Artificial lakes and ponds attract animals and their parasites over vast distances and provide optimal breeding grounds, especially for mosquitoes. Increasingly warm and moist winters in the Northern Hemisphere favor the propagation of parasites, especially ticks. Stray animals, usually infected with various pathogens, are reservoirs for infectious agents, not only in developing countries, but also in developed countries.

Worldwide tourism, especially trekking tours to remote areas and so-called adventure challenges (e.g., "survival training" with camping in open areas and consumption of raw or insufficiently cooked food) has encouraged contact of humans from industrialized countries who grew up under nearly aseptic conditions and agents and vectors that they have never encountered before.

Zoonotic agents of low virulence may cause fatal infections in immunosuppressed humans (e.g., patients infected with HIV).

A further potential source of infection is transport of breeding and slaughter animals over vast distances and across borders, often with insufficient inspection for disease control. New disease agents may be introduced to a country by legal, or, even worse, illegal importation of exotic animals for zoos, research purposes, or private homes. Isolated animal organs (xenotransplants) and cultures of animal cells may contain dangerous zoonotic agents. Furthermore, several zoonotic pathogens, for example, *Francisella tularensis, Yersinia pestis, Brucella* spp., *Bacillus anthracis, Coxiella burnetii*, and hemorragic fever viruses, are considered possible bioterrorism weapons.

The problem of diseases transmitted between animals and humans has many aspects, especially as it is not uncommon for animals serving as reservoir or intermediate hosts to be clinically inapparent carriers and/or excreters of an agent. Undoubtedly, currently unknown zoonoses will emerge in future. New methods for direct or indirect detection of microorganisms contribute to the detection of new zoonoses. When human invasion of hitherto uninhabited areas results in voluntary or involuntary environmental changes, new and potentially dangerous zoonoses may become evident. Severe acute respiratory syndrome, caused by a newly emerged coronavirus, is one of the latest examples of the threat of dangerous infections, although its possible zoonotic background has not yet been clarified.

In the study of zoonoses, medical experts and veterinarians should cooperate closely to study the etiology, epidemiology, and frequently complex developmental cycles and modes of transmission of pathogens and their vectors, as well as the clinical presentation, diagnosis, differential diagnosis, therapy, and prophylaxis of the attendant diseases. Our book is based on such cooperation, which since recently, is also postulated under the concept "One World – One Health."

REFERENCES

Barras V, Greub G, History of biological warfare and bioterrorism. *Clin. Microbiol. Infect.* 20(6), 497–502, 2014.

Christian MD, Biowelfare and bioterrorism. *Crit. Care Clin.* 29, 717–756, 2013.

Hamele M, Poss WB, Sweney J, Disaster prepardness, pediatric considerations in primary blast injury, chemical, and biological terrorism. *World J. Crit. Care Med.* 3, 15–23, 2014.

Klietmann WF, Ruoff KL, Bioterrorism: implications for the clinical microbiologist. *Clin. Microbiol. Rev.* 14, 364–381, 2001.

Rotz LD et al., Public health assessment of potential biological terrorism agents. *Emerg. Infect. Dis.* 8, 225–230, 2002.

Abbreviations

ACA	Acrodermatitis chronica atrophicans
AIDS	Acquired immunodeficiency syndrome
ARDS	Acute respiratory distress syndrome
a.s.l.	Above sea level
AV	Atrioventricular
BSL	Biosafety level
CD4	Cluster of differentiation 4 (glycoprotein on the surface of several immune cells)
CDC	Centers for Disease Control and Prevention
cDNA	Complementary DNA
CF test	Complement fixation test
CFU	Colony forming units
CIN	Agar cefsulodin-irgasan-novobiocin agar
CMV	Cytomegalovirus
CNS	Central nervous system
CPK	Creatine phosphokinase
CSD	Cat scratch disease
CSF	Cerebrospinal fluid
CT	Computed tomography
DNA	Deoxyribonucleic acid
EDTA	Ethylenediaminetetraacetate/etylenediaminetetraacetic acid
EHEC	Enterohemorrhagic *Escherichia coli*
EIA	Enzyme immunoassay
ELISA	Enzyme linked immunosorbent assay
EPEC	Enteropathogenic *Escherichia coli*
ETB	Ethambutol
FDA	US Food and Drug Administration
HAART	Highly active antiretroviral therapy
HACCP	Hazard analysis critical control point
HAT	Human African trypanosomiasis
HE	Hektoen enteric (agar)

HGA	Human granulocytic anaplasmosis
HGE	Human granulocytic ehrlichiosis
HIV	Human immunodeficiency virus
HLA	Human leukocyte antigen
HME	Human monocytic ehrlichiosis
HUS	Hemolytic-uremic syndrome
IARC	International Agency for Research on Cancer (WHO)
ICU	Intensive care unit
IF(A)	Immunofluorescence (assay)
Ig(A,G,M)	Immunoglobulin(A,G,M)
IGR	Insect growth regulator
IHA	Indirect hemagglutination assay
IIFT	Indirect immunofluorescence test
IL	Interleukin
i.m.	Intramuscular
INH	Isonicotinic acid hydrazide/isoniazide
i.p.	Intraperitoneal
i.v.	Intravenous
kbp	Kilobase pairs
kDa	Kilodalton
LAMP	Loop-mediated isothermal amplification
LEE	Locus of enterocyte effacement
LPS	Lipopolysaccharide
MAA	*Mycobacterium avium* subsp. *avium*
MAH	*Mycobacterium avium* subsp. *hominissuis*
MAI	*Mycobacterium avium-intracellulare*
MALDI-TOF	Matrix-assisted laser desorption ionization-time-of-flight mass spectrometry
MAP	*Mycobacterium avium* subsp. *paratuberculosis*
MAT	Microagglutination test
mb	Megabases
MHC	Major histocompatibility complex
MID	Minimum infective dose
mio	Million
MPS	Mononuclear phagocytic system
MRI	Magnetic resonance imaging
mRNA	Messenger RNA
MMT	Mendel-Mantoux test
MOMP	Mitochondrial outer membrane protein
MRSA	Methicillin-resistant *Staphylococcus aureus*
NSF	National Science Foundation
NNN	Novy-McNeal-Nicolle medium
NTM	Non-tuberculous mycobacterium
PAHO	Pan American Health Organization
PCR	Polymerase chain reaction
PFGE	Pulse field gel electrophoresis
PFU	Plaque forming unit
p.i.	Post infection
PI-IBS	Post infectious irritable bowel syndrome

p.o.	Peroral
p.p.	Post partum
RES	Reticuloendothelial system
RFLP	Restriction fragment length polymorphism
RMP	Rifampicin
RMSF	Rocky Mountain spotted fever
RNA	Ribonucleic acid
rRNA	Ribosomal RNA
RT-PCR	Reverse transcription PCR
SAF	Sodium acetic acid formaldehyde
s.c.	Subcutaneous
SCV	Small cell variant
SIRS	Systemic inflammatory response syndrome
s.l.	Sensu lato
SMAC	Sorbitol-MacConkey agar
spf	Specific pathogen free
SS	Salmonella-Shigella (agar)
s.s.	Sensu stricto
SSG	Sodium stibogluconate
STEC	Shiga toxin producing *Escherichia coli*
STx	Shiga toxin
Th (1,2)	T helper cell (1,2)
Tir	Translocated intimin receptor
TNF	Tumor necrosis factor
Tris	Tris(hydroxymethyl)aminomethane
TTP	Thrombotic thombocytopenic purpura
USDA	United States Department of Agriculture
UV	Ultraviolet
VSG	Variant surface glycoprotein(s) of African trypanosomes
WHO	World Health Organization
XLD	Xylose-lysine-deoxycholate (agar)

Viral Zoonoses

1

1.1 Introduction

1.1.1 CLASSIFICATION PRINCIPLES

Viruses are usually classified according to structural principles and genetic homology. Agents causing zoonoses exist in various virus groups that have similarities in the disease patterns that they induce. There may also be similarities involved in hosts and vectors. In this chapter, we have chosen a sequential arrangement following viral classifications for the most part. This sequence makes it possible to point out similarities within individual virus groups. Tables include the geographical distribution and clinical signs that are important for differential diagnosis. Viral zoonoses are also compared with nonviral zoonotic diseases.

1.1.2 ZOONOTIC VIRUSES

Among the agents causing zoonotic disease, zoonotic viruses are the most abundant and the majority of zoonotic viruses have RNA as genetic material. DNA viruses, due to effective proofreading mechanisms of the DNA polymerases, have greater genetic stability, restricting their host range to a spectrum of closely interrelated host animals. Only poxviruses and some representatives of the herpes virus family are able to cross species barriers and cause zoonotic infections.

RNA viruses on the other hand do not have proofreading mechanisms; consequently, every reproductive cycle will produce a great number of genetic variants, which may often be unable to reproduce in their original host cells. By chance, new variants may be produced with the ability to extend the host range to other hosts. Of course, all these variants will have to overcome a selection process that will, in most cases, restrict, or in some cases, even improve their reproductive success.

Single point mutation is not the only mechanism that is responsible for the variability of RNA viruses. In addition, some groups of RNA viruses have powerful mechanisms to use genetic recombination or genetic reassortment to extend their genetic variability enabling them to change or enlarge their host range, an ideal preposition for the life cycle of a zoonotic virus. Regarding the genetic variability of RNA-bacteriophages, von Eigen has coined the term "quasispecies," which offers an ideal understanding of the variability of zoonotic RNA viruses. In consequence of these developments, it has become more difficult to explain and to understand the relative stability that is observed in some none zoonotic RNA virus species, for example, in measles, mumps or rubella.

- In most RNA viruses, the recognition of a "species" is defined by a great diversity of selective mechanisms or circumstances, too large to be discussed in this text. Some of these restrictions are due to human habits and to the mobility of human populations; others are due to geographic conditions. In many cases, the restricting circumstances are not understood at all. For example, the virus of Venezuelan horse encephalitis, an alpha virus, normally exists in enzootic cycles, where it is transmitted by mosquitoes. From time to time, variants of this virus appear which cause epizootic disease in horses with a high rate of fatal encephalitis. Next to horses, humans are affected by the virus. These epizootic or epidemic variants of the virus are not detectable in the interepidemic periods, although the host reservoir of the enzootic variants is well known. In the same way, hitherto unknown viruses may by chance infect the human population and they may cause outbreaks of severe disease. The unexpected appearance of new viruses, such as Marburg virus and Lassa virus, which have caused outbreaks in the sixties of the last century with an at that time completely unknown, extreme rate of fatalities has motivated Joshua Lederberg to coin the term of "emerging infections." This term describes nothing but a phenomenon. Since that time, a great number of "new" zoonotic agents have emerged, not only viruses but also bacteria and even protozoa. However, in each of these examples, the circumstances and reasons of emergence are different.

In some cases, viruses have established themselves in the human host so successfully that epidemics and epizootics can proceed independently of each other. In such cases, the classification as a zoonosis is justified if a host change from an animal to a human host can be proven. Examples are the influenza A viruses and the rotaviruses. Both viruses are widespread in animal hosts and cause epizootics that do not necessarily lead to epidemic spread. Influenza A viruses and rotaviruses have segmented genomes that allow genetic exchange by reassortment. New variants, differing from the original virus in respect to host range, pathogenicity, and contagiosity may result from genetic recombination. In hepatitis E, there is also coexistence of epidemic and epizootic spread. In this case, it has been shown that among the four viral subtypes, strains 1 and 2 cause epidemics that are spread via the fecal-oral route. Strains 3 and 4 are causing zoonotic infections that are not transmitted by human-to-human contacts.

The causal agents of AIDS, the human immunodeficiency (HI) viruses, have switched to epidemic spread in a short period of time. However, even in this case, the zoonotic origin is indisputable as HIV I and HIV II exhibit a close relationship with immunodeficiency viruses occurring in monkeys and sporadic transmission of the simian viruses to humans happens. HIV I is closely related to SIV-cpz, a chimpanzee virus (from *Pan troglodytes*), HIV II is most probably derived from a virus that persists in mangabeys (*Cercocebus torquatus*). Genetic analyses have shown that HIV I was transferred at a minimum of four different occasions from chimpanzees or gorillas to humans.

Narrow relatives exist in the animal kingdom of TT virus, a newly discovered parvovirus, which is transferred between humans via blood transfusions. As human infections result from contact with infected people, and not from animal contacts, we do not speak of a zoonosis. Foamy agent is a simian retrovirus that is transmitted to people working or living in close contact with monkeys but apparently does not cause disease. This virus does not meet the definition of a zoonotic virus. Borna-virus, a horse virus belonging to the *Negavirales*, is highly pathogenic for horses. Antibodies against Borna are also found in the human population, mainly in psychiatric patients. The meaning is unclear. As all viral isolates obtained from human specimens agree in their genomic base sequence and do not differ from the laboratory strain, there is no convincing proof that these viruses are transferred from animals to humans. Newer findings about a murine retrovirus, XMRV, which is supposed to be transferred with blood donations, are based on serological evidence that has not been confirmed by other investigators.

This book does not include virus infections primarily affecting humans that are normally transmitted from human-to-human and only under special circumstances are transmitted to animals. Herpes simplex virus and hepatitis A virus are examples, both of which can be transmitted to monkeys.

Clams have long been known to pick up and concentrate viruses pathogenic for humans from sewage. In particular, enteroviruses, calicivirus, reoviruses, and hepatitis A and B viruses can be found in clams. Hepatitis A virus and several agents causing gastroenteritis, such as the "Norwalk agent," have caused epidemics in humans after eating clams. These infections caused by food-borne viruses are, according to present knowledge, not considered to be zoonoses. They are mentioned only in the context of food-borne infections in this book.

Virus infections, such as Russian spring-summer encephalitis and Kyasanur Forest disease, which are spread by ticks but may be transmitted from milk of infected animals, are included as zoonoses.

New arboviruses (arthropod-borne viruses) with a potential for human and animal infection without causing disease (see "Cycles of Arbovirus Infections" below) are constantly being isolated. Any listing of these agents with doubtful pathogenicity for humans would be incomplete and would reach beyond the purpose of this book.

Zoonotic viruses have in some cases been transmitted to humans deliberately, for example, for the purpose of vaccination against smallpox, or inadvertently, as in the early poliomyelitis vaccines (before 1960), which are suspected to have introduced simian virus 40 (SV40) from cercopithecine monkeys to humans. This virus, a polyomavirus, is known to be oncogenic in unrelated hosts. There is, however, debate about whether a virus closely related to SV40 might have existed in humans before poliomyelitis vaccination was begun. Nevertheless, sequences of the gene coding for SV40 T antigen are found in 40% of non-Hodgkin's lymphomas but not in any other malignancies. At present, it cannot be determined whether non-Hodgkin's lymphomas constitute an example of an iatrogenic zoonosis. The intended usage of xenotransplantation, for example, the transplantation of porcine organs to humans, is criticized for the possible transmission of porcine viruses into humans. The immune suppressive therapy of the acceptor might enable a change of host species.

Some of the viruses covered in this section reflect the modern concept of emerging and reemerging infections. This concept gives the appearance of a secret, perhaps active role of the viruses when they reemerge. Mutations and changes in the host spectrum are supposed to play a role here. There are examples of the surprising and miraculous appearance of new diseases and new agents, which cannot be denied. The Rocio encephalitis virus and the equine morbillivirus (Hendra virus) should be mentioned here. The emergence of new influenza viruses pathogenic for humans has appeared as a puzzle. Nowadays, analysis of the basic molecular mechanisms of these viruses has offered a better understanding. In most instances, however, it is not the virus itself that plays the active part in its spread, but rather, it is humans, who advance into areas from which humans were formerly excluded. Oropouche virus and Kyasanur Forest virus are classical examples of this type of spreading. The violation of well-known rules in hygiene is often responsible in other cases (e.g., Lassa virus and Ebola virus) when the circumstances for the spreading of "new" viruses are clarified. The talk about "emerging and reemerging" in these cases covers up the facts and is not useful for avoiding the causes of the spread. An important causative factor, often neglected in discussions on the spectacular reemergence of arboviral diseases that we see at this time, is the interruption in the use of dichlorodiphenyltrichloroethane (DDT) as a pesticide. This effect is intensified by overpopulation in areas of endemicity and an increase in diagnostic facilities and public awareness.

1.1.2.1 Bat-borne viruses
In addition to arboviruses transmitted by arthropods and roboviruses transmitted from rodents

to humans, viruses that are transmitted from bats to animals and humans have recently been identified. They include known and newly recognized strains of rabies virus and paramyxoviruses, which are transmitted by flying foxes (suborder Megachiroptera) to horses (Hendra virus) and pigs (Nipah virus and Menangle virus). With the exception of Menangle virus, these agents can cause fatal infections in humans. Flying foxes are also believed to be the host species of filoviruses and of newly detected coronaviruses, severe acute respiratory syndrome associated coronavirus (SARS-CoV) and Middle East respiratory syndrome coronavirus (MERS-CoV). Analogous to tick-borne viruses, which are transmitted by ticks, one could describe those transmitted by bats as "bat-borne viruses." Transmission of Hendra virus is facilitated by pregnancy in the bat, and pregnant horses are highly susceptible to the disease.

The connection between varying population densities of reservoir animals or vectors of some viruses and the frequency of their manifestation is interesting and often poorly understood. Changes in climatic conditions can explain the frequency of ticks and the spreading of tick-transmitted infections. The relationship is unknown between the changing population density of some rodents, which serve as reservoirs for viruses (e.g. Arena- and Hantaviruses), and the frequency of human infections. The weather phenomenon *El Niño* has been held responsible for the fluctuation in the mouse populations. Arena- and Hantaviruses do not seem to influence the survival chances of their reservoir animals because they are not pathogenic for them. It remains a possibility, however, that the virus infection itself could influence the population density of its host animals. If only one part, but not another, of the host population is resistant to the virus, it is easy to speculate that viruses themselves control the population density by eliminating sick individuals. Any animal surviving an epizootic will be protected. In this way, the chances for a new epizootic will be reduced, until a new generation of susceptible individuals is born or there is a variation in the viral agent.

It is important to know whether a person or an animal grew up in an area of endemicity in order to assess their susceptibility to zoonotic viral infections. Children living in areas of endemicity are often protected by maternal antibodies and are latently infected, or they are less susceptible at an early age. Based on serological studies, the relative frequency of clinically apparent diseases may be underestimated. The potential danger of contracting tick-borne meningoencephalitis or Japanese encephalitis is much greater for people who have not lived in an area of endemicity. This should be taken into consideration, for example, when giving vaccination advice for travelers.

1.1.2.2 Zoonotic viruses as B-weapons

Some of the most dangerous pathogens for humans must be discussed in this chapter. It seems to be inevitable that specialists who are interested in biological warfare are attracted by pathogens that have an extremely high case fatality rate, such as the Ebola virus. Yet, by way of compensation, the contagiousness of these pathogens is low as a rule, rendering them less suitable for military use. Influenza A viruses of human origin are feared for their pandemic potential. However, influenza virus strains of avian origin, which may cause fatal infections in humans, lack the ability to spread in the human population. Nevertheless, by way of genetic engineering, viruses of low pathogenicity could be transformed into dangerous pathogens, as has been experienced in the case of the ectromelia virus, an orthopoxvirus pathogenic for mice.

1.1.2.3 Global distribution of zoonotic agents

A potential risk of spreading zoonotic infections results from deliberate or inadvertent liberation of imported animals. Importation of exotic animals can be connected with the introduction of zoonotic viruses and should be controlled. The foot-and-mouth disease (FMD) virus can be imported with frozen meat or with latently infected sheep. Crimean Congo virus and Rift Valley virus were imported to Yemen, to Saudi Arabia, and to the United Emirates with fat stock. Raccoons, which were transported from Florida to the State of New York, have introduced raccoon rabies. Raccoon dogs imported from Iran have reintroduced rabies to Scandinavia. The most probable explanation for the introduction of West Nile Virus to North America is the importation of exotic birds. Giant rats, imported from Ghana have introduced monkey pox virus into the United States, where the virus was transmitted to prairie dogs, which were kept as pets.

For survival and transmission, arboviruses are dependent on the availability of competent arthropod vectors; the global distribution of arthropods is facilitated by climatic change and international traffic. The global migration of the Asian "tiger mosquito" (*Stegomyia albopicta*) is especially alarming. This vector is competent for the propagation of the Dengue virus, yellow fever, Chikungunya, and other arboviruses. Eggs of this mosquito were detected in used automobile tires that were shipped from South East Asia to the USA. The tires contained pools of rainwater sufficient for development and survival of the mosquito larvae. Since that time, the vector has settled in the south of the USA and in southern Europe.

Diagnostic Procedures. Approved diagnostic procedures for virus infections that are rare are not easily available. As a rule, ELISA techniques and PCR techniques are displacing older approaches for detection of viruses, e.g. virus-specific antigens, nucleic acids and antibodies.

The advantage of this displacement is that specialization is losing its importance. Anybody who is trained to do an ELISA or a PCR can learn to do it for any purpose. However, compared to those for non-zoonotic virus infections, the diagnostic reagents for many zoonotic infections are not commercially available. References to the literature are included, and it is stressed that the original papers must be consulted for the correct conditions to perform the tests. Most of these PCR techniques have not been evaluated in large numbers of diagnostic cases.

REFERENCES

Bányai K, Martella V, Molnár PJ, Genetic heterogeneity in human G6P [14] rotavirus strains detected in Hungary suggests independent zoonotic origin. *J Infect.* 59, 213–215, 2009.

Biebricher CK, Eigen M. "What is a Quasispecies". In Esteban Domingo. *Quasispecies: Concept and Implications for Virology.* Springer. p. 1. ISBN 978-3-540-26395-1, 2006.

Carbone KM et al., Pletnikov: Borna disease: virus-induced neurobehavioral disease pathogenesis. *Curr. Opin. Microbiol.* 4, 467–475, 2001.

Cong ME et al., Related TT viruses in chimpanzees. *Virology.* 274, 343–355, 2000.

Cooksley WG, What did we learn from the Shanghai hepatitis A epidemic? *J. Viral. Hepat.* Suppl. 1, 1–3, Review, 2000.

Eigen M, Schuster P, *The Hypercycle: A Principle of Natural Self-Organization.* Berlin: Springer-Verlag. ISBN 0-387-09293-5, 1979.

Eigen Manfred (October 1971). "Selforganization of matter and the evolution of biological macromolecules". *Die Naturwissenschaften* 58 (10): 465–523. doi:10.1007/BF00623322. PMID 4942363.

Holmes EC, On the origin and evolution of the human immunodeficiency virus (HIV). *Biol. Rev. Camb. Philos. Soc.* 76, 239–254, 2001.

Lederberg J, Infectious disease as an evolutionary paradigm. *Emerg. Infect. Dis.* 3, 417–423, 1997.

Lederberg J, Medical science, infectious disease, and the unity of mankind. *JAMA* 260, 684–685, 1988.

Martella V, Bányai K, Matthijnssens J, Zoonotic aspects of rotaviruses. *Vet Microbiol.* 140, 246–255, 2010.

Meertens L et al., Molecular and phylogenetic analysis of 16 novel T-cell leukemia virus type 1 from Africa: close relationhip of STLV-a from Allenopithecus nigroviridis to HTLV-1 subtype B strains. *Virology* 278, 275–285, 2001.

Morse SS (ed.), *Emerging Viruses.* Oxford University Press, New York, 1993.

Okamoto H et al., Genomic and evolutionary characterization of TT virus (TTV) in tupaias and comparison with species-specific TTVs in humans and non-human primates. *J. Gen. Virol.* 82, 2041–2050, 2001.

Robertson BH, Viral hepatitis and primates: historical and molecular analysis of human and nonhuman primate hepatitis A, B, and the GB-related viruses. *J. Viral. Hepat.* 8, 233–242, 2001.

Staeheli P, Lieb K, Bornavirus and psychiatric disorders – fact or fiction? *J. Med. Microbiol.* 50, 579–581, Review, 2001.

Suleman MA et al., An outbreak of poliomyelitis caused by poliovirus type I in captive black and white colobus monkeys (Colobus abyssinicus kikuyuensis) in Kenya. *Trans. R. Soc. Trop. Med. Hyg.* 78, 665–669, 1984.

1.1.3 CYCLES OF ARBOVIRUS INFECTIONS

Arboviruses (arthropod-borne viruses) exist in maintenance cycles between vertebrate hosts and primary vectors (Fig. 1.1). Mosquitoes are the most important vectors. Ticks, sand flies (*Phlebotomus* spp.), and gnats (*Culicoides* spp.) play a role as vectors of certain arboviruses.

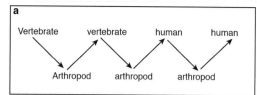

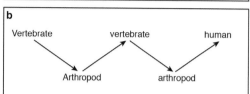

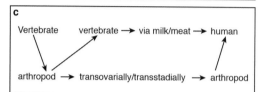

Figure 1.1(a, b, c) | Arboviral Transmission cycles (a) Urban infectious cycles where humans are the source of infection for mosquitoes have been demonstrated, or are possible, if the level of viremia is sufficient. Infected people have to be protected from mosquito bites. This type of infection cycle has been found for yellow fever, dengue, St. Louis encephalitis, Venezuelan equine encephalitis, and Chikungunya fever. It is possible for O'nyong-nyong, Mayaro, Ross River, Oropouche, Rift Valley, and Wesselsbron fevers. (b) Humans are the dead-end hosts in the infection chain and do not serve for amplification. This type of infection chain exists for eastern and western equine encephalitides and Rocio, West Nile, and Sindbis fevers. (c) A vertical transmission (transovarial and transstadial) exists in arthropods and is of importance epidemiologically. This type of transmission is found in the following tick-transmitted virus infections: spring-summer meningoencephalitis, Russian spring-summer meningoencephalitis, louping ill, Kyasanur Forest fever, Omsk hemorrhagic fever, Crimean-Congo hemorrhagic fever, and Colorado tick encephalitis. It is found in the following mosquito-transmitted infections: California and Japanese encephalitides and Murray Valley fever.

There is a close dependence between the virus and the vector. However, different mosquitoes may act as vectors for the same virus in different vertebrates depending on different geographical or ecological situations. Besides a few exceptions, humans are usually the dead-end host and not important as intermediate hosts in the maintenance cycle. Infection of humans by means other than vectors (e.g., via aerosols) is possible, especially in laboratories or as nosocomial infections if the level of viremia is sufficiently high.

The epidemiology of arbovirus infections is regulated by a number of independent factors. They include the number and immune status of the vertebrates that represent the agent reservoir, as well as climatic conditions under which the vector population can reproduce with changing efficiency. Different kinds of mosquitoes with changing host specificity are involved in the complex maintenance cycles with multiple host changes. The seasonal increase in frequency of virus infections is regulated by breeding conditions and the survival rate of the vectors.

In areas with temperate climatic conditions, the question has to be resolved whether arboviruses survive the winter or if they are reintroduced. It is important to know whether a vector maintains its role as reservoir by transovarial and transstadial virus transmission.

La Crosse virus is the most important virus among the agents causing California encephalitis. It is transmitted by its main vector, *Aedes (Stegomyia) triseriatus*, not only by transovarial and transstadial routes but also sexually. Bunyaviruses, similar to influenza viruses, are directly dependent on the viral gene expression and the metabolic activity of the host. Replication of bunyaviruses is controlled by a transnucleotidase, which transcribes the 5′ cap of the mRNA to the viral message (5′-end scavenging). Blood meals activate the cellular gene activity in the ovaries of the mosquitoes and simultaneously stimulate virus replication. Two different cap sequences, CS1 and CS2, are available for the activation of the viral messenger. Viral gene expression can be demonstrated during the hibernation of the eggs (diapause). However, 5′- end structures with CS2 sequences are used almost exclusively for the viral mRNA. After completion of the diapause, 100% of CS1-carrying viral messengers are used.

This special kind of viral gene expression of a gene recombination with intermolecular and intramolecular reassortment is facilitated if an egg is infected with two different bunyaviruses. This could contribute to the genetic multiplicity of the Bunyaviruses.

For viruses transmitted by ticks, it is important to remember that the tick development from egg to larva to nymph to the adult stage takes at least 2 years in a temperate climate. The tick needs a blood meal during each stage, which can cause transmission of an agent. The population density of ticks is influenced not only by atmospheric conditions of the present year but also by the climate of previous years.

Sometimes, entirely different viruses use the same maintenance cycles between virus reservoir and vector. A close epidemiological connection can be the result; for example, the western equine encephalitis virus, an alphavirus, and the St. Louis encephalitis virus, a flavivirus, are spread by the same cycle between wild birds and the mosquito species *Culex tarsalis*. In fact, both diseases frequently appear concurrently. A similar connection exists in Africa and Asia Minor between Sindbis virus, an alphavirus, and West Nile virus, a flavivirus. Both use a cycle between birds and *Culex* species (e.g., *Culex univittatus*). In Australia *Culex annulirostris* is the main vector for Murray Valley encephalitis virus, a flavivirus, and in addition it spreads Ross River virus (RRV), an alphavirus. The urban cycles of yellow fever, dengue, and Chikungunya fever depend upon the vector activity and competence of *Aedes (Stegomyia) aegypti. Anopheles gambiae*, the vector of the O'nyong-nyong virus, also transmits malaria.

The same sand fly species (*Phlebotomus papatasii, P. perniciosus,* and *P. perfilieri*) that transmit the agents of phlebotomus fever also spread *Leishmania* spp., the causative agents of Kala-azar and Oriental boil (Aleppo sore), and *Bartonella* spp.

Kemerovo virus, an orbivirus, is transmitted by *Ixodes persulcatus*, as is the Russian spring-summer (tick-borne) meningoencephalitis virus. Another member of the Kemerovo virus complex, Lipovnik virus, was found in *Ixodes ricinus*. This tick is also the vector of the western type of tick-borne encephalitis virus, a flavivirus, and of *Borrelia burgdorferi*, the causative agent of Lyme borreliosis. *Dermacentor marginatus*, a vector for *Coxiella burnetii*, can also transmit the viruses of the western and eastern types of tick-borne encephalitis.

The simultaneous presence of bacteria and viruses in the same arthropod might be a disadvantage for the viruses and could offer a possibility for vector control. It was shown that *Aedes aegypti* mosquitoes, infected with an intracellular bacterium (strain wMel from *Drosophila melanogaster*), can lose the vector competence for Dengue virus. As Wolbachia infected male mosquitoes can spread the Wolbachia infection in a mosquito-population, even under natural conditions, this principle might be a promising means for vector control.

New transmission cycles were recently found for dengue, dengue hemorrhagic fever, and sandfly fever caused by arboviruses. Maintenance cycles for these agents involving mosquitoes and lower vertebrates were recently identified. These sylvan or "jungle" cycles exist parallel to the urban infectious cycles (insect-human-insect-human). The urban transmission cycle appears to be independent because of a long-lasting viremia with high titers of virus in humans. It is possible, however, that the sylvan cycle is needed as a reservoir.

Rift Valley fever apparently has no sylvan cycle. Several *Aedes* species, so called "floodwater *Aedes*," can transmit the virus vertically and transstadially. The eggs are deposited in floodwater areas, where they survive long periods of drought. The larvae hatch after intensive flooding. Thus, the conditions for a new epizootic (virus amplification in sheep goats, and cattle) and for human infection are provided.

The spreading of arbovirus infections across continents is remarkable. Recent examples for this capacity to travel are the appearance of West Nile virus in the state of New York and the appearance of Rift Valley fever in Saudi Arabia. The persistence of the imported West Nile virus in the eastern United States was apparently not influenced by St. Louis encephalitis virus, which is endemic in the area. In contrast, the spreading of the agent of Japanese encephalitis in Australia is possibly hindered by the fact that feral pigs frequently have neutralizing antibodies against antigenically related flaviviruses, the Murray Valley encephalitis virus, and the Kunjin virus.

Zoonoses caused by arbovirus vector-transmitted zoonotic viruses can be found in the following families: (i) *Togaviridae*, genus *Alphavirus*; (ii) *Flaviviridae,* genus *Flavivirus*; (iii) *Bunyaviridae*, all genera except *Hantavirus*; and (iv) *Orbiviridae, Coltiviridae and Thogotoviridae*. See the sections on alphaviruses, flaviviruses, bunyaviruses, and reoviruses for more details. In 2014 a novel *Thogotovirus*, presumably transmitted by ticks, has caused a case of febrile disease with *thrombozytopenia* in Kansas, USA. The patient died with *multiorgan* failure.

REFERENCES

Beaty BJ et al., LaCrosse encephalitis virus and mosquitoes: a remarkable relationship. *ASM News* 66, 349–357, 2000.

Dobie DK et al., Analysis of LaCrosse virus S mRNA 5'termini in infected mosquito cells and Aedes triseriatus mosquitoes. *J. Virol.* 71, 4395–4399, 1997.

Mackenzie JS, Emerging viral diseases: an Australian perspective. *Emerg. Infect. Dis.* 5, 1–8, 1999.

Nash D et al., The outbreak of West Nile virus infection in the New York City area in 1999. *New Engl. J. Med.* 344, 1807–1814, 2001.

Porterfield JS (ed.), *Exotic viral infections.* Chapman and Hall Medical, London, New York, Tokyo, 1995.

Tsai TF, Chandler LJ, Arboviruses. In: Murray PR, Baron JE, Jorgensen JH, Candry MS, Pfaller AM, Yolken RH (ed.), *Manual of Clinical Microbiology*, 9th ed. ASM Press, Washington, 2007.

1.2 Zoonoses Caused by Alphaviruses

1.2.1 AGENTS

Approximately 25 species belong to the genus *Alphavirus* in the family *Togaviridae*. Alphavirus virions have a diameter of 45 to 75 nm. They have a cubic nucleocapsid and an envelope with three viral glycoproteins: E1, E2, and 6K. E2 is the receptor binding protein. E1 is associated with hemagglutination and determines the complex-specific reactivity. The host specificity includes a wide spectrum of vertebrate and invertebrate cells. The genome is single-stranded RNA and has a plus-strand polarity. The 5' end carries the information for four non-structural proteins that are directly translated from the genome and then immediately undergo proteolytic cleavage. The genes for the structural proteins, the capsid protein and the three membrane proteins, are located at the 3' end of the genome. They are translated by a subgenomic polycistronic mRNA (26S RNA), which is transcribed postreplicatively. As soon as the capsid protein is translated along with the signal peptide, which is needed for the insertion into the endoplasmic reticulum, the former is cleaved proteolytically. The translation of the glycoproteins follows connected to the endoplasmic reticulum. The virus maturation is completed by budding.

1.2.2 ALPHAVIRAL ZOONOSES

The following zoonoses are caused by alphaviruses:

- Eastern equine encephalitis (EEE) in North, Central, and South America
- Western equine encephalitis (WEE) in North and South America
- Venezuelan equine encephalitis (VEE) in Central and South America and the Southern United States
- Semliki Forest fever in Africa and possibly in Europe
- Sindbis fever in Africa, Europe, Asia, and Australia
- Ross River fever in Australia and Oceania
- Barmah Forest fever in Australia and Oceania
- Chikungunya fever in Africa south of the Sahara, in Southern Asia and Southeast Asia
- O'nyong-nyong fever in Africa
- Mayaro fever in South America

Transmission. All clinically relevant alphaviruses are transmitted by mosquitoes. The question of survival during winter remains unanswered for the alphaviruses in temperate climates. Bird migration plays an important role in the annual import of alphaviruses into countries in the Northern Hemisphere. More than one mosquito species is usually involved in the distribution cycle. Urban infectious cycles with human-to-human transmission by *Aedes* (new name *Stegomyia*) *aegypti* are known for Chikungunya fever. Urban transmission cycles are believed to be possible in VEE and Ross River fever as well as in Sindbis, Mayaro, and O'nyong-nyong fevers, since competent vectors (*Stegomyia* spp.) are found in urban environments and the viremia in humans reaches high titers.

The survival of alphaviruses in a certain region depends on the presence of vectors (mosquitoes) and of vertebrates that develop viremic infections with low pathogenicity. Important amplification hosts are birds [for EEE virus, WEE virus, Sindbis virus, and Semliki Forest virus (SFV)], rodents (for RRV, VEE virus, and Barmah Forest virus), and monkeys (for Chikungunya, Mayaro, and O'nyong-nyong viruses).

Occurrence. The occurrence of alphaviruses is predominantly limited geographically to the Southern Hemisphere. Bird migration is partially blamed for the introduction into countries in the Northern Hemisphere. However, different variants of EEE and WEE viruses are found in South and North America, suggesting over wintering might be possible for these viruses. The presence of antibodies in Europe and Asia could be interpreted as a worldwide distribution of alphaviruses (e.g., WEE virus). Sindbis virus strains isolated in Scandinavia were different from those isolated in Southern Europe or Africa.

Clinical Manifestations. Included in the group of zoonoses caused by alphaviruses are encephalitides and febrile diseases where *arthropathies* may be dominant. The spectrum of diseases caused by alphaviruses includes the diseases caused by the agents of American encephalitides (EEE, WEE, and VEE viruses). Encephalitis in these infections is only seen after a febrile non-characteristic prodromal period. Exanthemas are not a part of the signs. The disease signs of the second group of alphaviruses (RRV, Barmah Forest virus, Sindbis virus, Chikungunya virus, O'nyong-nyong virus, and Mayaro virus) are characterized by mild to severe arthropathy and maculopapular rashes. A disease course with encephalitis is occasionally seen in RRV, Sindbis virus, and Chikungunya virus infections. Subclinical infections are possible with all alphavirus infections. There is no indication for prenatal infections. Diseases caused by alphaviruses

tend to be more severe in children than in adults, whereas the opposite applies for the flaviviruses.

Diagnosis. Sporadic cases of alphavirus infections are difficult to diagnose. A high lethality in horses may indicate an epidemic with encephalitis viruses. Virus isolation or demonstration in EEE and WEE is difficult because the virus is only present in blood at low titers before the onset of encephalitis. Demonstration of virus by culture, animal inoculation, *immunohistology*, and, in most cases, PCR, is therefore only attempted with brain specimens obtained postmortem. SFV can be isolated from the blood and from the cerebrospinal fluid (CSF). VEE virus can be isolated from blood, throat washes, tissue samples, and the CSF. RRV, as well Chikungunya, Sindbis, Mayaro, and O'nyong-nyong viruses, can be isolated from blood during febrile episodes. The virus disappears after the febrile phase with the beginning of seroconversion.

Newborn mice (2 to 4 days old), baby hamster kidney cells (BHK21), Vero cells, LLC-MK, primary chicken or duck embryo cells, and mosquito cell cultures (C6/36 or AP61) are recommended for the isolation of alphaviruses. Alphaviruses cause cytopathic effects in primary cultures and cell lines from vertebrates. Mosquito cells are highly susceptible; however, the infection does not cause cytopathic effects but persistent infection. A marked auto-interference is present in alphavirus infections. False-negative results can be induced by inoculation of test material with high-titer virus. This can be avoided by using smaller or diluted inocula. Immunofluorescence, antigen capture ELISA, and RT-PCR can be used for detection and identification of new isolates.

A direct demonstration of the virus can be accomplished by hemagglutination with chicken or goose erythrocytes, by antigen capture ELISA with monoclonal antibody, or by RT-PCR. The roles of these modern techniques (i.e., antigen capture and RT-PCR) in a clinical evaluation remain to be established.

Primers for the genus-specific detection of alphaviruses by RT-PCR in combination with a seminested PCR were designed by M. Pfeffer and coworkers. They were selected from the aligned protein sequences of the 5' end of the nsP1 gene of six genotypes.

The serological techniques to demonstrate antibodies to alphaviruses and to identify isolates have the disadvantage of cross-reacting antibodies, interfering in the classical methods [complement fixation, hemagglutinin inhibition (HI), and serum neutralization] and in the modern ELISAs. All existing alphaviruses have to be included in serological tests in regions where more than one alphavirus is endemic. For practical purposes, the immunoglobulin M (IgM) capture ELISA has been introduced recently for diagnosis of acute alphavirus infections and the IgG ELISA for determining the immune states of all alphaviruses. Monospecific antigens are not yet available for these tests.

Therapy. Specific antiviral therapy for alphaviruses does not exist. Treatment, therefore, is symptomatic. Efficacious inactivated vaccines (for EEE, WEE, and Chikungunya fever) and attenuated live vaccines (for VEE) have been developed for immunization against some alphaviruses. However, they have not been sufficiently tested in field trials due to the nature of alphavirus epidemiology. Epidemics are difficult to forecast. Nevertheless, modified SFVs that also carry protective genes of other viruses have been produced by reverse genetics. These variants are not pathogenic under experimental conditions and are recommended to protect people at risk for laboratory infections.

Prophylaxis. During epidemics of Chikungunya virus or RRV, mosquito nets and repellents should be used in order to prevent an urban infection cycle. A promising prophylactic measure would be to vaccinate domestic animals to prevent virus amplification in these hosts. The chances for predicting outbreaks are improving with increasing knowledge of the natural cycles. In some cases, sentinel animals are employed to monitor for the presence of the virus.

REFERENCES

Gould et al., Understanding the alphaviruses: recent research on important emerging pathogens and progress towards their control. *Antivir. Res.* 87, 111–124, 2010.

Johnson AJ et al., Roehrig: Detection of antiarboviral immunoglobulin G by using a monoclonal antibody-based capture enzyme-linked immunosorbent assay. *J. Clin. Microbiol.* 38, 1827–1831, 2000.

Linssen B et al., Development of reverse transcription-PCR assays specific for detection of equine encephalitis viruses. *J. Clin. Microbiol.* 38, 1527–1535, 2000.

Martin DA et al., Standardization of immunoglobulin M capture enzyme linked immunosorbent assays for routine diagnosis of arboviral infections. *J. Clin. Microbiol.* 38, 1823–1826, 2001.

Paredes A et al., Structural biology of old world and new world alphaviruses. *Arch. Virol.* (Suppl.) 19, 179–185, 2005.

Pfeffer MB et al., Genus-specific detection of alphaviruses by a semi-nested reverse transcriptionpolymerase chain reaction. *Am. J. Trop. Med. Hyg.* 57, 709–718, 1997.

Pittmann PR et al., Immune interference after sequential vaccine vaccinations. *Vacc.* 27, 4879–4882, 2009.

Quetglas JI et al., Alphavirus vectors for cancer therapy. *Virus Res.* 153, 179–196, 2010.

Rulli NE et al., The molecular and cellular aspects of arthritis due to alphavirus infections: lesson learned from Ross Rivervrus. *Ann. N.Y. Acad. Sci.* 1102, 96–108, 2007.

Steele KE, Twenhafel NA, Pathology of animal models of alphavirus encephalitis. *Vet. Pathol.* 47, 790–805, 2010.

Zacks MA, Paessler S, Encephalitic alphaviruses. *Vet. Microbiol.* 140, 281–286, 2010.

1.2.3 EASTERN EQUINE ENCEPHALITIS

EEE is a zoonosis transmitted by mosquitoes, which originated in birds. It mainly causes a disease of the CNS in humans and horses. It is important to differentiate EEE from WEE and VEE. The last two of these are also zoonotic, with similar clinical signs and similar epidemiology. However, the etiological agents are clearly different from the agent of EEE.

Etiology. The agent of EEE is a member of the family *Togaviridae*, genus *Alphavirus*. A variant of EEE virus exists in Central America and parts of South America. It can be differentiated serologically and seems to be less harmful.

Occurrence. The distribution of the EEE virus is restricted to swamps in the coastal areas of the eastern United States and Canada. The prevalence of EEE is highest in Florida and Georgia. A variant of the EEE virus exists in Mexico and South America and is less harmful for humans. There is serological evidence for the existence of the EEE virus in the former Czechoslovakia, Poland, the former USSR, Thailand, and the

Philippines. The EEE virus persists in North America in a natural infectious cycle between *Culiseta melanura* and a large number of different wild birds. Freshwater swamps in forested coastal areas along the east coast of the United States play a major role in the infectious cycle between *C. melanura* and wild birds. Each spring, the occurrence of EEE is associated with birds migrating from the southern United States to northern Canada. The infection is always found first in wild birds, then in pheasants, and afterwards in horses and humans. The question of survival of the virus during winter is unresolved. Re-importation is believed to occur.

Transmission. Reptiles, bats, pheasants, rodents, and horses are additional hosts of the EEE virus. Pheasants develop viremia and disease following infection from latently infected wild birds. Diseased pheasants in turn are the source for the infection of horses and humans. Direct transmission from pheasants has been documented. *Aedes sollicitans* and *Aedes vexans*, not *C. melanura*, are vectors for the transmission from pheasants to horses and humans. In 1990, the EEE virus was isolated for the first time in the United States from a newly imported mosquito, *Aedes (Stegomyia) albopictus (a)*.

Clinical Manifestations. Encephalitic courses of EEE in humans are rare. Inapparent infection or nonfatal systemic disease is the rule; encephalitis is the exception. Only 6% of infected children and 2% of infected adults develop encephalitis; 166 cases have been diagnosed in the United States in 30 years and one-third of the reported cases occurred in Florida. Overlapping EEE and WEE have been reported only from Texas, Indiana, Wisconsin, and Michigan. The fatality rate of hospitalized patients is 50% or more. Many survivors have persistent neurological defects and deficits, regardless of age.

After an incubation period of 7 to 10 days, the disease begins abruptly with a sudden temperature elevation, headaches, conjunctivitis, nausea, and vomiting. The signs of disease in adults advance quickly from dizziness to delirium and coma. Patients express neck stiffness

and increased irritability. Sometimes Kernig's sign is positive. Reflexes can be hyperactive or absent. The limb muscles are spastic. Patients are unable to speak or to swallow, even when conscious. There is usually excessive salivation. The disease is terminal within 2 weeks, often within 7 days. In survivors, signs of CNS involvement with changing symptoms may persist for several weeks before patients slowly return to consciousness. During the recovery phase, it becomes obvious which centers and regions of the brain are permanently damaged. In children, the disease course is often biphasic. A leukocytosis with neutrophilic counts up to 50,000 cells/μl is a characteristic laboratory finding. The CSF pressure is increased, and the cell count can be increased to >1,000 cells/μl.

Fifty percent of infected horses show clinical manifestations and fatality can be up to 90%. Pheasants and ducks, but not other birds, can show symptoms of disease.

Diagnosis. Demonstration of the virus in blood or CSF is successful only in exceptional cases. Postmortem, the virus can be readily isolated from brain tissue. In cell cultures and in postmortem specimens, the virus can be detected by direct IFA or by RT-PCR. Papers describing oligonucleotide primers for a group-specific RT-PCR for all alphaviruses, targeting the nsP1 gene, are listed in the references chapter. Primers for a nested EEE virus-specific RT-PCR (E2 gene) were published by Linssen et al.

Demonstration of virus-specific IgM antibodies in serum and in CSF confirms the diagnosis in most cases. Virus-specific oligoclonal immunoglobulins can be found in the CSF of survivors. The Reiber quotient (plotting Q_{IgG} against Q_{Alb}) is an indicator of intrathecal immunoglobulin production. Because of a close serological relationship between WEE, EEE, and other alphaviruses, it is important to include other alphaviruses as controls.

Differential Diagnosis. The differential diagnosis is not difficult to make in typical epidemiological situations (dead pheasants and horses in a hot and humid summer near freshwater swamps). Sporadic cases with a mild disease are usually not diagnosed, or they have to be differentiated from several other *meningoencephalitides*, including rabies.

Therapy. There is no specific therapy for EEE. Once signs of disease are present, passive antibody transfusion has no beneficial effect. The treatment is symptomatic and is restricted to maintaining vital functions. Passive and active physical therapy is important during the recovery phase.

Prophylaxis. The rare occurrence of EEE does not justify the introduction of a vaccine. A formalin-inactivated vaccine is available for laboratory personnel and other people at high risk. A similar vaccine is available for horses.

Prophylactic provisions are limited to mosquito control in hatching areas. The population needs to be instructed to avoid mosquito bites by use of nets and repellents. Prediction of outbreaks early enough to prevent human infections is an important goal of epidemiologists.

REFERENCES

Armstrong PM, Andreadis TG, Eastern equine encephalitis virus in mosquitoes and their role as bridge vectors. *Emerg. Infect. Dis.* 16, 1869–1874, 2010.

Arrigo NC et al., Cotton rats and house sparrows as hosts for North and South American strains of eastern equine encephalitis virus. *Emerg. Infect. Dis.* 16, 1373–1380, 2010.

Brault AC et al., Genetic and antigenic diversity among eastern equine encephalitis viruses from North, Central, and South America. *Am. J. Trop. Med. Hyg.* 61, 579–586, 1999.

Calisher CH, Alphavirusinfections (family Togaviridae). In: Porterfield JS (ed.): *Exotic Viral Infections*, 1–18. Chapman and Hall Medical, London NewYork Tokyo, 1995.

Cupp EW et al., Transmission of eastern equine encephalomyelitis virus in central Alabama. *Am. J. Trop. Med. Hyg.* 68, 495–500, 2003.

Davis LE, Beckham JD, Tyler KL, North American encephalitic arboviruses. *Neurol. Clin.* 26, 727–757, 2008.

Deresiewicz et al., Clinical and neuroradiographic manifestations of eastern equine encephalitis. *New Engl. J. Med.* 336, 1867–1874, 1997.

Garen PD, Tsai TF, Powers JF, Human eastern equine encephalitis: immunohistochemistry and ultrastructure. *Mod. Pathol.* 12, 646–652, 1999.

Harvala H et al., Eastern equine encephalitis virus imported to the UK. *J. Med. Virol.* 81, 305–308, 2009.

Hull R et al., A duplex real-time reverse transcriptase polymerase chain reaction assay for the detection of St. Louis encephalitis and eastern equine encephalitis viruses. *Diagn. Microbiol. Infect. Dis.* 62, 272–279, 2008.

Linssen B et al., Development of reverse transcription-PCR assays specific for detection of equine encephalitis viruses. *J. Clin. Microbiol.* 38, 1527–1535, 2000.

Pittmann PR et al., Immune interference after sequential vaccine vaccinations. *Vacc.* 27, 4879–4882, 2009.

Sotomayor EA, Josephson SL, Isolation of eastern equine encephalitis virus in A549 and MRC-5 cell cultures. *Clin. Infect. Dis.* 29, 193–195, 1999.

Wang E et al., Reverse transcription-PCR-enzyme-linked immunosorbent assay for rapid detection and differentiation of alphavirus infections. *J. Clin. Microbiol.* 44, 4000–4008, 2006.

Young DS, Kramer LD, Maffei JG et al., Molecular epidemiology of eastern equine encephalitis virus, New York. *Emerg. Infect. Dis.* 14, 454–460, 2008.

1.2.4 WESTERN EQUINE ENCEPHALITIS

WEE is an arbovirus disease that predominantly infects horses and humans.

Etiology. The causative agent of WEE is a member of the family *Togaviridae* in the genus *Alphavirus,* which is cross-reactive serologically with other mosquito-transmitted alphaviruses. Five subtypes (WEE, Buggy Creek, Fort Morgan, and Highlands J in North America and Aura in South America) are found in the WEE complex. Sindbis virus with its four subtypes, found in Africa, Asia, Australia, and Europe, is regarded as a member of the WEE complex.

Occurrence. The areas of distribution of WEE virus include large regions in North and South America. It is not present in the tropical regions of Central America. Major human epidemics have only occurred between the Mississippi River delta and the Rocky Mountains and in Brazil. In Colorado and Utah, 10.9% and 8.6% of the population, respectively, had antibodies against WEE when tested. WEE and EEE overlap only in Texas, Indiana, Wisconsin, and Michigan.

Although the WEE virus is highly virulent for horses and humans, these hosts are not important for the distribution of the agent because the level of viremia is insufficient to infect mosquitoes. Domestic fowl, pigs, cattle, and feral rodents become infected without developing disease. They also are not important as reservoirs for the agent.

The most important amplification hosts appear to be wild birds, especially young birds. When the environment was tested, wild birds (e.g., nesting swallows) were most often virus positive. How WEE survives the winter in regions with moderate temperatures is not known. WEE virus can be found in wildlife in June and July. However, disease in horses and humans occurs only in August. Most WEE epidemics occur in regions where the June isotherm is higher than 21.1 °C. Heavy rain during the summer supports the occurrence of the disease because of an increased vector population.

No cases of WEE have occurred in the United States since 1994. The reduced number of cases may be due to the use of pesticides and repellents or to the adoption of air conditioning in the United States, whereas in Central and South America cases of WEE continue to occur.

Transmission. Numerous mosquito species, other insects, and mites can be infected with the WEE virus under natural conditions. The most important vector is *Culex tarsalis*. The same vector is responsible for the distribution of St. Louis encephalitis virus, a flavivirus. Both diseases appear under equal epidemiological conditions.

Clinical Manifestations. The virulence of WEE depends on the age of the host. It is most virulent in children. One in 58 children, but only 1 in 1,150 adults, develops clinical disease after infection. In some epidemics, 30% of children under 1-year of age showed clinical manifestation.

After a nonspecific prodromal period, the disease begins with fever and myalgia. Adults may not have prodromal signs. Diseased children have spasms, pathological reflexes, and flaccid and spastic pareses. Fifty percent of diseased children suffer permanent damage with mental retardation, emotional instability, and spastic paresis. With increased age, spasms and pareses occur less frequently. The apparent signs are dizziness, lethargy, coma, neck stiffness, headaches, visual disturbances, and photophobia. Permanent damage is rare in diseased adults. The fatality rate of WEE infections in children is between 3% and 4%.

For horses, the WEE virus is less virulent than the EEE virus. The incubation period is 1 to 3 weeks. Clinical signs include fever, somnolence, excitability, disturbed coordination and equilibrium, difficulties in swallowing, paresis of the lips, and an inability to stand up. The fatality rate in horses is 20% to 30% (in some epidemics up to 50%).

Diagnosis. Earlier sporadic cases (up to 3 weeks before an epidemic) or simultaneous cases of horse encephalitis may indicate an epidemic of WEE. The virus as a rule is not detectable in clinical specimens (blood or CSF).

The virus can be isolated in cell culture from the brain tissue of deceased patients. A genus-specific capture ELISA test exists for the demonstration of antigen, and RT-PCR is useful for the identification of isolated virus. Details on oligonucleotide primers for RT-PCR, group specific for all alphaviruses and targeting a domain of the nsP1 gene can be found in the references! Primers for a WEE virus-specific nested RT-PCR (two-step protocol) targeting the E2 gene, were published by Linssen et al.

In most cases, the diagnosis is confirmed by using an IgM capture ELISA specific for detection of IgM antibodies in serum and in CSF. Because of a close serological relationship between WEE, EEE, and other alphaviruses, it is important to include other alphaviruses as controls. Virus-specific IgG is detectable in the CSF of survivors.

Differential Diagnosis. Because of the clinical signs, it is essential in the differential diagnosis to consider diseases caused by other agents that cause meningitis and encephalitis, especially St. Louis encephalitis (which may occur at the same time and location), West Nile fever, California encephalitis, and EEE, but also diseases caused by enteroviruses depending on the season.

Therapy. Specific therapy for WEE does not exist. Treatment is symptomatic. Fluids and electrolytes have to be kept under control. Physical means should be used to reduce fever rather than antipyretics, which reduce interferon production.

Prophylaxis. Formalin-inactivated vaccines have been developed experimentally for the protection of laboratory workers and other people at high risk. In epidemics and epizootics, it is especially important to protect young children and pregnant women from mosquito bites by using mosquito nets, repellents, and insecticides. A formalin-inactivated vaccine is available for the protection of horses, which reduces their value as disease indicators.

Vector control is most important for the prophylaxis of humans and animals. However, it is limited by the available methods.

REFERENCES

Das D et al., Evaluation of a Western equine encephalitis recombinant E1 protein for protective immunity and diagnostics. *Antiviral Res.* 64, 85–92, 2004.

Forrester NL et al., Western equine encephalitis submergence: lack of evidence for a decline in virus virulence. *Virology* 380, 170–172, 2008.

Linssen B et al., Development of reverse transcription-PCR assays specific for detection of equine encephalitis viruses. *J. Clin. Microbiol.* 38, 1527–1535, 2000.

Nagata LP et al., Infectivity variation and genetic diversity among strains of Western equine encephalitis virus. *J. Gen. Virol.* 87, 2353–2361, 2006.

Pittmann PR et al., Immune interference after sequential vaccine vaccinations. *Vacc.* 27, 4879–4882, 2009.

Wang E et al., Reverse transcription-PCR-enzyme-linked immunosorbent assay for rapid detection and differentiation of alphavirus infections. *J. Clin. Microbiol.* 44, 4000–4008, 2006.

1.2.5 VENEZUELAN EQUINE ENCEPHALITIS

VEE is a mosquito-transmitted infectious disease of horses and humans. There are two forms of VEE: an epizootic form in horses and an enzootic or sylvatic variant with rodents as hosts. Humans and horses are only accidentally affected by the enzootic form. There is no direct connection with the epizootic form.

Etiology. The causative agent of VEE, the VEE virus, is a member of the genus *Alphavirus* in the family *Togaviridae*. The virus is not homogeneous. There are at least six subtypes in the VEE complex: subtype I (original), subtype II (Everglades, Fla.), subtype III (Mucambo), subtype IV (Pixuna), subtype V (Cabassou), and subtype VI (AG 80-636). The original VEE subtype exists in both the epizootic and the sylvan forms. There is a partial cross-immunity between VEE and EEE.

Occurrence. The VEE virus exists in Central and South America and there have been outbreaks in southern North America. VEE epizootics occur usually in regions where the enzootic form is common. However, the epizootic type of the virus has never been isolated between outbreaks.

The enzootic VEE persists in maintenance cycles. Large numbers of small rodents of various types are involved, depending on the geographic region and virus type. *Culex* mosquitoes are vectors in these cycles. The question of agent reservoirs of the epizootic variant between outbreaks is unresolved.

Transmission. Horses are the main hosts for the amplification of epizootic VEE. In addition, humans, dogs, pigs, cats, cattle, goats, bats, and birds can be infected during an epizootic. They develop a viremia that can be the source of mosquito infections. Numerous mosquito species as well as birds, especially herons, play a role in the distribution of the epizootic variant of VEE over distances of several thousand kilometers.

Direct transmission from horse-to-horse can occur during epizootics. However, it appears not to be important. Transplacental transmission of VEE infections has been observed in horses.

An unusually long rainy period occurred in September 1995 in the north of Venezuela, extending into Colombia (La Guajira Peninsula). A VEE epidemic, in which an estimated 13,000 people were affected, followed. Spasms occurred in 4% of the diseased; the fatality rate was 0.7%. More than 70,000 unvaccinated horses and donkeys were kept in the La Guajira region. They contributed to the maintenance cycle.

Infections of humans via aerosols in laboratories have occurred. Broken centrifuge bottles have played a major role in these accidental infections. However, human-to-human transmission is not known to occur. A strain with a high pathogenicity has been developed into a weapon for biological warfare with an intended use for aerosol infection.

Clinical Manifestations. After a bite from an infected mosquito, the incubation period for VEE is 2 to 3 days. It may be as short as 24 h after infection via high-titer aerosol.

In contrast to EEE and WEE, the VEE virus causes a systemic infection with viremia rather than a localized infection of the brain. In most cases, the disease appears with mild to severe signs of respiratory tract disease, with severe frontal headaches, myalgia and high fever, photophobia, conjunctival injection, and prostration. Pharyngeal hyperemia and vomiting are frequent. The disease is less severe in adults than in children. Signs of encephalitis are rare and are more frequently seen in children: 0.4% of adults and 4% of children show signs of encephalitis. Encephalitis occurs with the second peak of a biphasic fever. Signs are abnormal reflexes, spastic pareses, spasms, and coma. Laboratory findings of the CSF are unremarkable, with a slight pleocytosis. Permanent damage (paralysis, epilepsy, tremor, and/or emotional instability) is possible in children and adults. Patients with encephalitis have a fatality rate of 20%; in children under 5 years of age, the fatality rate is 35%. Approximately 150 animal species may become infected under natural conditions. Infection remains subclinical in most domestic animals. Dogs and pigs may become clinically ill. The disease in dogs may be fatal after infection with epizootic VEE virus.

Horses are most severely affected by the VEE infection. The severity of the disease varies. A subclinical and mild course of the disease is possible. In most cases, the disease is fulminant, with a picture of a generalized infection or encephalitis with lethal outcome or incomplete healing. Half of all cases of VEE disease in horses include encephalitis. Lethal outcomes without encephalitic signs are possible.

Diagnosis. Because 97% of cases of VEE in humans are mild and uncharacteristic, the proper diagnosis frequently is not made unless suspicion of VEE infection is aroused by other circumstances, for example, sojourn in an area where disease is epizootic or enzootic or where there is encephalitis in horses.

The virus can be isolated from blood, throat washes, tissue samples, and CSF. Reverse transcription polymerase chain reaction (RT-PCR) is replacing methods that demonstrate viral antigen with monoclonal antibody. A nested RT-PCR group specific for all alphaviruses, targeting the nsP1 gene, can be carried out with oligonucleotide primers. See the references!

Primers for a PCR specific group for the VEE virus (E1 gene) (two-step protocol) were designed and evaluated by Linssen et al. and are cited in the literature.

The serological diagnosis today is based on immunoenzymatic methods (IgM capture ELISA) with the detection of virus-specific IgM in serum and CSF. The Reiber quotient (plotting $Q._{IgG}$ against $Q._{Alb.}$) is used to demonstrate intrathecal production of immunoglobulins.

Differential Diagnosis. Cases of encephalitis have to be differentiated from numerous virus-induced encephalitides, especially those caused by enteroviruses, mumps virus, measles virus, varicella viruses, and other arboviruses, depending on season and epidemic situation.

Therapy. The course of VEE disease is frequently mild. There is no specific therapy. As for other viral encephalitides, supportive therapy is used in cases with encephalitis.

Prophylaxis. Experimental formalin-inactivated vaccines for prophylaxis in humans are available. They are not commonly used but are very effective at protecting exposed laboratory personnel. Formalin-inactivated vaccines have been available for horses for 30 years. More recently, live attenuated vaccines, which protect horses for life, have been used.

There are additional methods to limit and contain epizootics: restriction in horse transportations, vaccination of horses, and mosquito control. It is important to keep mosquitoes away from infected humans and animals because infected horses and humans can be a source for mosquito infections during the viremia phase.

REFERENCES

Aguilar PV et al., Endemic Venzuelan equine encephalitis in northern Peru. *Emerg. Infect. Dis.* 10, 880–888, 2004.

Brault AC et al., Positively charged amino acid substitutions in the E2 envelope glycoprotein are associated with the emergence of Venezuelan equine encephalitis virus. *Virol.* 76, 1718–1730, 2002.

Dai X et al., Microbead electrochemiluminescence immunoassay for detection and identification of Venezuelan equine encephalitis virus. *J. Virol. Meth.* 169, 274–281, 2010.

Estrada-Franco JG et al., Venezuelan equine encephalitis virus, southern Mexico. *Emerg. Infect. Dis.* 10, 2113–2121, 2004.

Gardner CL et al., Eastern and Venezuelan equine encephalitis viruses differ in their ability to infect dendritic cells and macrophages: impact of altered cell tropism on pathogenesis. *J. Virol.* 82, 10634–10646, 2008.

Linssen B et al., Development of reverse transcription-PCR assays specific for detection of equine encephalitis viruses. *J. Clin. Microbiol.* 38, 1527–1535, 2000.

Meissner JD et al., Sequencing of prototype viruses in the Venezuelan equine encephalitis antigenic complex. *Virus Res.* 64, 43–59, 1999.

Moncayo AC et al., Genetic diversity and relationships among Venezuelan equine encephalitis virus field isolates from Colombia and Venezuela. *Am. J. Trop. Med. Hyg.* 65, 738–746, 2001.

Navarro JC et al., Postepizootic persistence of Venezuelan equine encephalitis virus, Venezuela. *Emerg. Infect. Dis.* 11, 1907–1915, 2005.

O'Brien LM et al., Development of a novel monoclonal antibody with reactivity to a wide range of Venezuelan equine encephalitis virus strain. *Virol. J.* 6, 206, 2009.

Paessler S, Weaverm SC, Vaccines for Venezuelan equine encephalitis. *Vaccine* 27 (suppl. 4), D80–D85, 2009.

Quiroz E et al., Venezuelan equine encephalitis in Panama: fatal endemic disease and genetic diversity of etiologic viral strains. *PLoS Negl. Trop. Dis.* 3, e472, 2009.

Rosenbloom M et al., Biological and chemical agents: a brief synopsis. *Am. J. Ther.* 9, 5–14, Review, 2002.

Smith DR et al., Venezuelan equine encephalitis virus transmission and effect on pathogenesis. *Emerg. Infect. Dis.* 12, 1190–1196, 2006.

Yanoviak SP et al., Transmission of a Venezuelan equine encephalitis complex alphavirus by culex (melanoconion) gnamatos (dipteral: culicidae) in northeastern Peru. *J. Med. Entomol.* 42, 404–408, 2005.

Vilcarromero S et al., Venezuelan equine encephalitis and upper gastrointestinal bleeding in a child. *Emerg. Infect. Dis.* 15, 323–325, 2009.

1.2.6 SEMLIKI FOREST FEVER

Semliki Forest fever (African horse sickness) is an arbovirus infection, which in humans, is almost always inapparent. However, it may produce disease in humans under specific circumstances. Variants of SFV are presently used extensively in research for eukaryotic expression and for gene therapy, as well as the development of new vaccines.

Etiology. SFV is a member of the genus *Alphavirus* in the family *Togaviridae*.

Occurrence. SFV was isolated in 1942 from *Aedes (Stegomyia) abnormalis* mosquitoes in Uganda. Later it was isolated in different African countries from numerous mosquito species and from wild birds. Virus specific antibodies were found in wild rodents, in domestic animals, and in people of numerous African and Asiatic countries as well as the former Yugoslavia. It was also found in laboratory personnel working with SFV.

Transmission. Transmission of SFV is by mosquito bite. It is also possible by aerosol of contaminated material. In three cases, virus has been isolated from humans after laboratory infection. A major outbreak in the Central African Republic with more than 20 clinical cases was described for the first time in 1990. Hightiter antibodies against SFV were found in Senegal in five of six horses during an epizootic of horse encephalitis.

Clinical Manifestations. Patients with SFV in the Central African Republic had fever, headaches, arthralgias, and myalgias. Some patients had diarrhea, abdominal pain, and conjunctivitis. Uncharacteristic febrile disease for 4 to 7 days is the predominant feature, headaches may persist for 2 weeks, and convalescence may be protracted, with marked asthenia. Several cases of laboratory infection have been described. A fatal encephalitis occurred in one case in an individual infected in the laboratory.

Diagnosis. SFV can be isolated in cell culture (chick embryo fibroblasts). It was isolated from the CSF of the patient with fatal encephalitis who was infected in the laboratory. A group-specific RT-PCR (seminested PCR), targeting the nsP1 gene, has been described for the group-specific demonstration of alphaviruses. The primers can be found in the literature.

Demonstration of virus-specific IgM and IgG antibodies by ELISA techniques would, in analogy to other alphaviruses, constitute the most appropriate technique for serodiagnosis. Cross-reactivity between alphaviruses has to be considered.

Differential Diagnosis. Other arbovirus infections have to be considered in the differential diagnosis. As with other equine encephalitides, epidemic disease in equines is an important epidemiological indicator.

Prophylaxis. Regulations for protection and hygiene in laboratory settings have to be strictly followed, even when working with so-called apathogenic arboviruses. There is always the possibility of infection followed by disease. Vaccines for SFV have not been developed.

REFERENCES

Fazakerley JK, Semliki forest virus infection of laboratory mice: a model to study the pathogenesis of viral encephalitis. *Arch. Virol.* (suppl), 18, 179–190, 2004.

Lundstrom K, Semliki forest virus vectors for gene therapy. *Expert Opin. Biol. Ther.* 3, 771–775, 2003.

Morris-Downes MM et al., Semliki Forest virusbased vaccines: persistence, distribution and pathological analysis in two animal systems. *Vaccine.* 19, 1978–1988, 2001.

Willems WR, Kaluza G, Boschek CB, Semliki Forest virus: cause of a fatal case of human encephalitis. *Science* 203, 1127–1129, 1979.

1.2.7 SINDBIS FEVER

Sindbis fever in humans is a mild febrile disease with a vesicular exanthem and arthralgia. Clinically inapparent infections are not uncommon. This statement is based on seroprevalence studies.

Etiology. The causative agent of Sindbis fever is Sindbis virus, a member of the genus *Alphavirus* in the *Togaviridae* family. It is antigenically related to WEE virus. Subtypes of Sindbis virus are Babanki in Africa, Kyzylagach in Asia, Ockelbo and Pogosta in Europe, and Whataroa in Australia.

Occurrence. The virus was first isolated in 1955 from *Culex* mosquitoes in Sindbis, Egypt. Since that time, reports have been made of virus isolation and serological demonstration from numerous African countries and from Asia, Australia, and Europe (Czech Republic and Russia). Wild birds appear to be the reservoir. There is usually a latent infection with Sindbis virus in cloven-hoofed animals. Wild birds can be latently infected with several species of Sindbis virus. Virus can be found in the CNS, blood, or liver.

A high percentage of the human population may be infected in certain areas, especially in the Nile Valley and in other parts of Africa. Antibodies have also been found in domestic animals in Togo. Diseases caused by the Sindbis virus or related agents are known to occur in more than 20 countries in Africa, Asia, Europe, and Australia.

Sindbis virus infections in Scandinavia have been reported under different names, such as Ockelbo disease in Sweden, Pogosta disease in Finland, and Karelian fever. The agents are not identical to Sindbis virus but are closely related to it. These diseases are believed to be associated with chronic arthritis and rheumatism.

Transmission. Sindbis virus is transmitted by numerous ornithophilic mosquito species (*Anopheles, Mansonia, Aedes,* and *Culex* species). *Culex univittatus* is an ornithophile mosquito species that has been identified as the main vector in Southern Africa. This mosquito species attacks humans during humid periods after rapid replication. There is a close epidemiological relationship between infection with West Nile virus, a flavivirus, and Sindbis virus. They have a common maintenance cycle in wild birds and *Culex* species. Epidemics with both viruses may appear at the same time [such as the epidemiologic association between Western equine encephalitis virus and St. Louis encephalitis virus in the USA (see p. 49)]. In Israel, the presence of antibody to the West Nile virus was much more frequent in sera with the Sindbis virus antibody than in sera without it. Infections in humans occur only tangential to the natural infection cycle. They are of no importance in the epidemiology of the Sindbis virus since Humans are dead-end hosts.

Clinical Manifestations. Sindbis fever is similar to mild courses of West Nile fever. The incubation period is less than 1-week. The disease begins with low-grade fever, headaches, and arthralgia, mainly of the smaller joints on hands and feet. A maculopapular, later vesicular, rash develops on the body and limbs. Occasionally, there is throat inflammation. The acute disease lasts for 10 days. However, several weeks may pass before complete recovery. Persistent joint problems for up to 2 years after the onset of the disease have been reported in Scandinavia.

Diagnosis. The diagnosis is only rarely made by virus isolation from blood or more frequently from vesicle fluid. A nested RT-PCR for the species-specific demonstration of the virus is available today. A group-specific RT-PCR (semi-nested PCR, targeting the nsP1 gene) has been described for the recognition of alphaviruses. The oligonucleotide primers are to be found in the references. Primers for a type-specific nested RT-PCR including two amplification rounds were derived from the E2 region of Edsbyn and the Ockelbo subtypes.

An IgM capture ELISA is available for the demonstration of virus-specific IgM antibody and is mostly used for the diagnosis.

Differential Diagnosis. West Nile, Chikungunya, and O'nyong-nyong fevers have to be considered in the differential diagnosis as well as Ross River fever and Barmah fever in Australia and Oceania. Rubella and *Erythema Infectiosum* will most often be misdiagnosed in cases of Sindbis fever.

Therapy. Treatment of Sindbis virus is symptomatic. In cases of persistent arthritis, corticosteroids and acetylsalicylic acid are to be avoided. Nonsteroidal antiphlogistics, for example, diclofenac, should be used instead.

Prophylaxis. Mosquito nets and repellents may be used prophylactically. No vaccine is available.

REFERENCES

Assuncao-Miranda I, Bozza MT, Da Poian AT, Pro-inflammatory response resulting from Sindbis virus infection of human macro-phages: implications for the pathogenesis of viral arthritis. *J. med. Virol.* 82, 164–174, 2010.

Brummer-Korvenkontio M et al., Epidemiology of Sindbis virus infections in Finland 1981–1996: possible factors explaining a peculiar disease pattern. *Epidemiol. Infect.* 129, 335–345, 2002.

Horling J et al., Detection of Ockelbo virus RNA in skin biopsies by polymerase chain reaction. *J. Clin. Microbiol.* 31, 2004–2009, 1993.

Kurkela S et al., Causative agent of Pogosta disease isolated from blood and skin lesions. *Emerg. Infect. Dis.* 10, 889–894, 2004.

Kurkela S et al. (2005), Clinical and laboratory manifestations of Sindbis virus infection: prospective study, Finland, 2002–2003. *J. Infect. Dis.* 191, 1820–1829.

Kurkela S et al. (2008), Sindbis virus infection in resident birds, migratory birds, and humans, Finland. *Emerg. Infect. Dis.* 14, 41–47.

Kurkela S et al. (2008), Arthritis and arthralgia three years after Sindbis virus infection: clinical follow-up of a cohort of 49 patients. *Scan. J. Infect. Dis.* 40, 167–173.

Laine M et al. (2003), Prevalence of Sindbis-related (Pogosta) virus infections in patients with arthritis. *Clin. Exp. Rheumatol.* 21, 213–216.

Manni T et al., Diagnostics of Pogosta disease: antigenic properties and evaluation of Sindbis virus IgM and IgG enzyme immunoassays. *Vector Born Zoo. Dis.* 8, 303–311, 2008.

Pfeffer et al., Genus-specific detection of alphaviruses by a semi-nested reverse transcriptionpolymerase chain reaction. *Am. J. Trop. Med. Hyg.* 57, 709–718, 1997.

Turell MJ et al., Isolation of West Nile and sindbis viruses from mosquitoes collected in the Nile Valley of Egypt during an outbreak of Rift Valley fever. *J. Med. Entomol.* 39, 248–250, 2002.

1.2.8 EPIDEMIC POLYARTHRITIS (ROSS RIVER FEVER) AND BARMAH FOREST FEVER

Epidemic polyarthritis or Ross River fever is caused by an arbovirus infection in Australia and Oceania. It is characterized by polyarthralgia and rash. There are close clinical and serological relationships with Chikungunya, O'nyong-nyong, and Mayaro fevers.

Etiology. The causative agent, Ross River virus (RRV), is a member of the genus *Alphavirus* in the *Togaviridae* family. Barmah Forest virus is a closely related virus that has been isolated from mosquitoes in Western Australia. It causes a disease in humans that is similar to Ross River fever but has less severe symptoms.

Occurrence. From meteorological data (rainfall and temperature), it is possible to predict epidemics of RRV and Barmah Forest virus. Disease outbreaks are registered each year between January and May in Australia in Queensland, New South Wales, and Victoria. A total of 5,516 clinical cases were registered in Australia between early 1992 and May 1993.

Epidemics have also occurred in the Murray Valley region in southern Australia. Carriers of the antibody were found in New Guinea, Fiji, and Samoa. An epidemic with 30,000 to 40,000 cases occurred in Fiji in 1979.

Inapparent infections have been disclosed in many wild and domestic mammals in Australia, especially in cattle, sheep, horses, pigs, kangaroos and other marsupials, rodents, and dogs. The virus has also been found in wild birds.

A maintenance cycle of the agent between mosquito and mammals can be assumed. It is unknown how RRV survives the dry season in a mosquito-free time.

Transmission. The virus has been isolated from a variety of mosquitoes that may transmit the disease. *Aedes vigilax* and *Culex annulirostris* are the most important epidemic vectors. Vertical transmission in the mosquitoes seems to be possible. As in dengue, Chikungunya fever, yellow fever, and Venezuelan encephalitis, arthropod-borne human-to-human transmission (urban cycle) is believed to occur.

Clinical Manifestations. Clinical signs of Ross River fever are seen in 20% to 30% of infected persons. The epidemic polyarthritis is a benign disease with a slight temperature elevation. Patients complain about throat aches and arthralgias, especially in the small joints of the hands and feet. Joints may be slightly swollen. A transition from arthralgic into chronic polyarthritis has not been observed.

Many patients develop a generalized maculopapular rash on the body and limbs. Enanthemas and petechiae may be present. Enlarged lymph nodes, and plantar and palm pain, as well as paresthesiae, have been observed. The acute disease lasts for 2 weeks maximally. Recurrent signs of disease may cause problems, as has been seen with Chikungunya and Mayaro fevers. Recently cases of encephalitis in humans have been found in association with Ross River fever. Simultaneous infections with Japanese encephalitis or with Murray Valley disease virus were not detected in these cases.

Although 75% of patients complain about joint problems, only one-third of them have a true arthritis. The joint problems decline within 1 to 3 months but may persist for up to 3 years in exceptional cases. A high percentage of arthritis patients have a major histocompatibility complex antigen type of HLA DR7 or B12. Antigen type HLA B27 patients do not experience joint pain preferentially.

Persistent arthritis is less common in patients with obvious exanthem. Infection of macrophages is an important step in the pathogenesis of epidemic polyarthritis. Macrophages can be infected through virus receptors or through Fc receptors in the presence of the antibody. Upon infection via Fc receptors, the virus suppresses the expression of genes that are important for antiviral mechanisms, such as tumor necrosis factor, and for the inducible NO synthetase.

RRV crosses the placenta; murine and human fetuses are often infected following maternal infection. However, the prenatal infection rate in humans is only 3.5%, and in contrast to mice, there are no critical sequelae in human newborns.

Diseases caused by RRV in nonhuman animals are not known. Serological findings have indicated the occurrence of encephalitis and polyarthritis in horses after RRV infections.

Another alphavirus, Barmah Forest virus, causes a disease similar to the epidemic polyarthritis of RRV, with the following symptoms: polyarthritis, arthralgias, myalgias, fever, rash, and somnolence. The virus was isolated in 1989 in Western Australia from the mosquito *C. annulirostris*, which is the vector for this virus. The disease in humans occurs frequently after a RRV epidemic. There are more clinically inapparent Barmah Forest virus infections than inapparent RRV infections. Barmah Forest virus causes arthralgia less frequently and exanthema more frequently than RRV. Encephalitis occurs occasionally in Ross River fever. Both viruses have the same vector. Marsupials are possible vertebrate hosts of Barmah Forest virus.

Diagnosis. An attempt to isolate or demonstrate the virus from serum is only successful as long as antibodies are not present. Most patients seek medical treatment late because they have few complaints early on. The optimal method to isolate the virus is in C6/36 cells, a mosquito cell line. Virus isolation from joint fluid has not been described; however, the presence of viral antigen has been demonstrated.

A species-specific RT-PCR is available for RRV, and a group-specific RT-PCR (seminested PCR) for alphaviruses, targeting the nsP1 gene, has been reported. Papers describing the oligonucleotide primers are listed in the references. Isolation of RRV can be confirmed by RT-PCR (E2 gene; nested PCR, single-tube assay), which can also be used for virus detection in blood and synovial fluid.

Diagnosis of the disease in most cases is made by serology. Newer methods include an ELISA with the IgM capture method. The most specific test is a neutralization assay, in which plaque reduction of 80% is measured. This test differentiates between antibodies against RRV and against Barmah Forest virus. Serological cross-reactions with Chikungunya, O'nyong-nyong, and Mayaro viruses are not important because of geographically different distributions.

Differential Diagnosis. There are no problems in diagnosing the disease in epidemics with fully developed disease with rash and polyarthritis. The diagnosis is frequently missed in sporadic and abortive cases and in travelers. To be considered in the differential diagnosis are acute arthritides due to other causes: rubella, *erythema infectiosum*, Lyme borreliosis, Chikungunya fever, drug intolerance, and rheumatic fever. Dengue fever causes muscle pain without joint involvement. Varicella and Sindbis fever have to be ruled out in cases of vesicular exanthems. In cases with CNS involvement, Murray Valley encephalitis and other causes of encephalitis have to be ruled out.

Therapy. A specific therapy is not needed. Aspirin or nonsteroidal antirheumatics, but never steroids, should be given in cases of severe joint problems. Diclofenac can be given to alleviate pain and to reestablish mobility.

Prophylaxis. A vaccine does not exist. The importance of epidemic polyarthritis is considered to be minimal in Australia. Special regulations, therefore, have not been necessary.

REFERENCES

Azuolas JK et al., Isolation of Ross River virus from mosquitoes and from horses with signs of muskulo-skeletal disease. *Aust. Vet. J.* 81, 344–347, 2003.

Jacups SP, Whelan PI, Currie BJ, Ross River virus and Barmah Forest virus infections: a review of history, ecology, and predictive models, with implications for tropical northern Australia. *Vector Borne Zoo. Dis.* 8, 283–297, 2008.

Johnson AJ et al., Detection of anti-arboviral immunoglobulin G by using a monoclonal antibody-based capture enzyme-linked immunosorbent assay. *J. Clin. Microbiol.* 38, 1827–1831, 2000.

Kelly-Hope LA et al., Ross River virus disease in Australia, 1886–1998, with analysis of risk factors associated with outbreaks. *J. Med. Entomol.* 41, 133–150, 2004.

Klapsing P et al., Ross River virus disease reemergence, Fiji, 2003–2004. *Emerg. Infect. Dis.* 11, 613–615, 2005.

Lidbury BA, Mahalingam S, Specific ablation of antiviral gene expression in macrophages by antibody-dependent enhancement of Ross River virus infection. *J. Virol.* 74, 8376–8381, 2000.

Lindsay M et al., An outbreak of Ross River virus disease in Southwestern Australia. *Emerg. Infect. Dis.* 2, 117–120, 1996.

Linn ML, Aaskov JG, Suhrbier A, Antibodydependent enhancement and persistence in macrophages of an arbovirus associated with arthritis. *J. Gen. Virol.* 77, 407–411, 1996.

Martin DA et al., Standardization of immunoglobulin M capture enzyme linked immunosorbent assays for routine diagnosis of arboviral infections. *J. Clin. Microbiol.* 38, 1823–1826, 2001.

Pfeffer MB et al., Genus-specific detection of alphaviruses by a semi-nested reverse transcriptionpolymerase chain reaction. *Am. J. Trop. Med Hyg.* 57, 709–718, 1997.

Poidinger M et al., Genetic stability among temporally and geographically diverse isolates of Barmah Forest virus. *Am. J. Trop. Med. Hyg.* 57, 230–234, 1997.

Proll S et al., Persistierende Arthralgien bei Ross-River-Virus-Erkrankung nach Ozeanien- Reise. *Dtsch. Med. Wochenschr.* 124, 759, 1999.

Rulli NE et al., The molecular and cellular aspects of arthritis due to alphavirus infections: lesson learned from Ross River vrus. *Ann. N.Y. Acad. Sci.* 1102, 96–108, 2007.

Soden M et al., Detection of viral ribonucleic acid and histologic analysis of inflamed synovium in Ross River virus infection. *Arthritis Rheum.* 43, 365–369, 2000.

Suhrbier A, La Linn M, Clinical and pathologic aspects of arthritis die to Ross River virus and other alphaviruses. *Curr. Opin. Rheumatol.* 16, 374, 2004.

Woodruff RE, Early warning of Ross River virus epidemics: combining surveillance data on climate and mosquitoes. *Epidemiology* 17, 569–575, 2006.

1.2.9 CHIKUNGUNYA FEVER

Chikungunya fever is a mosquito-transmitted alphavirus infection that occurs in Africa and southern and southeastern Asia. In humans, it causes severe arthralgias and a maculopapular rash. The infection in monkeys causes a disease similar to dengue fever. It is clinically inapparent in birds. The name Chikungunya comes from Swahili and means "what bends."

Etiology. The causative agent of Chikungunya fever is a member of the family *Togaviridae*, genus *Alphavirus*. The virus is serologically closely related to O'nyong-nyong, Mayaro, Ross River, and Semliki Forest viruses but not other alphaviruses.

Occurrence. Virus isolation and demonstration of antibodies have been reported from Uganda, Tanzania, Zimbabwe, Angola, Zaire, and South Africa. It can be assumed that Chikungunya virus is present in all African countries south of the Sahara. In addition, there have been epidemics in numerous countries in southern and southeastern Asia (see Fig. 1.2).

Wild primates (galagos), bats, birds, and other animals appear to be agent reservoirs in Africa. Antibodies have been found in green monkeys, orangutans, and chimpanzees.

Recently (2014) it was reported that Chikungunya virus has reached South America. In Columbia, 1,900 cases were registered at the border with Venezuela. A baby aged 11 months died from the disease.

Besides the urban infection cycle, there is possibly a rural or rainforest cycle, as there is in yellow fever. Chikungunya virus has a wide distribution in Southeast Asia, similar to that of dengue but unlike that of yellow fever. In Southern Asia, outbreaks of Chikungunya fever may be epidemiologically associated with dengue fever. In 2004, an epidemic of Chikungunya

was spread to countries around the Indian Ocean. Finally, the virus was introduced from Reunion to Italy, where the outbreak culminated in 2007 and established autochthonic infections.

Transmission. *Aedes (Stegomyia) aegypti* was found to be the main vector in epidemics in large cities in Asia. It is assumed that humans are the main source of infection for mosquitoes and that vector-borne human-to-human transmission is the rule in urban outbreaks. Direct transmission between humans was not observed. There is no vertical virus transmission in mosquitoes.

In African epidemics, vectors besides *A. aegypti* are *Culex pipiens fatigans, Aedes africanus, A. furcifer taylori,* and *Mansonia* species, *A. furcifer taylori* and *A. africanus,* are found in tropical rainforests and prefer wild primates as hosts. As was shown by the outbreak in Italy in 2007, *Aedes albopictus* (new name: *Stegomyia albopicta*) has gained considerable importance in distributing the Chikungunya virus.

Clinical Manifestations. The incubation period for Chikungunya virus is considered to be 6 to 10 days. It was only 22 and 80 h in two laboratory infections resulting from mosquito bites.

The disease begins suddenly with fever and joint pain that immediately causes patients to be unable to move. Back and limb pain can be so extensive that morphine is required. Other symptoms are myalgias, nausea, vomiting, headaches, nasal discharge, conjunctivitis, retrobulbar pain, photophobia, and lymphadenopathy. Fever lasts for 3 to 10 days and is often biphasic. A maculopapular rash develops around days 2 to 5. It can become hemorrhagic.

Hemorrhagic disease has not been reported in African epidemics. Hemorrhagic disease has been observed in 5% to 7% of cases in Asia. The average fatality rate is 0.4% (2.8% in children and 1.6% in elderly people). Subclinical infections were not included in these data.

Arthralgias are often clinically recognizable, with reddening, swelling, and sensitivity to pressure of joints. Periarticular nodules may be present as seen in rheumatoid arthritis. Problems with arthralgias and edemas may persist

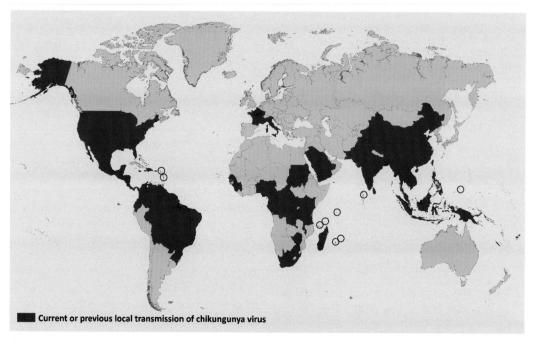

Current or previous local transmission of chikungunya virus

Figure 1.2 | Countries and territories, where cases of Chikungunya disease have been reported. http://www.cdc.gov/chikungunya/pdfs/ChikungunyaWorldMap_03-10-2015.pdf. Courtesy CDC.

for weeks after the acute disease. Eventually, there is complete healing. Permanent damage does not occur.

Similar clinical symptoms are caused by related alphaviruses: O'nyong-nyong, Mayaro, Ross River, and Sindbis viruses. Rubella virus, a Togavirus of the genus *Rubivirus*, also causes arthritis.

Diagnosis. For up to 6 days after the first symptoms, the virus can be isolated from patient blood, which is to be injected into animals or cell culture. In mice, the Chikungunya virus is pathogenic after injection by the peripheral route, O'nyong-nyong virus is not. Cross-reactions with O'nyong-nyong, Mayaro, and Ross River viruses may be difficult to eliminate. RT-PCR is used today in specialized laboratories for demonstrating and typing of the agent.

A group-specific RT-PCR (seminested PCR, targeting the nsP1 gene) has been described for the recognition of alphaviruses. Papers describing the primers are listed in the references chapter. Papers describing primers for a type-specific detection of Chikungunya virus by

nested RT-PCR (E2 gene) are also to be found in the references.

Serodiagnosis for Chikungunya virus infections is unreliable because a definite differentiation from O'nyong-nyong virus is not possible, at least in sera from Africa. The same holds true for Mayaro and Ross River virus infections. However, they affect different geographic regions. A neutralization test based on 80% plaque reduction can be used for serodiagnosis. It is reliable only when O'nyong-nyong virus is tested in parallel.

Differential Diagnosis. Dengue infections may be difficult to rule out if myalgias are misdiagnosed as arthritis. There is no arthritis in dengue fever. In addition, hemorrhagic manifestations are common with dengue fever, unlike Chikungunya fever. Other diseases to be considered in the differential diagnosis are O'nyong-nyong, Sindbis, and West Nile fevers.

Therapy. Therapy for Chikungunya virus is symptomatic. Strong analgesics may be required for severe joint pain. Diclofenac can be given to alleviate pain and to reestablish mobility. The use of steroids should be strictly avoided.

Prophylaxis. A commercial vaccine for humans does not exist. An experimental attenuated live virus vaccine is available for exposed laboratory personnel. Protection against mosquitoes is important. They are active shortly after sunset. Mosquito nets and repellents are recommended especially during epidemics. Control actions against malaria may influence the epidemiology of Chikungunya. Mosquitoes should not get access to viremic patients to avoid the initiation of an urban infection cycle by *A. aegypti*. The control of *A. aegypti* is essential in habitats near cities to prevent epidemics.

REFERENCES

Arankalle VA et al., Genetic divergence of Chikungunya viruses in India (1963–2006) with special reference to the 2005–2006 explosive epidemic. *J. Gen. Virol.* 88, 1967–1976, 2007.

Borgherini G et al. (2007), Outbreak of Chikungunya on Reunion Island: early clinical and laboratory features in 157 adult patients. *Clin. Infect. Dis.* 44, 1401–1407, 2007.

Borgherini G et al. (2008), Persistent arthralgia associated with Chikungunya virus: a study of 88 adult patients on Reunion Island. *Clin. Infect. Dis.* 47, 469–475

Brouard CP et al., Estimated risk of Chikungunya viremic blood donation during an epidemic on Reunion Island in the Indian Ocean, 2005–2207. *Transfusion* 48, 1333–1341, 2008.

Chen LH, Wilson ME, Dengue and Chikungunya infections in travelers. *Curr. Opin. Infect. Dis.* 23, 438–444, 2010.

Collao X et al., Different lineages of Chikungunya virus in Equatorial Guinea in 2002- 2006. *Am. J. Trop. Med.Hyg.* 82, 505–507, 2010.

Economopoulou A et al., Atypical Chikungunya virus infections: clinical manifestations, mortality and risk factors for severe disease during 2005–2006 outbreak on Reunion. *Epidemiol. Infect.* 137, 534–541, 2009.

Fritel X et al., Chikungunya virus infection during pregnancy, Reunion, France, 2006. *Emerg. Infect. Dis.* 16, 418–425, 2010.

Gould LH et al., An outbreak of yellow fever with concurrent chikungunya virus transmission in South Kordofan, Sudan, 2005. *Trans. R. Soc. Trop. Med. Hyg.* 102, 1247–1254, 2008.

Gould EA, Higgs S, Impact of climate change and other factors on emerging arbovirus diseases. *Trans. R. Soc. Trop. Med. Hyg.* 103, 109–121, 2009.

Grivard P et al., Molecular and serological diagnosis of Chikungunya virus infection. *Pathol. Biol. (Paris)* 55, 490–494, 2007.

Guilherme JM et al., Seroprevalence of five arboviruses Her Z et al., Chikungunya: a bending reality. *Microbes Infect.* 11, 1165–1176, 2009.

Johnson AJ et al., Detection of anti-arboviral immunoglobulin G by using a monoclonal antibody-based capture enzyme-linked immunosorbent assay. *J. Clin. Microbiol.* 38, 1827–1831, 2000.

Kariuki-Njenga M et al., Tracking epidemic Chikungunya virus into the Indian Ocean from East Africa. *J. Gen. Virol.* 89, 2754–2760, 2008.

Lanciotti RS et al., Emergence of epidemic O'nyong-nyong fever in Uganda after a 35- year absence: genetic characterization of the virus. *Virology.* 252, 258, 1998.

Liumbruno GM et al., The Chikungunya epidemic in Italy and its repercussion on the blood system. *Blood Transf.* 6, 199–210, 2008.

Martin DA et al., Standardization of immunoglobulin M capture enzyme linked immunosorbent assays for routine diagnosis of arboviral infections. *J. Clin. Microbiol.* 38, 1823–1826, 2001.

Massad E et al., The risk of chikungunya fever in a dengue-endemic area. *J. Travel. Med.* 15, 147–155, 2008.

McClain DJ et al., Immunologic interference from sequential administration of live attenuated alphavirus vaccines. *J. Infect. Dis.* 177, 634–641, 1998.

Moro ML et al., Chikungunya virus in North- Eastern Italy: a seroprevalence survey. *Am. J. Trop. Med. Hyg.* 82, 508–511, 2010.

Pfeffer M et al., Genus-specific detection of alphaviruses by a semi-nested reverse transcriptionpolymerase chain reaction. *Am. J. Trop. Med. Hyg.* 57, 709–718, 1997.

Pile JC et al., Chikungunya in a North American traveler. *J. Travel. Med.* 6, 137–139, 1999.

Pistone T et al., Cluster of chikungunya virus infection in travelers returning from Senegal, 2006. *J. Travel. Med.* 16, 286–288, 2009.

Powers AM et al., Re-emergence of Chikungunya and O'nyong-nyong viruses: evidence for distinct geographical lineages and distant evolutionary relationships. *J. Gen. Virol.* 81, 471–479, 2000.

Powers AM, Chikungunya. *Clin. Lab. Med.* 30, 209–219, 2010.

Ramful D et al., Mother-to-child transmission of Chikungunya virus infection. *Pediatr. Infect. Dis.* 26, 811–815, 2007.

Sissiko D et al. (2008), Outbreak of chikungunya fever in Mayotte, Comores archipelago, 2005–2006. *Trans. R. Soc. Trop. Med. Hyg.* 102, 780–786.

Sissoko D et al. (2009), Post-epidemic Chikungunya disease on Reunion Island: course of rheumatic manifestions and associated factors over a 15-month period. *PLos Negl. Trop. Dis.* 3, e389, 2009.

Smith DR et al., Development of field-based real-time reverse transcription-polymerasechain reaction assays for detection of Chikungunya and O'nyong-nyog viruses in mosquitoes. *Am. J. Trop. Med. Hyg.* 81, 679–684, 2009.

Staples JE, Breiman RF, Powers AM, Chikungunya fever: an epidemiological review of a re-emerging infectious disease. *Clin. Infect. Dis.* 49, 942–948, 2009.

Talbalaghi A et al., Are aedes albopictus or other mosquito species from northersn Italy competent to sustain new arboviral outbreaks? *Med. Vet. Entomol.* 24, 83–87, 2010.

Telles JN et al., Evaluation of real-time nucleic acid sequence-based amplification for detection of Chikungunya virus in clinical samples. *J. Med. Microbiol.* 58, 1168–1172, 2009.

Tsai TF, Chandler LJ, Arboviruses. In: Murray PR, Baron JE, Jorgensen JH et al. (eds.), *Manual of Clinical Microbiology*, 1553–1569, 8th ed. ASM Press, Washington, 2003.

Yap G et al., Evaluation of Chikungunya virus diagnostic assays: differences in sensitivity of serology assays in two independent outbreaks. *PLos Negl. Trop. Dis.* 4, e753, 2010.

1.2.10 O'NYONG-NYONG FEVER

O'nyong-nyong fever is an arbovirus infection in East Africa. In humans, infection causes fever, arthralgias, exanthemas, and lymphadenitis. The name comes from the Acholi language and means "very painful and weak."

Etiology. The agent of O'nyong-nyong fever is a member of the genus *Alphavirus* and is serologically closely related to Chikungunya virus, SFV, Mayaro virus, and RRV. The virus could be considered to be a subtype of the Chikungunya virus.

Occurrence. A major epidemic was registered in Uganda in 1959, which extended into Kenya, Tanzania, and Malawi. O'nyong-nyong fever was found in these countries for several years afterwards.

The natural agent reservoir is not known. There is no definite proof, therefore, that the disease is zoonotic. Under experimental conditions, the virus is only pathogenic after intracerebral injection in mice. In infected areas, the disease spreads quickly and affects many people.

Transmission. O'nyong-nyong fever is transmitted by the mosquitoes *Anopheles gambiae* and *Anopheles funestus*. O'nyong-nyong virus is one of the few arboviruses transmitted by the *Anopheles* species. There is no knowledge about an epidemiological connection with malaria.

Clinical Manifestations. The incubation period of O'nyong-nyong virus is about 8 days. The disease begins abruptly with fever, shivering chills, and epistaxis. Additional symptoms are pain and stiffness of the back and joints, headache, and ophthalmalgia. An itchy rash migrates from face to body. A considerable lymphadenitis especially affects the cervical lymph nodes. The fever lasts for 4 to 5 days. The outcome is always benign.

During an epidemic in Uganda in 1996 and 1997, the disease was monitored. A morbidity of 40% to 70% of the population was found. The duration of arthritic disease was between 1 and 14 days, with a mean of 4 days. Joints in the knees and feet were mainly affected.

Diagnosis. The O'nyong-nyong virus, like the Chikungunya virus, can be isolated in cell culture from blood during the febrile phase. Differentiating between the O'nyong-nyong virus and the Chikungunya virus isolates in the laboratory is difficult. There is predominantly a one-way cross-reaction: Chikungunya antisera react with the O'nyong-nyong virus; the reverse reaction is less pronounced. Peripheral inoculation of mice is important for the diagnosis because the O'nyong-nyong virus is not pathogenic by this route.

A group-specific RT-PCR (seminested PCR) has been described for the recognition of alphaviruses. Papers describing the primers are to be found in the references chapter.

The serodiagnosis for O'nyong-nyong virus infections is unreliable because a definite differentiation from Chikungunya virus is not possible, at least in sera from Africa. The same holds true for Mayaro and Ross River infections. However, they affect different regions. A neutralization test based on 80% plaque reduction can be used for serodiagnosis. It is reliable only when the Chikungunya virus is tested in parallel.

Differential Diagnosis. O'nyong-nyong fever is difficult to clinically differentiate from Chikungunya fever. However, there is usually no lymphadenitis in Chikungunya fever. Sindbis fever, rubella, Lyme borreliosis, *erythema infectiosum*, and classical causes of arthritis (rheumatic arthritis) have to be ruled out. Less severe cases of Marburg or Ebola virus disease may present diagnostic problems.

Therapy. Therapy for O'nyong-nyong fever is symptomatic. Diclofenac can be used for the alleviation of pain and to regenerate mobility. Corticosteroids should be avoided.

Prophylaxis. Protection against mosquitoes (repellents and mosquito control) is important as prophylaxis.

REFERENCES

Posey DL et al., O'nyong-nyong fever in West Africa. *Am. J. Trop. Med. Hyg.* 73, 32, 2005.

Powers AM, Re-emergence of Chikungunya and O'nyong-nyong viruses: evidence for distinct geographical lineages and distant evolutionary relationships. *J. Gen. Virol.* 81, 471–479, 2000.

Smith DR et al., Development of field-based real-time reverse transcription-polymerasechain reaction assays for detection of Chikungunya and O'nyong-nyog viruses in mosquitoes. *Am. J. Trop. Med. Hyg.* 81, 679–684, 2009.

Vanlandingham DL et al., Determinants of vector specificity of O'nyong nyong and chikungunya viruses in anopheles and aedes mosquitoes. *Am. J. Trop. Med. Hyg.* 74, 663–669, 2006.

1.2.11 MAYARO FEVER

Mayaro fever is a benign arbovirus infection that is known to occur only in tropical regions in South America. The disease is characterized by fever, arthralgia, and rash.

Etiology. The causative agent of Mayaro fever is a member of the genus *Alphavirus* and is serologically closely related to Chikungunya, Ross River, and O'nyong-nyong viruses.

Occurrence. The virus has been isolated from diseased people in Brazil, Trinidad, Bolivia, and Suriname. The disease has been diagnosed serologically in Guyana, Colombia, Peru, and Panama. Epidemics have been observed in humans living in tropical rainforests in Brazil and Bolivia.

A high percentage of several South American monkey species have antibodies to the Mayaro virus. They are believed to be reservoirs for the agent. There are also serological indications of Mayaro virus infection in wild birds.

Knowledge about Mayaro fever was originally based on observations during three epidemics with fewer than 100 cases each. Only people with close contact to forests were affected. More recently, epidemics in rural regions of South America with up to 4,000 people infected have been noticed repeatedly. Viremia as high as >105 50% infective doses (ID50) per ml of blood might be an indication that humans may serve as amplification hosts.

Transmission. The Mayaro virus has been isolated from different mosquito species (*Haemagogus* spp., *Culex* spp., and others). Transmission by mosquitoes has been documented experimentally. *Haemagogus*

Janthinomys appears to be the main vector for yellow fever (ratio of infected to uninfected mosquitoes, 1:386) and for Mayaro virus (1:82) in Brazil. Marmosets (*Callithrix argentata*) are assumed to be amplification hosts for the Mayaro virus in the tropical rainforest.

Clinical Manifestations. The incubation period of the Mayaro virus in humans is around 6 days. Clinical signs are fever, headaches, pain in the epigastric region, back pain, arthralgias, chills, nausea, photophobia, rash, and lymphadenitis. Arthralgias include hand and foot joints, predominantly of the fingers and toes. All diseased people are affected, but joint swelling is only found in 20% of cases. Arthralgias can persist for weeks and months, sometimes causing major distress, and they can be recurrent. A maculopapular rash affects the upper part of the body, especially the limbs; it may be generalized. Exanthemas were found in two-thirds of confirmed cases, more frequently in children than in adults. Some patients have an inguinal lymphadenopathy. Thrombocytopenia and leukopenia were found in most cases. The infection in animals (New World monkeys) is usually asymptomatic.

Diagnosis. The Mayaro virus can readily be isolated at the beginning of the disease from blood plasma in Vero cells or mosquito cell cultures. For virus typing, cross-reactions with Chikungunya virus, O'nyong-nyong virus, RRV, and SFV have to be considered. Usually there are no problems because of the different geographical distributions of these viruses. A group-specific RT-PCR (seminested PCR) has been described for alphaviruses. Descriptions of the oligonucleotide primers are to be found in the literature, cited in the references chapter.

Older serological methods have been replaced by an IgM capture ELISA to demonstrate IgM antibody.

Differential Diagnosis. Clinically, Mayaro fever is similar to Chikungunya, O'nyong-nyong, and Ross River fevers. However, it is the only one occurring in South America. Besides rubella, *erythema infectiosum*, and Lyme borreliosis, drug-induced exanthemas and chronic polyarthritis have to be ruled out in the differential diagnosis.

Therapy. A specific therapy for Mayaro virus is not known and usually not needed because of the benign course of the disease. Diclofenac may be used to alleviate pain and to regenerate mobility.

Prophylaxis. No specific prophylaxis is available.

REFERENCES

Azevedo RS et al., Mayaro fever virus, Brazilian Amazon. *Emerg. Infect. Dis.* 15, 1830–1832, 2009.

Bronzoni RV et al., Multiplex nested PCR for Brazilian alphavirus diagnosis. *Trans. R. Soc. Trop. Med. Hyg.* 98, 456–461, 2004.

De Thoisy BJ et al., Mayaro virus in wild animals, French Guiana. *Emerg. Infect. Dis.* 9, 1326–1329, 2003.

Hassing RJ, Leparc-Goffart I, Blank SN et al., Imported Marayo virus infection in the Netherlands. *J. Infect.* 61, 343–345, 2010.

Lavergne A et al., Complete nucleotide sequence and phylogenetic relationships with other alphaviruses. *Virus Res.* 117, 283–290, 2006.

Torres JR et al., Family cluster of Mayaro fever, Venezuela. *Emerg. Infect. Dis.* 10, 1304–1306, 2004.

1.3 Zoonoses Caused by Flaviviruses

Viruses in the family *Flaviviridae*, genus *Flavivirus* (formerly group B arboviruses), include agents pathogenic for humans that are transmitted by mosquitoes or ticks. The prototype of this family is yellow fever. Typical diseases caused by flaviviruses range from encephalitides to hemorrhagic fevers. There are at least eight different virus complexes with 66 virus types within the genus *Flavivirus*. They are related serologically, genetically, and ecologically. Only those virus complexes that include important agents pathogenic for humans are described here.

1.3.1 AGENTS

Flaviviruses, like alphaviruses, are enveloped RNA viruses with a cubic nucleocapsid and a single-stranded genome with plus polarity. The particles have a diameter of 37 to 50 nm. They have three structural proteins: the capsid protein (C), the matrix protein (M), and the envelope protein (E). The last two are glycosylated membrane proteins. The E protein is the receptor binding protein. In contrast to those for alphaviruses, the genes for the structural proteins of flaviviruses are located on the 5′ end of the genome. There are seven nonstructural proteins with their genes on the 3′ end of the genome. The complete genome functions as a polycistronic messenger and is the template for the translation of a polyprotein that needs to be cleaved proteolytically *in statu nascendi*. A subgenomic mRNA, as in alphaviruses, is not made. The budding of flaviviruses occurs on the membranes of cytoplasmic vesicles, not on the cytoplasmic membrane. Virus release is induced by lysis of cells.

Flaviviruses of clinical importance fall into three antigenic complexes, which are determined by vector usage and pathogenicity. As is the case in other virus families, the genus-specific immune reactivity is associated with the capsid protein. Flaviviruses have only one glycoprotein, which expresses group-specific, complex-specific, and subtype-specific determinants. As a rule, group-specific reactivity is associated with domain A of the E protein, complex-specific reactivity is associated with domain B, and the subtype-specific reactivity is associated with domain C, but these reactivities are not strictly separated, and therefore, any flavivirus infection can result in a broad spectrum of heterotypic reactions.

The early immune response against a given virus will yield protection immunity against related flaviviruses. Some weeks later, subtype-specific neutralizing antibodies are prevalent, but the group-specific reactivity is not abolished, and anamnestic immune reactions can be induced by any adventitious flavivirus infection. This heterotypic anamnestic response against a second infecting flavivirus is believed to explain the increased pathogenicity. It can be shown that virus titers are elevated in the presence of "enhancing" antibodies. Antibody-mediated macrophage infection does not occur, for example, in a primary dengue (DEN) virus infection, but may occur upon infection with a second dengue virus type. Geographic compartmentalization has in former times prevented an overlap of different flaviviruses in the same geographic location. But modern traffic has disrupted the original conditions and has led to globalization, resulting in increased pathogenicity. The complicated antigenic structure is unique to the flaviviruses, creating problems with respect to pathogenicity and the production of safe vaccines.

1.3.2 COMPLEXES OF THE *FLAVIVIRIDAE* WITH CLINICAL IMPORTANCE

Typical clinical pictures caused by Flaviviruses range from encephalitis to hemorrhagic fever. The genus flaviviridae comprises 66 different virus species in eight complexes, which are characterized by serologic ecologic and genetic relationships. Only virus complexes will be mentioned in which important human pathogens are contained.

1.3.2.1 Virus Complex Transmitted by Ticks

In the virus group transmitted by ticks [tick-borne encephalitis (TBE) complex], rodents are the most important vertebrate hosts. Hedgehogs, deer, and livestock may also be latently infected. *Ixodes, Dermacentor,* and *Haemaphysalis* ticks are the principal transmitters. The following flaviviral zoonoses are transmitted by ticks:

- TBE, European subtype [Central European encephalitis (CEE)]

- TBE, Eastern subtype [Russian spring summer encephalitis (RSSE)]
- Louping ill (LI) in Scotland and Negishi virus encephalitis in Japan
- Powassan encephalitis (PE) and Modoc virus encephalitis in North America
- Kyasanur Forest disease (KFD) in India
- Alkhurma hemorrhagic fever in Saudi Arabia
- Omsk hemorrhagic fever (OHF) in Siberia

1.3.2.2 Virus Complex Transmitted by Mosquitoes: Japanese Encephalitis Virus and Related Encephalitis Viruses

Birds are the most important vertebrate hosts in this group of viruses. Pigs [in Japanese encephalitis (JE)] and horses may also be involved and may develop disease. *Culex* mosquitoes are the main transmitters. The following flaviviral zoonoses are members of this group:

- JE in Southeast Asia
- Murray Valley encephalitis (MVE) in Australia and New Guinea
- Kunjin virus encephalitis in Australia
- St. Louis encephalitis (SLE) in North and South America
- Rocio encephalitis (RE) in South America
- West Nile fever (WNF) in Africa, Europe, Asia, and North America
- Usutu virus in Africa and Europe

1.3.2.3 Agents Causing Yellow Fever and Dengue, Forming Two Closely Related Virus Complexes

Simians and humans are viremic hosts. *Aedes* mosquitoes are the transmitters. The zoonotic diseases in this group are as follows:

- Wesselsbron fever in Africa
- Yellow fever (YF) in Central Africa and South America
- Dengue fever (DEN) type 1 (DEN-1) to DEN-4 in Asia, Africa, and Central and South America and DEN hemorrhagic fever (DHF)

Occurrence. Flaviviruses have a worldwide distribution. There is little overlap between areas of endemicity because specific antibodies can neutralize other flaviviruses, not only the homologous virus type. For example, the distribution of JE in Australia appears to be limited by the fact that wild boars carry antibodies to the autochthonous flaviviruses, Murray Valley and Kunjin viruses. These antibodies can neutralize JE virus.

In comparison to alphaviruses, flaviviruses are more dynamic epidemiologically. For example, DEN in Central America was almost extinct in the 1960s and 1970s. It was rare in Africa and only occasional cases were seen in Southeast Asia. Between 1959 and 1998, there was an increase from 1,000 reported cases to more than 500,000. Better diagnostic facilities and recognition may explain some but not all of the increase. Meanwhile, DEN has regained its old territories in South and Central America. DEN follows the reappearance of malaria by 1 or 2 decades. Global warming is held responsible by some for this recurrence and for the increased activity of yellow fever. There is a more likely explanation: previously, the use of DDT (*dichlordiphenytrichlorethane*) as a pesticide in Asia, Africa, and South America controlled the main vector of DEN and YF (*Stegomyia aegypti*), as well as *Anopheles* spp. for malaria. Since the use of DDT was prohibited, populations of mosquitoes have reached former levels. Urban epidemics of YF, DEN, and Chikungunya virus have the same vector, *A. (Stegomyia) aegypti*. The absence of YF in Asia has been tentatively explained by an incompatibility of DEN and YF. Conversely, DEN coexists with YF in Africa and in North and South America. The reason for this incompatibility, especially the responsible sequence in the transmission cycle, has not been explained. It cannot be denied that not only the use of DDT or its cessation has influenced the epidemiology of vectorborne diseases. Changes of climate, which have a direct impact on the survival of arthropod vectors and on reservoir animals, must necessarily influence the global distribution of many zoonotic diseases. However, in a complex network of action and reaction it will always be difficult to find convincing evidence of causal relationships.

JE is another example for the strong epidemiological dynamics as a consequence of ecological manipulations. The virus needs herons but may also use pigs as an amplification host. Consequently, JE is far less common in Muslim countries than in others. The main vector for JE is *Culex tritaeniorhynchus,* which replicates in rice fields. It has been found that its larvae develop faster and are more numerous in rice fields fertilized with nitrogen compounds than in unfertilized fields. That may explain the increased distribution of JE in India and Indochina. In Japan, as well as in Korea, JE is totally eradicated.

JE is the most important disease of this group. It is widely distributed in the Far East. There is an overlap between JE and the West Nile virus (WNV), another flavivirus in the same antigen group, on the west coast of India. WNV is predominant in the Near East, Southern Europe, and Africa. The SLE virus in North and South America and the RE virus in South America are additional members of this virus group. In 1999, the West Nile virus invaded the east coast of North America, where it now over-laps with the SLE virus.

Transmission. All members of the genus *Flavivirus* that are pathogenic for humans are arboviruses transmitted either by ticks (TBE complex) or by mosquitoes. Vertical virus transmission is possible both in ticks and in mosquitoes by transovarial and transstadial routes. Infection of vertebrates is needed for the maintenance cycle. In spite of high levels of viremia, these vertebrates do not necessarily develop clinical diseases but serve as the amplification hosts of the virus from which ticks and mosquitoes become infected. There are similarities in the dependence on viremic hosts and in vector usage in each of the antigenic complexes mentioned above.

In human flavivirus infections, transmission by direct contact does not occur. However, virus transmission by transfusion of blood and blood products, as well as by organ transplantation and breast-feeding, was recently observed with WNV infections. The DEN virus can also be transmitted by blood transfusion.

As a rule, the donor is in the preclinical phase of the infection. The viremia is low but is sufficient for virus transmission in a large volume. Due to the high infectious volume and the acceptor's preexisting disease, such cases have a severe prognosis.

Clinical Manifestations. The disease course of flavivirus infections is marked by biphasic fever and a distinct prodromal period. Diseases of the CNS are predominant in tick-transmitted Togavirus infections (CEE, RSSE, LI, and PE) and in mosquito-transmitted Togavirus infections. Generalized disease, hepatitis, and hemorrhagic fever are predominant in YF, in DHF, and in the tick-transmitted KFD. However, encephalitis in these diseases is not uncommon. The same is true for DEN. Myalgia is the main symptom in DEN, and therefore DEN is difficult to differentiate from alphavirus-induced arthropathies. A careful clinical examination is important. Mixed infections with DEN virus and Chikungunya virus have been reported. The same vector, *Stegomyia aegypti*, can distribute DEN viruses and Chikungunya virus in an urban environment.

The pathogenesis of flavivirus infections involves virus antibody complexes that attach to mononuclear leukocytes via the Fc receptor. Cross-reacting flavivirus antibodies may recognize a related viral antigen without neutralizing the virus and without inactivating the virus by complement-dependent lysis. Once the macrophages are infected, their NO *synthetase* is inhibited and intracellular virus inactivation is prevented. Infected leukocytes release cytokines in addition to increasing virus titers by 2 or 3 log10 units. Life-threatening complications can occur during DEN virus infections. DEN shock syndrome (DSS) and DHF occur frequently when cross-reacting antibodies are present from another DEN infection with a different virus subtype. These antibodies bind to the virus but do not neutralize it. DSS has been observed in newborn babies who had maternal antibodies to one of the DEN subtype viruses and who were infected with a heterologous subtype. With the exception of the West Nile Virus, no flavivirus-associated prenatal infection or embryopathy in human fetuses has been reported. Infection during pregnancy may result in chorioretinitis in the fetus. In general, flavivirus infections are less severe in children than in adults, which might be based on children's lack of immunologic experience with other flaviviruses. In alphavirus infections, pediatric disease is more severe than adult disease.

Animal Infections with Flaviviruses. The question of whether an animal is infected by an arbovirus seems to be mainly a problem of the host range and species specificity of the vectors. Animals that undergo viremic infections can be amplifying hosts of the virus; non-viremic hosts cannot. Antibodies against indigenous flaviviruses are usually found in a high percentage of domestic animal species. Reports of the pathogenicity of some of these viruses for horses may be contradictory. It has not been determined whether antibody-mediated infection of macrophages may be involved in these contradicting reports on flavivirus pathogenicity for horses. WNV infection has been shown to be pathogenic for crows and for alligators.

Diagnosis. It is important to look at the seasonal preference of arbovirus infections, which is bound to the life cycle of the vectors. The diagnosis of sporadic flavivirus infections can be difficult. Isolation or demonstration of the virus usually is impossible; it is successful only during the first week of infection, when typical clinical signs are absent. That is especially true for the encephalitides. Dead animals (monkeys, horses, or birds) are sometimes important indicators of a disease outbreak.

Suckling mice (age, 2 to 4 days) and cell cultures from vertebrates are suitable for the isolation of the virus, for example, Vero, BHK21, and LLC-MK cells, primary chicken or duck embryo fibroblasts, or mosquito cell lines (C6/36 or AP 6/1). Mosquito cells are highly susceptible to infection but do not show cytopathic effects. Concentrated inocula or presence of antibody may cause pro zone effects with negative results. Diluted inocula may result in virus isolation. An isolated virus may be detected and identified by immunofluorescence, plaque neutralization, and RT-PCR.

Methods have been developed for the direct demonstration of the virus in clinical samples (blood, tissue, and CSF), but they can be used only for viruses that cause a sufficiently high titer in blood for a sufficient period of time. RT-PCR and antigen capture methods using monoclonal antibodies are available. As a rule, the neurotropic flaviviruses are not detected in the peripheral circulation.

A seminested RT-PCR has been developed for detection of all clinically relevant flaviviruses, using group-specific primers A and B to amplify the C-terminal one-fourth of the NS5 gene. Addition of a species-specific upstream amplimer C allows amplification of a species-specific amplicon in combination with the flavivirus group-specific downstream amplimer A. As an example, the combination of a group-specific RT-PCR and a virus-specific seminested PCR for detection of TBE viruses is to be found in the literature.

For direct virus documentation, it is important to have methods that have been proven experimentally. Standardization for clinical applications is not available. Due to the considerable problems connected with direct virus demonstration, it is not surprising that serology is still frequently used for the diagnosis of acute cases and for typing the agent. Most serological tests allow only a tentative diagnosis because of extensive cross-reactions between flaviviruses. All epidemiologically and geographically relevant antigens have to be included in the test. The neutralization test still has significance among the classical serological tests, because it is fairly type specific. It also indicates protective immunity after vaccination. If virus isolates do not produce typical cytopathic effects in cell culture, the fluorescent focus inhibition test can be used. Demonstration of IgM antibody by IgM capture ELISA is most important for the diagnosis of acute infections with flaviviruses. It can be improved by using type-specific antigens. Again, related antigens have to be included in the test. The best diagnostic evidence is a significant rise of IgG antibody titers after the switch from IgM antibodies.

Therapy. Antiviral therapy for flavivirus infections is not available. Treatment is symptomatic and is primarily directed towards maintaining homeostasis. Some infections are life threatening. Transport to a central competent hospital should be strictly avoided (patients should be treated in local hospitals), especially in cases with a hemorrhagic course. The positive or negative effects of hyperimmune serum for therapy and for prophylaxis are controversial. Controlled clinical studies are lacking.

Prophylaxis. Inactivated vaccines are available for a series of flaviviruses. They are especially used for the prevention of CEE, RSSE, and JE, but inadvertent reactions may occur. Vaccines should never be given after exposure to the virulent agents or too close to an exposure. Postexposure treatment of humans against TBE virus with hyperimmune serum resulted in severe cases of encephalitis. This prophylaxis, therefore, is no longer recommended for children less than 14 years old after tick bites.

To prevent virus transmission by blood transfusion or organ transplants, the donor's serum should be tested for the presence of class IgM antiviral antibody if the donation took place during the period of seasonal prevalence. Virus detection by RT-PCR is probably not adequate to detect a low-titer viremia.

Immunization against YF with the attenuated 17D strain developed by Theiler has been very successful for more than 50 years. Side effects, risks, and contraindications have been known since the introduction of this vaccine. On rare occasions, YF vaccination with the 17D strain may result in lethal infections with the vaccine virus. In some cases, a vaccine associated viscerotropic disease with multiorgan failure or a vaccine associated neurotropic disease is observed.

Recently, a series of six fatal cases following YF vaccination reported from Australia, Brazil, and the United States has raised attention to this problem.

Vaccination and the problem of immune enhancement in flavivirus infections. Attenuated live virus vaccines against JE and DEN have been produced or are under investigation. Recombinant viruses expressing the protective antigens of JE and DEN viruses are being developed based on the 17D vaccine strain of YF virus. Not one of these vaccines has been sufficiently clinically evaluated as of yet. Vaccine tolerance is difficult to evaluate, especially for DEN, because of the immune enhancement phenomenon and because of the uncontrollable epidemiology of the disease. It is well established that the reproduction of flaviviruses can be enhanced in the presence of antibodies. In animal experiments, it was shown that pre-existing antiviral antibodies, directed against epitopes of the E-protein but unable to neutralize or to lyse the virus, can mediate macrophage infection via the Fc-receptor. This phenomenon is held to be responsible for the development of DHF and DSS observed in individuals when they experience their second DEN infection with an antigenically related virus. In addition, this phenomenon was shown as early as 1981 to occur with the 17D strain used for YF vaccination. At present, no prediction of the individual risk for an antibody mediated macrophage infection can be made, and it is not known whether the generalized infections with the 17D strain of YF, which caused the death of vaccinees in 2001, were associated with immune enhancement. It is conceivable that the observed differences in the pathogenicities of flaviviruses that infect horses (e.g., JE virus, SLE virus, and WNV) might reflect the phenomenon of immune enhancement.

Laboratory infections with flaviviruses have occurred repeatedly. They should be prevented by vaccination and other protective measures. Nosocomial or hospital infections have not been reported. Patients with YF and DEN should be isolated if competent vectors (e.g., *S. aegypti*) have access to the patients which could initiate an urban cycle (human-to-human transmission). Mosquito nets and repellents should always be used prophylactically. Vaccines are not available for all arboviruses. Populations in equatorial Africa, which lack mosquito nets or vaccines in most instances, recently became exposed again to YF.

Immunization of amplification hosts of flaviviruses can reduce epidemics. Immunization of pigs against JE might reduce the frequency of human infections.

REFERENCES

Cavrini F et al., Usutu virus infection in a patient who underwent orthotropic liver transplantation, Italy, August-September 2009. *Euro Surveill* 14, ppii=19448.

CDC, Possible West Nile virus transmission to an infant through breast-feeding – Michigan, 2002. *JAMA*, 288, 1976–1977, 2002.

CDC, West Nile virus activity – United States, September 26 – October 2, 2002, and investigations of West Nile virus infections in recipients of blood transfusion and organ transplantation. *JAMA*, 288, 1975–1976, 2002.

Chan RC et al., Hepatitis and death following vaccination with 17D-204 yellow fever vaccine. *Lancet* 358, 121–122, 2001.

Chang GJ et al., Flavivirus DNA vaccines: current status and potential. *Ann. N. Y. Acad. Sci.* 951, 272–285, 2001.

Diamond MS, Progress on the development of therapeutics against West Nile virus. *Antivir. Res.* 83, 214–227, 2009.

Galler R et al., Phenotypic and molecular analyses of yellow fever 17DD vaccine viruses associated with serious adverse events in Brazil. *Virology.* 290, 309–319, 2001.

Fernandez-Garcia MD et al., Pathogenesis of flavivirus infections: using and abusing the host cell. *Cell Host Microbe* 5, 318–328, 2009.

Gardner CL, Ryman CD, Yellow fever: a reemerging threat. *Clin. Lab. Med.* 30, 237–260, 2010.

Harris E et al., Molecular biology of flavivirus. *Novartis Found. Symp.* 277, 23–39, 2006.

Jansen CC, Beebe NW, The dengue vector Aedes aegypti: what comes next. *Microbes Infect.* 12, 272–279, 2010.

Johnson AJ et al., Detection of anti-arboviral immunoglobulin G by using a monoclonal antibody-based capture enzyme-linked immunosorbent assay. *J. Clin. Microbiol.* 38, 1827–1831, 2000.

Kimura T et al., Flavivius encephalitis: pathological aspects of mouse and other animal models. *Vet. Pathol.* 47, 806–818, 2010.

Knauber M et al., Clinical proof of principle for ChimeriVax: recombinant live, attenuated vaccines against flavivirus infections. *Vaccine* 20, 1004–1018, 2002.

Kramer LD, Li J, Shi PY, West Nile virus. *Lancet Neurol.* 6, 171–181, 2007.

Kyle JL, Harris E, Global spread and persistence of dengue. *Annu. Rev. Microbiol.* 62, 71–92, 2008.

Lasala PR, Holbrook M, Tick-borne flaviviruses. *Clin. Lab. Med.* 30, 221–235, 2010.

Leong AS et al., The pathology of dengue hemorrhagic fever. *Semin. Diagn. Pathol.* 24, 227–236, 2007.

Malet H et al., The flavivirus polymerase as a target for drug discovery. *Antivir. Res.* 80, 23–35, 2008.

Marin M et al., Fever and multisystem organ failure associated with 17D yellow fever vaccination: a report of four cases. *Lancet* 358, 98–104, 2001.

Martin DA et al., Standardization of immunoglobulin M capture enzyme linked immunosorbent assays for routine diagnosis of arboviral infections. *J. Clin. Microbiol.* 38, 1823–1826, 2001.

Martina BE, Koraka P, Osterhaus AD, Dengue virus pathogenesis: an integrated view. *Clin. Microbiol. Rev.* 22, 564–581, 2009.

Miller N, Recent progress in dengue vaccine research and development. *Curr. Opin. Mol. Ther.* 12, 31–38, 2010.

Monath TP (2008), Treatment of yellow fever. *Antivir. Res.* 78, 116–124.

Olifant T, Diamond MS, The molecular basis of antibody-mediated neutralization of West Nile virus. *Expert Opin. Biol. Ther.* 7, 885–892, 2007.

Pattniak P, Kyasanur forest disease: an epidemiological view in India. *Rev. Med. Virol.* 16, 151–165, 2006.

Petersen LR, Hayes EB, West Nile virus in the Americas. *Med. Clin. North Am.* 92, 1307–1322, 2008.

Ruzek D et al., Omsk haemorrhagic fever. *Lancet* 376, 2104–2113, 2010.

Schlesinger JJ, Brandriss MW, Antibodymediated infection of macrophages and macrophage- like cell lines with 17D-yellow fever virus. *J. Med. Virol.* 8, 103–117, 1981.

Schlesinger JJ, Brandriss MW, Growth of 17D yellow fever virus in a macrophage-like cell line, U937: role of Fc and viral receptors in antibody-mediated infection. *J. Immunol.* 127, 659–665, 1981.

Stiasny K, Heinz FX, Flavivirus membrane fusion. *J. Gen. Virol.* 87, 2755–2766, 2006.

Tesh RB et al., Immunization with heterologous flaviviruses protective against fatal West Nile encephalitis. *Emerg. Infect. Dis.* 8, 245–251, 2002.

Trent DW, Chang GJ, Detection and identification of flaviviruses by reverse transcriptase polymerase chain reaction. In: Becker Y, Darai G (eds.): *Diagnosis of Human Viruses by Polymerase Chain Reaction Technology*, Chapter 27, 355–369. Springer, Berlin, Heidelberg, New York, 1992.

Urcuqui-Inchima S et al., Recent developments in understanding dengue virus replication. *Adv. Virus Res.* 77, 1–39, 2010.

Van den Hurk AF, Ritchie SA, Mackenzie JS, Ecology and geographical expansion of Japanese encephalitis virus. *Annu. Rev. Entomol.* 54, 17–35, 2009.

Van der Schaar HM, Wilschut JC, Smit JM, Role of antibodies in controlling dengue virus infection. *Immunobiol.* 214, 613–629, 2009.

Vasconcelos PFC et al., Serious adverse events associated with yellow fever 17D vaccine in Brazil: a report on two cases. *Lancet* 358, 91–97, 2001.

Weissenbock H et al., Emergence of Usutu virus, an African Mosquito-borne flavivirus of the Japanese encephalitis virus group, Central Europe. *Emerg. Infect. Dis.* 8, 652–656, 2002.

1.3.3 ZOONOSES CAUSED BY TICK-BORNE FLAVIVIRUSES

1.3.3.1 Tick-Borne Encephalitis (TBE) European Subtype (Central European Encephalitis) and TBE Eastern Subtype (Russian Spring-Summer Meningoencephalitis)

Central European tick encephalitis (CEE, also known as the European or western subtype of TBE), or spring-summer meningoencephalitis, is the most important human arbovirus infection in Central Europe. It is transmitted by a tick bite. In full-blown cases, it develops into a meningoencephalitis with a biphasic clinical course.

Closely related to CEE is the eastern subtype of TBE, Russian spring-summer meningoencephalitis (RSSE), also called Far Eastern Encephalitis. The disease is transmitted by different ticks and it causes a disease even more severe than CEE.

Etiology. The causative agents of CEE and RSSE are flaviviruses, family *Flaviviridae*, genus *Flavivirus*. Together with other tick-transmitted flaviviruses they are classified in a subgroup known as the TBE complex.

Occurrence. TBE virus has been isolated in Bulgaria, Germany, Finland, France (Vosges Mountains), Greece, Italy, the former Yugoslavia, Austria, Poland, Romania, Sweden, Switzerland, Slovakia, the Czech Republic, the former USSR, and Hungary. Closely related to TBE virus are the tick-transmitted agents of LI, KFD, and OHF. Powassan virus, which occurs in North America, rarely causes encephalitis. The distribution areas of CEE and RSSE include not only Europe but also large parts of Asia (Fig. 1.3.). The prevalence of TBE was shown in 20 to 30 countries in Eurasia. The geographical distribution and the vectors of the arboviruses in the genus *Orbivirus* (e.g., Kemerovo virus) are the same as those for agents causing TBE (European and eastern subtypes). There is a close epidemiological and possibly pathogenetic correlation between these viruses.

Ixodid ticks are also vectors of *Borrelia burgdorferi*. Double infections with Lyme borreliosis occur in regions of endemicity.

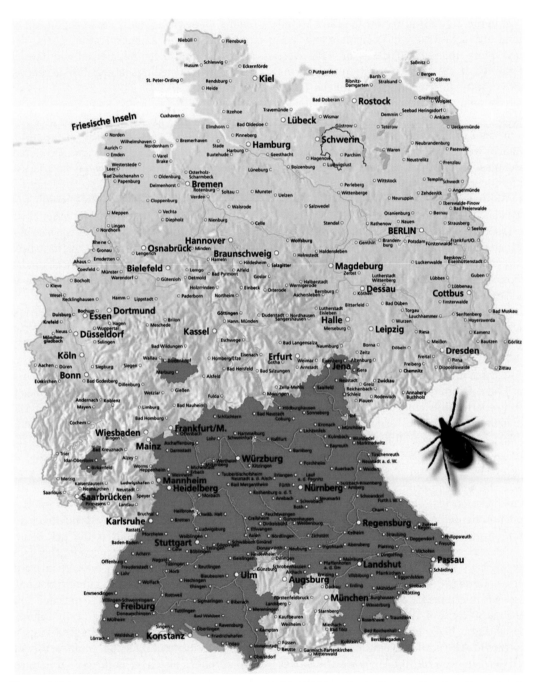

Figure 1.3 | Areas in Germany where tick-borne encephalitis (TBE) is endemic. The transition from the eastern to the western type of TBE is indicated. Outside the areas of endemicity, sporadic autochthonous TBE infections have been found. (Courtesy of Chiron Behring.)

Serologically, the existence of the TBE virus infection in feral animals has been found in Denmark, Spain, and Turkey. In the western part of Germany, the northern limit of the disease approximately follows the Main River. In central Germany, cases of TBE are known to exist in the Thuringian Forest, the Harz Mountains, and occasionally in Pomerania and Saxony. More than 1,000 cases of TBE were registered in the former East Germany in the early 1960s. Infected ticks can still be found in the area, but human disease no longer exists.

In cases of TBE that appear north of the river Main or west of the river Rhine, imported infection must be ruled out before a local source of infection can be assumed. There is a gradual transition in Eastern Europe between the European and the eastern subtypes of TBE. The eastern subtype was described in Russia in 1937 and recognized as a health hazard. In contrast, the European subtype was recognized first in Czechoslovakia in 1948 and later in Austria. Migration to the north of Europe was registered during the last decade. Endemic infections were found not only in Sweden and Finland but also in Norway.

The first cases of TBE in the Baltic countries (791 cases in Lithuania and 166 cases in Estonia) were reported in 1993. In 1994, 1,366 cases were reported from Lithuania (52.4 per 100,000 inhabitants). Climatic, economic, and even political changes were discussed as causes of a dramatic increase in TBE infections in the former eastern bloc countries after 1990. The use of DDT and other insecticides in agriculture may have been an important factor in causing the low prevalence of TBE in countries behind the Iron Curtain.

Ten cases of CEE have been documented serologically within the last 5 years in central Hesse, Germany. They have to be considered endemic infections for epidemiological reasons. Among 30 cases of TBE which had been diagnosed since 1970, no endemic infection was diagnosed. The northern limit for CEE in western Germany now lies 100 km north of the river Main. More recently, autochthonous cases of CEE were found in Rhineland-Palatinate, in Thuringia around the city of Jena, and in the Vosges.

Hedgehogs, shrews, and moles are important reservoirs for CEE and RSSE. The virus persists in hibernating hedgehogs. In addition, waterfowl and bats have been identified as hosts.

Among domestic animals, the infection can be found in grazing animals (cattle, goats, and sheep). Dogs also can be infected and develop clinical signs of meningoencephalitis, in contrast to ruminants.

Transmission. CEE is transmitted predominantly by *Ixodes ricinus,* and RSSE is transmitted predominantly by *Ixodes persulcatus, Dermacentor marginatus,* and *Dermacentor silvarum* as well as some *Haemaphysalis* species. Undeveloped tick nymphs are infected by engorging on viremic animals and then can infect other hosts. Ticks not only serve as vectors, they can also play a role as reservoirs. Vertical infections have been demonstrated with transovarial and transstadial virus passage from egg to larva to nymph to adult and again to eggs (Fig. 1.4).

The role of ticks as vectors explains some epidemiological peculiarities. Reported human cases are between 100 and 500 per year. For their maturation, ticks need a temperature of 15 °C during their development. If the temperature exceeds 15 °C, the relative humidity needs to be almost saturated. The biting activity of ticks is restricted to periods of weekly temperatures averaging between 7 °C and 15 °C. For climatic reasons, infections with CEE are restricted to May and June. RSSE infections typically peak in the spring and fall.

People are infected by a bite of an infected tick. As far as CEE is concerned, tick bites are only considered dangerous if the tick comes from an area with natural infection, that is, if 0.1% to 1% of the ticks in the area are infected.

CEE can be transmitted to humans not only by tick bites but also through fresh milk and non-pasteurized milk products (Fig. 1.4). Latently infected cattle, goats, and sheep shed virus in milk are a source of infection. Multiple laboratory infections also have occurred. Virus transmission is possible by direct contact or by aerosol.

Clinical Manifestations
The incubation period is 1 to 2 weeks, but it can be shorter or last up to 4 weeks. The infection results in clinical manifestation in 10% to 30% of cases. In an area of endemicity, only 0.1% to

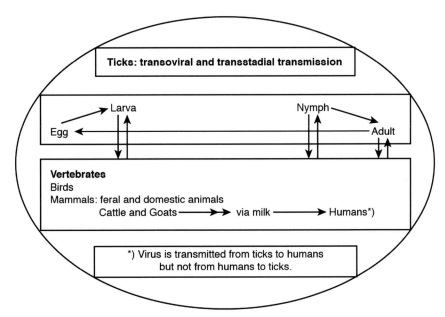

Figure 1.4 | Infectious cycle of the tick-borne encephalitis virus complex.

0.3% of tick bites result in CEE. Clinically apparent infections are less common in children. The rate of clinical manifestation in adults who have not grown up in areas of endemicity appears to be higher than the calculated rate.

The typical clinical course is biphasic, with a prodromal stage of 1 to 6 days seen in 71% of all cases with clinical manifestation. In two-thirds of all clinical cases, the disease is restricted to the prodromal stage. In the remaining cases, a disease-free interval of 7 to 10 days follows the first disease phase. Meningoencephalitis with another fever elevation follows thereafter.

Clinical signs in the prodromal stage are nonspecific. They are flu-like with catarrhal appearance, fever up to 39 °C, limb pain, headaches, and gastrointestinal problems. There is leukopenia. The disease in humans is frequently seen in the spring, with farmers and foresters in most cases, and occasionally, there is meningism. The second phase begins with a fever up to 40°C or more with severe signs of disease. An increase in protein in the CSF, as well as a mononuclear pleocytosis, is found in many cases of meningitis (47%) and encephalitis (42%). Asymptomatic convalescence may occur after 2 to 14 days. However, it may develop into a long phase of increased weakness of the autonomic nervous system and tendency towards severe headaches (23% within 1 to 5 years). Severe cases manifest as encephalomyelitis with paresis and paralysis or as meningoencephalomyelitis (11%). Complete recovery is possible even in these cases. Frequently, spinal paralysis may remain or the patient may die with a bulbar paralysis. In patients with encephalomyelitis, the fatality rate for CEE is 1% to 5%; the fatality rate for RSSE is up to 20%. Myopericarditis has also been described to occur in cases of CEE infection.

Simultaneous infections of CEEV with Lyme Borreliosis (*B. burgdorferi*, *B. afzelii*, or *B. garinii*) can occur and require special diagnostic and therapeutic measures. In children, if they are free of constitutional problems, severe courses of CEE with encephalomyelitis and residua occur less frequently than in adults.

Diagnosis

The record of a tick bite or previous presence in an area of endemicity (Fig. 1.2) is essential for a tentative diagnosis. A tick bite could have happened up to 4 weeks previously. The ingestion of raw sheep or goat milk can also raise a suspicion if it happened in an area of endemicity.

Presence of a virus can be demonstrated by isolation, antigen detection, or PCR. Virus detection by direct or indirect techniques is successful only during the prodromal phase, not later. For the same reason, RT-PCR is not used in the diagnosis of clinical cases. It is applicable for the demonstration of virus in ticks and in postmortem examinations. An RT-PCR is available for the group-specific amplification of the C-terminal one-fourth of the flaviviral NS5 gene. Addition of the virus-specific up-amplimer C allows species-specific amplification: a seminested PCR is carried out with a virus-specific up-amplimer in combination with the flavivirus group-specific down amplimer (for details, see the references).

Demonstration of virus-specific IgM antibodies in serum and in CSF is useful for an early and fast diagnosis. Because of the small success rate in isolating the virus after CNS signs are present, the demonstration of virus-specific IgM antibody is more practical for the diagnosis.

Serological cross-reactions among flaviviruses, not only in the TBE complex, limit the value of serological tests. In Central Europe, vaccination against YF has to be considered as a cause of cross-reacting antibodies since other flavivirus infections do not exist. In patients recovering from CEE or RSSE, antibodies are present not only in serum but also in the CSF. The Reiber quotient (plotting $Q._{IgG}$ against $Q._{Alb}$.) is used for demonstration of intrathecal antibody production. A new fluorescent focus inhibition test has been developed for the detection of protective antibodies. Successful vaccination can only be confirmed by determination of neutralizing antibodies. A positive signal in the IgG ELISA is not sufficient.

Differential Diagnosis

In the prodromal stage, influenza-like diseases and poliomyelitis should be considered for a differential diagnosis. In the meningoencephalitic stage, the spectrum narrows towards causative agents of serous meningitis or encephalitis, for example, the mumps virus and many enteroviruses. Garin-Bujadoux-Bannwarth meningopolyneuritis (*Borrelia garinii*) should be considered, especially after a tick bite. Dual infections with *B. burgdorferi* and CEE virus should be kept in mind in areas of endemicity. After a tick bite has been found, human granulomatous Ehrlichiosis should be considered during the early phase of the disease. In the absence of evidence of infection, tick paresis or tick paralysis should be considered.

Therapy

Specific therapy for CEE and RSSE does not exist, and treatment is symptomatic. Extended bed rest is important to ameliorate the autonomic system instability and to shorten the recovery period. Paralysis in the second phase can be reduced if the patient stays in bed even during the disease-free interval. Early physical therapy is important to avoid muscle atrophy and to enhance regeneration.

Prophylaxis

Foresters and forest workers as well as tourists in light clothing are at risk. In areas of endemicity, raw milk, especially from goats and sheep, should not be consumed.

Anti-TBE hyperimmunoglobulin (FSME-Bulin) was in former times recommended for pre-exposure prophylaxis (0.05 ml of solution/kg) and for postexposure prophylaxis (0.2 ml of solution/kg). Postexposure treatment should be given earlier than 92 h after a tick bite, if the bite happens in a region of endemicity. Recently, children have developed severe disease following immunoprophylaxis. Therefore, pre-exposure prophylaxis by passive immunization is no longer recommended. The same applies for postexposure treatment with hyperimmunoglobulin.

Active immunization is effective and is recommended for individuals with a high exposure to ticks in areas of endemicity. An inactivated virus vaccine is available [Encepur® CEE vaccine for adults (Novartis vaccines, Marburg, Germany), three doses of 0.5 ml i.m. on days 0, 7, and 28; repeat after 12 months]. A special preparation for infants is also available. The Encepur vaccine can be given at short intervals (0, 7, and

21 days) or at long intervals (0, 28, and 300 days). Protective antibodies should be present 3 weeks after the second vaccination. A booster vaccination should be administered 3 years after the basic vaccination. Adverse vaccine effects, which were observed in children, were caused by allergic reactions against gelatin, which had been used as a stabilizer of the vaccine. This stabilizer has now been replaced. Special vaccines with a lower dose are available for children. Severe cases of CEE with encephalomyelitis and permanent damage or lethal outcome are rare in physically healthy children without immunologic deficiencies. CEE vaccination also protects vaccinees from an infection with the virus that causes RSSE. There are also Russian vaccines containing far Eastern strains of RSSE.

Postexposure vaccination, that is, vaccination after a tick bite in the area of endemicity, is contraindicated. Likewise, vaccination should not be given during the stage of generalized disease and CNS disease. Severe neuritis and egg white allergies present contraindications.

Vaccination campaigns have drastically reduced the occurrence of CEE in Austria and Bavaria. The rate of undesirable side effects for the Encepur vaccine is less than 10^{-6}. After active immunization against TBE, neuritis and neuralgia have been described. In several cases, it was recognized as an adverse effect of vaccination. At most 1 in 200 to 300 tick bites produces CEE, which remains clinically harmless in two-thirds of patients. Vaccination of people vacationing in areas of endemicity, therefore, is not urgently recommended by the vaccination board. The same holds true for immunoglobulin prophylaxis. Active immunization is recommended for seronegative inhabitants of areas of endemicity, especially for people professionally at high risk.

If antibodies against other flaviviruses (e.g., DEN or YF) are present in a person, the initiation of protective immunity can be delayed after active immunization against CEE.

REFERENCES

Alkadhi H, Kollias SL, MRI in tick-borne encephalitis. *Neuroradiology* 42, 753–755, 2000.

Arras C, Fescharek R, Gregersen JP, Do specific hyperimmunoglobulins aggravate clinical course of tick-borne encephalitis? *Lancet* 347, p1331, 1996.

Bakhvalova VN et al., Tick-borne encephalitis strains of Western Siberia. *Virus Res.* 70, 1–12, 2000.

Bröker M, Kollaritsch H, After a tick bite in a tick-borne encephalitis virus endemic area: current positions about post-exposure treatment. *Vaccine*, 26, 863–868, 2008.

Dobler G, Zoonotic tick-borne flaviviruses. *Vet. Microbiol.* 140, 221–228, 2010.

Duppenthaler A, Pfammatter JP, Aebi C, Myopericarditis associated with central European tick-borne encephalitis. *Eur. J. Pediatr.* 159, 854–856, 2000.

Heyman P et al., A clear and present danger: tick-borne diseases in Europe. *Expert Rev. Anti. Thera.* 8, 33–50, 2010.

Holzmann et al., Correlation between ELISA, hemagglutinin inhibition, and neutralization tests after vaccination against tickborne encephalitis. *J. Med. Virol* 48, 102–107, 1996.

Kaiser R, Tick-borne encephalitis. *Infect. Dis. Clin. North Am.* 22, 561–575, 2008.

Latric-Furlan S et al., Clinical distinction between human granulocytic ehrlichiosis and the initial phase of tick-borne encephalitis. *J. Infect.* 40, 55–58, 2000.

Lindquist L, Vapalathi O, Tick-borne encephalitis. *Lancet* 371, 1861–1871, 2008.

Logar M et al., Comparison of the epidemiological and clinical features of tick-borne encephalitis in children and adults. *Infection* 28, 74–77, 2000.

Lu Z, Bröker M, Liang G, Tick-borne encephalitis in mainland China. *Vector Borne Zoonotic Dis.* 8, 713–720, 2008.

Özdemir FA et al., Frühsommermeningoenzephalitis (CEE) – Ausweitung des Endemiegebietes nach Mittelhessen. *Der Nervenarzt* 70, 119–122, 1999.

Rendi-Wagner P, Persistence of antibodies after vaccination against tick-borne encephalitis. *Int. J. med. Microbiol.* 296 (suppl. 40), 202–207, 2006.

Rendi-Wagner P, Advances in vaccination against tick-borne encephalitis. *Expert Rev. Vacc.* 7, 589–596, 2008.

Treib J et al., Tick-borne encephalitis in the Saarland and the Rhineland-Palatinate. *Infection* 24, 242–244, 1996.

Waldvogel et al., Severe tick-borne encephalitis following passive immunization. *Eur. J. Paediatr.* 155, 775–779, 1996.

1.3.3.2 Louping Ill

LI is caused by an arbovirus infection transmitted by ticks. It is similar to spring-summer meningoencephalitis (CEE). However, in contrast to CEE, LI is rarely found in humans. The name "louping" is derived from a Scottish dialect and it indicates the hyperactivity and jumping gait of infected sheep.

Etiology. The agent of LI is a flavivirus (family *Flaviviridae*, genus *Flavivirus*). It belongs to the TBE virus complex together with CEE virus, OHF virus, KFD virus, and some other viruses.

Negishi virus is similar to the agent of LI. It was isolated from two fatal cases of human encephalitis in Tokyo. The virus is also known to cause encephalitis in China.

Occurrence. LI has been found in sheep and cattle in Scotland, northern England, Wales, and Ireland. It has also been seen in France, Sweden, Finland, Poland, Portugal, Bulgaria, and the former USSR. More recently, it has been seen in Norway. In eastern Scotland, the disease in sheep has the character of an enzootic. In contrast, periodic epizootics are the rule in western Scotland. The tick *I. ricinus* has a key role in the epidemiology of LI, similar to CEE. The tick serves as vector and reservoir. Of epidemiological importance besides sheep are grouse, red deer, hares, rabbits, bats, and hedgehogs.

Transmission. The occurrence of LI in humans is exceptional. Of 35 known cases in humans, 26 have been caused by laboratory infection. The others were infected from direct contact with diseased sheep or from tick bites. Aerogenic infections (transmitted via dust) are not known to occur. In contrast to CEE, transmission of LI via milk or cheese appears not to occur.

Clinical Manifestations. In humans, the clinical disease has a biphasic course. After an incubation period of 4 to 7 days, the disease begins with an influenza-like prodromal phase, which lasts 2 to 11 days. A symptom-free interval of 1 to 2 weeks follows. Another fever then initiates the manifestation in the CNS. The disease is rarely fatal. Clinically inapparent infections have been found frequently in humans.

In sheep, the infection with LI virus causes a viremia of short duration with fever. Nervous signs follow several days later. They include incoordination (jumping disease) and then paralysis. The fatality rate is 20% to 50%. Dogs can also develop CNS disease after infection.

Diagnosis. The diagnosis of LI is based on demonstration of the agent in the CSF as well as on rising antibody titers in paired serum samples. A group- specific RT-PCR is available for the demonstration of flavivirus infections. The species-specific flavivirus genome can be identified with specific primers.

Differential Diagnosis. For differential diagnosis, the agents of other meningitides and meningoencephalitides, including Lyme borreliosis and enteroviruses, have to be considered.

Therapy. Specific therapy for LI does not exist. The therapy is supportive.

Prophylaxis. This is a rare disease in humans and it does not justify the introduction of a vaccine for general use. Laboratory personnel, shepherds, and veterinarians are especially at risk. A formalin-inactivated vaccine prepared in sheep kidney cell cultures has been used widely in sheep.

REFERENCES

Gilbert L et al., Role of small mammals in the persistence of Louping Ill virus: field survey and tick co-feeding studies. *Med. Vet. Entomol.* 14 (3), 277–282, 2000.

Laurenson MK et al., The role of lambs in Louping Ill amplification. *Parasitology* 120, 97–104, 2000.

1.3.3.3 *Powassan Virus Encephalitis*

Powassan virus was isolated in 1957 from a fatal human case of encephalitis. It is a tick-transmitted flavivirus that causes encephalitis in humans in the northern United States, Canada, and Russia.

Etiology. The virus is a member of the TBE complex in the family *Flaviviridae*, genus *Flavivirus*. Together with Modoc virus, it is the American addition to the TBE complex. Their RNA base sequences are markedly different from CEE and RSSE base sequences.

Occurrence. Human disease with Powassan virus is known to occur in Canada (Ontario), Russia, the northeastern United States (New York and Pennsylvania), and Wisconsin. Juvenile males ≤20 years of age involved in outdoor activities are mostly affected. The disease is rare in the remaining population, affecting only 0.5% to 4%. On the basis of serological analysis, it can be assumed that all of North America is affected, including British Columbia, California, and Mexico.

Transmission. Squirrels and groundhogs (woodchucks) are important in the transmission cycle of Powassan virus. Infection with Powassan virus has been demonstrated by virus isolation and serology in rabbits, dogs, skunks, and foxes. Experimentally infected goats shed the virus in their milk.

Ixodes ticks (*I. marxi, I. cookei, I. spinnipalpus,* and *I. andersoni*) are believed to be responsible for transmission. Experimentally, *I. scapularis* is a competent host. The epidemiology of Powassan virus is similar to those of Lyme borreliosis and Ehrlichiosis. The virus has been isolated in Russia from *Haemaphysalis neumanni* ticks and from mosquitoes.

Clinical Manifestations. Considering the seroprevalence, human disease with the Powassan virus begins with a nonspecific influenza-like prodromal period followed by meningitis and encephalitis. The encephalitis resembles herpesvirus encephalitis and may be fatal.

Diagnosis. A tentative clinical diagnosis of PE can only be made after signs of encephalitis are evident. Virus isolation from human cases is usually possible only from biopsy specimens or from brain tissue (postmortem). A group-specific RT-PCR is available for the demonstration of flavivirus infection. The species-specific flavivirus genome can be identified with specific primers.

Commonly, evidence of virus-specific IgM in serum (IgM capture ELISA) is used for diagnosis. Cross-reactivity with other flaviviruses has to be considered.

Differential Diagnosis. The differential diagnosis includes all agents causing encephalitis in North America, especially arboviruses but also herpesvirus. The disease is rare. Besides viruses, bacteria causing encephalitis should be considered. If a tick exposure has occurred, Lyme borreliosis and Ehrlichiosis have to be ruled out.

Therapy. There is no specific therapy for PE and treatment is symptomatic.

Prophylaxis. Protection from tick exposure and prompt removal of ticks after attachment is the best prophylaxis.

REFERENCES

CDC, Outbreak of Powassan encephalitis – Maine and Vermont, 1999–2001. *MMWR Morb. Mortal Wkly. Rep.* 50, 761–764, 2001.

CDC, Outbreak of Powassan encephalitis – Maine and Vermont, 1999–2001. *JAMA* 286, 1962–1963, 2001.

Ebel GD, Update on Powassan virus: emergence of a North American tick-borne flavivirus. *Annu. Rev. Entomol.* 55, 95–110, 2010.

Ford-Jones EL et al., Human surveillance for West Nile virus infection in Ontario in 2000. *CMAJ* 166, 29–35, 2002.

Romero JR, Simonson KA, Powassan encephalitis and Colorado tick fever. *Infect. Dis. Clin. North Am.* 22, 545–559, 2008.

1.3.3.4 Kyasanur Forest Disease and Alkhurma Virus Hemorrhagic Fever

KFD is a disease transmitted by tick bites. Symptoms include fever and CNS disturbances, and, at times, a hemorrhagic course. The Alkhurma virus is closely related to the KFD virus. It was isolated from human cases of severe hemorrhagic fever in Saudi Arabia.

Etiology. The causative agent is a flavivirus (family *Flaviviridae*, genus *Flavivirus*). It belongs to the TBE complex.

Occurrence. The disease occurs in districts of India [Shimoga and North and South Kanara districts as well as the Chikamagaloor district in the state of Karnataka (formerly Mysore)]. The area of distribution of the virus in India is much larger than the area where the disease occurs. Besides humans, monkeys may develop encephalitis. Latently infected cattle and monkeys (Rhesus and Langur) are considered to be reservoirs, as are small rodents and birds. There is a seasonal prevalence. The disease does not occur during the monsoon season (second half of the year). The lumber workers are especially at risk. Fatal cases in monkeys often indicate the beginning of an epidemic. The disease is frequently seen in connection with cattle farming in recently cleared areas.

Transmission. The bite of infected *Haemaphysalis* ticks (several species) results in human infection. As with CEE, drinking raw milk can cause an infection via the mucous membranes of the oropharynx and the gastrointestinal tract.

Clinical Manifestations. The incubation period is 8 days. The disease course is biphasic. The first phase, which lasts approximately 1 week, includes fever, headache and myalgia, conjunctivitis, bronchitis, gastrointestinal signs with diarrhea, and maculopapular exanthemas. Hemorrhages may be seen on mucous membranes. Signs then subside. Encephalitis may appear 1 to 3 weeks later. The mortality rate may be 5% to 10%. Fatal cases present as hemorrhagic fever.

Monkeys (*Presbytis entellus* and *Macaca radiata*) can show disease and may die from encephalitis. The infection in other animals is subclinical.

Diagnosis. Especially during the early phase of the disease, the agent can be isolated from blood, CSF, or organs from sick people by the use of cell culture, embryonating hen eggs, or experimental animals (newborn mice). A group-specific PCR (nested PCR) is available for the demonstration of flavivirus infections. The species-specific flavivirus genome can be identified with specific primers in a seminested PCR protocol.

ELISA and indirect immunofluorescence are commonly used today for the demonstration of antibodies. The quotient of IgM antibodies in serum and in CSF is indicative of acute infection. Intrathecal immunoglobulin production is demonstrated using the Reiber quotient (plotting $Q_{.IgG}$ against $Q_{.Alb.}$). Group-specific reactions with other flaviviruses (JE virus, WNV, and DEN virus) have to be considered.

Differential Diagnosis. Other TBEs and hemorrhagic fevers should be included in the differential diagnosis, as well as Lyme borreliosis, JE, and enterovirus infections.

Therapy. Therapy is symptomatic.

Prophylaxis. Tick repellents, protective clothing, and treatment of cattle with acaricides are the recommended means of prophylaxis. Vaccination is used to immunize people in areas of endemicity. Cattle are vaccinated to break the chain of infection.

REFERENCES

Charrel RN et al., Complete coding sequence of the Alkhurma virus, a tick-borne flavivirus causing severe hemorrhagic fever in humans in Saudi Arabia. *Biochem. Biophys. Res. Commun.* 287, 455–461, 2001.

Mehla R et al., Recent ancestry of Kyasanur Forest disease virus. *Emerg. Infect. Dis.* 15, 1431–1437, 2009.

Pattnaik P, Kyasanur Forest disease: an epidemiological view in India. *Rev. Med. Virol.* 16, 151–165, 2006; oerratum: *Rev. Med. Virol.* 18, 211, 2008.

Venugopal K et al., Analysis of the structural protein gene sequence shows Kyasanur forest disease virus as a distinct member in the tickborne encephalitis virus serocomplex. *J. Gen. Virol.* 75, 227–232, 1994.

1.3.3.5 Omsk Hemorrhagic Fever

OHF is an acute but benign disease caused by an arbovirus. The disease was described for the first time in 1944 near Novosibirsk and Kurgansk, Russia. Virus transmission to humans is by tick bite.

Etiology. The causative agent of OHF is a flavivirus that belongs to the TBE complex, an antigenically and biologically closely related group. Among others, the agents of LI, CEE, and KFD belong to this complex.

Occurrence. The geographical distribution of OHF is limited to the forest and steppe regions of western Siberia. The disease in humans is usually seen in spring and summer.

The natural maintenance cycle of the virus is not well defined. Ticks (*Dermacentor reticulatus* and *Dermacentor apronophorus* among others) are the vectors. Small water rats, especially *Arvicula terrestris*, are considered to be viremic hosts. Muskrats (*Ondatra zibethica*) are epizootic hosts with high mortality.

Transmission. Transmission from muskrats to humans is usually not by ticks but by direct contact with blood, urine, or feces. Muskrat hunters are especially at risk.

The virus may persist in monkey kidneys. If kidneys from infected monkeys are used for the preparation of cell cultures, the virus can be found in these cultures.

Clinical Manifestations. The incubation period is 3 to 12 days. The disease begins suddenly with head and limb aches, malaise, vomiting, and fever, which lasts for 2 to 15 days. Biphasic courses are possible. However, they are the exception in contrast to other diseases caused by agents of the TBE complex.

The face of patients is red. Conjunctivitis, gingivitis, pharyngitis, and hyperemia with reddening of the mucous membranes and face are common. A hemorrhagic diathesis is manifested by epistaxis, hematemesis, and urogenital bleeding.

The disease course is usually benign. There is a case fatality rate of 0.5% to 3%. Convalescence can be delayed. Complications of the autonomic nervous system, headaches, sweating, and nausea are common.

Diagnosis. Mild cases of OHF are often not diagnosed. Virus can be isolated from blood and urine at the onset of fever. The PCR primers that are designed for species-specific detection of TBE virus can also be used for the detection of the OHF virus (see the list of references).

The diagnosis is most frequently made by demonstration of virus-specific IgM antibodies. IgM capture is the preferred technique. Cross-reactions with the closely related virus of CEE and RSSE can cause problems.

Differential Diagnosis. Crimean-Congo hemorrhagic fever and Korean hemorrhagic fever with renal syndromes have to be excluded in cases of OHF with extensive hemorrhagic syndromes.

Therapy. There is no specific therapy for OHF, and treatment is symptomatic. The hemorrhagic diathesis can be treated with clotting factors, fresh blood transfusion, or blood plasma.

Prophylaxis. A specific vaccine does not exist. However, there is cross-protection between CEE or RSSE and OHF. Therefore, vaccines for CEE or RSSE can be used for populations at risk.

REFERENCES

Holbrrok MR et al., An animal model for the tickborne flavi-Omsk hemorrhagic fever virus. *J. Infect. Dis.* 191, 100–108, 2005.

Li L et al., Molecular determinants of antigenicity of two subtypes of tick-borne flavivirus Omsk haemorrhagic fever virus. *J. Gen. Virol.* 85, 1619–1624, 2004.

Lin D et al., Analysis of the complete genome of the tick-borne flavivirus Omsk haemorrhagic fever virus. *Virology* 313, 81–90, 2003.

Yoshii K, Hoolbrook MR, Sub-gennmic replicon and virus-like particles of Omsk hemorrhagic fever virus. *Arch. Virol.* 154, 573–580, 2009.

1.3.4 ZOONOSES CAUSED BY MOSQUITO-BORNE FLAVIVIRUSES

1.3.4.1 Japanese Encephalitis

JE, formerly called Japanese B encephalitis, is caused by a flavivirus transmitted by mosquitoes.

Etiology. The causative agent, JE virus, is a flavivirus (family *Flaviviridae*, genus *Flavivirus*) and is closely related to the agents of SLE, WNF, and MVE.

Occurrence. The disease is endemic and epidemic in wide areas of Asia (Fig. 1.5 infection. WHO 2007). JE virus has been found in the

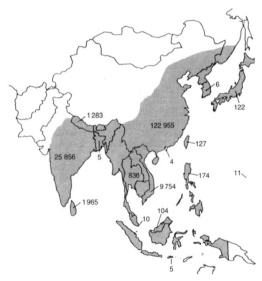

Figure 1.5 | Countries in which Japanese encephalitis has been identified. Status Nov. 2012. Courtesy CDC.

maritime regions of Siberia, as well as in China, Japan, Korea, Taiwan, the Philippines, Vietnam, Thailand, Cambodia, Laos, Indonesia, Burma, Malaysia, Bangladesh, Pakistan, and southern and eastern India, more recently it has been found in Bali and Australia (Torres Strait Islands). In tropical areas of Asia, the disease occurs throughout the year. In areas with a temperate climate, the winter is free of disease.

The spread of JE in Australia is limited due to the fact that 80% of wild boars have antibodies against the MVE and Kunjin viruses. These antibodies protect against infection with the JE virus.

Up to 70% of adults in tropical regions of Asia have JE antibodies. Children are primarily affected in epidemics. The manifestation rate in children is estimated to be 0.2%; in American soldiers in Vietnam, it was 4%.

Under natural conditions, several vertebrates are infected: pigs, cattle, goats, cats, dogs, birds, bats, snakes, and toads. Pigs and herons develop a viremic infection, amplify their viral load, and play an important role in the natural infection cycle.

JE occurs frequently in Malaysia but not in Indonesia. Reduced pig farming in the Islamic country may be an explanation. Introduction of the JE virus into formerly JE-free areas is possible. An outbreak of the disease occurred on the island of Saipan for the first time in 1990. Between 1989 and 1993, three tourists became infected in Bali and developed JE, with one tourist dying. More recently, visitors to Bali are advised to be vaccinated against JE, even if they spend only short time periods in tourist areas. In 5 years, between 1986 and 1990, 126,000 cases were registered in China, 26,000 were registered in India, 836 were registered in Thailand, and 122 were registered in Japan.

Transovarial virus transmission in mosquitoes has been proven. Therefore, they can serve as virus reservoirs for overwintering, even in areas with a temperate climate.

Transmission. *Culex* mosquitoes of the Vishnui complex *(C. tritaeniorhynchus, C. annulus,* and *C. annulirostris)* and *Aedes* mosquitoes are the vectors of JE virus. Different species may be involved in different geographical regions. The combination of rice crops and pig farming gives the JE virus an epidemiological advantage. The increase in JE cases in India can be explained by the increased use of fertilizers in rice fields. The main vector of JE virus, *C. tritaeniorhynchus,* hatches in rice fields. Its multiplication is increased by 50% in fertilized fields. The seasonal occurrence of the disease in northern regions is caused by migrating birds, especially herons. Transmission from human-to-human or animal-to-animal has not been shown occur.

Clinical Manifestations. Most infections are clinically inapparent. The rate of clinical manifestation is in the range of 0.1% to 4%. The incubation period is 4 to 14 days. A prodromal period of 2 to 3 days begins with fever, headaches, nonspecific malaise, and nonspecific respiratory and gastrointestinal disturbances. Palatal vesicles are found in some cases. Thrombocytopenia and leukocytopenia are often detected. Hemorrhages, consisting of petechiae, bleeding gums, epistaxis, hemoptysis, and melena, are seen occasionally. The full clinical picture develops with meningeal irritation, reduced consciousness, seizures (especially in children), rigidity, ataxia, tremor, uncontrolled movements, central nerve paralysis, paresis, and pathological reflexes. In a favorable course, the temperature returns to normal levels after 7 to 9 days, and the neurological signs subside. In an unfavorable course, the fever remains, the neurological signs worsen, and death occurs after cardiac and respiratory complications. Biphasic courses of fever and disease reminiscent of TBE are often seen. Fatality in children with clinical manifestations is around 20%; in adults more than 50 years old, it is 50%. The recovery is prolonged. In 30% to 40% of survivors, remaining disturbances in the form of motor or sensory deficits occur in addition to choreoathetosis, Parkinsonism, and psychopathological symptoms. A disease with predominantly myelitic or bulbar deficits is possible. Transplacental infection results in fetal death and abortion.

Fifty thousand cases occur annually in Eastern Asia, with 11,000 fatalities. Fifteen cases imported to the United States were monitored, with four patients experiencing recovery, five experiencing permanent impediment, and six meeting with a lethal outcome. In the state of Andhra Pradesh in India, JE epidemics occur every 2 to 3 years. In September 1999, a JE epidemic of 965 cases resulted in 200 deaths (20.7%). In 1997, an epidemic of 267 cases mostly affected children, with 32 fatalities.

The infection in nonhuman animals is subclinical; however, it causes abortion in pregnant sows and death in newborn piglets. Under natural conditions, viremic infections have been detected in pigs and frogs. JE causes inapparent infection in horses, but occasionally neurotropic virus infections were observed with a high fatality rate.

Diagnosis. A tentative diagnosis can only be made in connection with the epidemiological situation (history of traveling or epidemiology). A definite diagnosis is confirmed by seroconversion or demonstration of virus-specific IgM antibodies in the CSF. Intrathecal antibody production is demonstrated with the Reiber quotient. Cross-reactions with other flaviviruses should be considered.

Attempts to isolate the virus from the CSF or blood are rarely successful. Postmortem, the virus can be isolated from brain tissue or can be demonstrated by fluorescence microscopy. More recently, RT-PCR has been recommended to confirm the diagnosis postmortem, but it has not been recommended in antemortem diagnoses. PCR can also be used to detect the agent in mosquitoes for disease control. A group-specific RT-PCR, targeting the NS5 gene, is available for the demonstration of flavivirus infections. It can be combined with a virus-specific PCR in a seminested protocol.

Differential Diagnosis. The differential diagnosis includes a broad spectrum of virus encephalitides. MVE and Kunjin virus encephalitis have to be considered in Australia. At the west coast of India, WNF, also caused by a flavivirus, may occur. In Malaysia, Nipah virus encephalitis, which is transmitted by bats from pigs, can cause problems in the differential diagnosis. In Southeast Asia, meningoencephalitis caused by enterovirus 71 has increased considerably in recent years, while the eradication of poliomyelitis has been successful in that region.

Therapy. Special therapy for JE virus does not exist, and treatment is symptomatic. Vital functions have to be supported in comatose patients. Anticonvulsive drugs are used for seizures, and mannose infusions are given in cases of increased intracranial pressure.

Prophylaxis. Inactivated virus vaccines prepared in mouse brain or cell culture with a good immunogenicity and efficacy are available in China and Japan for individual prophylaxis. These vaccines are based on the strain Beijing 1 of the JE virus. They also protect against the MVE virus. Two immunizations are recommended with a 2-week interval and booster vaccinations after 1-year and every 3 or 4 years thereafter. The vaccines are mostly free of undesirable effects. However, a series of side effects happened recently (July 2002) in Chinese children. There are no reports about postvaccinal demyelinating encephalitis.

Nowadays, a virus vaccine (strain SA 14-14-2), which is propagated in Vero cells is available (Ixiaro®; Novartis Vaccines, Frimley Business Park, Frimley, Camberley, Surrey, GU16 7SR The ground immunization consists of two doses applied intramusculary into the upper arm. After 12 months, 83% of the vaccinees are protected. Headaches, muscular pain or itching pain at the vaccination site may occur after the vaccination. This vaccine is the only JE vaccine, which is licensed for use in Europe and in the USA.

In several Asian countries, the vaccination was included into the vaccination calendar of children.

It was recently announced that a chimeric vaccine based on the 17D YE vaccine will be available soon.

Delayed-type hypersensitivity reactions have been observed in connection with immunizations in 3 to 10 cases per 100,000. The indication for vaccination, therefore, should be carefully considered. A Chinese live attenuated vaccine has been used successfully and without serious side effects in 150 million cases since 1989.

In Germany, vaccines against JE were not licensed until recently. Modern vaccines based on recombinant DNA technique have been developed but have not been widely used. The possibility of inducing an antibody-mediated infection of macrophages is a general problem in flavivirus vaccinations.

Changes in pig farming, use of insecticides, reduced rice crops, and mass vaccination of the population are responsible for the reduced occurrence of JE in Japan and Korea. Theoretically, one could expect JE to be successfully controlled by keeping rice crops and pig farming in separate locations.

REFERENCES

Appaiahgari MB, Vrati S, IMOJEV®: a yellow-fever virus-based novel Japanese encepghalitis vaccine. *Expert Rev. Vacc.* 9, 1371–1384, 2010.

Arroyo et al., Molecular basis for attenuation of neurovirulence of a yellow fever virus/Japanese encephalitisvirus chimera vaccine (ChimeriVax-JE). *J. Virol.* 75, 934–942, 2001.

Ashok MS, Rangarajan PN, Evaluation of the potency of BIKEN inactivated Japanese encephalitis vaccine and DNA-vaccines in an intracerebral Japanese encephalitis virus challenge.*Vaccine.* 19, 155–157, 2000.

Beecham III HJ et al., A cluster of severe reactions following improperly administered Takeda Japanese encephalitis vaccine. *J. Travel. Med.* 4, 8–10, 1997.

Chung CC et al., Acute flaccid paralysis as an unusual presenting symptom of Japanese encephelatits: a case report and review of the literature. *Infection* 35, 30–32, 2007.

Dubischar-Kastner K et al., Safety analysis of a Vero-cell culture derived Japanese encephalitis vaccine, IXIARO (IC51), in 6 months of follow-up. *Vaccine* 28, 6463–6469, 2010.

Dubischar-Kastner K et al., Long-term immunity and immune response tio a booster dose following vaccination with the inactivated Japanese encephalitis vaccine. *Vaccine* 28, 5197–5202, 2010

Fischer M, Lindsay N, Staples JE, Centers for Disease Control and Prevention: Japanese encephalitis vaccine: recommendations of the Advisory Committee on Immunization Practices (ACIP). *Morb. Mort. Wkly. Rep.* 59, 1–27, 2010.

Halstead SB, Thomas SJ, Japanese encephalitis: new options for active immunization. *Clin. Infect. Dis.* 50, 1155–1164, 2010.

Jellinek T, Ixiaro: a new vaccine against Japanese encephalitis. *Expert Rev. vacc.* 8, 1501–1511, 2009.

Kaltenböck A et al., Immunogenicity and safety of IXIARO (IC51) in a phase II study in healthy Indian children between 1 and 3 years of age. *Vaccine* 28, 834–939, 2010.

Kanesa-Thasan N et al., Safety and immunogenicity of NYVACJEV and ALVAC-JEV attenuated recombinant Japanese encephalitis virus–poxvirus vaccines in vaccinia-nonimmune and vaccinia-immune humans. *Vaccine.* 19, 483–491, 2000.

Karunaratne SH, Hemingway J, Insecticide resistance spectra and resistance mechanisms in populations of Japanese encephalitis vector mosquitoes, Culex tritaeniorhynchus and Cx. gelidus, in Sri Lanka. *Med. Vet. Entomol.* 14, 430–436, 2000.

Kurane I, Takasaki T, Yamada KI, Trends in flavivirus infections in Japan. *Emerg. Infect. Dis.* 6, 569–571, 2000.

Liu W et al., Risk factors for Japanese encephalitis: a case-control study. *Epidemiol. Infect.* 138, 1292–1297, 2010.

Mackenzie JS, Gubler DJ, Petersen LR, Emerging flaviviruses: the spreas and resurgence of Japanese encephalitis, West Nile and dengue viruses. *Nat. Med.* 10, S98–S109, 2004.

Ogata A, Tashiro K, Pradhan S, Parkinsonism due to predominant involvement of substantia nigra in Japanese encephalitis. *Neurology* 55, 602, 2000.

Oya A, Kurane I, Japanese encephalitis for a reference to international travelers. *J. Travel Med.* 14, 259–268, 2007.

Robinson JS et al., Evaluation of three commercially available Japanese encephalitis virus IgM enzyme-linked immunosorbent assays. *Am. J. Trop. Med. Hyg.* 83, 1146–1155, 2010.

Takahashi H et al., Adverse events after Japanese encephalitis vaccination: review of post-marketing surveillance data from Japan and the United States. The VAERS Working Group. *Vaccine* 18, 2963–2969, 2000.

Victor TJ, Reuben R, Effects of organic and inorganic fertilisers on mosquito populations in rice fields of southern India. *Med. Vet. Entomol.* 14, 361–368, 2000.

Wilder-Smith A, Halstead S, Japanese encephalitis: update on vaccines and vaccine recommendations. *Curr. Opin. Infect. Dis.* 23, 426–431, 2010.

Yeh JY et al., Fast duplex one-step reverse transcriptase PCR for rapid differential detection of West Nile and Japanese encephalitis viruses. *J. Clin. Microbiol.* 48, 4010–4014, 2010.

1.3.4.2 Murray Valley Encephalitis and Kunjin Virus Disease

MVE is an arbovirus infection in Australia and New Guinea and is closely related to JE. It is a life-threatening disease. The Kunjin virus shares the same geographic distribution with MVE but causes milder cases of human febrile illness with rash and occasionally mild encephalitis.

Etiology. The MVE virus belongs to the family *Flaviviridae*, genus *Flavivirus*. It is antigenically related to other mosquito-transmitted flaviviruses, forming a closely related complex with the agents of JE, SLE, and WNV. Kunjin virus is closely related to WNV.

Wild boars in Australia have neutralizing antibodies to the MVE and Kunjin viruses. These immunoglobulins neutralize the virus of JE, explaining in part the absence of JE in Australia.

Occurrence. Between 1917 and 1974, eight major epidemics of MVE occurred in Australia. On the basis of serological investigations, it can be assumed that the virus is endemic in Australia and New Guinea. Epidemics occur in late summer (February to April). The agent persists in a maintenance cycle between waterfowl (herons and pelicans) and mosquitoes.

Transmission. The MVE virus is transmitted to humans by mosquitoes. The main vector is *C. annulirostris*, which hatches in ponds. The Kunjin virus was first isolated from *C. annulirostris* mosquitoes. It may cause neurological disease in horses, whereas MVE virus is not pathogenic for horses.

Clinical Manifestations. Serological investigations indicate that only 0.2% of cases develop clinical manifestations. The disease begins suddenly with headaches, photophobia, anorexia, vomiting, severe malaise, irritability, numbness, fever, and meningismus. Severe cases result in cramps, coma, and death. Paralysis of the upper or lower motor neurons can disturb swallowing and breathing. The disease lasts for 2 weeks. Severe psychological and neurological deficits remain in some patients. The fatality rate, 60% in earlier epidemics, has been reduced to 20% by modern intensive care. However, the percentage of persisting deficits has increased.

Diagnosis. A tentative diagnosis can be based on clinical signs and epidemiological circumstances. It must be confirmed by laboratory diagnostics. The diagnosis ante-mortem is possible by demonstrating IgM antibodies by IgM capture ELISA. Cross-reactions with other flaviviruses should be considered, especially with Kunjin virus, JE virus, and DEN virus. Attempts to isolate the MVE virus from blood or CSF have not been successful. The virus can be isolated from brain and spinal cord postmortem. PCR is likewise of no use for *in vivo* diagnosis.

A group-specific RT-PCR, targeting the *NS5* gene, is available for the demonstration of flavivirus infections. It can be combined with a virus-specific PCR in a seminested protocol (see the references).

Differential Diagnosis. Other known encephalitides should be considered in the differential diagnosis, especially JE and meningoencephalitis caused by enterovirus

For people who had contact with pigs while traveling in Malaysia, Nipah encephalitis should be kept in mind.

Therapy. Treatment is symptomatic. Intensive treatment is essential.

Prophylaxis. A specific vaccine is not available. Vaccines against the JE virus have a protective effect for MVE. Prophylactic mosquito control can be conducted with larvicidal and adulticidal drugs.

REFERENCES

Broom AK et al. (1995), Two possible mechanisms for survival and initiation of Murray Valley encephalitis virus activity in the Kimberley region of Western Australia. *Am. J. Trop. Med. Hyg.* 53, 95–99.

Broom et al. (2000), Immunisation with gamma globulin to Murray valley encephalitis virus and with an inactivated Japanese encephalitis virus vaccine as prophylaxis against Australian encephalitis: evaluation in a mouse model. *J. Med. Virol.* 61, 259–265.

Broom et al. (2003), Epizootic activity of Murray Valley encephalitis and Kunjin viruses in an aboriginal community in the southeast Kimberley region of Western Australia: results of mosquito fauna and virus isolation studies. *Am. J. Trop. Med. Hyg.* 69, 277–283.

Brown A et al., Reappearance of human cases due to Murray Valley encephalitis and Kunjin virus in central Australia after an absence of 26 years. *Commun. Dis. Intell.* 26, 39–44, 2002.

Hall RA, Scherret JH, Mackenzie JS, Kunjin virus: an Australian variant of West Nile? *Ann. N. Y. Acad. Sci.* 951, 153–160, 2001.

Huppatz C et al., Encephalitis in Australia, 1979–2006: trends and aetiologies. *Commun. Dis. Intell.* 33, 192–197, 2009.

Johansen CA et al., Genetic and phenotypic differences between isolates of Murray Valley encephalitis virus in Western Australia, 1972–2003. *Virus Genes* 35, 147–154, 2007.

Joy J et al., Biochemical characterization of Murray Valley encephalitis virus proteinase. *FEBS Lett.* 584, 3149–3152, 2010.

Lobigs M et al., Live chimeric and inactivated Japanese encephalitis virus vaccines differ in their cross-protective values agianst Murray Valley encephalitis virus. *J. Virol.* 83, 2436–2445, 2009.

McMinn PC, Carman PG, Smith DW, Early diagnosis of Murray Valley encephalitis by reverse transcriptase-polymerase chain reaction. *Pathology.* 32, 49–51, 2000.

Mancini EJ et al., Structure of the Murray Valley encephalitis virus RNA helicase at 1.9 Angstrom resolution. *Protein Sci.* 16, 2294–2300, 2007.

Matthews V et al., Morphological features of Murray Valley encephalitis virus infection in the central nervous system of Swiss mice. *Int. J. Exp. Pathol.* 81, 31–40, 2000.

Pyke AT et al., Detection of Australasian flavivirus encephalitic viruses using rapid fluorogenic TaqMan RT-PCR assays. *J. Virol. Meth.* 117, 161–167, 2004.

Stich G et al., Clinical and laboratory findings on the first imported case of Murray Valley encephalitis in Europe. *Clin. Infect. Dis.* 37, e19–e21, 2003.

Studdert MJ et al., Polymerase chain reaction tests for the identification of Ross River, Kunjin and Murray Valley encephalitis virus infections in horses. *Aust. Vet. J.* 81, 76–80, 2003.

1.3.4.3 St. Louis Encephalitis

SLE is the most important arbovirus infection in North America. The disease was first described in 1933. About 10,000 human cases, with approximately 1,000 fatalities, have been recorded since that time (4,453 human cases between 1964 and 1997).

Etiology. The SLE virus belongs to the family *Flaviviridae*, genus *Flavivirus*. Serologically, it shows cross-reaction with other mosquito-borne flaviviruses, especially with the viruses of JE and WNF, the latter being of special importance since its introduction to the Eastern United States in 1999.

Occurrence. Epidemics of SLE have occurred all over North America, including Mexico and Canada, with the exception of some New England states. The seasonal occurrence of SLE is restricted to the presence of mosquitoes. The highest prevalence of infection is found in the Ohio-Mississippi Valley. Between 1964 and 1993, 931 cases of SLE were diagnosed in Texas, 540 cases were diagnosed in Illinois, and 358 cases were diagnosed in Florida. The most recent outbreak in the United States occurred in Florida in 1993, when 223 clinical cases and 11 fatalities were reported.

An average of 128 cases of SLE is reported in the United States annually. The rate varies considerably. Infections with the virus are occasionally seen in the Caribbean and in South America (Brazil). Urban infection cycles from humans to mosquitoes to humans have been suspected.

Epidemics occur predominantly south of the 21 °C June isotherm, most frequently in years with hot summers. In years with SLE epidemics, the virus is the most frequent cause of all identified encephalitides in the United States. In other years, it accounts for less than 5% of cases. The frequency of clinically overt infection in humans is estimated to be between 1 per 425 infections and 1 per 20 infections. Clinically obvious infections are less frequent in children than in adults. SLE occurs three to five times more often rurally than in urban populations.

Most vertebrates are infected without developing a viremia. The exceptions are wild and domestic birds, in which the infection produces a long-lasting viremia. Sparrows and pigeons are believed to be responsible for the distribution of the disease in human populations.

Transmission. In the United States, several *Culex* species are responsible for the transmission of SLE virus. The number of virus-infected mosquitoes and young sparrows serves as a predictor of epidemics.

Culex tarsalis is the main vector for SLE virus in the western United States. The virus in the western United States occurs frequently in close epidemiological relation to western equine encephalitis (WEE). *Culex pipiens* and *Culex quinquefasciatus* are the main vectors in the rest of the United States.

Transmission from human-to-human or animal-to-animal does not occur, and infected humans are not a source for mosquito infection.

Clinical Manifestations. Clinical signs occur in 10% of humans infected with the SLE virus. Most cases are mild, with fever, photophobia, sore throat, myalgia, and headaches that last for only a few days. Occasionally, an aseptic meningitis or meningoencephalitis can lead to life-threatening conditions.

The onset of the disease is sudden after an incubation period of a few days and consists of up to 2 weeks with reduced consciousness. Seizures are more frequent in children than in adults. The most common neurological signs are neck stiffness, tremor, *dysdiadochokinesis*, and nystagmus. Cranial nerves are involved in 20% of the cases. Other signs are myalgias, photophobia, conjunctivitis, and indications of moderate kidney failure with urea retention. Encephalitis cases in adults have a 10% to 25% fatality rate. Persistent fever of >40 °C is a grave symptom. Most terminal cases occur when signs of encephalitis are declining. Convalescence may take a long time. Changes in personality and emotional lability may persist.

Diagnosis. A diagnosis of SLE is suspected only during an epidemic. The SLE virus cannot be isolated from blood or CSF of patients. It can be demonstrated in the brain in autopsies. The laboratory diagnosis, therefore, is based on serology. Demonstration of virus-specific IgM antibodies by IgM capture allows an early diagnosis with one serum sample. Intrathecal antibody formation is detected by applying the Reiber quotient. Cross-reactions with other flaviviruses (Powassan virus and WNV) have to be considered.

PCR is of no use for *in vivo* diagnosis. A group specific RT-PCR is available for the detection of all flavivirus infections (see the references at the end of this section). It can be combined with a virus-specific PCR in a seminested protocol. The virus-specific up-amplimer for SLE virus is to be used in conjunction with group-specific primers A and B.

For control purposes, a specific primer for detection of WNV should be included in SLE virus-specific RT-PCR.

Cross-reactions with WNV and YF, JE, MVE, and RE viruses may complicate the serological diagnosis.

Differential Diagnosis. All encephalitides caused by viruses, bacteria, rickettsiae, chlamydiae, fungi, and parasites should be considered in the differential diagnosis. Arboviruses (Eastern, Western, and Venezuelan encephalitis viruses; WNV; Powassan virus; and California encephalitis virus) have to be considered only in summer. Cerebral vascular processes, tumors, and metabolic diseases also have to be kept in mind.

Therapy. Treatment for SLE is symptomatic. There is no vaccine available.

Prophylaxis. Prophylaxis should concentrate on vector control and early recognition of epidemics.

Survival of the agent over winter in zones with temperate climates appears to be the weakest link in the infection cycle. Ultra-low-volume sprays of organophosphate insecticides are used in late fall and spring in breeding areas of the vector. Immune enhancement, a widespread phenomenon often seen in flavivirus infections, is a serious problem and a drawback in the development of vaccines.

REFERENCES

Auguste AJ, Pybus OG, Carrington CV, Evolution and dispersal of St. Louis encephalitis virus in the Americas. *Infect. Genet. Evol.* 9, 709–715, 2008.

Baillie GJ et al., Phylogenetic and evolutionary analyses of St. Louis encephalitis virus genomes. *Mol. Phylogenet. Evol.* 47, 717–728, 2008.

Chandler LJ, Parsons R, Randle Y, Multiple genotypes of St. Louis encephalitis virus (Flaviviridae: Flavivirus) circulate in Harris County, Texas. *Am. J. Trop. Med. Hyg.* 64, 12–19, 2001.

Chang GJ et al., Flavivirus DNA vaccines: current status and potential. *Ann. N. Y. Acad. Sci.* 951, 272–285, 2001.

Day JF, Stark LM, Frequency of Saint Louis encephalitis virus in humans from Florida, USA: 1990–1999. *J. Med. Entomol.* 37, 626–633, 2000.

Day JF, Predicting St. Louis encephalitis virus epidemics: Lessons from recent, and not so recent, outbreaks. *Ann. Rev. Entomol.* 46, 111–138, 2001.

Day JF, Sharman J, Severe winter freezes enhance St. Louis encephalitis virus amplification and epidemic transmission in peninsular Florida. *J. Med. Entomol.* 46, 1498–1506, 2009.

Flores FS et al., Vertical transmission of St. Louis encephalitis virus in culex quinquefasciatus (dipteral: culicidae) in Cordoba, Argentina. *Vector Borne Zoo. Dis.* 10, 999–1002, 2010.

Gruwell JA et al., Role of peridomestic birds in the transmission of St. Louis encephalitis virus in southern California. *J. Wildl. Dis.* 36, 13–34. 2000.

Hull R et al., A duplex real-time reverse transcriptase polymerase chain reaction assay for the detection of St. Louis encephalitis and eastern equine encephalitis viruses. *Diagn. Microbiol. Infect. Dis.* 62, 272–279, 2008.

Lanciotti RS, Kerst AJ, Nucleic acid sequencebased amplification assays for rapid detection of West Nile and St. Louis encephalitis viruses. *J. Clin. Microbiol.* 39, 4506–4513, 2001.

May FJ et al., Genetic variation of St. Louis encephalitis virus. *J. Gen. Virol.* 89, 1901–1910, 2008.

Meehan PJ et al., Epidemiological features of and public health response to a St. Louis encephalitis epidemic in Florida, 1990–1. *Epidemiol. Infect.* 125, 181–188, 2000.

Ottendorfer CL et al., Isolation of genotype V St. Louis encephalitis virus in Florida. *Emerg. Infect. Dis.* 15, 604–606, 2009.

Patz JA, Reisen WK, Immunology, climate change and vector-borne diseases. *Trends Immunol.* 22, 171–172, 2001.

Pesko K, Mores CN, Effect of sequential exposure on infection and dissemination rates for West Nile and St. Louis encephalitis viruses in culex quinquefasciatus. *Vector Borne Zoo. Dis.* 9, 281–286, 2009.

Phillpotts RJ, Venugopal K, Brooks T, Immunisation with DNA polynucleotides protects mice against lethal challenge with St. Louis encephalitis virus. *Arch Virol.* 141, 743–749, 1996.

Pond WL et al., Carter: Heterotypic serologic responses after yellow fever vaccination; detection of persons with past St. Louis encephalitis or dengue. *J. Immunol.* 98, 673–682, 1967.

Rahal JJ et al., Effect of interferon-alpha2b therapy on St. Louis viral meningoencephalitis: clinical and laboratory results from a pilot study. *J. Infect. Dis.* 190, 1084–1087, 2004.

Reisen WK et al., Patterns of avian seroprevalence to western equine encephalomyelitis and Saint Louis encephalitis viruses in California, USA. *J. Med. Entomol.* 37, 507–527, 2000.

Rodrigues SG et al., Molecular epidemiology of Saint Louis encephalitis in Brazilian Amazon: genetic divergence and dispersal. *J. Gen. Virol.* 91, 2420–2427, 2010.

Sanago YO et al., A real-time TaqMan polymerase chain reaction for the identification of culex vectors of West Nile and Saint Louis encephalitis viruses in North America. *Am. J. Trop. Med. Hyg.* 77, 58–66, 2007.

Shaman J et al., Seasonal forecast of St. Louis encephalitis transmission, Florida. *Emerg. Infect. Dis.* 10, 802–809, 2004.

Spinsanti LI et al., Human outbreak of St. Louis encephalitis detected in Argentina, 2005. *J. Clin. Virol.* 42, 27–33, 2008.

Wotton SH et al., St. Louis encephalitis in early infancy. *Pediatr. Infect. Dis.* 23, 951–954, 2004.

1.3.4.4 Rocio Encephalitis

RE is an arbovirus infection only known to occur in southeastern Brazil. The infection in domestic animals does not result in clinical signs.

Etiology. Rocio virus belongs to the family *Flaviviridae*, genus *Flavivirus*. It is serologically closely related to the agents of SLE and JE. The Rocio virus is an example of an emerging virus. It is assumed to be a pathogenic variant of the Ilheus virus.

Occurrence. In 1975 and 1976, approximately 1,000 cases were seen in the coastal area south of Santos in the state of São Paulo, Brazil, the only area where the disease has occurred. Young men with outdoor activities in rural areas were predominantly affected. The infection cycle is not yet known. Humans appear to be dead-end hosts.

Transmission. It is assumed that wild birds are involved in the cycle and mosquitoes are the vectors. Under experimental conditions, *Aedes (Stegomyia) scapularis* and *Psorophora ferox* can transmit RE virus.

Clinical Manifestations. The incubation period for Rocio virus is 7 to 14 days. The disease begins abruptly with fever, headaches, malaise, vomiting, pharyngitis, photophobia, and conjunctivitis. Meningitis develops later, with neck stiffness and hyperactive and pathological reflexes. The gait becomes atactic. The sense of equilibrium is impaired. Loss of motor and sensory functions is rare. The consciousness becomes cloudy and patients frequently become comatose. The fatality of hospitalized patients is 4%. Neurological and neuropsychiatric changes have been observed in 20% of survivors.

Diagnosis. Detection of IgM antibodies by the IgM capture method is the most commonly used serodiagnosis today. Serological cross-reactions with the SLE virus, which also occurs in this region, can obfuscate the correct diagnosis.

A viremia in humans cannot be found. The virus can be isolated postmortem from the brain in biosafety level 3 (BSL-3) laboratories. A group specific RT-PCR targeting the NS5 gene is available for the demonstration of flavivirus infections (see the references at the end of this section). Special RT-PCR techniques and sets of primers are recommended for the newly emerged problem of discriminating between the SLE virus and WNV, two closely related flaviviruses that occur in the United States.

Differential Diagnosis. The differential diagnosis includes a large number of *meningoencephalitides* caused by viruses and other agents (see "St. Louis Encephalitis" above). WNV should now be included in the differential diagnosis, after its appearance in horses and humans in the state of New York in 1999.

Therapy. There is no specific therapy for RE.

Prophylaxis. A formalin-inactivated virus vaccine prepared from infected suckling mouse brains was found to be ineffective.

REFERENCES

Aviles G et al., Secondary serologic responses to Dengue epidemic in 1998 in Salta, Argentina, where other flavivirus co-circulate, *Medicina (B Aires)*. 61, 129–136. Spanish, 2001.

Coimbra TL et al., Iguape: a newly recognized flavivirus from Sao Paulo State, Brazil. *Intervirology* 36, 144–152, 1993.

Figueiredo LT et al., Identification of Brazilian flaviviruses by a simplified reverse transcriptionpolymerase chain reaction method using flavivirus universal primers. *Am. J. Trop. Med. Hyg.* 59, 357–362, 1998.

Figueiredo LT, The Brazilian flaviviruses. *Microbes Infect.* 2, 1643–1649, 2000.

Medeiros DB et al., Complete genome characterization of Rocio virus (flavirirus, flaviviridae), a Brazilian flavivirus isolated from a fatal case of encephalitis during an epidemic in Sao Paulo state. *J. Gen. Virol.* 88, 2237–2246, 2007.

1.3.4.5 West Nile Fever

WNF is a virus disease marked by fever, pharyngitis, muscle and limb pain, rash, and lymphadenopathy. WNV infecting older patients causes severe disease with encephalitis. Wild birds, horses, and ornithophile mosquitoes are involved in the maintenance cycle of the virus. The name of the disease was derived from a district in Uganda where the virus was first isolated.

Etiology. WNV is an arbovirus in the *Flaviviridae* family, genus *Flavivirus*. There is a close relation with the virus complex consisting of agents of SLE, JE, and MVE. The Usutu virus is another member of the JE complex of flaviviruses that is transmitted by mosquitoes and may cause fatal disease in birds. It is restricted to the African continent but in 2001 was isolated from dead birds in Austria. Human infections were recognized in 2 cases.

Occurrence. The agent of WNF has been found not only in Uganda but also in Egypt, the Democratic Republic of the Congo (formerly Zaire), South Africa, India, Borneo, Israel, Cyprus, the former USSR, and southern France. About 450 cases of meningitis and meningoencephalitis were caused by WNV in Romania in late summer 1996, with a fatality rate of 8.7%. WNV appeared for the first time in August 1999 on the east coast of the United States. There were 62 patients with encephalitis with seven deaths in Queens, New York. In 2000, there were 14 patients diagnosed with WNF, and two of these cases were fatal. Meanwhile, the virus appears to have found a natural distribution cycle in the northeastern United States. Wild birds (crows) and birds in zoological gardens become viremic and may die from the disease. Mosquitoes (*Aedes (Stegomyia) japonicus*) act as vectors. WNV was found in mosquitoes in pools in Central Park in New York City and on Staten Island, New York. Horses and other vertebrates besides humans are involved in the infection cycle of WNF in the United States. By November 2002, a total of 3,737 human cases of WNV infection, including 202 fatalities, were noted in 39 states and in Washington, DC. Evidence of animal infection [birds, mosquitoes, and other animals (primarily horses)] was obtained from 43 states.

The unexpected appearance of WNV in the center of New York City has raised speculation on bioterrorism. However, multiple events of "airport malaria" have proven that pathogens and their vectors can travel with ease on intercontinental routes.

Like DEN virus, WNV is now an arbovirus with global distribution. In Asia, it touches the regions where JE virus is endemic on the west coast of India. It has even been found in Australia. In the Western Hemisphere, it reaches the zone where SLE is endemic.

In Southern Africa, WNF is considered to be the most frequent arbovirus infection in humans. In Israel and Egypt, the virus causes epidemics between May and October. Up to 60% of the population may develop disease, as evidenced by serology.

The virus persists in a maintenance cycle between numerous ornithophilic *Culex* species and wild birds, similar to the Sindbis virus, an alphavirus. Epidemics with both viruses frequently occur together. They share the same vector, *Culex univittatus*. In wild birds, a persistent viremia can be found. Domestic fowl become infected without a pronounced viremia and, therefore, are not a source for the infection of mosquitoes. Humans are not an important source for the distribution of the virus. Humans seropositive for Sindbis virus are positive for antibodies against WNV in a significantly higher proportion compared to Sindbis virus seronegative individuals.

Transmission. *C. univittatus* has been identified as the principal vector in epidemics in southern Africa. This vector is an ornithophile mosquito, which attacks birds and also humans in periods of high humidity, with an explosion-like replication. WNV was isolated from *A. (Stegomyia) japonicus* on the North American east coast after its recent introduction. This vector transmits the virus to humans.

Numerous laboratory infections have occurred, sometimes with aerogenic virus transmission. In human flavivirus infections, transmission by direct contact does not occur. However, virus transmission by transfusion of blood and blood products, as well as by organ transplantation and breast-feeding, was recently observed with WNV infections.

Clinical Manifestations. In 80% of cases, the WNV infection does not cause overt disease. In 20% of cases, symptoms reminiscent of Dengue are observed.

The severity of WNV disease depends on the age of the patient. Children develop a mild disease, while adults frequently show severe symptoms. Meningoencephalitis develops in adults only.

The incubation period is 3 to a maximum of 6 days. The disease begins with an abrupt, sometimes biphasic fever, malaise, headache, myalgia and arthralgia, lymphadenopathy, and a macular rash, which is restricted to the torso. The exanthema disappears after 5 to 7 days without a desquamation. Arthritis and myocarditis occur occasionally. Neurologic signs may be seen in 25% of cases in elderly people. The fatality rate in these cases may reach 10%. Of 151 patients in an epidemic in Israel in 2000, 76 had to be hospitalized, and 12 died with encephalitis. Cases resulting from WNV transmission by way of blood transfusion or organ transplants often have unfavorable prognoses as large volumes are transfused and the acceptors often have impaired resistance due to their underlying disease.

WNV can cause encephalitis in cattle, horses, and other mammals. Latent infections are possible. WNV causes fatal infections in birds (crows) and even in alligators.

Diagnosis. In 77% of cases, the virus can be isolated from the blood of patients on the first day of the disease and all through the febrile phase with viremia. In that respect, WNV behaves differently from the related agents of SLE, JE, and MVE. A group specific RT-PCR targeting the NS5 gene is available for the demonstration of flavivirus infections (for literature see the end of this section). It can be combined with a virus-specific PCR in a seminested protocol.

The diagnostic significance of rises of antibody titers or seroconversion is limited to people without a previous infection with a flavivirus or vaccination against YF because of wide cross-reactions. The IgM capture ELISA method is used today to detect IgM antibodies. In encephalitic courses, intrathecal immunoglobulin production is detectable.

Differential Diagnosis. Sindbis fever, caused by an alphavirus, has to be ruled out because of its clinical picture being similar to that of WNF and because of similarities in its epidemiology and geographical distribution. In North America, a broad range of arboviral encephalitides (EEE, WEE, VEE, SLE, PE, and California encephalitis) has to be considered in addition to non-zoonotic causes of encephalitis and fevers.

Therapy. Treatment of WNF is purely symptomatic. Development of protease inhibitors for Proteases WNV NS2B/NS3 and of polymerase inhibitors is underway.

Prophylaxis. Vaccine options, a formalin-inactivated vaccine resembling the CEE vaccine or a live attenuated chimeric vaccine based on the 17D YF vaccine as a vector are in preparation. At present, no licensed vaccine is available. Elderly people should avoid vector exposure in situations of endemicity. In New York, a pesticide (Anvil with a *pyrethroid* basis) has been used as a spray to control mosquitoes.

Slaughtered chickens may be a source of infection. Conversely, domestic fowl kept near human housing may protect humans from the attack of ornithophile vectors.

To prevent virus transmission by blood transfusion or organ transplants, the donor's serum would have to be tested for the presence of class IgM antiviral antibody if the donation took place during the period of seasonal prevalence. Virus detection by RT-PCR is probably not adequate to detect a low-titer viremia.

REFERENCES

Asnis DS et al., The West Nile virus encephalitis outbreak in the United States (1999–2000): from Flushing, New York, to beyond its borders. *Ann. N. Y. Acad. Sci.* 951, 161–171, 2001.

CDC, Intrauterine West Nile virus infection – New York, 2002. *Morb. Mort. Wkly. Rep.* 51, 1135–1136, 2002.

Baqar S et al., Vertical transmission of West Nile virus by culex and aedes species mosquitoes. *Am. J. Trop. Med. Hyg.* 48, 757–762, 1993.

Biedenbender R et al., Phase II, randomized, double-blind, placebo-controlled, multicenter study to investigate the immunogenicity and safety of a West Nile virus vaccine in healthy adults. *J. Infect. Dis.* 203, 75–84, 2011.

Biggerstaff BJ, Petersen LR, Estimated risk of West Nile transmission through blood transfusion during an epidemic in Queens, New York City. *Transfusion* 42, 1019–1026, 2002.

Bin H et al., West Nile fever in Isreal 1999–2000: from geese to humans. *Ann. N. Y. Acad. Sci.* 951, 127–142, 2001.

Campbell GL, Ceianu CS, Savage HM, Epidemic West Nile encephalitis in Romania: waiting for history to repeat itself. *Ann. N. Y. Acad. Sci.* 951, 94–101, 2001.

Castillo-Olivares J, Wood J, West Nile virus infection of horses. *Vet. Res.* 35, 467–483, 2004.

CDC, Laboratory-acquired West Nile virus infections – United States, 2002. *Morb. Mort. Wkly. Rep.* 51, 1133–1135, 2002.

CDC, West Nile transmission via organ transplantation and blood transfusion – Louisianna, 2008. *Morb. Mort. Wkly. Rep.* 58, 1263–1267, 2009.

CDC, West Nile virus activity – United States, 2009. *Morb. Mort. Wkly. Rep.* 59, 769–772, 2010.

Chappell KJ et al., West Nile NS2B/NS3 protease as an antiviral target. *Curr. Med. Chem.* 15, 2771–2784, 2008.

Cook RL et al., Demographic and clinical factors associated with persistent symptoms after West Nile virus infection. *Am. J. Trop. Med. Hyg.* 83, 1133–1136, 2010.

Couissinier-Paris P, West Nile in Europe and Africa: still minor pathogen, or potential threat to public health? *Bull. Soc. Pathol. Exot.* 99, 348–354, 2006.

Dauphin G, Zientara S, West Nile virus: recent trends in diagnosis and vaccine development. *Vaccine* 25, 5563–5576, 2007.

Davis LE et al., West Nile virus neuroinvasive disease. *Ann. Neurol.* 60, 286–300, 2006.

Eiden M et al., Two new real-time quantitative reverse transcription polymerase chain reaction assays with unique target sites for the specific and sensitive detection of lineages 1 and 2 Wets Nile virus strains. *J. Vet. Diagn. Invest.* 22, 748–753, 2010.

Granwehr BP et al., West Nile virus: where are we now? Lancet *Infect. Dis.* 4, 547–556, 2004.

Gray RR et al., Evolutionary characterization of the West Nile virus complete genome. *Mol. Phylogenet.* 56, 195–200, 2010.

Gubler DJ, The continuing spread of West Nile virus in the western hemisphere. *Clin. Infect. Dis.* 45, 1039–1046, 2007.

Guy B, Guirakhoo F, Barban V et al., Preclinical and clinical development of YFV 17D-based chimeric vaccines against dengue, West Nile and Japanese encephalitis viruses. *Vaccine* 28, 632–649, 2010.

Hayes CG, West Nile virus: Uganda, 1937, to New York, 1999. *Ann. N. Y. Acad. Sci.* 951, 25–37, 2001.

Hayes EB, Looking the other way: preventing vector-borne disease among travelers to the United States. *Travel Med. Infect. Dis.* 8, 277–284, 2010.

Hunsperger EA et al., West Nile virus from blood donors, vertebrates, and mosquitoes, Puerto Rico, 2007. *Emerg. Infect. Dis.* 15, 1298–1300, 2009.

Johnson N et al., Assessment of a novel realtime pan-flavivirus RT-polymerase chain reaction. *Vector Borne Zoo. Dis.* 10, 665–671, 2010.

Jupp PG, The ecology of West Nile virus in South Africa and the occurrence of outbreaks in humans. *Ann. N. Y. Acad. Sci.* 951, 143–152, 2001.

Kauffman EB et al., Detection of West Nile virus. *Meth. Mol. Biol.* 665, 383–413, 2011.

Komar N, Clark GG, West Nile virus activity in Latin America and the *Caribbean. Rev. Panam. Salud Pub.* 19, 112–117, 2006.

Kramer LD, Li J, Shi PY, West Nile virus. *Lancet Neurol.* 6, 171–181, 2007.

Loeb M et al., Prognosis after West Nile virus infection. *Ann. Intern. Med.* 149, 232–241, 2008.

Mehlhop E, Diamond MS, The molecular basis of antibody protection against West Nile virus. *Curr. Top. Microbiol. Immunol.* 317, 125–153, 2008.

Monaco F et al., Re-emergence of West Nile virus in Italy. *Zoo. Pub. Health* 57, 476–486, 2010.

Monge Maillo B et al., Importation of West Nile virus infection from Nicaragua to Spain. *Emerg. Infect. Dis.* 14, 1171–1173, 2008.

Nash D et al., The outbreak of West Nile virus infection in the New York City area in 1999. *N. Engl. J. Med.* 344, 1807–1814, 2001.

Papin JF et al., Genome-wide real-time PCR for West Nile virus reduces the false-negative rate and facilitates new strain discovery. *J. Virol. Meth.* 169, 103–111, 2010.

Petersen LR, Hayes EB, West Nile virus in the Americas. *Med. Clin. North Am.* 92, 1307–1322, 2008.

Planitzer CB et al., West Nile virus infection in plasma of blood and plasma donors, United States. *Emerg. Infect. Dis.* 15, 1668–1670, 2009.

Posadas-Herrera G et al., Development and evaluation of a formalin-inactivated West Nile virus vaccine (WN-VAX) for a human vaccine candidate. *Vaccine* 28, 7939–7946, 2010.

Rossi SL, Ross TM, Evans JD, West Nile virus. *Clin. Lab. Med.* 30, 47–65, 2010.

Sejvar JJ, Marfin AA, Manifestations of West Nile neuroinvasive disease. *Rev. Med. Virol.* 16, 209–224, 2006.

Shi PY, Wong SJ, Serologic diagnosis of West Nile virus infection. *Expert Rev. Mol. Diagn.* 3, 733–741, 2003.

Smith HL et al., Development of antigen-specific memory CD8+ T cells following live-attenuated chimeric West Nile virus vaccination. *J. Infect. Dis.* 203, 513–522, 2011.

Tardei G et al., Evaluation of immunoglobulin M (IgM) and IgG enzyme immunoassays in serologic diagnosis of West Nile virus infection. *J. Clin. Microbiol.* 38, 2232–2239, 2000.

Trevejo RT, Eidson M, Zoonosis update: West Nile virus. *J. Am. Vet. Med. Ass.* 232, 1302–1309, 2008.

Unlu I et al., Evidence of vertical transmission of West Nile virus in field-collected mosquitoes. *J. Vector Ecol.* 35, 95–99, 2010.

Venter M et al., Transmission of West Nile virus during horse autopsy. *Emerg. Infect. Dis.* 16, 573–575, 2010.

Zou S et al., West Nile characteristics among viremic persons identified through blood donor screening. *J. Infect. Dis.* 202, 1354–1361, 2010.

1.3.4.6 Usutu Virus

Usutu virus is a flavivirus, which was isolated in South Africa from mosquitoes in 1959. It is present in wide parts of Sub-Saharan Africa and was detected in 2001 in Austria as the cause of lethal infections in blackbirds (*Turdus merula*).

In humans, the virus causes clinical inapparent infections. In one case, it was isolated from a patient suffering from mild disease with fever and rash. In 2009, the Usutu virus caused severe meningoencephalitis in a patient with a B-cell lymphoma, who had received a liver transplant.

Etiology. The Usutu virus, belonging to the group of mosquito-borne encephalitis agents, is closely related with the viruses of JE and WNV.

REFERENCES

Cavrini F et al., Usutu virus infection in a patient who underwent orthotropic liver transplantation, Italy, August-September 2009. *Euro Surveill* 14: pii=19448.

Weissenbock H et al., Emergence of Usutu virus, an African mosquito-borne Flavivirus of the Japanese encephalitis group, Central Europe. *Emerg Infect Dis* 2002; 8: 652–656.

1.3.4.7 Wesselsbron Fever

Wesselsbron fever is an acute infectious disease of sheep. Mosquitoes can transmit the disease to humans. It appears sporadically with signs of fever, headaches, muscle aches, and exanthema. It is not fatal.

Etiology. The causative agent is an arbovirus in the family *Flaviviridae,* genus *Flavivirus.*

Occurrence. Wesselsbron fever occurs mainly in southern and central Africa. Infections have been reported from Madagascar and Thailand. The virus has been isolated from several *Aedes* species, as well as from sheep, cattle, and humans. It was also found in ducks and coyotes. The true virus reservoir is not known.

Transmission. Viremic sheep and cattle are the source for infection of mosquitoes, which transmit the Wesselsbron virus to humans. Other sources of infection for farmers and veterinarians are obstetrics for sheep and autopsies of cadavers of infected sheep. Numerous laboratory infections have occurred.

Clinical Manifestations. The incubation period in laboratory infections is 2 to 4 days. It is believed to be longer after mosquito infections. The disease begins with rigors, fever, myalgia, arthralgia, *ophthalmalgia*, and dermal hyperesthesia. A macular rash, lymphadenopathy, and hepatosplenomegaly are often found. In severe cases, encephalitis with a dimmed consciousness, visual disturbances, and photophobia may be seen. The prognosis in cases of human disease is favorable.

Wesselsbron disease in sheep is similar to Rift Valley fever. An intrauterine infection in pregnant sheep leads to fetal death, mummification, and abortion. The infection in lambs is fatal.

Diagnosis. The signs of disease in humans are uncharacteristic. A tentative diagnosis, therefore, has to be based on the epidemiology: professional contact with sheep and/or fetal death in sheep. The virus can be isolated from blood and throat secretions during the febrile phase.

A group-specific RT-PCR is available for the demonstration of flavivirus infections. The diagnosis can only be confirmed by serology if the patient has not been exposed to another flavivirus. There is a close antigenic relationship, especially to YF.

Differential Diagnosis. Infections in humans with influenza-like diseases have to be ruled out. If there is contact with diseases in sheep and cattle, Rift Valley fever has to be considered.

Therapy. Treatment for Wesselsbron fever is symptomatic.

Prophylaxis. Although the reservoir of the agent is not known, mosquito control may be useful prophylactically.

REFERENCES

Bollati M et al., Recognition of RNA cap in the Wesselsbron virus NS5 methyltransferase domain: implications for RNA-capping mechanisms in flavirus. *J. Mol. Biol.* 385, 140–152, 2009.

Diallo M et al., Mosquito vectors of the 1998-1999 outbreak of Rift Valley fever and other arboviruses (Bagaza, Sanar, Wesselsbronn and West Bile) in mauritania and Senegal. *Med. Vet. Entomol.* 19, 119–126, 2005.

Johnson AJ et al., Detection of anti-arboviral immunoglobulin G by using a monoclonal antibody-based capture enzyme-linked immunosorbent assay. *J. Clin. Microbiol.* 38, 1827–1831, 2000.

1.3.4.8 Yellow Fever

YF is an arbovirus infection in humans and primates and is characterized by icterus and fever in humans. Several mosquito species with breeding grounds close to human housing or in the rainforest transmit the disease. YF virus persists in a constant jungle cycle between mosquitoes and monkeys. Humans take the place of the vertebrate in the urban cycle. Both cycles exist in parallel and are intermittent.

Etiology. The causative agent, YF virus, is the prototype of the family *Flaviviridae*, genus *Flavivirus* (formerly group B arboviruses).

Occurrence. The YF zone in Africa reaches from 15°N to 10°S. This zone includes 33 countries with numerous large cities and with 468 million inhabitants, many of them living in urban slums. Most are not vaccinated and do not have mosquito nets. Many are HIV infected. Several monkey species are vertebrate hosts in Africa.

The YF zone in the Americas reaches from 20°N to 25°S. The health situation of the population in this zone is only slightly better than that in Africa. There is always the potential danger of epidemics, with a high degree of fatality, in Africa or the Americas.

The urban cycle of YF has disappeared in areas where mosquitoes in urban areas are under control. YF persists in rural areas, especially among forest workers in West, Central, and East Africa and in South and Central America (Fig. 1.6). The jungle cycle of YF includes monkeys in the wild.

There has been little change in the YF situation in South America in recent years, especially in comparison to DEN. The WHO reports approximately 150 YF infections per year in South America, 80% of them in Bolivia and Peru. The fatality rate in these cases is 55% to 58%. There has been a considerable increase of *Stegomyia* (*Aedes*) species, especially *Stegomyia albopicta*, which serve as vectors for the YF virus in rural and urban regions. An increase of YF, therefore, must be expected. There is a potential danger of urban cycles in socially disadvantaged border zones of South American large cities.

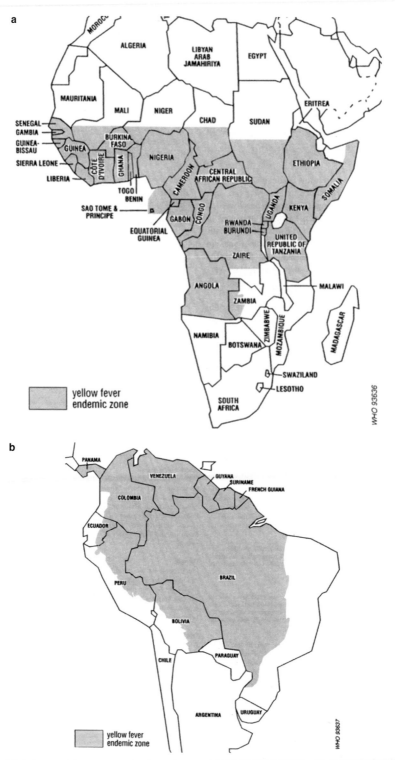

Figure 1.6(a, b) | Areas with risk of Yellow Fever transmission in South America. http://www.cdc.gov/yellowfever/maps/south_america.html. Courtesy CDC

Officially, the last urban epidemic of YF in the Americas was in 1954 in Trinidad. Six cases of YF were documented in urban residents in Santa Cruz, Bolivia, in 1997 and 1998. These people had not traveled to areas of endemicity and, therefore, they were infected in the city. There were some suspected cases in Brasilia, Brazil, and Sao Paulo, Brazil.

The official WHO report of 1991 lists 2,561 YF cases in 12 African countries. The morbidity in this report was underestimated by a factor of 100. An increase of cases of YF was noticed in Kenya and in some countries in West and East Africa. Ten years ago, a certificate of vaccination was only required from travelers coming from areas of endemicity. The epidemics now affect a largely unvaccinated population without protection from mosquito nets. There are new indications that urban YF cycles are reappearing.

A partial cross-immunity between YF virus and DEN virus may explain the lack of YF in Asia, in spite of the widely distributed main vector, *Aedes (Stegomyia) aegypti*. A reduced vector competence of Asiatic *A. aegypti* for YF virus might be another explanation.

The increase of YF in South America and in Africa has had a consequence for travelers. The first cases since 1924 were diagnosed in the United States in two travelers returning from Venezuela in 1996 and 1999. In Germany, a traveler returning from the Ivory Coast came back with YF in 1999. The two American patients and the German patient traveled unvaccinated. In all three cases, the disease ended fatally with kidney failure and encephalitis. YF virus and DEN virus coexist in Africa and in South America.

Transmission. The urban cycle of YF is solely maintained by *Stegomyia,* formerly *Aedes aegypti* and *Stegomyia simpsoni.* In the jungle, several *Haemagogus* species are responsible for the transmission of the YF virus.

Clinical Manifestations. The clinical picture in humans may reach from an unknown percentage of inapparent infections to severe disease with lethal outcome.

The incubation period is 3 to 6 days. Mild cases are restricted to the prodromal stage of the disease with an influenza-like syndrome displaying sudden fever, bradycardia, head and back aches, myalgia, nausea, epistaxis, and conjunctival injection that lasts for 1 to 3 days. In severe and fatal cases, a remission that lasts for hours or days is observed. Thereafter, a second rise of fever occurs with bradycardia, jaundice, epistaxis, melena, hematemesis (black, coffee-like vomit), urogenital bleeding, and signs of kidney failure with albuminuria and oliguria. Gastric and duodenal ulcers may cause severe hemorrhages. In terminal cases, the patient becomes delirious, highly agitated, and comatose. The fatality rate is 10% to 50%. There are presently no reports available on dual infections with YF and HIV infection in patients. The risk of YF in pregnant women has not been systematically investigated.

Oliguria, anuria, and albuminuria with urea retention, as well as hyperbilirubinuria and prolonged prothrombin time, are common laboratory findings with YF.

Diagnosis. Oliguria, anuria, albuminuria and a prolonged prothrombin time are typical laboratory findings in Yellow fever. The clinical picture of YF is similar to those of numerous other tropical infectious diseases. A diagnosis based on clinical signs, therefore, can only be made during epidemics. Vaccinated people are protected from YF.

Virus isolation from blood or CSF taken during the first fever phase confirms the diagnosis. The virus is detected in cell culture by immunofluorescence or by cytopathic effects. Mosquito cell cultures from *Aedes* species (AP 6/1) are well suited for isolation of the virus. A group-specific RT-PCR targeting the NS5 gene is available for the demonstration of flavivirus infections. It can be combined with a virus-specific PCR in a seminested protocol.

A real-time PCR technique (TaqMan) for quantification of YF virus in clinical and experimental specimens was published by Preiser et al. This technique is sensitive enough to detect 4 PFU of strain D17 or Asibi per ml of cell culture supernatants.

An increase of antibody titers can be used for the diagnosis. Serodiagnosis and demonstration of virus-specific immunity are not complicated, provided the patient has not previously been infected with another flavivirus.

The IgM capture ELISA is the best method to detect IgM antibodies. IgM antibodies can be found for up to 18 months after vaccination with the 17D strain of YF virus. Previous vaccinations or infections with other flaviviruses should always be kept in mind in the serological diagnosis of YF. Currently, the neutralization test is still the preferred method for seroepidemiological studies.

Differential Diagnosis. Based on the course of the disease, the predominant symptoms should be addressed in the differential diagnosis. Epidemiology is an additional tool. Numerous infectious diseases have to be kept in mind: malaria, the hemorrhagic form of DEN, hemorrhagic fevers (Marburg, Lassa, Ebola, and Crimean-Congo fevers), meningococcal sepsis, Hantavirus diseases, viral hepatitis, leptospirosis, and recurrent fever. The first febrile phase in YF appears to be shorter than in other virus-induced hemorrhagic fevers. Hemorrhages and death can occur before the second week of the disease.

Therapy. A specific therapy for YF does not exist; treatment is symptomatic. It is important to control fluids and electrolytes as well as blood clotting and thrombocyte numbers. Fresh blood transfusions from vaccinated donors can be useful if possible. Exchange transfusions should be avoided. Hemodialysis is indicated in cases with progressive liver and kidney failure. Unfortunately, there is still no clear answer to the question if and when anti-YF immunoglobulin would be useful for the patient. Although many people are vaccinated against YF, a serum pool for such indications does not exist.

Patients with a clinical manifestation of YF should be treated in a local hospital if possible. There is no need to keep patients in isolation if vectors (*Aedes* species) have no access to the facility. Transportation of the patient would be too dangerous and the risk of infection for the hospital personnel is minimal in the absence of mosquitoes.

Prophylaxis. Active immunization is legally required for travelers visiting areas of endemicity or traveling from areas of endemicity into countries presently free of YF. There are two types of legal regulations: (i) countries in the zone of endemicity require vaccination certificates from visitors and immigrants; (ii) countries that are free of YF but have potential vectors require vaccination certificates from citizens of countries in the zone of endemicity and from people who have visited such a country before. The most important technique of individual prophylaxis is active vaccination for travelers in endemic regions and in Asian countries hitherto free of yellow fever.

There are two attenuated live YF virus vaccines available. The neurotropic French Dakar vaccine is produced in mouse brain. The other is the 17D-204 strain of Theiler, raised in chick embryos. The 17D vaccine is applied subcutaneously or by intramuscular route. The risk of producing encephalitis is considerably lower than that with the Dakar vaccine. The only exceptions for vaccination with the 17D vaccine are children under 9 months of age and pregnant women. Vaccination produces a long-lasting immunity that can be confirmed by the virus neutralization test.

There could be problems with vaccination of immunesuppressed people. The immune status and the need to vaccinate should be carefully tested before vaccination. Two HIV-positive patients without significant immunosuppression were successfully vaccinated with the 17D vaccine without complications. Recently a series of six fatal cases following YF vaccination was reported from Australia, Brazil, and the United States. After an incubation of a few days, the vaccinated individuals fell ill and showed clinical signs of YF. The vaccine strain was isolated from their organs. Five of the vaccinees were elderly people (>60 years). It is not yet known whether preexisting flavivirus antibodies were present in these cases. A girl, 5 years of age, had been vaccinated with mumps-measles-rubella vaccine a few days before 17D vaccination. The old rule that a minimum of 4 weeks must be allowed between the applications of two live, attenuated virus vaccines needs to be reinforced, at least for the 17D vaccine. As of July 2002, it seems that the 17D strain, which had caused adverse effects in Brazilian vaccinees, is genetically stable. Therefore, it seems to be more probable that rare constellations in the individual genetic or immunological background of the vaccinees may have influenced the outcome.

Neurologic complications of the YF vaccine, the yellow fever vaccine associated neurologic disease (YELAND) is mainly encountered in babies <9 months of age. The yellow fever vaccination associated visceral disease may occur in elderly (>60 years old) or in immunosuppressed people. Between 1996 and 2005, 34 cases of YELAND were reported; 50% of these patients died from the complications.

Pregnant women and babies <9 months should never be vaccinated against YF. There have been complications in about 10% of cases where vaccination was performed. The possibility to induce protective immunity with hyperimmune globulin has not been tested systematically. Preparations are not commercially available.

The 17D vaccine has recently been tested as a gene shuttle in experimental vaccines against DEN and JE.

REFERENCES

Arroyo J et al., Molecular basis for attenuation of neurovirulence of a yellow fever virus/Japanese encephalitis virus chimera vaccine (ChimeriVax-JE), *J. Virol.* 75, 934–942, 2001.

Barnett ED, Yellow fever: epidemiology and prevention. *Clin. Infect. Dis.* 44, 850–856, 2007.

CDC, Fatal yellow fever in a traveler returning from Venezuela, 1999. *MMWR Morb. Mortal Wkly. Rep.* 49, 303–305, 2000.

CDC, Fenner F, Candidate viral diseases for elimination or eradication. *MMWR Morb Mortal Wkly. Rep.* 48, Suppl., 186–190, 1999.

Chan RC et al., Hepatitis and death following vaccination with 17D-204 yellow fever vaccine. *Lancet* 358, 121–122, 2001.

Chang GJ et al., Flavivirus DNA vaccines: current status and potenzial. *Ann. N. Y. Acad. Sci.* 951: 272–285, 2001.

Galler R et al., Phenotypic and molecular analyses of yellow fever 17D vaccine viruses associated with serious adverse events in Brazil. *Virology.* 290, 309–319, 2001.

Gardner CL, Ryman KD, Yellow fever: a reemerging threat. *Clin. Lab. Med.* 30, 237–260, 2010.

Gould LH et al., An outbreak of yellow fever with concurrent chikungunya virus transmission in South Kordofan, Sudan, 2005. *Trans. R. Soc. Trop. Med. Hyg.* 102, 1247–1254, 2008.

Gubler D, The changing epidemiology of yellow fever and dengue, 1900 to 2003: full circle? *Comp. Immunol. Microbiol. Infect. Dis.* 27, 319–330, 2004.

Hayes EB, Acute viscerotropic disease following vaccination against yellow fever. *Trans. R. Soc. Trop. Med. Hyg.* 101, 967–971, 2007.

Marianneau P, Georges-Courbot M, Deubel V, Rarity of adverse effects after 17D yellowfever vaccination. *Lancet* 358, 84–85, 2001.

Marin M et al., Cetron Fever and multisystem organ failure associated with 17D yellow fever vaccination: a report of four cases. *Lancet* 358, 98–104, 2001.

Munoz J et al., Yellow fever-associated visverotropic disease in Barcelona, Spain. *J. Travel Med.* 15, 202–205, 2008.

Mutebi JP, Barrett AD, The epidemiology of yellow fever in Africa: Microbes Infect. 4, 1459–1468, 2002.

Oyelami SA, Olaleye CO, Oyejide O et al., Severe post-vaccination reaction to 17D yellow fever vaccine in Nigeria. *Rev. Roum. Virol.* 45, 25–30, 1994.

Pond WL et al., Heterotypic serologic responses after yellow fever vaccination; detection of persons with past St. Louis encephalitis or Dengue. *J. Immunol.* 98, 673–682, 1967.

Querec TD, Pulendran B, Understanding the role of innate immunity in the mechanism of action of the live attenuated yellow fever vaccine 17D. *Adv. Exp. Med. Biol.* 590, 43–53, 2007.

Receveur MC et al., Yellow fever vaccination of human immunedeficiency virus-infected patients: report of 2 cases. *Clin. Inf. Dis.* 31, E7–8, 2000.

Schlesinger JJ, Brandriss MW, Antibodymediated infection of macrophages and macrophage-like cell lines with 17D-yellow fever virus. *J. Med. Virol.* 8, 103–117, 1981

Schlesinger JJ, Brandriss MW, Growth of 17D yellow fever virus in a macrophage-like cell line, U937: role of Fc and viral receptors in antibody-mediated infection. *J. Immunol.* 127, 659–665, 1981.

Schoub BD et al., Encephalitis in a 13-year-old boy following 17D yellow fever vaccine. *J. Infect.* 21, 105–106, 1990.

Tesh RB et al., Immunization with heterologous flaviviruses protective against fatal West Nile encephalitis. *Emerg. Infect. Dis.* 8, 245–251, 2002.

Van Der Most RG et al., Chimeric yellow fever/dengue virus as a candidate dengue vaccine: quantitation of the Dengue virusspecific CD8 T-cell response. *J. Virol.* 74, 8094–8101, 2000.

Vasconcelos PFC et al., Serious adverse events associated with yellow fever 17D vaccine in Brazil: a report on two cases. *Lancet* 358, 91–97, 2001.

WHO, Fever, jaundice, and multiple organ system failure associated with 17D-derived yellow fever vaccination, 1996–2001. *MMWR Morb. Mortal Wkly. Rep.* 50, 643–645, 2001.

1.3.4.9 Dengue Fever (Dengue Hemorrhagic Fever and Dengue Shock Syndrome)

DEN is the most important and most frequent mosquito-transmitted virus infection of humans. It is marked by a biphasic fever, myalgias, lymphadenopathy, rash, and leukopenia with a benign outcome. Fewer than 1,000 cases per year were reported between 1955 and 1959. There were 1.2 million cases reported in 1998. According to an estimate from the WHO, over 2 billion people in more than 100 countries are at risk for DEN. It is assumed that up to 50 million infections with DEN virus occur worldwide per year; 400,000 of them are in the form of DHF or DSS. The risk of DHF is about 0.2% after the primary infection but reaches 20% upon consecutive infection with a second DEN virus. Children are mainly affected. Their mortality is about 15% under unfavorable conditions. DEN is the most frequent virus infection imported by tourists into countries of temperate climate zones.

The name "denga" or "dyenga" was used in the 19th century in West Africa as a name for the very characteristic picture of disease and was transformed to "Dengue," when the disease was introduced to South America with the slavery shipments. The name "dandy fever" is also used, making reference to the "dandylike" walk of the patients.

Etiology. The causative agent is the DEN virus, a flavivirus with four closely related serotypes, DEN-1 to DEN-4. The closest antigenic relationship exists between types 1 and 4. People who recover from a type 1 infection are protected against type 4 for a short time, and vice versa.

Occurrence. DEN fever exists on all continents except Europe and Antarctica. More than 2 billion people are exposed to DEN in tropical regions, with 30 million to 50 million cases of disease annually (see Fig. 1.7). Seventy percent of all DEN infections imported into Germany come from Southeast Asia, especially Thailand. Large outbreaks of Dengue or Dengue-like disease with an estimated up to 10^6 cases were reported from Brazil. (999.688 cases were registered in 2010.) In 1990, 102 imported and confirmed DEN cases were reported in the United States, and 46 such cases were reported in 1993 and 1994. A 12-year-old patient developed DSS. Endemic infections were reported in Texas. The urban vector, *Stegomyia* (formerly *Aedes*) *aegypti*, has re-colonized the south coast of the United States. In addition, *Stegomyia albopicta*, which was only recently imported to the USA, is also competent as a vector for dengue and for yellow fever.

In Japan. ca. 200 cases of Dengue are diagnosed per year in travelers returning from journeys. In 2014, Dengue infection was for the first time diagnosed in 20 Japanese patients who had not been traveling abroad but they had been infected by mosquitoes in a small park in central Tokyo. Dengue had been absent from Japan for 70 years.

The course of DEN fever is almost always benign in countries or regions such as Central America, large parts of South America, equatorial Africa, and northern Australia. However, the feared complications of DHF and DSS are known to occur in Venezuela, the Caribbean, and especially in India, Indochina, Indonesia, and the Philippines, where 1% to 2% of the hospitalized patients die. It is believed that widespread distribution of the DEN subtypes occurred during Pacific-theater battles of World War II and as a result of modern air traffic. As a consequence of this global distribution, consecutive outbreaks of infections with two different DEN virus subtypes may appear within short intervals of time in the same town and may cause DHF and DSS. These diseases were for the first time observed in Manila, Philippines, in 1952.

After infection, clinical disease only occurs in humans. Monkeys, especially chimpanzees, gibbons, and macaques, become infected and develop viremia that is high enough and lasts long enough to allow mosquitoes to become infected. Other species of monkeys only develop a low grade and short-lasting viremia. A high percentage of the monkey population becomes infected with the DEN virus in Africa and Indonesia. It is not clear whether the rainforest cycle

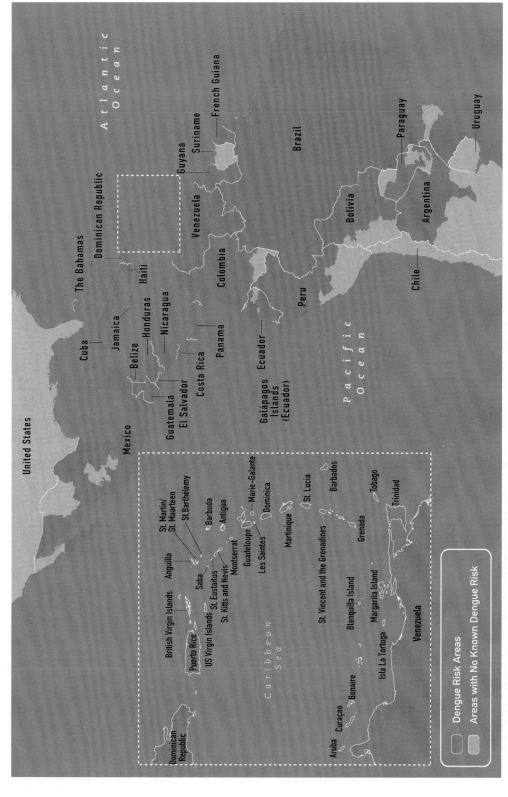

Figure 1.7 | Distribution of Dengue virus infection. CDC 2012

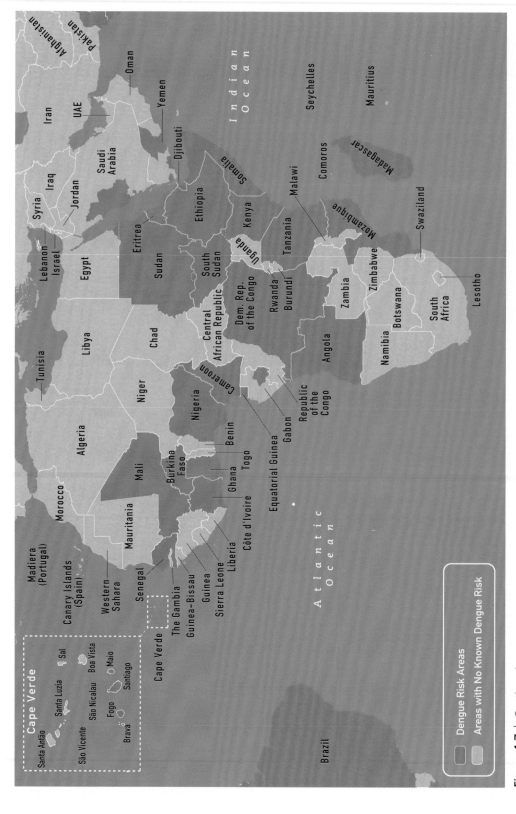

Figure 1.7 | *Continued*

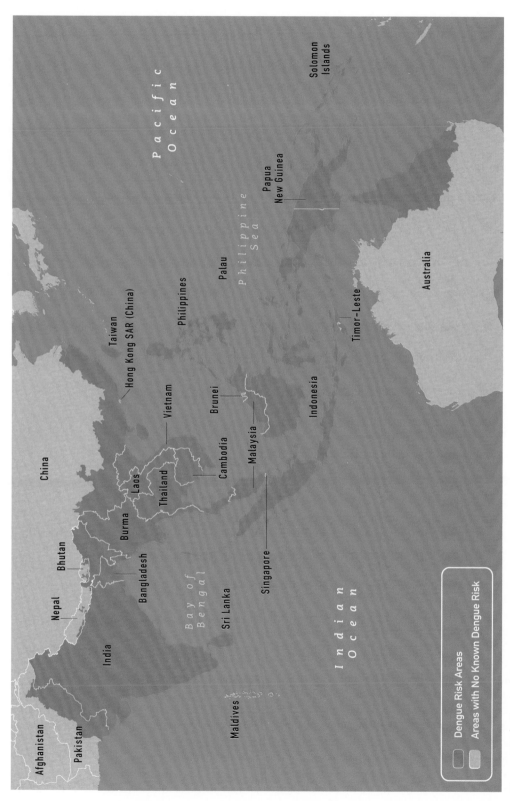

Figure 1.7 | *Continued*

is essential for maintenance of the DEN virus in regions where urban infectious cycles exist.

Transmission. For a long time only the urban cycle of transmission was known, with *A. (Stegomyia) aegypti* being responsible for transmission, similar to YF and Chikungunya fever. Transovarial transmission maintained the reservoir. In rural regions, DEN virus is predominantly transmitted from human to human by *Stegomyia albopicta*, *S. scutellaris*, and *S. africana* (rural transmission cycle). More recently, a jungle cycle has been identified besides the two other cycles, in which the virus is transmitted by rainforest *Stegomyia* (*Aedes*) species between monkeys (sylvan cycle). The connection of the sylvan and urban cycles is made possible by *Stegomyia nivea,* which attacks monkeys and humans (e.g., in Malaysia). DEN, therefore, is a zoonosis that is restricted to humans in the urban cycle but may cause epidemics across regions near rainforests. Insect control in the 1950s nearly succeeded in eliminating *S. aegypti* and DEN in America. However, since the 1960s, DEN has been spreading again in South and Central America and in the Caribbean. A nosocomial transmission of DEN-2 by a needle injury was documented in France in 1998. DEN can also be transmitted by way of donated blood.

Clinical Manifestations. The incubation period is 4 to 7 days, with an extreme range of 3 to 14 days. Mild cases last for 2 to 3 days with fever, headaches, and myalgias. The most common sign of "classical" DEN fever is sudden fever with severe headache, epigastric pain, and retro-orbital pain, which becomes worse after movement. A transient macular rash and a painless lymphadenopathy may be seen. Additional signs are nausea, vomiting, lack of appetite, taste disturbances, cutaneous hyperesthesia, insomnia, and general weakness; occasionally petechial bleeding, epistaxis, hematuria, and melena; and rarely myocarditis and encephalopathy. Granulocytopenia and thrombocytopenia are characteristic, as is hemoconcentration with an increased hematocrit. Signs are resolved after 2 to 5 days. There is a second phase with clinical signs after a 2-day remission that is milder than those in the first phase. A biphasic disease is typical but not always seen. During the recovery phase patients complain about fatigue and depression for a long time.

The complications of DHF and DSS according to WHO criteria are defined by four clinical manifestations: high fever, hemorrhagic diathesis, hepatomegaly, and shock. Depending upon the severity, milder courses, grades 1 and 2, are defined as DHF and the more severe courses, grades 3 and 4, are defined as DSS. In DEN-1 and DEN-2 epidemics in Venezuela between 1989 and 1993, the percentage of DHF was 24% to 66%, with a fatality rate of 0.2% to 0.7%.

Non-neutralizing circulating immune complexes (immune enhancement) are believed to be responsible for the occurrence of DHF and DSS. Immune complexes of that nature are found in patients with two sequential DEN virus infections of different types. Antibodies against the first virus do not neutralize the second virus. However, they attach to the virus and enhance productive infections of macrophages via the Fc-receptor. Six risk factors are known for DHF and DSS.

1. Infection in the presence of non neutralizing antibodies is a risk factor.

2. The source of the second virus being Southeast Asia is a risk factor.

3. Women are more frequently affected than men.

4. Caucasians and Asiatic people are frequently affected, while black people rarely are.

5. Children under the age of 15 years are most frequently affected.

6. Newborn children with maternal antibody who acquire a heterotypic DEN virus are at risk.

The severity of a DEN virus infection correlates with the level of viremia after the second infection, especially with DEN-2. AIDS or a compensated HIV infection does not appear to cause further problems during the course of DEN. Gastric and duodenal ulcers may be sources of life-threatening hemorrhages.

DEN fever during pregnancy can be life threatening for the fetus or for both mother and fetus, especially in the case of DHF. Prenatal infections are possible (3.5% of pregnancies in exposed populations) and may lead to early delivery. However, most pregnancies complicated by DEN infection are known to take a normal course, with delivery of healthy children. The differences may be explained by the epidemiological situation and the immune status of the mother. Newborn children are protected by maternal antibodies against a homotype DEN virus but they may die from DHF or DSS upon first exposure to a heterotypic DEN virus.

Diagnosis. A tentative diagnosis is based on classical clinical symptoms and on a history of travel. A documentation of hypovolumemia (increasing hematocrit) and an altered hemostasis (thrombocyte count below 100,000) is important for the diagnosis of DHF or DSS.

Virus isolation from blood confirms the etiological diagnosis. Infected humans have a viremia of 10^8 mosquito ID_{50} for 4 to 5 days, and sometimes up to 12 days. Live mosquitoes, mosquito cell cultures from *A. albopictus*, or monkey kidney cell lines are suitable for virus isolation. Viral antigen can be found by immunofluorescence in tissue samples from liver, lung, kidney, spleen, and lymph nodes. Antigen capture test as well as RT-PCR are suitable for direct virus detection.

A group-specific PCR targeting the *NS5* gene is available for the demonstration of flavivirus infections (see the references at the end of this section). It can be combined with a virus-specific PCR in a seminested protocol.

IgM detection by the IgM capture method is recommended for serodiagnosis. Serum is IgM positive by 7 days after infection in 97% of the cases. A simultaneous quantitative testing of IgG titers predicts the IgM/IgG quotient for the differentiation of primary and secondary antibody responses.

Cross-reactions with antibodies to agents causing other flavivirus infections (JE, WNF, and YF vaccine) may lead to misinterpretations of serological results.

DEN infections are frequently found in travelers to tropical countries, especially when cases with suspected but unconfirmed malaria are routinely tested for DEN.

Differential Diagnosis. Respiratory and influenza-like syndromes should be taken into consideration in the differential diagnosis, as well as hepatitis, leptospirosis, early phases of malaria, and Tsutsugamushi fever. Rashes similar to the ones induced by DEN virus can be seen in Chikungunya and O'nyong-nyong fevers (both caused by alphaviruses) as well as WNF (another flavivirus). If exanthemas are not evident, DEN-like syndromes can be induced by other arbovirus infections, such as Colorado tick fever, sandfly fever, and mild forms of Rift Valley fever.

All viruses, rickettsiae, and bacteria, which may induce hemorrhagic fever, should be taken into consideration in the differential diagnosis of DHF and DSS: Machupo, Junin, and Lassa viruses; Ebola and Marburg viruses; Hantaviruses; the agents of YF, Crimean-Congo hemorrhagic fever, and Rift Valley fever; *Rickettsia prowazekii*; leptospires; and meningococci.

Therapy. A specific antiviral therapy for DEN does not exist. Blood transfusions and replacement of fluids and plasma proteins are essential for DHF and DSS, with constant testing and balancing of electrolytes. Solutions with Dextran 70 have been especially helpful to overcome shock.

Prophylaxis. A tetravalent attenuated live virus vaccine has been developed for DEN that induces neutralizing antibodies to all four serotypes. However, this vaccine has not yet been sufficiently tested. Live attenuated vaccines against DEN are presently being tested that contain recombinants of Theiler's 17D strain of YF. Considering the recent reports of fatalities after 17D vaccination against YF, introduction of these recombinant vaccines appears doubtful at least.

Presently, methods for vector control dominate. Yellow fever has been successfully controlled by eliminating breeding sites of *S. aegypti* and by vaccination. Vector control has been successful in cities in Southeast Asia to reduce DEN and Chikungunya fever, both of which are disseminated by *S. aegypti*.

For travelers in tropical countries, especially Venezuela and Southeast Asia, it is recommended to use personal protection such as covering exposed skin with clothing at dusk, mosquito nets, and repellents. Special precautions are recommended to people who have already had their first experience with DEN.

REFERENCES

Angibaud G et al., Brain involvement in Dengue fever. *J. Clin. Neurosci.* 8, 63–65, 2001.

Anonymous, Case definitions. Dengue fever. *Epidemiol. Bull.* 21, 14–15, 2000.

Anonymous, Dengue/Dengue haemorrhagic fever. *Wkly. Epidemiol. Rec.* 175, 193–196, 2000.

Carles G et al., Dengue et grossesse. Etude de 38 cas en Guyane française. *J. Gynécol. Obstet. Biol. Réprod.* (Paris). 29, 758–762, 2000.

Centers for Disease Control and Prevention. 2012. CDC Health Information for International Travel. Oxford University Press, New York, NY.

Chen LH, Wilson ME, Dengue and Chikungunya infections in travelers. *Curr. Opin. Infect. Dis.* 23, 438–444, 2010.

Clement J, Colson P, van Ranst M, Dengue versus hantavirus in CNS infections. *Lancet* 355, 2163–2168, 2000.

Conceicao TM, da Poian AT, Sorgine MH, A real-time PCR procedure for detection of dengue virus serotypes 1, 2, and 3, and their quantitation in clinical and laboratory samples. *J. Virol. Meth.* 163, 1–9, 2010.

Das S et al., Detection and serotyping of dengue virus in serum samples by multiplex reverse transcriptase PCR-ligase detection reaction assay. *J. Clin. Microbiol.* 46, 3276–3284, 2008.

Gubler D, The changing epidemiology of yellow fever and dengue, 1900 to 2003: full circle? *Comp. Immunol. Microbiol. Infect. Dis.* 27, 319–330, 2004.

Guzman MG et al., Epidemiologic studies on Dengue in Santiago de Cuba, 1997. *Am. J. Epidemiol.* 152, 793–799, 2000.

Guzman MG, Kouri G, Halstead SB, Do escape mutants explain rapid increases in Dengue case-fatality rates within epidemics? *Lancet* 355, 1902–1903, 2000.

Guzman MG, Kouri G, Dengue and dengue hemorrhagic fever in the Americas: lessons and challenges. *J. Clin. Virol.* 27, 1–13, 2003.

Halstead SB, Dengue. *Lancet* 370, 1644–1652, 2007.

Halstead SB et al., Intrinsic antibody-dependent enhancemant of microbial infection in macrophages: disease regulation by immune complexes. *Lancet Infect. Dis.* 10, 712–722, 2010.

Haritoglou C et al., Okuläre Manifestation bei Dengue-Fieber. *Ophthalmologe* 97, 433–436. 2000.

Huang KJ et al., Manifestation of thrombocytopenia in Dengue-2virus-infected mice. *J. Gen. Virol.* 81, 2177–2182, 2000.

Jain A, Chaturvedi UC, Dengue in infants: an overview. *FEMS Immunol. Med. Microbiol.* 59, 119–130, 2010.

Jansen CC, Beebe NW, The dengue vector Aedes aegypti: what comes next. *Microbes Infect.* 12, 272–279, 2010.

Jelinek T, Dengue fever in international travelers. *Clin. Infect. Dis.* 31, 144–147, 2000.

Kyle JL, Harris E, Global spread and persistence of dengue. *Annu. Rev. Microbiol.* 62, 71–92, 2008.

Kuno G, Emergence of the severe syndrome and mortality associated with dengue and dengue-like illness: historical records (1890 to 1950) and their compatibility with current hypothesis on the shift of disease manifestations. *Clin. Microbiol. Rev.* 22, 186–201, 2009.

Martina BE, Koraka P, Osterhaus AD, Dengue virus pathogenesis: an integrated view. *Clin. Microbiol. Rev.* 22, 564–581, 2009.

McGready R, Paw E, Nosten F, Menorrhagia caused by Dengue fever. *Aust. N. Z. J. Obstet. Gynaecol.* 40, 354–355, 2000.

Miller N, Recent progress in dengue vaccine research and development. *Curr. Opin. Mol. Ther.* 12, 31–38, 2010.

Monroy V, Ruiz BH, Participation of the Dengue virus in the fibrinolytic process. *Virus Genes.* 21, 197–208, 2000.

NN, Case definitions. Dengue fever. *Epidemiol. Bull.* 21, 14–15, 2000.

NN, Dengue/Dengue haemorrhagic fever. *Wkly. Epidemiol. Rec.* 175, 193–195, 2000.

Noble CG et al., Strategies for development of dengue virus inhibitors. *Antivir Res.* 85, 450–462, 2010.

Pouliot SH et al., Maternal dengue and pregnancy outcomes: a systematic review. *Obstet Gynecol. Surv.* 65, 107–118, 2010.

Rawlinson SM et al., Dengue virus RNA polymerase NS5: a potential therapeutic target? *Curr. Drug Targets* 7, 1623–1638, 2006.

Rodenhuis-Zybert IA, Wilschut J, Smit JM, Dengue virus life cycle: viral and host factors modulating infectivity. *Cell. Mol. Life Sci.* 67, 2773–2786, 2010.

Ross TM, Dengue virus. *Clin. Lab. Med.* 30, 149–160, 2010.

Schlesinger JJ, Brandriss MW, Growth of 17D yellow fever virus in a macrophage-like cell line, U937: role of Fc and viral receptors in antibody-mediated infection. *J. Immunol.* 127, 659–665, 1982.

Schlesinger JJ, Brandriss MW, Antibodymediated infection of macrophages and macrophage like cell lines with 17D-yellow fever virus. *J. Med. Virol.* 8, 103–117, 1981.

Schwartz E et al., Changing epidemiology of Dengue fever in travelers to Thailand. *Eur. J. Clin. Microbiol. Infect. Dis.* 19, 784–786, 2000.

Schwartz E et al., Evaluation of ELISA-based serodiagnosis of Dengue fever in travelers. *J. Clin. Virol.* 19, 169–173, 2000.

Seed CR et al., The risk of dengue transmission by blood during a 2004 outbreak in Cairns, Australia. *Transfusion* 49, 1482–1487, 2009.

Stevens AJ et al., The medicinal chemistry of dengue fever. *J. Med. Chem.* 52, 7911–7926, 2009.

Teles FR, Prazeres DM, Lima-Filho JL, Trends in dengue diagnosis. *Rev. Med. Virol.* 15, 287–302, 2005.

Swaminathan S, Batra G, Khanna N, Dengue vaccines: state of the art. *Expert Opin. Ther. Pat.* 20, 819–835, 2010.

Ter Meulen J et al., Isolation and partial characterization of Dengue virus type 2 and 4 strains from Dengue fever and Dengue haemorrhagic fever patients from Mindanao, Republic of the Philippines. *Trop. Med. Int. Health.* 5, 325–329, 2000.

Torres JR, Liprandi F, Goncalvez AP, Acute parotitis due to Dengue virus. *Clin. Infect. Dis.* 31, E28–29, 2000.

Trent DW, Chang GJ, Detection and identification of flaviviruses by reverse transcriptase polymerase chain reaction. In: Becker Y, Darai G (eds.), *Diagnosis of human viruses by polymerase chain reaction technology.* Chapter 27, 355–369, Springer, Berlin, Heidelberg, New York, 1992.

Trung DT, Wills B, Systemic vascular leakage associated with dengue infections – the clinical perspective. *Curr. Top. Microbiol. Immunol.* 338, 57–66, 2010.

Urcuqui-Inchima S et al., Recent developments in understanding dengue virus replication. *Adv. Virus Res.* 77, 1–39, 2010.

Van Der Most RG et al., Chimeric yellow fever/Dengue virus as a candidate dengue vaccine: quantitation of the dengue virusspecific CD8 T-cell response. *J. Virol.* 74, 8094–8101, 2000.

Vasilakis N, Weaver SC, The history and evolution of the human dengue emergence. *Adv. Virus Res.* 72, 1–76, 2008.

Whitehead SS et al., Prospects for a dengue virus vaccine. *Nat. Rev. Microbiol.* 5, 518–528, 2007.

WHO, Dengue: Guidelines for diagnosis, treatment, prevention and control. New edn. Geneva: World Health Organisation, 2009.

Wichmann O, Jelinek T, Dengue in travelers: a review. *J. Travel Med.* 11, 161–170, 2004.

Wu JY et al., Dengue fever in mainlnd China. *Am. J. Trop. Med. Hyg. Am. J. Trop. Med. Hyg.* 83, 664–671, 2010.

1.4 Zoonoses Caused by Bunyaviruses

The bunyavirus family includes more than 300 RNA viruses that can be differentiated serologically. They all have a segmented genome with large (L), medium (M), and small (S) segments. Bunyaviruses are divided into four genera (*Orthobunyavirus*, *Hantavirus*, *Nairovirus*, and *Phlebovirus*) according to structure, genetics, and ecology. They also include the genus *Tospovirus*, with viruses that are predominantly phytopathogenic and not pathogenic for animals. Most bunyaviruses, including the tospoviruses, have been isolated from arthropods and therefore, are arboviruses. Only the genus *Hantavirus* includes viruses that are spread by rodents and have not yet been found in arthropods. Viruses from all four genera are pathogenic for humans.

However, no more than about 20 of them cause a defined disease entity in humans.

Similar to Orthomyxoviruses, all Bunyaviruses are dependent on the 5′ caps (m7GpppNm caps) of cellular mRNA molecules to initiate their mRNA synthesis. Uninterrupted expression of host cell genes is needed for viral replication. For the S segment, the phleboviruses and tospoviruses use an ambisense technique by encoding the gene for the N protein (the capsid protein) in the complementary RNA (plus strand) and the gene for the nonstructural (NS) protein in the genomic RNA (minus strand). Bunyaviruses of the genus *Bunyavirus* encode both genes in the genomic RNA (minus strand). No NS protein has yet been found in H antaviruses and Nairoviruses. Their gene for the N protein is encoded in the genomic RNA. The negative strand of the M segment codes for the glycoproteins G1 and G2. These are transcribed polycistronically and are split proteolytically posttranslation. The L segment codes for the polymerase. A genetic recombination of the Bunyaviruses by reassortment is possible, similar to that in orthomyxoviruses. A reassortment under natural conditions has been documented for Rift Valley fever (RVF) virus and for other Bunyaviruses. Bunyaviruses implicated in zoonoses are listed in Tab. 1.1.

Other Bunyaviruses may occasionally cause uncharacteristic human disease worldwide in many countries. The names of these viruses are listed as follows without additional remarks: Apeu, Batai, Bunyamwera, Bwamba, Cache Valley, Caraparu, Catou, Fort Sherman, Germiston, Guama, Ilesha, Itaqui, Lumbo, Madrid, Marituba, Marutucu, Ngari, Nepuyo, Nyando, Oriboca, Ossa, Restan, Shokwe, Shuni, Tacaiuma, Tataguine, Tensaw, and Wyeomyia viruses.

Syndromes caused by these infections include febrile illness, myalgia, photophobia, and conjunctivitis; some viruses may cause rash, arthralgia, vomiting, diarrhea, cough, and meningitis or myocarditis. Many species of mosquitoes are the vectors for these viruses.

The arthropod-transmitted bunyaviruses are closely adapted to their vectors. They can survive by vertical transmission under unfavorable climatic conditions (cold or dry periods). La

Table 1.1 | Zoonotic bunyaviruses

VIRUS	HOST(S)	VECTOR(S)	DISEASE	GEOGRAPHICAL OCCURRENCE
Genus *Bunyavirus*[1] (mosquitoes as vectors)				
La Crosse virus	Squirrels, rabbits	*Aedes triseriatus*	California (La Crosse) encephalitis	North America (Ohio, Wisconsin, Minnesota)
Snowshoe hare virus			California encephalitis	North America
Tahyna virus			California encephalitis	Old World
Oropouche virus[2]	Sloths, primates	Culicoid flies (*Aedes* spp.)	Oropouche fever	Brazil
Genus *Nairovirus* (ixodid ticks as vectors)				
Crimean-Congo hemorrhagic fever virus	Herbivores	*Hyalomma* ticks	Crimean-Congo hemorrhagic fever	Southern Europe, Asia, Africa
Genus *Phlebovirus* (*Phlebotomus* spp. as vectors)				
Rift Valley fever virus	Rodents (?), herbivores	Mosquitoes (*Culex* spp.)	Rift Valley fever	Africa, Asia Minor
Sandfly fever virus	Gerbils, bats (?)	Sand flies (*Phlebotomus* spp.)	Sandfly fever	Southern Europe, Northern Africa, South America, West and Central Asia
Genus *Hantavirus*[3]				
Subgroup A (HFRS)[4]				
Puumala virus	Bank vole (*Clethrionomys glareolus*)		NE Europe	North and Central
Hantaan virus	Striped field mouse (*Apodemus agrarius*)		Korean hemorrhagic fever	East Asia
Dobrava virus	Yellow-necked (*Apodemus flavicollis*) and striped (*A. agrarius*) field mice		Balkan hemorrhagic fever	Southern Europe
Seoul virus	Norwegian rat (*Rattus norvegicus*)		Hemorrhagic fever with renal syndrome	Worldwide
Subgroup B (HPS)[5]				
Sin Nombre virus	Deer mouse (*Peromyscus maniculatus*)		Hantavirus pulmonary syndrome	North America, Northern Mexico
Laguna Negra	Laucha chica (*Calomys laucha*)		Hantavirus pulmonary syndrome	Argentina

continued

Table 1.1 *continued*

VIRUS	HOST(S)	VECTOR(S)	DISEASE	GEOGRAPHICAL OCCURRENCE
Andes virus	Rice rat (*Oligoryzomys longicaudatus*)		Hantavirus pulmonary syndrome	South America
Bayou virus	Rice rat (*Oryzomys palustris*)		Hantavirus pulmonary syndrome	North America (Louisiana)
Black Creek	Cotton rat (*Sigmodon hispidus*)		Hantavirus pulmonary syndrome	North America Canal virus (Florida)
Subgroup C (no importance as human pathogens)[6]				
Prospect Hill virus	Vole (*Microtus pennsylvanicus*)			North America
Tula virus	Vole (*Microtus arvalis*)			Northern Europe
Lemming virus	Lemming (*Lemmus lemmus*)			Northern Europe

[1] Only selected members of the genus are listed.
[2] *Simbu* subgroup.
[3] Hosts of hantaviruses serve as virus reservoirs and are the sources of human infections.
[4] Viruses found in Eurasia with hosts from the subfamily Murinae.
[5] New World hantaviruses with hosts from the family Cricetidae.
[6] Viruses with hosts from the subfamily Arvicolinae.

Crosse virus, the most important agent in the California encephalitis group, is transmitted in its main vector, *Aedes triseriatus*, by transovarial and sexual routes. Similar to influenza viruses, bunyaviruses are directly dependent for their gene expression on the metabolic activity of their host. The 5' cap (m7GpppNm cap) of the cellular mRNA is needed for initiation of the viral mRNA synthesis (5' cap snatching). Blood meals activate the cellular gene activity in the ovaries of mosquitoes, which stimulates viral replication. Two different 5'-end sequences of the host (CS1 and CS2) are available for the activation of the viral message. Viral gene expression can be found in mosquito eggs during winter (diapause). However, 5' cap structures with CS2 sequences are used almost exclusively as primers for viral RNA. After the diapause, 100% of CS1-carrying viral messengers are used. If an egg is infected with two different bunyaviruses, the special mode of viral gene expression facilitates a gene recombination with intermolecular and intramolecular reassortment, a possible explanation for the multiplicity of bunyaviruses.

An ELISA using recombinant antigen for the demonstration of virus-specific IgM antibodies is generally used for the diagnosis of bunyavirus infections. Virus-specific IgM antibodies can usually be found at the onset of the disease.

RT-PCR is usually not used for the clinical diagnosis of bunyavirus infections, especially La Crosse virus and hantavirus infections. However, it can be used for the postmortem diagnosis to solve epidemiological questions. S-RNA coding for the N protein and, if present, the NS protein are usually used for the RT-PCR for bunyaviruses. A combination of three pairs of primers was recommended for a group-specific detection of the genomes of bunyaviruses of groups A and C and the Simbu group by RT-PCR and nested PCR techniques. Recently RT-PCR techniques were used for the detection of the Oropouche virus and the RVF virus.

Ribavirin has been used successfully for the treatment of some bunyavirus infections, especially with Hantaviruses, the Crimean-Congo hemorrhagic fever (CCHF) virus, and the RVF virus.

REFERENCES

Aleksandrowicz P et al., Viral haemorrhagic fever and vascular alterations. *Haemostasiol* 28, 77–84, 2008.

Blair CD, Adelman ZN, Olson KE, Molecular strategies for interrupting arthropodborne virus transmission by mosquitoes. *Clin. Microbiol. Rev.* 13, 651–661, 2000.

Bouloy M, Flick R, Reverse genetics technology for Rift Valley fever virus: current and future applications for the development of therapeutics and vaccines. *Antivir. Res.* 84, 101–118, 2009.

Elliott RM, Bunyaviruses and climate change. *Clin. Microbiol. Infect.* 15, 510–517, 2009.

Johnson AJ et al., Detection of anti-arboviral immunoglobulin G by using a monoclonal antibody-based capture enzyme-linked immunosorbent assay. *J. Clin. Microbiol.* 38, 1827–1831, 2000.

Lambert AJ, Lanciotti S, Molecular characterization of medically important viruses of the genus orthobunyavirus. *J. Gen. Virol.* 89, 2580–2585, 2008.

Lozach PY et al., *Cell Host Microbe* 25, 488–499, 2010.

Martin DA, Standardization of immunoglobulin μ-capture enzyme linked immunosorbent assays for routine diagnosis of arboviral infections. *J. Clin. Microbiol.* 38, 1823–1826, 2001.

Moreli ML, Aquino VH, Figueiredo LTM, Identification of Simbu, California and Bunyamwera serogroup bunyaviruses by nested RT-PCR. *Trans. R. Soc. Med. Hyg.* 95, 108–113, 2001.

Morikawa S, Saijo M, Kurane I, Recent progress in molecular biology of Crimean-Congo hemorrhagic fever. *Comp. Immunol. Microbiol. Infect. Dis.* 30, 375–389, 2007.

Nichol ST, Bunyaviruses. In: Knipe DM, Howley PM, Griffin DE (eds.), *Fields Virology*, 931–960, Lippincott, Williams & Wilkins, Philadelphia. 4th ed., 2001.

Tsai TF, Chandler LJ, Arboviruses. In: Murray PR et al. (eds.), *Manual of Clinical Microbiology*, 1553–1569, 8th ed. ASM Press, Washington, 2003.

1.4.1 LA CROSSE (CALIFORNIA ENCEPHALITIS) VIRUS, SNOWSHOE HARE VIRUS, AND TAHYNA VIRUS

La Crosse or California encephalitis is an acute disease of the CNS transmitted by mosquitoes. It appears during the summer in various parts of the United States. Most cases are reported from Ohio, Wisconsin, and Minnesota. La Crosse encephalitis is virtually nonexistent west of Oklahoma. The name "California encephalitis" is misleading.

Etiology. The causative agents are bunyaviruses, genus *Bunyavirus*. The viruses of the California encephalitis complex (14 serotypes) have common antigens but can be differentiated serologically. The La Crosse virus is one of the subtypes; another, the Tahyna virus, has been isolated in Slowakia, where it caused influenza-like diseases in humans.

The Tahyna virus and other viruses of the California encephalitis group also exist in Central Europe. Neutralizing antibodies have been found in individuals in rural areas, and the virus has been isolated from mosquitoes in Franconia, Germany. No human disease attributable to Tahyna virus has been observed.

Occurrence. Between 30 and 160 cases of California encephalitis are recognized annually in the United States. Children under 15 years are especially affected. The La Crosse virus is the most commonly reported cause of pediatric arboviral encephalitis in the United States. The number of inapparent infections is high: 40% of the population in Wisconsin has antibodies. Epidemics are frequent in Wisconsin, Minnesota, Iowa, Ohio, Illinois, and Indiana. There are sporadic cases in North Carolina, Texas and Florida.

Transmission. The agents are transmitted by numerous mosquitoes. Small mammals, such as feral rabbits and squirrels, serve as reservoirs and sources for amplification. Survival of the agents during winter is possible through vertical, transovarial, and transstadial transmission. Virus latency in diapause mosquito eggs is directed by the dependence of viral gene expression on the cellular mRNA synthesis.

The La Crosse virus, the most important agent of this group, uses *Stegomyia triseriata* as vector and squirrels as a reservoir. *Stegomyia albopicta* is also a potential vector. Men are more frequently affected than women by California encephalitis, possibly because the infection takes place during outdoor activities.

Clinical Manifestations. The incubation period is 5 to 10 days. Subclinical infections are much more common than clinical manifestations, and summer flu-like illness is predominant. The onset of the disease is slow with subfebrile temperatures and headaches. Confusion and seizures bring the patient to a physician. Patients may show signs of meningitis and may become comatose. Pathological reflexes or paralysis does not occur. Fever lasts 2 weeks on average. Recovery can be slow, especially in children. In 10% of patients, epileptic episodes may persist as well as pareses and learning difficulties (2%), especially in children. Fatal cases are rare (1%). Congenital infections may occur.

Diagnosis. The disease cannot be diagnosed from clinical signs alone. Virus isolation from living patients has never been accomplished; the virus has only been isolated from brain tissue postmortem. The viruses of this group cause productive cytopathic infections in BHK21 cells and Vero cells. Persistent, but not cytopathic infections are seen in mosquito cell cultures. Usually, the diagnosis is confirmed by seroconversion, increased antibody titers, or demonstration of virus-specific IgM antibodies. Intrathecal antibody production can be proven by the Reiber quotient.

RT-PCR is not important for the clinical diagnosis but is useful for the postmortem diagnosis, for testing mosquitoes and for monitoring cell cultures. A group-specific RT-PCR exists for the Simbu-California-Bunyamwera serogroup. The S segment is amplified by using primers BUN-S and BUN-C, which are complementary to the 3′ and 5′ ends of the RNA. Amplicons have a length of 700 to 1,300 bp. A type-specific diagnosis of La Crosse virus can then be completed with a nested PCR using specific primers BBC-S and BBC-C.

Differential Diagnosis. Other encephalitides caused by arboviruses or by more commonly occurring viruses and bacteria are to be considered. Posttraumatic subdural hematomas should also be excluded in the differential diagnosis. West Nile fever must be considered because of its introduction into the United States in 1999.

Therapy. Specific therapy and a vaccine for active immunization are not available. Treatment is symptomatic. Treatment with ribavirin may be indicated in severe cases. Under experimental conditions ribavirin blocks viral replication of some bunyaviruses, for example, CCHF virus. If administered early, ribavirin (4 g/day loading dose, and then 16 mg/kg every 6 h i.v. or per infusion) can ameliorate the course of hantavirus disease. A systematic study to test the efficacy on bunyavirus infections, especially on California encephalitis, has not been performed.

Prophylaxis. The control of vectors is very difficult because of the habit of mosquitoes to hatch in trees. Individual protection is possible against mosquito bites with sufficient clothing and repellents.

REFERENCES

Balkhy HH, Schreiber JR, Severe La Crosse encephalitis with significant neurologic sequelae. *Pediatr. Infect. Dis. J.* 19, 77–80, 2000.

Beaty BJ, Rayms-Keller A, Borucki MK, Blair CD, La Crosse encephalitis virus and mosquitoes: a remarkable relationship. *ASM News* 66, 349–351, 2000.

Boyce TG et al., Fever and encephalopathy in two school age boys. *Pediatr. Infect. Dis. J.* 17, 939–940, 1998.

CDC, Possible congenital infection with La Crosse encephalitis virus, West Virginia, 2006-2007. *Morb. Mort. Wkly. rep.* 58, 4–7, 2009.

Chandler LJ et al., Characterization of La Crosse virus RNA in autopsied central nervous system tissue. *J. Clin. Microb.* 36, 3332–3336, 1998.

Haddow AD, Odoi A, The incidence risk, clustering, and clinical presentation of La Crosee virus infections in the eastern United States, 2003–2007. *PLos One* 4, e6145, 2009.

Jones TF et al., Serological survey and active surveillance for La Crosse virus infections among children in Tennessee. *Clin. Infect. Dis.* 31, 1284–7, Nov 2000.

Joy JE, Hildreth-Whitehair A, Larval habitat characterization for Aedes triseriatus (Say), the mosquito vector of La Crosse encephalitis in West Virginia. *Wilderness Environ Med.* 11, 79–83, 2000.

Lambert AJ et al., Nucleic acid amplification assays for the detection of La Crosse virus RNA. *J. Clin. Microbiol.* 43, 1885–1889, 2005.

Lambert AJ et al., La Crosse virus in Aedes albopictus mosquitoes, Texas, USA, 2009. *Emerg. Infect. Dis.* 16, 856–858, 2010.

Moreli ML, Aquino VH, Figueiredo LT, Identification of Simbu, California and Bunyamwera serogroup bunyaviruses by nested RT-PCR. *Trans. R. Soc. Trop. Med. Hyg.* 95, 108–113, 2001.

Nichol ST, Bunyaviruses. In: Knipe DM, Tatum LM et al. Canine LaCrosse viral meningoencephalomyelitis with possible public health implications. *J. Vet. Diagn. Invest.* 11, 184–188, 1999.

1.4.2 OROPOUCHE FEVER

Oropouche fever is a mild febrile disease that occurs epidemically. There are few characteristic symptoms. The disease is also called *febre de Mojui*, after the village of Mojui in northern Brazil. The Oropouche virus belongs to the emerging viruses. The first epidemic occurred after a clearing of tropical rainforest for human settlements.

Etiology. The causative agent, the Oropouche virus, belongs to the Simbu-California-Bunyamwera serogroup of the genus *Bunyavirus*. It is presently the only virus in this serogroup that is pathogenic for humans.

Occurrence. Evidence of Oropouche virus activity is found in Brazil, Colombia, Panama, Peru, Tobago, and Trinidad. The virus was first isolated in 1955 from a forest worker in Trinidad with a febrile disease, although epidemics with this virus have never been observed in Trinidad. Numerous urban epidemics occurred in the Amazon region between 1961 and 1991. There were probably more than 300,000 cases; children and juveniles were predominantly affected. Fatal cases do not occur. The invasion of urban settlements by mosquitoes and the migration of susceptible persons from regions of nonendemicity (e.g., soldiers and laborers) into regions of endemicity have caused extensive outbreaks, affecting a high percentage of the population.

Monkeys in Colombia have antibodies to the Oropouche virus. The virus was isolated from four sloths in the Amazon region. The animals did not show signs of disease.

Transmission. In urban epidemics, the virus is transmitted by *Culicoides paraensis*. The cycle of urban infections can be maintained by vector-human-vector-human transmission. A sylvan cycle appears to exist, with monkeys and sloths (family Bradypodidae) as reservoirs and forest mosquitoes as vectors. *Aedes albopictus* and *Culex quinquefasciatus* are also potential vectors based on experimental evidence.

Clinical Manifestations. The incubation period is 4 to 8 days with a range of 3 to 12 days. The onset of disease is sudden without a prodromal phase. Fever (up to 40 °C) is common, with rigors, headaches, myalgias (neck and back), arthralgias, daze, and photophobia. Additional signs are conjunctival injections, bronchitis, nausea, vomiting, diarrhea, epigastric pain, and a burning sensation in many body regions. Meningoencephalitis has been seen in a few cases. Blood counts reveal leukopenia.

The disease lasts for 2 to 7 days, but recovery may be slow. Cases with repeated recurrent symptoms are known to occur. No fatalities have been documented in the known epidemics.

Diagnosis. A presumed diagnosis of Oropouche fever based on clinical signs can only be made in areas of endemicity during epidemics, because of the lack of characteristic symptoms. The serological diagnosis is based on the detection of IgM antibodies.

The virus can be isolated from heparinized blood or from serum by inoculation of newborn mice or hamsters; it also replicates in cell cultures from hamsters and monkeys. The virus can be detected by a nested RT-PCR in cell cultures, blood, or in mosquitoes.

A group-specific RT-PCR exists for the Simbu-California-Bunyamwera serogroup. The S segment is amplified by using primers BUN-S and BUN-C, which are complementary to the 3' and 5' ends of the RNA. Amplicons have a length of 700 to 1,300 bp. A type-specific diagnosis can then be completed with a nested PCR using specific primers BS-S and BS-C. For references see the end of this section.

Differential Diagnosis. Malaria has to be excluded first in the differential diagnosis. Otherwise, a large number of febrile diseases without characteristic symptoms that exist in South America or worldwide, including dengue, Rocio and Mayaro fever, have to be considered.

Therapy. A specific therapy does not exist. Treatment is symptomatic, but patients frequently have to be hospitalized. Specific antiviral therapy is not needed in most cases. Treatment with ribavirin could be attempted in severe cases with a defined diagnosis based on the experience with the treatment of other bunyavirus infections. Under experimental conditions ribavirin blocks viral replication of some bunyaviruses, for example, CCHF virus. If administered early, ribavirin (4 g/day initially, and then 16 mg/kg every 6 h i.v. or per infusion) can ameliorate the course of the disease. A systematic study to test the efficacy of ribavirin has not been carried out.

Prophylaxis. An antiviral vaccine is not available. Mosquito nets and repellents can be used in epidemic situations. Because a high percentage of the population is affected in epidemics, the supply for the population has been problematic in small municipalities.

There is not yet sufficient evidence for the role of specific arthropods as vectors to control the epidemics with vector control.

REFERENCES

Baisley KJ et al., Wilson: Epidemiology of endemic Oropouche virus transmission in upper Amazonian Peru. *Am. J. Trop. Med. Hyg.* 59, 710–716, 1998.

Livonesi MC et al., In vitro and in vivo studies of ribavirin action on Brazilian orthobunyavirus. *Am. J. Trop. Med. Hyg.* 75, 1011–1016, 2006.

Moreli ML et al., Diagnosis of Oropouche virus infection by RT-nested-PCR. *J. Med. Virol.* 66, 139–142, 2002.

Moreli ML, Aquino VH, Figueiredo LT, Identification of Simbu, California and Bunyamwera serogroup bunyaviruses by nested RT-PCR. *Trans. R. Soc. Trop. Med. Hyg.* 95, 108–113, 2001.

Saeed MF et al., Jatobal virus is a reassortant containing the small RNA of Oropouche virus. *Virus Res.* 77, 25–30, 2001.

Saeed MF et al., Diagnosis of Oropouche virus infection using a recombinant nucleocapsid protein-based enzyme immunoassay. *J. Clin. Microbiol.* 39, 2445–2452, 2001.

Vasconcelos HB et al., Oropouche fever epidemic in Northern Brazil: epidemiology and molecular characterization of isolates. *J. Clin. Virol.* 44, 129–133, 2009.

Walsh JF, Molyneux DH, Birley MH, Deforestation: effects on vector-borne disease. *Parasitology* 106 Suppl: S55–S75, 1993.

Watts DM et al., Venezuelan equine encephalitis and Oropouche virus infections among Peruvian army troops in the Amazon region of Peru. *Am. J. Trop. Med. Hyg.* 56, 661–667, 1997.

1.4.3 CRIMEAN-CONGO HEMORRHAGIC FEVER

CCHF is an acute disease caused by an arbovirus that is transmitted to humans by ticks. The disease was first described in 1944 on the Crimean peninsula. The viral etiology was confirmed in 1945. An identical or serologically similar agent has been identified in sporadic cases of hemorrhagic fever in the Asian part of the former USSR, in Bulgaria, and in the former Yugoslavia. Virus isolates from the Democratic Republic of the Congo (formerly Zaire) and other Western and Central African regions were serologically identical to the agent of CCHF.

Etiology. CCHF virus belongs to the family *Bunyaviridae*, genus *Nairovirus* (from the Nairobi sheep disease virus). There are at least three subtypes of the CCHF virus.

Occurrence. Human CCHF is known to occur in 38 countries. During the past decade, it was reported from Bulgaria, Albania, Serbia, Greece Russia, Turkey, the United Arab Emirates, Oman, Iraq, Kuwait, Iran, Afghanistan, Pakistan, the People's Republic of China, Mauritania, Burkina Faso, Senegal, the Democratic Republic of the Congo, Australia (Tasmania), Sierra Leone, and South Africa.

In the former USSR, CCHF is seasonally restricted. It appears in Astrakhan in May and June and around Rostov from May until August. However, in Iraq sporadic cases occur throughout the year. Numerous disease and fatal cases due to CCHF with the symptoms of hemorrhagic fever have been reported from southern and west Africa.

In areas of endemicity, infections with the CCHF virus can be found in humans and domestic animals, more frequently in cattle than in sheep or goats. Birds living on the ground are infected. Farm-raised ostriches are more frequently infected than chickens. Hedgehogs, horses, and mouse-like rodents serve as reservoirs for the agent.

The CCHF virus has been isolated from more than 30 different tick species, predominantly *Hyalomma* but also *Ixodes* species. Transovarial and transstadial virus transmission was demonstrated in ticks. However, the cycle between ticks and vertebrates appears to be important for the maintenance of the virus. The distribution of CCHF roughly coincides with the occurrence of ticks of the genus *Hyalomma*, indicating that these are the most efficient vectors and reservoir hosts of CCHF virus.

Human infections occur in rural areas, with livestock, rendering plants, slaughterhouses, ostrich farms, and dairy cattle the source of epidemics. The CCHF virus was introduced by camels into the United Arab Emirates from Afghanistan and by cattle from Somalia. Steak from farmed ostriches is imported to the Northern Hemisphere and it might be infected with the CCHF virus.

Transmission. Contact with ticks or infected livestock causes human infections. When a tick, sucking on a cow, is brushed with the hand, the virus can be transmitted. Activities such as slaughter, castrations, and branding of animals, as well as birth support and work in rendering plants in rural areas, may be hazardous. Nosocomial infections are frequent. They occur in patient caretakers under hygienically unfavorable conditions. Distribution by aerosol cannot be ruled out, especially in laboratories. The CCHF virus might be a candidate virus for bioterrorism, but infectivity is low in cell culture systems and consecutive passages will end in attenuation of the virus.

Clinical Manifestations. The incubation period after a tick bite is 1 to 3 days. Depending on the virus dose it may be 5 to 6 days or up to 9 days following nosocomial exposure or exposure to viremic animal blood, tissues, and excreta. The disease begins abruptly with fever, then shivering, malaise, irritability, and head, limb, and backaches. Patients are anorexic and complain about nausea and abdominal pain. Vomiting is common. Fever usually lasts for 5 to 12 days, but recurrent or biphasic courses are seen. The skin on the face and neck is red and swollen. The conjunctiva and mucous membranes are congested and edematous. Patients usually are depressed and somnolent. A hemorrhagic diathesis may be seen in 75% of the patients on day 4 or 5. Petechial bleedings on the skin of the entire body, bleeding on mucosal

membranes, hematemesis, melena, and urogenital bleeding are seen. The lethality is dependent on the virus variant and its degree of attenuation. It may amount to 30% to 50% but is lower in patients without hemorrhagic diathesis. Patients usually die in hemorrhagic shock or from secondary infections.

Diagnosis. There is no difference in the course of CCHF between cases in the Russia and those in Africa. A diagnosis cannot be made during the noncharacteristic prodromal phase. Information on tick bites (predominantly of the genus *Hyalomma* and acquired in Russia, the near or Middle East, and Africa) and a report on agricultural work in areas of endemicity may give a hint. If CCHF is suspected, diagnostic tests should be performed in BSL-4 laboratories. The virus can be isolated in Vero cells from blood of severely affected patients. Chilled EDTA-treated blood (around 4 °C) should be sent. Virus-infected Vero cells do not show cytopathic effects. The virus in Vero cells or in the brain of intracerebrally injected mice has to be demonstrated with immunofluorescence or by PCR. In addition to virus isolation, a direct RT-PCR (two-step nested PCR) can be performed on patient blood.

Virus culture, testing for virus-specific IgM antibodies (IgM capture method with recombinant antigen) should be made alternatively or in addition to virus isolation in all suspected cases.

Differential Diagnosis. Patients give the impression of a septic disease resembling typhoid fever. Causes of hemorrhagic fevers have to be included in the differential diagnosis, for example, rickettsiosis (typhus), leptospirosis, borreliosis (relapsing fever), meningococcal infections, malaria, yellow fever, dengue, Omsk hemorrhagic fever, and Kyasanur Forest disease. Patients infected with hanta-, filo-, or arenaviruses (e.g., Lassa, Marburg, or Ebola virus) may present with similar clinical signs.

Therapy. Intensive care has to be delivered in negative-pressure units using safety clothing. High pressure protective suits for the staff are preferable to wards with negative pressure. Vital functions must be controlled, and packed red cells, platelets, clotting factors, and albumin are required for the treatment of hemorrhagic shock. The therapeutic value of hyperimmune globulin has not been proven. Under experimental conditions, ribavirin blocks viral replication. If administered early, ribavirin (4 g/day initially, and then 16 mg/kg every 6 h i.v. or per infusion) can ameliorate the course of the disease. A systematic study to test the efficacy of the approach has not been performed.

Transport of patients with hemorrhagic fever to a hospital with isolation quarters is not recommended, because patients are usually in a critical stage at the time of the diagnosis. It has been recommended that these patients be attended locally by experienced personnel.

Prophylaxis. An inactivated virus vaccine from mouse brain was prepared in Russia. As the disease is relatively rare, there is no urgent need for the development of a modern vaccine.

It is advisable to use gloves in contact with patients suspected of suffering from viral hemorrhagic fever and in contact with potentially infected cattle, sheep, goats, and camels. Treatment to prevent tick infestation in domestic animals has not been practical. To prevent nosocomial infections, any laboratory work has to be done under safety conditions. Safe handling of virus-infected clinical specimens in a normal clinical laboratory may present a special challenge. Wherever feasible, the specimens should be inactivated by fixation or by thermal (56 °C, 30 min) or chemical treatment before being removed from the isolation ward. Addition of detergent to a serum specimen will reduce the virus titer. Running infected specimens in a centrifuge is the most dangerous of all manipulations. Sticks with infected needles and cuts with infected knives should be avoided.

REFERENCES

Deyde JL et al., Crimean-Congo haemorrhagic fever virus genomics and global diversity. *J. Virol.* 80, 8834–8842, 2006.

Duh D et al., Viral load as a predictor for Crimean-Congo haemorrhagic fever outcome. *Emerg. Infect. Dis.* 13, 1769–1772, 2007.

Ergonul O, Treatment of Crimean-Congo haemorrhagic fever. *Antivir. Res.* 78, 125–131, 2008.

Flick R et al., Reverse genetics for Crimean-Congo haemorrhagic fever virus. *J. Virol.* 77, 5997–6006, 2003.

Flick R, Whitehouse CA, Crimean-Congo haemorrhagic fever. *Curr. Mol. Med.* 5, 753–760, 2005.

Khan AS et al., An outbreak of Crimean-Congo hemorrhagic fever in the United Arab Emirates, 1994–1995. *Am. J. Trop. Med. Hyg.* 57, 519–525, 1997.

Leblebicioglu H, Crimean-Congo haemorrhagic fever in Eurasia. *Int. J. Antimicrobiol. Agents* 36 (suppl. 1), S43–S46, 2010.

Mardani M, Rahnavardi M, Sharifi-Mood B, Current treatment of Crimean-Congo haemorrhagic fever in children. *Expert Rev. Anti Infect. Ther.* 8, 911–918, 2010.

Ozkaya E et al., Molecular epidemiology of Crimean-Congo haemorrhagic fever virus in Turkey: occurrence of local topotype. *Virus Res.* 149, 64–70, 2010.

Soares-Weiser K et al., Ribavirin for Crimean-Congo haemorrhagic fever: a systemic review and meta-analysis. *BMC Infect. Dis.* 10, 207, 2010.

Tang Q et al., A patient with Crimean-Congo haemorrhagic fever serologically diagnosed by recombinant nucleoprotein-based antibody detection systems. *Clin. Diagn. Lab. Immunol.* 10, 489–491, 2003.

Tarantola A et al., Lookback exercise with imported Crimean-Congo haemorrhagic fever, Senegal and France. *Emerg. Infect. Dis.* 12, 1424–1426, 2006.

Tsai TF, Chandler LJ, Arboviruses. In: Murray PR et al. (eds.), *Manual of Clinical Microbiology, 1553–1569*, 8th ed. ASM Press, Washington, 2003.

Williams RJ et al., Crimean-Congo haemorrhagic fever: a seroepidemiological and tick survey in the Sultanate of Oman. *Trop. Med. Int. Health*. 5, 99–106, 2000.

1.4.4 RIFT VALLEY FEVER

RVF is a virus infection transmitted to humans by mosquitoes in connection with enzootic and epizootic infections of sheep, goats, and cattle. The disease is named after the Rift Valley in East Africa.

Etiology. The RVF virus is an arbovirus in the family *Bunyaviridae*. Because of its genetic relationship it is classified in the genus *Phlebovirus*, although it is not transmitted by sand flies. There is little information about the pathogenicity of different isolates.

Occurrence. RVF virus activity is well documented in more than 30 countries. The virus is distributed by mosquitoes in Africa south of the Sahara after rainy periods. Based on virus isolation and serological tests, the virus exists in Kenya, Uganda, Namibia, Angola, and

Nigeria. More recently, epidemics have occurred in Madagascar and Egypt. The RVF virus amplifies in sheep, goats, cattle, buffaloes and camels. It is highly pathogenic for sheep and goats. Epizootic and enzootic infections of domestic animals are prerequisites for an epidemic distribution in humans. RVF was seen for the first time in Saudi Arabia and Yemen, where it caused epidemics in the fall of 2000. The mechanism of this distribution is not clear. Perhaps sheep transported from Africa have played a role. The RVF virus can be transmitted by more than 40 species of mosquitoes, and therefore, is one of the few arboviruses with a potential for worldwide distribution. There have been no imported infections with RVF virus in Europe or North America.

Possibly more than 18,000 people developed the disease during an epidemic in Aswân, Egypt, in 1977 following a severe epizootic with multiple losses of cattle and sheep. At least 600 people died with hemorrhagic fever. The disease reappeared in June of 1993 without causing an epizootic in the same area. The epidemic was remarkable because many people complained about a loss of vision after a noncharacteristic virus infection. Intensive searches for the virus in the area between 1981 and 1993 failed. It is assumed that the reintroduced virus caused the 1993 epidemic.

Transmission. Handling of diseased animals during slaughter or parturition is partly responsible for human infections. Sleeping outdoors without mosquito nets is an important risk factor. While the vector responsible for the transmission to humans is not known, more than 40 *Stegomyia* and *Culex* mosquito species are potential vectors for the RVF virus. They play a role in the transmission cycle in enzootics and epizootics, where sheep, goats, and cattle serve as amplification hosts and may also transmit RVF to the human population.

Transovarial RVF virus transmission has been documented in some vectors. Floodwater *Aedes (Stegomyia)* species play a role as reservoirs and as vectors. They lay infected eggs that are resistant to desiccation and survive long dry periods. Repeated heavy rain periods in arid regions initiate epizootics of RVF.

A pandemic distribution of the RVF virus might be possible because of its lack of vector specificity. A mechanical transmission was documented by flies, mosquitoes, Phlebotomes, and blood-sucking mites. This transmission may add to the distribution of the virus. A sylvan transmission cycle is assumed but is not proven.

Clinical Manifestations. The incubation period is 3 to 7 days. The acute disease begins with fever, rigors, severe malaise, myalgias, back pain, maculopapular rash, and gastrointestinal symptoms. There is a complete recovery after 2 to 7 days, sometimes after a biphasic fever.

A hemorrhagic manifestation with icterus and renal failure develops in 1% to 3% of cases, with a fatality rate of 50%. One to 4 weeks following the acute disease, severe encephalitis with fever may develop, along with headaches, coma, focal CNS deficits, and spasms. There may be a fatal outcome or a complete recovery without residual symptoms. The most frequent complication is a severe bilateral vascular syndrome of the retina, with bleeding into the macula, exudates, and infarcts. This retinal disease is seen in 1% of patients within 4 weeks after the acute disease. The severity of the lesion determines the remaining loss of function. The fatality rate is 0.1%. There are probably subclinical infections caused by less- pathogenic variants of the virus. In an endemic area 10% to 15% of the population are found seropositive after an episode of epidemic or epizootic disease.

A total of 140 cases of RVF in humans were diagnosed between August and October 2000 in Saudi Arabia and Yemen. Men were affected in 78% of the cases. The average age was 47 years, and the fatality rate was 19%. The calculation of the fatal outcome was probably high because less severe cases were not included. The source of infection could be confirmed in 64% of the cases: close contact with animals (sheep or goats) or contact with dead or aborted animals. All patients claimed mosquito bites. Infected mosquitoes were found (*Aedes caspius* and *Culex tritaeniorhynchus*). Complications were retinitis, hepatitis, renal failure, hemorrhages, and encephalitis.

Sheep and goats, especially pregnant animals, are highly susceptible to RVF. Abortions with the death of the dam are common. The RVF virus causes hepatitis and encephalitis in young livestock. The fatality rate of calves is 70%, while that of adult cattle is only 15%. Pregnant cattle abort.

Diagnosis. Suspicion of a case of RVF is raised by a history of illness in sheep and cattle in the same region and contact with sheep and cattle in the week preceding the onset of disease. Humans and domestic animals have a viremia during the acute phase of the disease, which can be detected by virus isolation, antigen capture assay, or PCR. IgM and IgG antibodies can be found during the recovery phase. Retinitis and encephalitis appear later when the viremia has ceased. These cases can only be diagnosed by an IgM capture assay. In cases of encephalitis, IgM antibodies to the RVF virus can be detected in the CSF. Cross-reactions with sandfly fever virus (Phlebovirus) may interfere in serologic reactions.

Differential Diagnosis. Uncomplicated febrile diseases have to be considered in the differential diagnosis, as well as hemorrhagic fever, encephalitis, and vascular retinopathy.

Abortions in sheep and cows, dead lambs and calves, and dead pregnant sheep and cows are important indications if human disease occurs in connection with an epizootic.

Therapy. Experimentally infected rhesus monkeys that have a low interferon production are prone to develop hemorrhagic symptoms. Monkeys with a late interferon response are more likely to develop severe disease. The NS protein has an interferon-antagonistic effect. The disease can be blocked with moderate doses of alpha interferon and viremia can be stopped with hyperimmune globulin. Experimental oral application of ribavirin has been beneficial in prophylaxis and therapy. Under experimental conditions, ribavirin blocks viral replication. If administered early, ribavirin (4 g/day initially, and then 16 mg/kg every 6 h i.v. or per infusion) can ameliorate the course of the disease. A systematic study to test the efficacy of ribavirin has not been performed. Clinical data of this approach are not yet available. A combination of ribavirin and interferon might be more efficient than a monotherapy with either alone.

Prophylaxis. Mosquito control and individual protection from mosquito bites are important means of prophylaxis. Caution should be taken when handling sick or dead animals. Slaughter, assisting parturition, and knackery work carry high risk. A formalin-inactivated vaccine is available for animals. It has been tested for safety and efficacy. An attenuated live virus vaccine has been developed too. Both vaccines have only been used to a limited extent in humans.

Prophylactic immunization of domestic animals is the best prophylactic measure to prevent epizootics and epidemics. The formalin-inactivated vaccine is used for cattle, while the attenuated live virus vaccine is used for sheep and goats.

REFERENCES

Al-Hazmi A et al., Ocular complications of Rift Valley fever outbreak inSaudi Arabia. *Ophthalmology* 112, 313–318, 2005.

Anyamba A et al., Prediction of a Rift Valley fever outbreak. *Proc. Natl. Acad. Sci. USA*, 106, 955–959, 2009.

Bouloy M et al., Genetic evidence for an interferon- antagonistic function of Rift Valley fever virus nonstructural protein NSs. *J. Virol.* 75, 1371–1377, 2001.

Bouloy M, Flick R, Reverse genetics technology for Rift Valley fever virus: current and future applications for the development of therapeutics and vaccines. *Antivir. Res.* 84, 101–118, 2009.

Bouloy M, Weber F, Molecular biology of Rift Valley fever virus. *Open Virol. J.* 4, 8–14, 2010.

CDC, Outbreak of Rift Valley fever – Yemen, August–October 2000. *MMWR Morb. Mortal Wkly. Rep.* 49, 1065–1066, 2000.

CDC, Outbreak of Rift Valley fever – Saudi Arabia, August–October, 2000. *JAMA.* 284, 2310–2311, 2000.

Chen JP, Cosgriff TM, Hemorrhagic fever virusinduced changes in hemostasis and vascular biology. *Blood Coagul. Fibrinolysis.* 11, 461–483, 2000.

Fisher-Hoch SP et al., Crimean-Congo-haemorrhagic fever treated with oral ribavirin. *Lancet* 346, 472–475, 1995.

Garcia S et al., Quantitative real-time PCR detection of Rift Valley fever virus and its application to evaluation of antiviral compounds. *J. Clin. Microbiol.* 39, 4456–4461, 2001.

Gerdes GH, Rift Valley fever. *Rev. Sci. Tech.* 23, 613–623, 2004.

Jost CC et al., Epidemiological assessment of the Rift Valley fever outbreak in Kenya and Tanzania in 2006 and 2007. *Am. J. Trop. Med. Hyg.* 83 (suupl. 2), 65–72, 2010.

Kahlon SS et al., Severe Rift Valley fever may present with a characteristic clinical syndrome. *Am. J. Trop. Med. Hyg.* 82, 371–375, 2010.

LaBeud AD, Kazura JW, King CH, Advances in Rift Valley fever research: insights for disease prevention. *Curr. Opin. Infect. Dis.* 23, 403–408, 2010.

Rweyemamu M et al., Emerging diseases of Africa and the Middle *East. Ann. N. Y. Acad. Sci.* 916, 61–70, 2000.

Sall AA et al., Singletube and nested reverse transcriptase-polymerase chain reaction for detection of Rift Valley fever virus in human and animal sera. *J. Virol. Methods* 91, 85–92, 2001.

1.4.5 SANDFLY FEVER

Sandfly fever (SFF), or phlebotomus or pappataci fever, is a mild arbovirus infection that occurs in Mediterranean countries, the Near East, Central Asia, and South America. It is transmitted by the bite of sand flies. The SFF-serotype Toscana may cause neurological disease (meningitis and encephalitis).

Etiology. The causative agent belongs to the family *Bunyaviridae*, genus *Phlebovirus*. Only eight of the 36 phleboviruses are transmitted by sand flies (*Phlebotomus* spp.). In Mediterranean countries, SFF is caused by serotypes Sicilia (SFS), Naples (SFN), Toscana (SFT), and Corfu. In addition, serotypes Alenquer, Arboledas, Bujaru, Cacao, Candiru, Chagres, Corfu, and Punta Toro cause sandfly fever in the New World, especially in Colombia, Panama, and Brazil.

RVF also belongs to the genus *Phlebovirus* because of its close serological relation, although it is not transmitted by sand flies.

Occurrence. The disease was first observed in 1886 in soldiers in Herzegovina. The causative agent was isolated from American soldiers in Italy after World War II. During World War II, more than 10,000 soldiers in southeastern Europe developed SFF. More recently, SFF has been diagnosed in military operations, for example, in Cyprus and Afghanistan. Based on serology and virus isolation, SFF has a distribution from the Mediterranean region to Southeast Asia and South America. Tourists returning from areas of endemicity may develop SFF.

SFS and SFN have a wide distribution in the Mediterranean and are less virulent than SFT, which has only been found in Italy, Portugal (Algarve), Spain (Castile), Greece, Turkey, and Cyprus. SFT is believed to be one of the most important agents causing aseptic meningitis in Tuscany.

Sheep, cattle, squirrels, and forest mice may be infected with SFF virus without developing disease. The most important amplification hosts are the great gerbil (*Rhombomys opimus*), the long-clawed ground squirrel (*Spermaphilopsis leptodactylus*), and the long-eared hedgehog (*Hemiechinus auritus*).

Transmission. Vectors for SFS and SFN are the species *Phlebotomus papatasii*, order Diptera, family Psychodidae. Vectors for SFT are *Phlebotomus perfilieri* and *Phlebotomus perniciosus*. The same vectors transmit leishmanias.

Until recently, only the urban transmission cycle was known, with sand flies as vectors as well as reservoirs by transovarial transmission. The sylvan cycle has now been elucidated, with gerbils, long-clawed ground squirrels, and hedgehogs shown to be amplification hosts. SFF, therefore, is considered to be a zoonosis.

Clinical Manifestations. The incubation period for SFF is 3 to 5 days. The disease begins abruptly with symptoms similar to dengue fever: high fever, frontal headaches, retrobulbar pain, photophobia, myalgias, arthralgias, nausea, vomiting, facial flush, anorexia, and leukopenia. Children are predominantly affected in areas of endemicity. Unprotected tourists may be infected.

The disease is not fatal. Only SFT is neuropathogenic. Infections with this virus may produce CNS manifestations with serous meningitis or meningoencephalitis following the acute phase and a symptom-free interval. A subdued consciousness, stiffness of the neck, nystagmus, tremor, and paralysis may be seen. Infections with SFT may have a biphasic course. Hearing loss may result from the disease, comparable to that observed with Lassa fever. It is assumed that up to one-third of undiagnosed cases of serous meningitis in children in Italy are caused by SFT. The New World SFF is not known to cause neurologic symptoms, sequelae, or fatality.

Diagnosis. Sand fly bites are seen predominantly on the lower extremities with inflammatory reactions. In tourists with this history and clinical signs, the diagnosis of SFF should be considered. For a specific diagnosis, virus isolation from blood is only possible on the first day of sickness. Virus in heparin-plasma inoculated onto Vero cells produces a cytopathic effect in 2 to 3 days. SFT can be isolated from the CSF in cases of meningitis.

The virus can be detected in the early phase by PCR. Because most cases of SFF begin with an influenza-like disease, this technique has little importance in diagnosis.

Detection of virus-specific IgM with the IgM capture method is used as serodiagnosis. It begins to be positive around the fifth day after the onset of disease. ELISA, hemagglutination inhibition (HI), and virus neutralization tests are used to detect IgG. A test kit for Western blotting using recombinant antigen is commercially available for serodiagnosis.

Viral RNA was amplified in serum specimens taken 3 and 7 weeks after the onset of disease and in a CSF specimen taken from a second patient at onset of disease. Oligonucleotide primers addressing the genomic S segment of SFT were designed for RT-PCR and nested PCR by Schwarz et al. (see the end of this section).

Differential Diagnosis. Children living in areas of endemicity are predominantly affected with an influenza-like disease. Only SFT causes meningitis and meningoencephalitis. Severe cases are more common in tourists, soldiers, and other people traveling in areas of endemicity.

Therapy. Antiviral therapy is possible but seldom indicated. The efficacy of ribavirin has been proven in volunteers. If administered early, ribavirin (4 g/day initially, and then 16 mg/kg every 6 h i.v. or per infusion) can ameliorate

the course of the disease. A systematic study to test the efficacy has not been performed. Clinical data for this approach are not yet available.

Prophylaxis. A vaccine for SFF is not available. Repeated infections are possible because the different serotypes of phleboviruses do not induce cross-protection. The commercial immunoglobulin preparations do not contain antibodies to phleboviruses.

Sand flies are active between May and October. The mesh of regular mosquito nets is too wide and does not protect against sand flies. The use of curtains as well as mosquito repellents may be indicated. Sand flies travel for only 200 m. Breeding places, for example, in dumps, which are close to sand fly habitats should be sanitized.

REFERENCES

Batieha A et al., Seroprevalence of West Nile, Rift Valley, and sandfly arboviruses in Hashimiah, *Jordan. Emerg. Infect. Dis.* 6, 358–362, 2000.

Brett-Major DM, Claborn DM, Sandfly fever: what have we learned inone hundred years? *Mil. Med.* 174, 426–431, 2009.

Charrel R et al., Emergence of Toscana virus in Europe. *Emerg. Infect. Dis.* 11, 1657–1663, 2005.

Collao X et al., Genetic diversity of Toscana virus. *Emerg. Infect. Dis.* 15, 574–577, 2009.

Cohen D et al., Prevalence of antibodies to West Nile fever, sandfly fever Sicilian, and sandfly fever Naples viruses in healthy adults in Israel. *Public Health Rev.* 27, 217–230, 1999.

Dionisio D et al., Encephalitis without meningitis due to sandfly fever virus serotype Toscana. *Clin. Infect. Dis.* 32, 1241–1243, 2001.

Dionisio D et al., Epidemiological, clinical and laboratory aspects of sandfly fever. *Curr. Opin. Infect. Dis.* 16, 383–388, 2003.

Perez-Ruiz M et al., Reverse transcription, realtime PCR assay for detection of Toscana virus. *J. Clin. Virol.* 39, 276–281, 2007.

RKI, Sandfliegenfieber. *Epidemiol. Bull.* 32/96, 222–223, 1996.

Sabin AB, Recent advances in our knowledge of dengue and sandfly fever. *Am. J. Trop. Hyg.* 4, 198–207, 1955.

Soldateschi D et al., Laboratory diagnosis of Toscana virus infection by enzyme immunoassay with recombinant viral nucleoprotein. *J. Clin. Microbiol.* 37, 649–652, 1999.

Schwarz TF, Gilch S, Schatzl HA, A recombinant Toscana vius nucleoprotein in a giagnostic immunoblot test system. *Res. Virol.* 149, 413–416, 1998.

Valassini M et al., Detection of neurotropic viruses circulating in Tuscany: the incisive role of Toscana virus. *J. Med. Virol.* 60(1), 86–90, 2000.

Valassina M, Cusi MG, Valensin PE, A Mediterranean arbovirus: the Toscana virus. *J. Neurovirol.* 9, 577–583, 2003.

Weidmann M et al., Rapid detection of important human pathogenic phleboviruses. *J. Clin. Virol.* 41, 138–142, 2008.

1.4.6 ZOONOSES CAUSED BY HANTAVIRUSES

1.4.6.1 Hemorrhagic Fever with Renal Syndrome (Old World Hantaviruses) and Hantavirus Pulmonary Syndrome (New World Hantaviruses)

Hemorrhagic manifestations combined with fever and kidney failure were reported from Asia, Russia, and northern Europe as early as the 1930s and 1940s. An etiological connection with the Hantaan virus, the causative agent of Korean hemorrhagic fever (KHF), was established only in 1978. Common antigens were found in a variety of diseases: KHF in the Far East; a hemorrhagic fever with renal syndrome (HFRS), nephrosonephritis or Tula fever, in Russia and the People's Republic of China; and nephropathia epidemica (NE) in Scandinavia. Cases of nephritis in the field (*Feldnephritis* in German) observed in World Wars I and II may have been caused by this agent. Hantavirus pulmonary syndrome (HPS) became known in May 1993 as a new Hantavirus disease in the United States. The disease is also called Four Corners disease, Sin Nombre disease, or Muerto Canyon virus disease.

Etiology. The causative agents of HFRS and HPS were added to the bunyavirus family in 1987 as the genus *Hantavirus*. Small rodents serve as reservoirs for the different hantaviruses. They are the source of infection for humans. The genus *Hantavirus* is exceptional in the bunyavirus family, as no arthropod vectors are included in the transmission cycle.

The type and genus specificity of Hantaviruses corresponds exactly to the taxonomy of different hosts, which indicates a long-lasting common evolution. By sequence homology, the Old World Hantaviruses are more closely related among themselves than to the New World viruses, reflecting the genetic relatedness of the host animals. Puumala, Prospect Hill, and Tula viruses have hosts in the subfamily Arvicolinae and form a separate genetic group. *Calomys laucha*, the host of Laguna Negra virus, is also a host for Junin virus, an arenavirus.

Hantaviruses together with arenaviruses are also called roboviruses (rodent-borne viruses) for ecological reasons. The prototype is the Hantaan virus, with its host *Apodemus agrarius* (the striped field mouse), causing KHF. Seoul virus, with its hosts *Rattus rattus* and *Rattus norvegicus,* causes a milder and urban form of KHF that occurs worldwide in harbor cities. Puumala virus with its host *Clethrionomys glareolus* (the bank vole) occurs in northern Europe and causes NE and possibly field nephritis. Dobrava virus was isolated in Belgrade, Serbia. It is associated with *Apodemus flavicollis* (the yellow-necked field mouse) and with *A. agrarius* and is closely related to Hantaan virus. Sin Nombre virus was discovered in 1993 as the causative agent of HPS. It is transmitted to humans predominantly by *Peromyscus maniculatus* (the deer mouse) but also by *Sigmodon* species (cotton rats). There are additional variants of the Sin Nombre virus with different hosts causing the same diseases: Black Creek Canal virus in cotton rats (*Sigmodon hispidus*) and Bayou virus in rice rats (*Oryzomys palustris*). Subclinical human infections are induced by the American Prospect Hill virus, with its host *Microtus pennsylvanicus*. The virus is similar to Puumala virus. Thai virus, with its host *Bandicota indicus,* is closely related to Seoul virus.

Occurrence. A disease caused by Hantaviruses and characterized as a virus disease was first described in the 1930s in the Amur basin and in Manchuria. Numerous cases with a fatality rate of up to 30% in hospitalized patients occurred in United Nations troops during the Korean War. At the same time, similar syndromes were described in Japan and, as NE, in Scandinavia. Based on serological findings, it can be assumed that diseases caused by Hantaviruses also occur in countries of the Balkan Peninsula and in Scotland, France, Greece, and Germany. A Hantaan-like virus, Dobrava virus, was isolated in Bosnia. It causes a severe disease similar to Hantaan virus. Its host is *Apodemus flavicollis*. Based on serology, there are indications that Dobrava virus also occurs in Central Europe.

Importation of the Seoul virus into harbor cities, possibly by ship rats, has been described. Strains of laboratory rats have carried Seoul virus and have transmitted it into animal houses, where animal caretakers and scientific staff were infected. Hantavirus was spread in an animal house, when a wild caught vole (*C. glareolus*) was kept there in addition to experimental animals.

The close association between different Hantavirus species with the corresponding host determines the virus species and its distribution. Human infections especially occur after a massive reproduction of host animals, when humans or food comes into contact with mouse excrement. A seasonal increase in human disease is characteristic for NE and KHF in early summer (maximum in June) and fall (maximum in November). An increased incidence in Siberia occurs in winter, when mice may invade houses in search of a warm place. In summer, predominantly men with outdoor activities are involved (farmers, forest workers, fishermen, sportsmen, and soldiers). The exposure in most cases occurs in damp meadows and in swamps. There are about 100,000 cases annually of Hantavirus disease (Seoul and Hantaan viruses) in the People's Republic of China. Up to 10% of the population in areas of hyperendemicity in Sweden may become infected with the Puumala virus.

Only one Puumala-like virus has been isolated in Germany. More than 400 recent infections with Puumala virus have been diagnosed serologically and, in some cases, with PCR. The antibody prevalence to the Puumala virus in western Germany is around 1.85%, and in eastern Germany it is 1.2%. Based on serology, it is assumed that not only the Puumala virus, but also a Hantaan-like virus, possibly Dobrava virus, exists in eastern Germany.

In Germany, HPS has recently been diagnosed in two women in Detmold in a wool-spinning factory. The agent appears to be related to the Puumala virus and not to the American virus isolates. Women are more frequently affected with HPS than men.

El Niño in the western United States and in South America caused a massive reproduction of rodents, which was probably the cause of transmission to humans of the Sin Nombre virus. Especially lightly built houses and cottages are infested by *P. maniculatus*, the host of the Sin Nombre virus.

Scientists and animal caretakers have been infected in experimental stations in Japan, South Korea, Russia, and Belgium by latently infected laboratory rats. Hantaviruses have also been found in birds and bats in South Korea. The significance of this observation for human disease is not clear.

Transmission. The source of human infection with Hantaviruses is water contaminated with mouse excrements or by aerosol. Typical infection risks are working or staying for long periods in rooms that are infested with rodents and their excrement, farm work, mining, boot camps in rodent-infested areas, and deposition of food or cigarettes in humid grass, for example, during fishing or playing golf. Recruits in their basic military training and soldiers during military operations are also at risk for HFRS.

Nosocomial and other human-to-human transmissions are rare. Human-to-human transmission was reported for the first time in southern Argentina during an outbreak of Andes virus. A chain of transmission with four links was observed.

Trapped field mice or rats, in most cases Wistar rats, were the source of infection in numerous laboratories in Japan, South Korea, the former USSR, and Belgium.

The old suspicion that mites might be involved in the epidemic of Hantaviruses seems to be confirmed now. In China, mites of the species *Leptobromidium scutellare* were found which were infected with the agent of Tsutsugamushi fever, *Orienta Tsutsugamishi*, and at the same time were carrying the Hantaan virus. Japanese researchers had obtained evidence for this already in the 1930s.

Clinical Manifestations. The incubation period of KHF is 5 to 35 days. The disease begins with a sudden fever, which lasts for 3 to 6 days. Patients complain about severe malaise, loss of appetite, nausea, and vomiting. There is a pronounced conjunctival inflammation and erythema (flush) on face, neck, and thorax. Thrombocytopenia (>50,000 thrombocytes/mm3), shift-to-the-left leukocytosis and lymphocytosis with immunoblasts (<30,000 immunoblasts/mm3), elevated levels of C-reactive protein, and elevated serum enzyme levels are typical laboratory results. The hemorrhagic diathesis appears as petechiae in axillary folds and on the face, neck, and soft palate. Later, the conjunctivitis becomes hemorrhagic. A sudden drop in blood pressure in this phase may lead into shock. One-third of all fatal cases end as a consequence of irreversible shock. Petechiae increase. Mild hematuria and proteinuria are present. Patients complain about lumbago. Between 3 and 7 days after the disease onset, patients develop oliguria and uremia, increase of blood pressure as well as hemorrhagic diathesis. This is followed by epistaxis and intracerebral, gastrointestinal, and urogenital bleeding. Renal functions become insufficient and have to be compensated on occasion by dialysis. A relative sinus bradycardia (50%) and a rapidly developing myopia (25% of cases) are suggestive of Hantavirus infection.

Signs of CNS involvement (rarely, encephalitis or Guillain-Barré syndrome) may occur in severe cases, and pulmonary edema may develop. Lethal cases usually end in oliguria or with lung edema. Failure of the tubules to concentrate leads to an increased diuresis after the oliguric phase. A disturbed electrolyte balance and secondary infections are typical complications during this phase. Recovery may take months but is complete in most instances. The fatality rate of KHF is around 5%, but it can increase to 30% under unfavorable conditions.

NE is a milder form of KHF without hemorrhagic manifestations. It is similar to the urban type of KHF in Southeast Asia after contact with infected rats. NE may mimic an acute abdomen, which in one case led to laparotomy and even to re-laparotomy. A shift-to-the-left leukocytosis may, in combination with high fever, be suggestive of septic disease. The fatality rate of the acute disease is about 0.1%. There are some reports of chronic renal disease with hypertension in patients with a history of Hantavirus disease.

The incubation period of HPS is 9 to 33 days (median, 14 to 17 days). Inhalation of contaminated aerosols in houses infested with deer mice is the most likely route of infection. Often, first signs are high fever with rigors, severe malaise, myalgias, nausea, vomiting, diarrhea, and headaches. Additional signs are respiratory distress, daze, arthralgias, sweating, back pain, retrosternal pain, and occasionally, rhinitis and pharyngitis. The tentative diagnosis is frequently pneumonia of other causes or ARDS, and sometimes the diagnosis is sepsis or pyelonephritis. Laboratory tests reveal hypoxia, leukocytosis with more than 30,000 cells, shift to the left with myelocytes, and a typical lymphocytosis with immunoblasts. Hemoconcentration with a hematocrit of >50%, thrombocytopenia, prolonged prothrombin time, elevated serum enzyme activities (lactate dehydrogenase and serum glutamic pyruvate transaminase) are characteristic findings. Generalized edema results from increased capillary leakage. A protein-rich pulmonary edema develops rapidly, with an 80% plasma protein concentration. Of 92 patients that have been observed, 62% have died. HPS was reported in five women in their 13th to 29th week of pregnancy. One woman and two fetuses died. Three children were born healthy without any indication of prenatal infection. The three placentas of the living children and organs from both dead fetuses did not show any signs of a virus infection. There was no evidence of vertical virus transmission.

Persistent infection and virus excretion without clinical symptoms were found in the mouse species that serve as reservoirs of Hantaviruses. The same is true for experimental infections. Wistar rats experimentally infected with Hantavirus do not show any clinical symptoms.

Diagnosis. A tentative diagnosis of KHF and NE should be made in patients with fever, increasing renal insufficiency, edema, and hemorrhagic diathesis. The epidemiological situation and possible exposure to rodents should be taken into consideration. HPS should be suspected in patients with high fever, rapidly increasing lung densities, and respiratory insufficiency. Shift-to-the-left leukocytosis of up to 38,000 leukocytes/mm3 may suggest septic disease or even leukemia, but in combination with thrombocytopenia (>40,000 thrombocytes/mm3) and finding of immunoblasts, Hantavirus infection should be suspected.

Neutralizing antibodies are present in serum at the onset of acute disease, which is in contrast to hemorrhagic fevers caused by arena-, flavi-, or filoviruses, where increasing neutralizing antibody titers are only found during the recovery phase. The chance of Hantavirus isolations, therefore, is small. Hantaviruses can be detected by RT-PCR, where the full reading frame for the nucleocapsid (S gene) is transcribed. A nested RT-PCR technique targeting conserved regions of the M gene (which codes for the G1 and G2 proteins) of three species of Hantaviruses allows virus detection in postmortem specimens and in environmental investigations.

PCR is not important for diagnosis in acute cases of NE and KHF. However, it is useful for postmortem examinations and examination of kidney specimens. In cases of HPS, viremia could be quantified in plasma specimens by means of RT-PCR between days 5 to 20 after onset of pulmonary edema. The method of choice in acute cases of KHF and NE is an IgM capture ELISA to demonstrate virus-specific IgM antibodies. A recombinant nucleocapsid antigen is available for the Old World Hantaviruses and can be used with Western blots.

Differential Diagnosis. Meningococcal sepsis, leptospirosis, and recurrent borreliosis should be considered in patients with high fever, hemorrhagic diathesis, shock, and renal failure. The high leukocyte count with a shift to the left may be misleading because it is common to both Hantavirus and bacterial infections. Cases of NE or KHF can be confused with acute abdominal pain. One example was a suspected case of appendicitis in a patient with severe abdominal pain, fever, and left-shifted

leukocytosis. A laparotomy was performed followed by a re-laparotomy because of persistent bleeding. Finally, the diagnosis of NE was made with positive serology. In another case, a Hantavirus infection was mistakenly diagnosed in a patient with a perforated gall bladder and with signs of renal insufficiency. A false-positive result of anti-Hantavirus IgM caused the misdiagnosis.

Depending on the epidemiological situation, other viral hemorrhagic fevers should be included in the differential diagnosis: yellow fever, CCHF, Marburg fever, Ebola fever, Lassa fever, and other arenavirus caused hemorrhagic fevers. Recently emerged zoonotic coronaviruses, SARS-CoV and MERS-CoV would also have to be considered.

For the differential diagnosis of HPS, all febrile diseases should be included that involve pneumonia, pulmonary edema, and ARDS. The high leukocyte count may confuse Hantavirus diseases with bacterial infections.

Therapy. The course of the disease can be improved by early administration of ribavirin (4 g/day initially, and then 16 mg/kg every 6 h i.v. or per infusion). A systematic study to test the efficacy of this approach has not yet been performed. The application of virus-specific hyper immunoglobulin is of no use, because antiviral antibodies are present at the onset of symptoms.

Symptomatic treatment should concentrate on support of circulation and kidney functions. Caution is recommended at the transition from hypotension to oliguria, because shock therapy at that stage may lead to fatal pulmonary edema. Dialysis should be initiated early in severe cases. During the polyuric phase, the electrolyte balance and prophylactic treatment for secondary infections are most important.

An extracorporeal CO_2 elimination system might be helpful for HPS, but only if the plasma volume can be controlled, because of the extreme capillary leakage.

The transport of patients with hemorrhagic fever to a hospital with isolation quarters is not recommended, because patients are usually in a critical stage at the time of the diagnosis.

Any mechanical stress during the transport would increase the capillary leakage. It is recommended to treat these patients locally, attended by experienced personnel. The safety of other patients and health care workers depends on the safe practice of barrier nursing techniques.

Prophylaxis. Personal hygiene in infected areas is important. If possible, patients and suspected patients should be kept in negative-pressure units to avoid nosocomial spread of Hantaviruses. Protective suits (positive pressure) with filtered air to be worn by the nursing staff are highly recommended, as negative-pressure tents are not comfortable for patients. Safe handling of virus-infected clinical specimens in a normal clinical laboratory may present a special challenge. Wherever feasible, the specimens should be inactivated by fixation or by thermal (56 °C, 30 min) or chemical treatment before introducing them to the laboratory. Addition of detergent to a serum specimen reduces the virus titer. Running infected specimens in a centrifuge is the most dangerous of all manipulations. Sticks with infected needles and cuts with infected knives should be avoided.

Special precautions are needed in laboratories working experimentally with laboratory animals that may be latently infected. They may shed virus that causes human infections via aerosol.

Control of mouse populations could be beneficial as prophylaxis. Human infections are closely linked to changes in rodent populations. There is no vaccine available for active immunization.

REFERENCES

Bausch DG, Ksiazekn TG, Viral hemorrhagic fevers including hantavirus pulmonary syndrome in the *Americas. Clin. Lab. Med.* 22, 981–1020, 2002.

Chu YK et al., Serological relationships among viruses in the Hantavirus genus, family Bunyaviridae. *Virology.* 198, 196–204. 1994.

Colby TV et al., Hantavirus pulmonary syndrome is distinguishable from acute interstitial pneumonia. *Arch. Pathol. Lab. Med.* 124, 1463–1466, 2000.

Drebot MA, Artsob H, Werker D, Hantavirus pulmonary syndrome in Canada, 1989–1999. *Can. Commun. Dis. Rep.* 26, 65–69, 2000.

Glass GE et al., Using remotely sensed data to identify areas at risk for hantavirus pulmonary syndrome. *Emerg. Infect. Dis.* 6, 238–247, 2000.

Heyman P et al., Hantavirus infections in Europe: from virus carriers to a major public- health problem. *Expert Rev. Anti Ther.* 7, 205–217, 2009.

Jones A, Setting a trap for hantavirus. *Nursing.* 30, 20, 2000.

Jonsson CB, Hopper J, Mertz G, Treatment of hantavirus pulmonary syndrome. *Antivir. Res.* 78, 162–169, 2007.

Jonsson CB, Figueiredo LT, Vapalathi O, A global perspective on hantavirus ecology, epidemiology, and disease. *Clin. Microbiol. Rev.* 23, 412–441, 2010.

Klempa B, Hantaviruses and climate change. *Clin. Microbiol. Infect.* 15, 518–523, 2009.

Klempa B et al., Serological evidence of human hantavirus infections in Guinea, West Africa. *J. Infect. Dis.* 201, 1031–1034, 2010.

Maes P et al., Hantaviruses: immunology, treatment, and prevention. *Viral Immunol.* 17, 481–497, 2004.

Makary P et al., Disease burden of Puumala virus infections, 1995–2008. *Epidemiol. Infect.* 138, 1484–1492, 2010.

Markotic A, Human-to-human transmission of hantaviruses. *Lancet* 350, 596, 1997.

McCaughey C, Hart CA, Hantaviruses. *J. Med. Microbiol.* 49, 587–599, 2000.

Nelson R et al., Confirmation of Choclo virus as the cause of hantavirus cardiopulmonary syndrome and high serum antibody prevalence in Panama. *J. med. Virol.* 82, 1586–1593, 2010.

Olsson GE, Leirs H, Henttonen H, Hantaviruses and their hosts in Europe: reservoirs here and there, but not everywhere? *Vector Borne Zoo. Dis.* 10, 549–561, 2010.

Park K, Kim CS, Moon KT, Protective effectiveness of hantavirus vaccine. *Emerg. Infect. Dis.* 10, 2218–2220, 2004.

Plyusina A et al., Co-circulation of three pathogenic hantaviruses: *J. med. Virol.* 81, 2045–2052, 2009.

Ramos MM, Hjelle B, Overturf GD, Sin nombre hantavirus disease in a ten-yearold boy and his mother. *Pediatr. Infect. Dis. J.* 19, 248–250, 2000.

Rhodes LV et al., Hantavirus pulmonary syndrome associated with monongahela virus, *Pennsylvania. Emerg. Infect. Dis.* 6, 616–621, 2000.

Schilling S et al., Hantavirus disease outbreak in Germany: limitations of routine serological diagnostics and clustering of virus sequences of human and rodent origin. *J. Clin. Microbiol.* 45, 3008–3014, 2007.

Schmaljohn CS, Hjelle B, Hantaviruses: a global disease problem. *Emerg. Infect. Dis.* 3, 95–104, 1997.

Schmaljohn CS, Lee HW, Dalrymple JM, Detection of hantaviruses with RNA probes generated from recombinant DNA. *Arch. Virol.* 95, 291–301. 1987.

Schmaljohn CS, Dalrymple JM, Analysis of Hantan virus RNA: evidence for a new genus of bunyaviridae. *Virology* 131, 482–491, 1983.

Schmaljohn CS, Vaccines for hantaviruses. *Vacc* 27 (suppl. 4), D61–64, 2009.

Schwarz AC et al., Risk factors for human infection with Puumala virus, southwestern Germany. *Emerg. Infect. Dis.* 15, 1032–1039, 2009.

Sibold C et al., Dobrava hantavirus causes hemorrhagic fever with renal syndrome in central Europe and is carried by two different Apodemus mice species. *J. Med. Virol.* 63, 158–167, 2001.

Simpson SQ et al., Hantavirus pulmonary syndrome. *Infect. Dis. Clin. North Am.* 24, 159–173, 2010.

Stuhlfauth K, Bericht über ein neues schlammfieberähnliches Krankheitsbild bei deutschen Truppen in Lappland. *Dtsch. Med. Wschr.* 69, 439–442, 1943.

Verity R et al., Hantavirus pulmonary syndrome in Northern Alberta, Canada: clinical and laboratory findings for 19 cases. *Clin. Infect. Dis.* 31, 942–946, 2000.

Vincent MJ et al., Hantavirus pulmonary syndrome in Panama: Identification of novel hantaviruses and their likely reservoirs. *Virology* 277, 14–19, 2000.

Wells RM et al., An unusual hantavirus outbreak in southern Argentina: person-toperson transmission? *Emerg. Inf. Dis.*, 3, 171–174, 1997.

Wichmann D et al., Hemorrhagic fever with renal syndrome: diagnostic problems with a known disease. *J. Clin. Microbiol.* 39, 3414–3416, 2001.

WHO, Hantavirus in the Americas: Guidelines for diagnosis, treatment, prevention and control. 1999.

Zhang Y et al., Hantavirus outbreak associated with laboratory rats in Yunnan, China. *Infect. Genet. Evol.* 10, 638–644, 2010.

1.5 Zoonoses Caused by Reoviruses (*Coltiviridae* and *Orbiviridae*)

Viruses in the family *Reoviridae* (reo=respiratory enteric orphan) are also called diplornaviruses, because they have double-stranded RNA genomes. The genomes are segmented, and most reoviruses have 10 segments. The virus particle has no lipid and no envelope. The capsid consists of an inner and an outer layer. The genetic program specifies four proteins that are associated with the outer capsid and four proteins associated with the inner capsid. There are two or three additional NS proteins.

There are numerous reoviruses pathogenic for animals, transmitted by arthropods or by the fecal-oral route. However, only a few are important as zoonotic diseases. They belong to the genera *Orbivirus* and *Coltivirus* and are transmitted by *Ixodes* ticks, in contrast to most orbiviruses, which are transmitted by mosquitoes. The genome of orbiviruses has 10 segments, while coltiviruses have 12 segments. These observations as well as additional structural differences have recently caused the two genera to be separated. The segmented genome allows frequent genetic recombinations.

The S2 segment of the genome is usually the target for a diagnostic RT-PCR because it is the smallest segment. Antigen detection for demonstration of viruses in this group has a high sensitivity.

Representatives of the genus Rotavirus are widely distributed in the animal kingdom and they mostly cause gastroenteritis with mild to severe and life-threatening diarrhea in young animals, in sucklings, and small children. According to serologic criteria, six groups are differentiated. Epidemiology and epizootiology are characterized by co-circulation of different virus strains giving rise to new strains due to genetic reassortment. The genome consists of 11 segments. Molecular techniques have revealed that genetic reassortment often occurs between rotaviruses of domestic animals and the human strains. Therefore, animal rotaviruses represent a genetic reservoir for the recruitment of new rotaviruses, which may spread in the human population.

1.5.1 GENUS *COLTIVIRUS*

The genus *Coltivirus* contains two zoonotic viruses, Colorado tick fever virus and Eyach virus.

1.5.1.1 Colorado Tick Fever

Colorado tick fever or Colorado fever is a nonfatal virus infection in the Rocky Mountains transmitted by ticks. The dominant symptoms are headaches, back pain, biphasic fever, and leukopenia.

Etiology. Colorado tick fever virus is the prototype of the genus *Coltivirus*. Coltiviruses have a double stranded RNA genome with 12 segments. Colorado tick fever virus is an arbovirus transmitted by ticks (*Dermacentor andersoni*). Eyach virus, another coltivirus, has been isolated in Central Europe.

Occurrence. Colorado tick fever virus exists in the Rocky Mountains, including the western provinces of Canada. Most human cases of disease are seen in Colorado. There is a seasonal occurrence in spring and summer. Numerous mammals can be infected, which has been documented by virus isolation and antibody tests. The most important reservoirs are ground squirrels, western chipmunks, wood rats, and *Peromyscus* species (deer mice). *Peromyscus maniculatus* is also the reservoir for Sin Nombre virus, the causative agent of the Hantavirus pulmonary syndrome.

The Colorado tick fever virus persists in a cycle between mammals and ticks. A transstadial viral persistence in *D. andersoni* has been detected, but there is no evidence for transovarial transmission.

Transmission. The most important vector is *D. andersoni*, a hard-shelled tick that can be found at elevations between 1,500 and 3,000 m, the same as the distribution of Colorado tick fever virus infections in humans and mammals. Human-to-human transmissions have occurred by blood transfusion several months after acute disease.

Clinical Manifestations. The disease incidence is four human cases per 100,000, with 50% of infected people developing clinical disease. After an incubation period of 3 to 7 days, the disease begins abruptly with fever up to 38 to 40 °C, headaches, retro-orbital pain, myalgias (especially in the back and legs), photophobia, and nausea. The objective signs of disease are nonspecific conjunctivitis, reddened mucous membranes of the throat, and slightly enlarged spleen and lymph nodes. Some of the patients have a spotty or maculopapular rash on the body and limbs. Half of the patients have a biphasic fever with a 2-day interval when patients feel well again. The second febrile phase comes with renewed malaise and more severe pain. A rare form of the disease, seen only in children, includes the CNS, with meningitis and encephalitis. Hemorrhagic manifestations have also been viremia is characteristic. The virus can be detected for up to 120 days within erythrocytes. Clinical pathology reveals leukopenia with a relative lymphocytosis. The virus has an affinity for the cells in the hemopoietic system, especially affecting granulocyte, thrombocyte, and erythrocyte development. Cells in the bone marrow undergo myelosuppression.

Diagnosis. Colorado tick fever should be suspected when patients in an area of endemicity, or after a stay in such a place, become sick 3 to 7 days after a tick bite. The diagnosis can be confirmed by virus isolation from heparinized blood inoculated intracerebrally into suckling mice. As the viremia lasts for up to 120 days, the virus can be detected in blood throughout the disease. A rapid diagnosis is possible by the demonstration of virus in erythrocytes by fluorescent antibody. A seminested RT-PCR for viral detection can be used for diagnosis before antibodies appear. It is also important to detect persistent infection in erythrocytes. Primers for a 528-bp fragment of the DNA of the S2 segment have been published by Johnson et al. They are also useful for the detection of other coltiviruses. RNA extraction is achieved with the QIAmp viral RNA kit. PCR is recommended also for detection of virus in blood donors. Relevant literature is cited at the end of this section.

Virus-specific IgM antibodies can be detected by ELISA. They disappear 6 weeks after the onset of disease.

Differential Diagnosis. Rocky Mountain spotted fever is the primary differential diagnosis. It is also transmitted by *D. andersoni* and it occurs in the same locale, in addition to other areas in the United States. Colorado tick fever is the more common disease in Colorado. A biphasic fever is typical for Colorado tick fever. A spotty exanthema is typical for Rocky Mountain spotted fever.

Therapy. The therapy for Colorado tick fever is symptomatic. The prognosis is almost always favorable.

Prophylaxis. Inactivated and attenuated virus vaccines have been developed and tested but have not been licensed and were not widely used because of the mildness of the disease. The most important prophylaxis is solid clothing and use of repellents at an altitude between 1,500 and 3,000 m in the Rocky Mountains.

Infected people should not donate blood for at least 6 months because of the persistent viremia.

1.5.2 GENUS *ORBIVIRUS* (KEMEROVO COMPLEX)

The genus *Orbivirus* contains two zoonotic viruses, Kemerovo virus and Lipovnik virus. Kemerovo virus (about 23 serotypes) exists in countries of the former USSR. Like Russian spring-summer encephalitis virus (a flavivirus), it is transmitted by *Ixodes persulcatus*. More recently, these viruses have been found in North America. Lipovnik virus is transmitted by *Ixodes ricinus,* mostly in Austria, the Czech Republic, and Slovakia.

The pathogenicity of these viruses for humans is minimal. Dual infections are not uncommon with tick-transmitted encephalitis viruses and orbiviruses. These dual infections may influence the course of TBE. Coinfections with *Borrelia* and *Ehrlichia* spp. are also possible.

REFERENCES

Attoui, H, P. De Micco, and X. de Lamballerie. 1997. Complete nucleotide sequence of Colorado tick fever virus segments M6, S1 and S2. *J. Gen. Virol.* 78:2895–2899.

Attoui, H, F. Billoir, P. Biagini, P. de Micco, and X. de Lamballerie. 2000. Complete sequence determination and genetic analysis of Banna virus and Kadipiro virus: proposal for assignment to a new genus (Seadornavirus) within the family Reoviridae. *J. Gen. Virol.* 81:1507–1515.

Attoui, H, F. Billoir, P. Biagini, JF Cantaloube, R. de Chesse, P. de Micco, and X. de Lamballerie. 2000. Sequence determination and analysis of the full- length genome of Colorado tick fever virus, the type species of genus Coltivirus (family Reoviridae). *Biochem. Biophys. Res. Commun.* 273:1121–1125.

Emmons, RW. 1988. Ecology of Colorado tick fever. *Annu. Rev. Microbiol.* 42:49–64.

Friedman, AD. 1996. Hematologic manifestations of viral infections. *Pediatr. Ann.* 25:555–560.

Hughes LE et al., Persistence of Colorado tick fever virus in red blood cells. *Am. J. Trop. Med. Hyg.* 23, 530–532, 1974.

Knudson DI, Monath TP, Orbiviruses. In: Fields BN et al. (eds.), *Virology.* 2nd edition. Raven Press, New York, 1405–1436, 1990.

Johnson, AJ, N. Karabatsos, and RS Lanciotti. 1997. Detection of Colorado tick fever virus by using reverse transcriptase PCR and application of the tech- nique in laboratory diagnosis. *J. Clin. Microbiol.* 35:1203–1208.

Libikova, H, F. Heinz, D. Ujhazyova, and D. Stunzner. 1978. Orbiviruses of the Kemerovo complex and neurological diseases. *Med. Microbiol. Immunol. (Berlin)* 166:255–263.

Miller, DS, DF Covell, RG McLean, WJ Adrian, M. Niezgoda, JM Gustafson, OJ Rongstad, RD Schultz, LJ Kirk, and TJ Quan. 2000. Serologic survey for selected infectious disease agents in swift and kit foxes from the western United States. *J. Wildl. Dis.* 36:798–805.

Miller DS et al., Serologic survey for selected infectious disease agents in swift and kit foxes from the western United States. *J. Wildl. Dis.* 36, 798–805, 2000.

Nuttall, PA, SC Jacobs, LD Jones, D. Carey, and SR Moss. 1992. Enhanced neurovirulence of tick- borne orbiviruses resulting from genetic modulation. *Virology* 187:407–412.

1.5.3 GENUS ROTAVIRUS

Rotaviruses occur in many avian and mammalian species. They cause mild to severe forms of gastroenteritis with heavy diarrhea resulting in death due to dehydration. As a rule, epidemic and epizootic spread and disease is only caused by the species specific rotavirus strains. Zoonotic rotaviruses are transmitted to children from domestic animals but they cause clinically inapparent infections or mild disease. The problem is that double infections with human and animal strains may create new virus variants by genetic reassortment.

Etiology. Having a bilayerd capsid and a double stranded RNA genome consisting of 11 segments, rotaviruses are diplornaviruses and are members of the family Reoviridae. According to serologic properties, they are separated into groups A to G out of which groups A, B, and C are causes of diarrhea in humans and in animals. Members of group A with under groups A1 and A2 are found all over the world. They cause diarrhea in young animals as well as in sucklings and small children. Group B is mainly encountered in China and causes diarrhea in adults. The pathogenic potential of group C is unclear. Members of groups D, E, and F are causes of diarrhea in mammals and in birds. Formation of reassortants is only observed between members of the same serologic group.

Two proteins of the outer capsid, glycoprotein VP 7 (G-types) and the protease sensitive protein VP 4 (P-types) are receptor binding proteins and induce formation of neutralizing antibodies. Nineteen G-types and 30 P-types are known and each virus contains in its outer capsid a G- and a P-protein in free combination resulting in 570 different virus species. In analogy to influenza A viruses a binary nomenclature was introduced for group A rotaviruses, in which numbers G1 to G19 are combined with numbers P1 to P30. As there is incomplete correspondence of genotypes and serotypes in group P proteins, an additional number for the genotype is added. The complete formula for an equine rotavirus would be: G12P12 [18].

As genome segments of two rotaviruses that infect the same cell may be freely reassorted, new serotypes can result, which may be able to cross species barriers. In addition, the individual genome segments underlie antigenic drift as a consequence of point mutations and in this way, new strains are created with new properties. Genetic reassortment has been shown to occur under natural conditions; however, the impact on epidemiology and epizootiology is not clear. It is believed that in Europe, 1.37% of all rotavirus infections may originate from zoonotic infections.

Occurrence. For human health, the rotaviruses of groups A1 and A2 are the most important. All over the world, these viruses account for 50% of all cases of diarrhea, which are admitted to hospitals making them the most frequent single cause of diarrhea on a worldwide scale. The highest incidence is in children after the weaning period; 80% to 100% of 3-year-old children have antibodies. In spite of a high seroprevalence, the susceptibility for rotavirus infections exists for life. Epidemics occur often in retirement homes. In third world countries, rotaviruses are among the most frequent causes of infant mortality. In the USA, nonbacterial forms of infectious gastroenteritis are looked at as the second most frequent human infection ranging directly after common colds. In livestock-breeding rotavirus, infections are causing great economic losses.

In the temperate climatic zones, rotavirus epidemics occur most often during winter, and they are restricted to people living in a certain geographic region. The same is true for epizootics, which are restricted to a certain region and a certain animal species. However, genome segments of "human" group A viruses are encountered in many mammalian species, even in bats, therefore, it must be assumed that a large gene-pool exists between human and animal strains. Calves, piglets, and rabbits among others are looked at as the sources and potential reservoirs of human rotavirus infections.

Transmission. Rotavirus infections are transmitted via the fecal-oral route from water, towels, food, and contaminated surfaces. In feces of infected humans $>10^{11}$ virus particles are found per ml. The infectious dose is ca. 100 plaque-forming units. Hospital infections are frequent especially in wards for neonates.

Clinical picture. The majority of infections is clinically inapparent or may cause mild clinical symptoms. The incubation time is 1 to 2 days. The fully developed picture of disease is characterized by nausea, vomiting, spasmodic epigastric pain, fever, and severe diarrhea, with frequent watery or bloody discharges. It will, in a short time, result in dehydration. Respiratory symptoms are also seen, although no virus replication is found in the respiratory epithelium. Epidemics with so-called nursery strains may have clinical inapparent courses. Virus persistence and hepatitis may occur in immunocompromised children. Disease is less frequent in breast fed children. Often parents develop the disease together with their children but have milder courses.

Virus replication occurs in the mature epithelial cells on top of the villi in the small intestine. In the cell, membrane integrins, N-acetyl neuraminic acid and the GM1-ganglioside were identified as viral receptors. The nonstructural viral protein NSP4 is very early secreted from the infected cells and is taken up by other epithelial cells in which it acts like an enterotoxin disturbing the membrane permeability, elevating the intracellular level of calcium and setting free chloride ions. Viral RNA and proteins are found in the serum of sick children.

The impact of this finding is not clear. Viremia is not found.

In piglets, calves, and foals, rotaviruses produce similar signs of disease like in humans. There are large economic losses in livestock breeding.

Diagnosis. Rotaviruses can easily be detected in stools by electronmicrosopic examination and they were originally discovered by this technique. They can be grown in cell cultures but this is not done in routine diagnosis. For routine diagnosis antigen capture, ELISAs are available. A type-specific diagnosis can be made with the RT-PCR. Normally diagnostic virology is only requested in outbreaks in neonate wards and in severe cases.

Differential diagnosis. Enteropathogenic bacteria, adenoviruses, caliciviruses, and astrovirus, as well as toxigenic coli and enteric parasites, are to be considered. In 30% to 50% of suspected cases, the diagnosis will not be successful.

Therapy. To replace losses of fluid and electrolytes is the most important measure. This can be achieved with "oral rehydration solutions" as recommended by the WHO. In severe cases, a spasmolytic therapy may be necessary. For neonates oral administration of specific immunoglobulins has been recommended.

Prophylaxis. Two live attenuated vaccines protecting against types G1P1 [8] (Rotarix$^{TM®}$) **Rotarix** Manufacturer: GlaxoSmithKline Biologicals, License #1617 or against types G1, G2, G3, G4 and G9 (Rota Teq$^®$) Merck & Co., Inc. Vaccine Customer Center 770 Sumneytown Pike WP97-A383 West Point, 19486-0004 are on the market destined for oral vaccination of newborn children at the age of 6 weeks. It is recommended to repeat the vaccination one to two times in 4-weeks intervals. The rate of protection is more than 90%. Side effects such as fever, diarrhea, vomiting and respiratory symptoms may occur. There is no licensed vaccine for protecting animals.

A strict regimen of hygiene with hand washing, disinfection of feces, vomit, cloth, and other objects is to be followed. Measures of isolation are inefficient due to asymptomatic virus excretion. In the case of outbreaks in hospitals, stables, or cowsheds, etc., closure of the wards and "cohort nursing" in small groups is inevitable. Rotaviruses are resistant against most hand wash solutions; 70% alcohol solutions are recommended for disinfecting surfaces.

REFERENCES

Angel J, Franco MA, Greenberg HB, Rotavirus vaccines: recent devepopemnts and future considerations. *Nat. Rev.* 2007, 5, 529–539.

Attoui et al., Complete sequence determination and genetic analysis of Banna virus and Kadipiro virus: proposal for assignment to a new genus (Seadornavirus) within the family Reoviridae. *J. Gen. Virol.* 81, 1507–1515, 2000.

Attoui H et al., Sequence determination and analysis of the fulllength genome of colorado tick fever virus, the type species of genus Coltivirus (Family Reoviridae). *Biochem. Biophys. Res. Commun.* 273, 1121–1125, 2000.

Awachat PS, Kelkar SD, Unexpected detection of simian SA11 in human reassortant strains of rotavirus G3P[8] genotype from diarrhea epidemic among tribal children in Western India. *J.Med. Virol.* 2005, 77: 128–135.

Blutt SE et al., Rotavirus antigenemia and viremia: a common event? *Lancet* 2003, 362: 1445–1449.

Emmons RW, Ecology of Colorado tick fever. *Ann. Rev Microbiol.* 42, 49–64, 1988.

Friedman AD, Hematologic manifestations of viral infections. *Pediatr. Ann.* 25, 555–560, 1996.

Hughes LE et al., Persistence of Colorado tick fever virus in red blood cells. *Am. J. Trop. Med. Hyg.* 23, 530–532, 1974.

Iturriza-Gómara M et al., Reassortment in vivo: driving force for diversity of human rotavirus strains isolated in the United Kingdom between 1995 and 1999. *J. Virol.* 2001, 75: 3696–3705.

Iturriza-Gómara M et al., Rotavirus surveillance in Europe, 2005–2008: web-enabled reporting and real-time analysis of genotyping and epidemiological data. *J Infect Dis.* 2009 Suppl 1: 215–21.

Johnson AJ, Karabatsos N, Lanciotti RS, Detection of Colorado tick fever virus by using reverse transcriptase PCR and application of the technique in laboratory diagnosis. *J. Clin. Microbiol.* 35, 1203–1208, 1997.

Knudson DI, Monath TP, Orbiviruses. In: **Fields BN et al.** (eds.), *Virology.* 2nd edition. Raven Press, New York, 1405–1436, 1990.

Libikova H et al., Orbiviruses of the Kemerovo complex and neurological diseases. *Med. Microbiol. Immunol. (Berl)* 166, 255–263, 1978.

Matthijinssens et al., Full analysis of human rotavirus strain B 4106 and lapine rotavirus strain 30/96 provides evidence for interspecies transmission. *J.Virol.* 2006, 80: 3801–3810.

Matthijinssens J et al., Full genome-based classification of rotaviruses reveals common origin between human

Wa-like and procine rotavirus strains and human DS-1- like and bovine rotavirus strains. *J. Virol.* 2008, 82: 3704–3719.

Matthijinsens J et al., Multiple reassortment and interspecies trasnmsission events contribute to the diversity fo feline, canine and felin/canine-like human group A rotavirus strains. *Infect.Genet. Evol.* 2011; 11(6): 1396–1406

Midgley SE et al., Suspected zoonotic transmission of rotavirus group A in Danish adults. *Epidemiol. Infect.* 2011: 27: 1–5.

Miller DS et al., Serologic survey for selected infectious disease agents in swift and kit foxes from the western United States. *J. Wildl. Dis.* 36, 798–805, 2000.

1.6 Zoonoses Caused by Arenaviruses

The name *Arenaviridae* is derived from the characteristic electron microscopic morphology of sand-like granules inside the virus particle surrounded by an envelope. These structures are host cell ribosomes. Arenaviruses are the only viruses that contain ribosomes and rRNA. Their segmented genome is a single-stranded RNA. The L segment codes for viral RNA polymerase, which is present in the virion in an active form. The L segment also codes for Z protein, a zinc finger protein that forms homo-oligomers and complexes with the G-protein and interacts with NP and L-protein. It is believed to modulate the activity of the L-protein. Interaction of NP and Z proteins is needed for genome packaging. The S segment codes for the N protein and for the G protein. Arenaviruses are special in their use of a so-called ambisense technique for gene expression and gene regulation. The information on the L segment for polymerase and on the S segment for the N protein are coded in negative polarity. The virus-specific polymerase, therefore, functions as a transcriptase and can read the message for the L and N proteins directly from the genomic RNA. The message on the genome is in plus polarity for the Z protein on the L segment and for the G protein on the S segment. The messages can only be read from a replicative intermediate. This genetic peculiarity is shared only with the Bunyaviruses.

After translation, the G protein is split proteolytically into G1 and G2, the receptor binding proteins in the virus envelope. The capsid structure of arenaviruses is not clearly defined. RNA polymerase and N protein are located inside the virus particle.

All known arenaviruses are associated with rodents as hosts, like Hantaviruses. The term Robovirus (rodent-borne viruses) is occasionally used for these viruses transmitted by rodents. Arenaviruses are usually not pathogenic for their hosts but induce a persistent infection after perinatal exposure. Similar to Hantaviruses, each Arenavirus has a single species as host. Lymphocytic choriomeningitis (LCM) virus, the prototype for Arenaviruses, induces immune tolerance in mice (*Mus musculus*) after perinatal infection. The lifelong carrier state in mice usually does not induce disease. This persistent infection can be eliminated with T cells from mice of the same haplotype and immune to LCM viruses. Circulating immune complexes may later induce immune complex disease in these treated mice. It may also occur spontaneously in some mouse strains that carry the virus.

When adult immunocompetent mice are experimentally infected with LCM virus, they develop severe and often fatal disease with hepatitis and encephalitis. The LCM virus induced disease can be blocked by simultaneous immunosuppressive treatment. It can be concluded that the disease in adult mice is an immunologic conflict with virus-infected mouse organs. Virus-infected and immunosuppressed mice remain virus carriers. If immunocompetence is reconstituted, severe lethal diseases develop.

Old World and New World arenaviruses (Tab. 1.2) are classified according to the distribution of host animals and based on group-specific reactions.

Arenaviruses are divided into Old World and New World viruses. The Eurasian arenaviruses are associated with mice. African arenaviruses are associated with multimammate "rats" (*praomys, mastomys*). New World arenaviruses are associated with species of the genera *oryzomys* (rice rat), *calomys*, *neotoma* (wood rats), and *sigmodon* (cotton rats). The common genetic origin of Old and New World arenaviruses is unanswered as is the common origin of the host animals.

Table 1.2 | Zoonotic arenaviruses

VIRUS	HOST	DISEASE	GEOGRAPHICAL OCCURRENCE
Arenaviruses of the Old World			
LCM virus	House mouse (*Mus musculus*)	LCM	Europe, America
Lassa virus[1]	Multimammate "rats" (*Mastomys spp.*)		West Africa
American hemorrhagic fever (arenaviruses of the New World, Tacaribe complex[2])			
Junin virus	Laucha chica (*Calomys laucha*)	AHF	Argentina, Paraguay
Machupo virus	Laucha grande (*Calomys callosus*)	BHF	Bolivia
Guanarito virus	Cotton rat (*Sigmodon alstoni*)?	VHF	Venezuela
Sabia virus	?	Brazilian hemorrhagic fever	Northern Brazil
Whitewater Arroyo virus[3]	Wood rat (*Neotoma albigula*)	US hemorrhagic fever	Colorado, New Mexico

LCM, lymphocytic choriomeningitis; AHF, Argentinian hemorrhagic fever; BHF, Bolivian hemorrhagic fever; VHF, Venezuelan hemorrhagic fever.
[1] Mopaia, Mobala, and Ippy viruses are closely related to Lassa virus. They infect other hosts and are not considered to be pathogenic for humans. *Praotomys huberti* and *P. erythroleucus* are host animals for Lassa virus.
[2] The Tacaribe complex includes at least six additional arenaviruses. They are not known to cause disease in humans.
[3] There are three different genetic lineages (A, B, and C) in the Tacaribe complex. The newly discovered Whitewater Arroyo virus is believed to be a natural recombinant from lineage A (the N gene) and lineage B (the GPC gene).

Transmission. Humans become infected with arenaviruses only after direct contact with infected animals or from food that is contaminated with infectious secretions from rodents. Human infections with arenaviruses can result in severe disease with hemorrhagic fever, hepatitis, and meningoencephalitis.

Clinical Manifestations. Arenavirus infections in humans cause a wide spectrum of disease from clinically inapparent and mild syndromes with fever and respiratory disease to severe cases characterized by meningitis and meningoencephalitis alone or in addition to hemorrhagic fever. LCM virus is mainly a cause of CNS disease. Lassa virus and the New World arenaviruses (Tacaribe complex) cause severe viral hemorrhagic fevers with high fatality rates but may also cause meningitis and meningoencephalitis. Laboratory infections as well as nosocomial and prenatal infections are quite common with arenaviruses.

Diagnosis. Arenaviruses can be isolated from blood or from CSF by inoculation of cell cultures or suckling mice. A group-specific RT-PCR technique can be used with a set of primers targeting the N gene of the Old World or the New World arenaviruses. For details, see the end of this section.

REFERENCES

Charrel RN, de Lamballerie X, Fulhorst CF, The White-water Arroyo virus: natural evidence for genetic recombination among Tacaribe de Manzione N, serocomplex viruses (family Arenaviridae). *Virology* 283, 161–166, 2001.

1.6.1 LYMPHOCYTIC CHORIOMENINGITIS

LCM is a zoonosis that occurs sporadically in humans. The disease is influenza-like with or without CNS involvement, sometimes with meningoencephalitis or encephalomyelitis.

Etiology. The causative agent is the LCM virus, an Arenavirus. Three distinct strains of the virus exist: WE, Armstrong, and Traub. They exhibit differences in mouse pathogenicity. Strain WE seems to be more virulent in mice, as is the case with humans in the case of laboratory infections. The Armstrong strain causes influenza-like disease and is rarely a cause of meningitis.

Occurrence. LCM virus occurs worldwide and is best documented in Europe and North America. The house mouse (*M. musculus*) is the natural reservoir for the agent.

Virus transmission in infected mouse colonies is vertical. The distribution of virus infected mice is focal as opposed to diffuse. Streets were found in which virus infected mouse colonies were living in houses on one side and non-infected animals on the opposite side. Human infections only occur in the houses in which LCM virus infected mice are living.

Perinatally infected mice remain virus carriers for life, unable to eliminate the virus. Infected hamster colonies were found to be the source for an epidemic occurrence of human LCM in the United States and Germany. Latent LCM infections have also been found in dogs, monkeys, guinea pigs, and several strains of laboratory mice.

In addition, LCM virus has repeatedly been found in cell cultures, in transplantable tumors, and in strains of *Toxoplasma gondii* or *Trichinella spiralis*, which are passaged on a regular basis in laboratory mice. Handling of such material is more frequently the cause of laboratory infections than handling virus cultures directly. Even monoclonal antibody preparations may contain LCM virus.

Transmission. Infected mice, hamsters, and other laboratory animals are the most important sources for human infection. An infection can be induced from infected animals by biting, by smear infections, or by aerosol. Nude mice were the source of a laboratory epidemic in a recent report. Food contaminated with murine excretions is an important source of human infections. Virus transmission by arthropods has been shown experimentally. However, it is not clear whether that route of infection plays a role under natural conditions. Several cases of prenatal infections have been documented, mainly in connection with hamsters that were kept as pets. Sexual virus transmission was not observed, either under natural or experimental conditions. Virus transmission via blood donations was not described. However, in two incidents eight patients who had received organ transplants were infected and died of the disease. In both cases, the organ donors had died under the picture of cerebral bleeding but LCM infection had not been diagnosed as the cause of death. Only one out of the organ acceptors survived the disease. He was treated with ribavirin and his immunosuppressive therapy was reduced.

Clinical Manifestations. The incubation period for LCM virus in humans is 6 to 13 days. The disease usually begins with an influenza-like prodromal period with high fever, severe malaise and headaches, spasm-like retrosternal pain resembling stenocardia, photophobia, sneezing, and bronchitis. The course of the disease does not progress further in many cases and may not be diagnosed, unless suspected as a result of a known exposure.

There is a brief recovery following the prodromal stage. One or 2 days later, CNS signs may appear. Meningitis may also appear without a prodromal stage marked by severe headaches and stiffness of the neck, confusion, and nausea. A meningoencephalitis or encephalitis may develop: patients become somnolent, reflexes are initially enhanced but later reduced, and paresthesia and paralysis may develop. This disease course can be lethal. Not infrequently, surviving patients have persistent headaches, paralysis, and personality changes. Convalescence may take weeks. Deafness may persist after LCM infection, as is the case after Lassa virus infection. Myelitis and tetraparesis may also be induced by LCM virus infection. Prenatal human infections have occurred in a few hamster-induced LCM epidemics. Hydrocephalus internus, uveitis, and chorioretinitis were found; the children were mentally retarded, and their visual capacity was reduced. According to newer studies in the United States and Europe, prenatal infection with the LCM virus may be underrated as a cause of congenital lesions of the CNS and impaired visual capacity. Chorioretinal scars should be an indication for testing for prenatal LCM virus infections. Laboratory infections with lethal outcome were observed in dual infections when cultures of LCM virus and *T. gondii* were simultaneously passaged. A LCM virus-induced hepatitis was reported in *Callithrix* monkeys.

Perinatally infected mice develop an asymptomatic persistent infection. They are unable to eliminate the virus due to immune tolerance. Intracerebral infection of adult mice induces a lethal infection. The disease is a result of an immune response to the virus; immunosuppressive therapy blocks the development of disease. Nude mice without a thymus carrying the *nu/nu* gene do not develop disease following infection with LCM virus.

Persistently infected carrier mice may develop an immune complex disease due to a simultaneous production of virus and the virus-specific antibody.

Diagnosis. LCM virus can be found in the blood during the febrile phase and in CSF when meningitis develops. Antigen capture tests can be used for the diagnosis. Sequences of the S segments of the genome, coding for the NP, are used for a nested RT-PCR. Virus-specific IgM antibodies are detectable early in the course of disease and persist for several months. They are also found in CSF. Indirect immunofluorescence, neutralization test, and immunoenzyme tests are available for serodiagnosis.

Differential Diagnosis. In cases of unexplained fever and malaise without signs of meningitis, a causal LCM virus infection will mostly remain unrecognized. Differential diagnosis is only required in cases with meningitis and meningoencephalitis. All forms of aseptic meningitis or meningoencephalitis have to be considered. A history of animal bites, pets, or professional contact with infectious material may serve as leads. Mumps, poliomyelitis and other enterovirus infections, listeriosis, brucellosis, leptospirosis, borreliosis, rickettsial diseases, and tuberculous meningitis are well-known causes of aseptic meningitis and have to be considered.

A differential diagnosis for LCM should be included for children born with hydrocephalus, for mentally retarded children, and for children with chorioretinal scars, especially when congenital cytomegalovirus infection, toxoplasmosis, and rubella can be excluded.

Therapy. Early administration of ribavirin has been highly beneficial for the treatment of human infections with other arenaviruses (Lassa, Junin, and Machupo viruses). There is not sufficient evidence for the treatment of LCM disease in humans because of its sporadic appearance. One can predict a beneficial effect from ribavirin based on experimental data of LCM infections in animals.

Lumbar CSF tap, which is used for diagnostic purposes, gives temporary relief for LCM patients because of pressure reduction, although the fluid removed is rapidly replaced during the acute phase. Lumbar puncture in the convalescence phase can cause severe problems due to delayed replacement of liquid (low pressure) and should be avoided.

Prophylaxis. Control of mice in households and testing of laboratory mice and hamsters are important for prophylaxis. Women of childbearing age and especially pregnant women should be informed about the potential danger of hamsters and mice.

Careful handling of laboratory mice and products derived from them, including production and use of monoclonal antibodies, is advisable. In cases of organ donations, the possibility of an infectious disease has to be carefully ruled out as the cause of the death of the donor.

REFERENCES

Ackermann R, Die Gefährdung des Menschen durch LCM-Virus verseuchte Goldhamster. *Dtsch. Med. Wschr.* 102, 1367–1370, 1977.

Ackermann R et al., Syrische Goldhamster als Überträger von Lymphozytärer Choriomeningitis. *Dtsch. Med. Wschr.* 97, 1725–1731, 1972.

Asper M et al., First outbreak of callitrichid hepatitis in Germany: genetic characterization of the causative lymphocytic choriomeningitis virus strains. *Virology* 284, 203–213, 2001.

Barton LL, Peters CJ, Ksiazek TG, Lymphocytic choriomeningitis virus: an unrecognized teratogenic pathogen. *Emerg. Infect. Dis.* 1, 152–153, 1995.

Brezin AP et al., Lymphocytic choriomeningitis virus chorioretinitis mimicking ocular toxoplasmosis in two otherwise normal children. *Am. J. Ophthalmol.* 130, 245–247, 2000.

Campo A et al., Impairment in auditory and visual function follows perinatal viral infection in the rat. *Int. J. Neurosci.* 27, 85–90 1985.

Gessner A, Lother H, Homologous interference of lymphocytic choriomeningitis virus involves a ribavirin-susceptible block in virus replication. *J. Virol.* 63, 1827–1832, 1989.

Gossmann J et al., Murine hepatitis caused by lymphocytic choriomeningitis virus. II. Cells involved in pathogenesis. *Lab. Invest.* 72, 559–570, 1995.

Hirsch E, Sensorineural deafness and labyrinth damage due to lymphocytic choriomeningitis. Report of a case. *Arch. Otolaryngol.* 102, 499–500, 1976.

Humbertclaude V et al., Les myélites aigues de l'enfant, à propos d'une cause rare: le virus de la chorioméningite lymphocytaire. *Arch. Pediatr.* 8, 282–285, 2001.

Lehmann-Grube F, Lymphocytic Choriomeningitis. In: Gard S, Hallauer C, Meyer KF (eds.), *Virology Monographs Bd. 10*, Springer, Wien, New York, 1971.

Lehmann-Grube F, Mechanism of recovery from acute virus infection. VI. Replication of lymphocytic choriomeningitis virus in and clearance from the foot of the mouse. *J. Gen. Virol.* 69, 1883–1891, 1988.

McCormick JB, King IJ, Webb PA, Lassa fever: Effective therapy with ribavirin. *New Engl. J. Med.* 314, 20–26, 1986.

Mets MB et al., Lymphocytic choriomeningitis virus: an underdiagnosed cause of congenital chorioretinitis. *Am. J. Ophthalmol.* 130, 209–215, 2000.

Müller S et al., Role of an intact splenic microarchitecture in early lymphocytic choriomeningitis virus production. *J. Virol.* 76, 2375–2383, 2002.

Park JY et al., Development of a reverse transcription-polymerase chain reaction assay for diagnosis of lymphocytic choriomeningitis virus infection and its use in a prospective surveillance study. *J. Med. Virol.* 51, 107–114, 1997.

Zeller W, Bruns M, Lehmann-Grube F, Lymphocytic choriomeningitis virus. X. Demonstration of nucleoprotein on the surface of infected cells. *Virology* 162, 90–97, 1988.

1.6.2 LASSA FEVER

Lassa fever is an infectious disease in West Africa that is transmitted to humans by mice of the *Mastomys* genus. The disease course is a hemorrhagic fever. The disease was first described in Lassa, Nigeria, in 1969, when three American missionary sisters became infected, and subsequently became ill.

Etiology. The causative agent is the Lassa virus, which belongs to the arenavirus family along with the LCM virus and the viruses causing South American hemorrhagic fevers.

There are additional African Arenaviruses related to Lassa virus: Mopaia, Mobala, and Ippy viruses. However, they infect different hosts. Human infections with these viruses occur but are usually subclinical.

Occurrence. The most important sources of infection for humans are the commensal-living multimammate rats of the genus *Mastomys*, the reservoir for the agent. These mice are widespread in Africa, south of the Sahara. Epidemics have occurred predominantly in West Africa, Nigeria, Liberia, and Sierra Leone. Thirteen percent of the human population in West Africa has antibodies to the Lassa virus. The Lassa virus has not yet been found in other African regions where *Mastomys* spp. are present.

Seventeen percent of trapped *Mastomys natalensis* mice in an area of endemicity in Sierra Leone were infected with the Lassa virus. *Rattus rattus* and *Mus minutoides* may also play a role as a source of human infection.

Human infections usually occur sporadically or in families living in *Mastomys* infested homes. The manifestation rate is 3%; the fatality rate is 15%. Probably more than 100,000 cases of Lassa fever occur in West Africa annually. Four tourists carried Lassa virus to Europe in 2000: two from Sierra Leone, one from Nigeria, and one traveling through Ghana, Burkina Faso, and Ivory Coast. All four patients died. The same is true for a patient who imported Lassa fever to the United States. Secondary cases did not occur on these occasions.

Transmission. There is no evidence for virus transmission to humans by insects. Rodent excrements cause human infections by way of contaminated dust or food. Sometimes rodents are killed and eaten. Infections within families are not uncommon. Virus transmission can occur while taking care of diseased individuals or sexually during the prodromal or recovery phase. Repeated use of hypodermic needles is a frequent source of hospital infections as well as contact with secretions, excrements, or blood from infected persons. Lassa fever patients spit and vomit blood, which contaminates the surroundings. Fetal infections were observed in 18 cases; all resulted in fetal death.

The fatality rate in nosocomial outbreaks was reported to be 52%. Human-to-human transmission is more frequent with Lassa fever than with other hemorrhagic fevers.

Clinical Manifestations. After a 6 to 21-day incubation period, the disease begins without a prodromal stage, but not abruptly; severe malaise with high fever, muscle aches, limb aches, and headaches, occasionally rigors, and retrosternal pain resembling angina pectoris occur. Ulcerations can be seen, with whitish deposits on the tonsils and mucous membranes of the mouth and throat. Cervical lymph nodes are enlarged. Additional symptoms are coughing, nausea, vomiting, diarrhea with colic, and conjunctivitis. Leukopenia, proteinuria, and hepatic dysfunction are seen. One-third of patients develop hemorrhagic diathesis with petechiae, hematomas, bleeding puncture holes, hemoptysis, melena, hematuria, and intracerebral hematoma. Hemorrhagic diathesis announces a fatal course. Myocardial and kidney damage, as well as bacterial pneumonias, have been seen. CNS involvement with tonic-clonic spasms and comatose conditions are present in some cases. Ephemeral residual symptoms are alopecia, deafness, tremor, and pronounced circulatory lability. Deafness often persists and is an important epidemiological marker. In villages where Lassa fever is endemic, hearing loss correlates well with presence of antibody to Lassa virus in the villagers.

Diagnosis. Only laboratories with biosafety level 4 facilities should perform diagnostic tests for Lassa virus. The virus can be isolated in Vero cells from blood. Infected cells can be identified by immunofluorescence. The use of antigen capture ELISA and RT-PCR can speed the diagnosis.

RT-PCR is of practical value for the diagnosis in imported cases. Virus isolation attempts are used to confirm the diagnosis. EDTA-treated blood is the best source for virus isolation.

Employing antigen detection and virus-specific IgM tests, the sensitivity is 88% and the specificity is 90% when compared with a combination of virus isolation and RT-PCR. A group-specific RT-PCR technique can be done with a set of primers targeting the N gene of the Old World or the New World arenaviruses.

The serological diagnosis can be confirmed by a significant titer rise using an indirect immunofluorescence test or the demonstration of virus-specific IgM.

Differential Diagnosis. To rule out yellow fever is most important for the differential diagnosis due to its more frequent occurrence in West Africa. In addition, other viral and nonviral hemorrhagic fevers have to be considered: Marburg and Ebola fever as well as Crimean-Congo hemorrhagic fever and dengue hemorrhagic fever, meningococcal sepsis, and infections by rickettsiae, salmonellae, leptospires, borreliae, and protozoa. Viral hepatitis is often initially suspected in cases of Lassa fever.

Therapy. Antiviral therapy with ribavirin produces good results in all stages of the disease and it can prevent a lethal outcome. While the fatality rate in untreated cases is between 20% and 47%, it is reduced to 5% to 9% by an early i.v. administration of ribavirin. The recommended treatment is 2 g of ribavirin i.v. the first day, four doses of 1 g/day for the following 4 days, and then three doses of 0.5 g per day for the next 6 days. A better alternative is the infusion of 16 mg of ribavirin/kg over 6 h per day. Attempts to treat Lassa fever with immunoglobulins or interferon have failed. A symptomatic treatment addresses the hemorrhagic diathesis and shock.

A blood transfusion with 2.5 liters of blood initially improved the clinical picture in an imported case of Lassa fever. However, the patient developed acute encephalopathy 2 weeks later and died.

Patients with hemorrhagic fever are usually in critical condition at the time the diagnosis is made. The transportation to a hospital with isolation facilities is not advisable despite the potential danger of transmission. Experienced personnel, wearing high-pressure protective suits, could treat the person in the local hospital. There is no danger of transmission if barrier nursing techniques are strictly implemented.

Prophylaxis. The most important prophylactic measure is the control of rodents in human dwellings. Rats should not be allowed to contaminate food. Trapped rats should not be eaten.

Experimental vaccines have been developed. It remains to be seen whether they will be of importance, considering the possibility to control the infection with hygiene and with the use of barrier nursing. It has been shown that in monkeys, Armstrong virus, a low-pathogenicity strain of LCM virus, can confer protective immunity against Lassa virus. It might serve as a live vaccine.

A strict isolation of patients is essential to avoid hospital infections. High-pressure suits for clinical staff and a strict implementation of safety regulations are required to avoid contact or airborne infections.

Experimental and diagnostic procedures with the virus have to be conducted in biosafety level 4 laboratories. Safe handling of virus infected clinical specimens in a normal clinical laboratory may present a serious challenge. Wherever feasible, the specimens should be inactivated by fixation or by thermal (56 °C, 30 min) or chemical treatment, before removing them from the ward. Addition of detergent to a serum specimen will reduce the virus titer. Running infected specimens in a centrifuge is the most dangerous of all manipulations. Sticks with infected needles and cuts with infected knives should be strictly avoided.

REFERENCES

Bausch DG al., Diagnosis and clinical virology of Lassa fever as evaluated by enzyme-linked immunosorbent assay, indirect fluorescent- antibody test, and virus isolation. *J. Clin. Microbiol.* 38, 2670–2677, 2000.

Bowen MD et al., Genetic diversity among Lassa virus strains. *J. Virol.* 74, 6992–7004, 2000.

Buckley SM, Casals J, Down WD, Isolation and antigenic characterization of Lassavirus. *Nature* 227, 174, 1970.

Casals J, Buckley SM, Lassa fever. *Progr. Med. Virol.* 18, 111–126, 1974.

Cummins D et al., Lassa fever encephalopathy: clinical and laboratory findings. *J. Trop. Med. Hyg.* 95, 197–201, 1992.

Cummins D, Bennett D, Machin SJ, Exchange transfusion of a patient with fulminant Lassa fever. *Postgrad. Med. J.* 67, 193–194, 1991.

Cummins et al., Acute sensorineural deafness in Lassa fever. *JAMA.* 264, 2093–2096, 1990.

Demby AH et al., Early diagnosis of Lassa fever by reverse transcription-PCR. *J. Clin. Microbiol.* 32, 2898–2903, 1994.

Djavani M et al., Mucosal immunization with Salmonella typhimurium expressing Lassa virus nucleocapsid protein cross-protects mice from lethal challenge with lymphocytic choriomeningitis virus. *J. Hum. Virol.* 4, 103–108, 2001.

Fisher-Hoch SP et al., Unexpected adverse reactions during a clinical trial in rural west Africa. *Antiviral Res.* 19, 139–147, 1992.

Fisher-Hoch SP et al., Effective vaccine for Lassa fever. *J. Virol.* 74, 6777–6783, 2000.

Fisher-Hoch SP, McCormick JB, Towards a human Lassa fever vaccine. *Rev. Med. Virol.* 11, 331–341, 2001.

Fisher-Hoch SP et al., Review of cases of nosocomial Lassa fever in Nigeria: the high price of poor medical practice. *BMJ.* 311, 857–859, 1995.

Fleischer K et al., Lassa-Fieber. *Med. Klin.* 95, 340–342, 2000.

Gunther S et al., Imported Lassa fever in Germany: molecular characterization of a new Lassa virus strain. *Emerg. Infect. Dis.* 6, 466–476, 2000.

Gunther S et al., Lassa fever encephalopathy: Lassa virus in cerebrospinal fluid but not in serum. *J. Infect. Dis.* 184, 345–349, 2001.

Ignatyev G et al., Experimental study on the possibility of treatment of some hemorrhagic fevers. *J. Biotechnol.* 83, 67–76, 2000.

McCormick JB, King IJ, Webb PA, Lassa fever: Effective therapy with ribavirin. *New Engl. J. Med.* 314, 20–26, 1986.

Monson MH et al., Pediatric Lassa fever: a review of 33 Liberian cases. *Am. J. Trop. Med. Hyg.* 36, 408–415, 1987.

Simonsen L et al., Unsafe injections in the developing world and transmission of blood-borne pathogens: a review. *Bull. WHO* 77, 789–800, 1999.

Ter Meulen J, Lassa fever: immuno-epidemiological approach to the study of an endemic viral haemorrhagic fever. *Med. Trop. (Mars).* 60, Suppl. 20–23, 2000.

Trappier SG et al., Evaluation of the polymerase chain reaction for diagnosis of Lassa virus infection. *Am. J. Trop. Med. Hyg.* 49, 214–221, 1993.

WHO, Lassa fever, Sierra Leone, *Wkly. epid. Rec.* 72, p. 145 and 162, 1999.

WHO, Lassa fever, imported case, Netherlands. *Wkly. epid. Rec.* 75, pp. 17–18 and 265. 2000.

WHO, Lassa fever, imported case, United Kingdom. *Wkly. epid.Rec.* 75, p. 85 and 189, 2000.

1.6.3 ZOONOSES CAUSED BY NEW WORLD ARENAVIRUSES (AGENTS OF HEMORRHAGIC FEVER)

Argentinian hemorrhagic fever (AHF), Bolivian hemorrhagic fever (BHF), and Venezuelan hemorrhagic fever (VHF) are acute virus-induced diseases. The causative agents are transmitted by rodents to humans, especially in rural regions in South America. The patients present with fever, myalgias, hemorrhagic diathesis, shock, and neurologic disease.

An additional arenavirus, Whitewater Arroyo virus, has recently been isolated from three patients with lethal hemorrhagic fever in Colorado.

Etiology. The causative agent of AHF is the Junin virus. BHF is caused by the Machupo virus. Guanarito virus, the agent of VHF, and a Brazilian agent, Sabia virus, have only recently been isolated. These viruses belong to the arenaviruses together with the LCM virus (the prototype) and the Lassa virus. There are 15 known viruses in this family. However, only six (LCM, Lassa, Junin, Machupo, Guanarito, and Sabia viruses) are known to be pathogenic for humans.

All known arenaviruses cause persistent infections in mice or other rodents that serve as reservoirs. Together with Hantaviruses, they are now known as roboviruses (rodent-borne viruses).

The recently discovered Whitewater Arroyo virus is probably a recombinant from two South American arenaviruses (lineage A and B of the Tacaribe complex).

Occurrence. AHF is endemic in the Argentinian provinces of Buenos Aires, Cordoba, Santa Fe, and La Pampa. Several hundred to several thousand cases are registered annually in these regions, especially among farm workers, which is probably because of a high exposure rate, men are affected four times as often as women.

BHF has only been seen in the Bolivian province of Beni between the Mamora and Branco Rivers. A hospital infection outside the province of Beni could be traced to an index case inside

Beni. BHF also occurs more frequently in men than in women.

The disease in humans is restricted to the dry season between April and September. The most important reservoirs for Junin virus are *Calomys laucha* mice living in cornfields, *Calomys musculinus*, and other mouse species. The reservoir for Machupo virus is *Calomys callosus*, which lives in houses, meadows, and around forests in eastern Bolivia. Fifty percent of *C. callosus* mice trapped in houses were infected with Machupo virus during epidemics of BHF. Guanarito virus has been isolated from cotton rats (*Sigmodon* spp.). *Sigmodon alstoni* is the reservoir of the virus. Antibodies were found in rice rats (*Oryzomys* spp.). Whitewater Arroyo virus appears to be associated epidemiologically with *Neotoma albigula*, the white-throated wood rat, an association that has been confirmed in Oklahoma and New Mexico. *Neotoma cinerea* and *Neotoma micropus* were found to be hosts in Utah.

Perinatal infection of rodents leads to persistent infection that is transmitted to the next generation. Considerable amounts of virus are excreted in saliva and excrements.

Transmission. Human infections with AHF occur during harvest time by direct contact with *C. laucha* or with their excrements. An increased occurrence of AHF was seen after new harvesting techniques led to killing of more mice with spreading of blood. Mouse excretions are also the most important source of infection of BHF and VHF.

Transmission from human-to-human is rare. Nosocomial epidemics and family infections are possible, similar to Lassa fever. Laboratory infections with Junin, Machupo, and Sabia viruses have been observed.

Clinical Manifestations. Signs of AHF, BHF, and VHF disease are almost identical and are similar to those of Lassa fever with the exception that CNS involvement is less frequent with Lassa fever.

The incubation period is 7 to 14 days. The disease begins gradually with fever, limb aches, stomachache, and headache. Conjunctival injection is seen in most cases, as is rash or rather a flush on the head, neck, and thorax. Nausea, vomiting, and diarrhea are seen in less than half of the cases, with a hemorrhagic diathesis in one-third. Petechial bleeding is seen on gums, with epistaxis and gastrointestinal and urogenital bleeding. Hemorrhagic diathesis announces a bad prognosis. A fine tremor of tongue and hands is seen in most patients. Less discrete signs of neurological disturbances are common. Between days 6 and 10, most patients experience a hypotonic crisis that indicates an unfavorable prognosis, often with a lethal outcome if not controlled.

The acute disease lasts 2 to 3 weeks. The recovery phase can be long lasting. Patients complain about fatigue. Alopecia is frequently seen, as in other arenavirus infections. The lethality is around 18% for BHF and 10% to 20% for AHF.

Clinically inapparent infections are rare. Leukopenia and thrombocytopenia are pronounced. In hospitalized patients with suspected AHF, the combination of thrombocytopenia (<100,000 thrombocytes/mm3) and leukopenia (<2,500 leukocytes/mm3) has a high predictive value (87% sensitivity and 88% specificity).

Diagnosis. Sixty percent of AHF cases are diagnosed clinically. Blood during the febrile phase is the best source for virus isolation. The virus can also be found in mucosal secretions. Virus isolation attempts are time-consuming, dangerous, and only partially successful.

A group-specific RT-PCR technique can be used for direct virus detection with a set of primers targeting the N gene of the Old World or the New World arenaviruses.

For serological diagnosis, the antigen capture ELISA is useful during the early phase of the disease. An IgM antibody test (IgM capture ELISA) can be used during the second week of the disease. A combination of antigen capture, RT-PCR, and IgM capture ELISA is optimal.

Differential Diagnosis. If the clinical course is not characteristic, arbovirus infections, typhus, rickettsiosis, leptospirosis, and parasitic infections have to be considered in the differential diagnosis. In severe cases with hemorrhagic diathesis and ARDS, Hantavirus pulmonary syndrome (the Andes virus and others) has to be ruled out.

Therapy. Early administration of neutralizing antibodies may reduce the lethality of AHF from 15% to 6%. The lethality of Machupo virus in monkeys was reduced with ribavirin. The recommended treatment is 2 g of ribavirin i.v. the first day, four doses of 1 g per day for the following 4 days, and then three doses of 0.5 g per day for the next 6 days. A better alternative is the infusion of 16 mg of ribavirin/kg over 6 h per day. Symptomatic treatment is essential to control the hemorrhagic diathesis and shock. Clotting factor preparations, either fresh blood or plasma, are recommended.

Prophylaxis. The administration of serum from recovered persons is recommended after exposure in the laboratory or while handling patients. Because of the danger of nosocomial infections, all suspected or diseased patients should be isolated in low-pressure isolation units. Alternatively, high-pressure protective suits could be used by health care workers. Patients with suspected VHF should not be transported to prevent any injury due to transportation.

Safety laboratories (BSL-4) are needed for diagnostic work, especially when virus cultivation is tried. Safe handling of virus-infected clinical specimens in a normal clinical laboratory may present a serious challenge. Wherever feasible, the specimens should be inactivated by fixation or by thermal (56 °C, 30 min) or chemical treatment, before introducing them to the laboratory. Addition of detergent to a serum specimen will reduce the virus titer. Running infected specimens in a centrifuge is the most dangerous of all manipulations. Sticks with infected needles and cuts with infected knives should be avoided.

The most important prophylactic measurement is the control of murine reservoirs and control of exposure during farm work.

A formalinized vaccine against AHF has been developed. Its protective value for BHF has been proven experimentally. More recently, an attenuated live virus vaccine for AHF was produced, which has been used in more than 100,000 people without problems.

REFERENCES

Calisher CH et al., Transmission of an arenavirus in white-throated woodrats (Neotoma albigula), southeastern Colorado, 1995–1999. *Emerg. Infect. Dis.* 7, 397–402, 2001.

Charrel RN, de Lamballerie X, Fulhorst CF, The Whitewater Arroyo virus: natural evidence for genetic recombination among Tacaribe de Manzione N, serocomplex viruses (family Arenaviridae). *Virology* 283, 161–166, 2001.

Fulhorst CF et al., Isolation and characterization of pirital virus, a newly discovered South American arenavirus. *Am. J. Trop. Med. Hyg.* 56, 548–553, 1997.

Fulhorst CF et al., Isolation and characterization of Whitewater Arroyo virus, a novel North American arenavirus. *Virology* 224, 114–120, 1996.

Fulhorst CF et al., Natural rodent host associations of Guanarito and Pirital viruses (Family Arenaviridae) in Central Venezuela. *Am. J. Trop. Med. Hyg.* 61, 325–330, 1999.

Fulhorst CF al., Geographic distribution and genetic diversity of Whitewater Arroyo virus in the southwestern United States. *Emerg. Infect. Dis.* 7, 403–407, 2001.

Fulhorst CF et al., Experimental infection of the cane mouse Zygodontomys brevicauda (family Muridae) with Guanarito virus (Arenaviridae), the etiologic agent of Venezuelan hemorrhagic fever. *J. Infect. Dis.* 180, 966–969, 1999.

Fulhorst CF et al., Experimental infection of Neotoma albigula (Muridae) with White water Arroyo virus (Arenaviridae). *Am. J. Trop. Med. Hyg.* 65, 147–151, 2001.

Garcia JB et al., Genetic diversity of the Junin virus in Argentina: geographic and temporal patterns. *Virology* 272, 127–136, 2000.

Harrison LH et al., Clinical case definitions for Argentine hemorrhagic fever. *Clin. Infect. Dis.* 28, 1091–1094, 1999.

Lopez N et al., Homologous and heterologous glycoproteins induce protection against Junin virus challenge in guinea pigs. *J. Gen. Virol.* 81, 1273–1281, 2000.

Lozano ME et al., A simple nucleic acid amplification assay for the rapid detection of Junin virus in whole blood samples. *Virus Res.* 27, 37–53, 1993.

Lozano ME et al., Rapid diagnosis of Argentine hemorrhagic fever by reverse transcriptase PCR-based assay. *J. Clin. Microbiol.* 33, 1327–1332, 1995.

McCormick JB, King IJ, Webb PA, Lassa Fever: Effective therapy with ribavirin. *New Engl. J. Med.* 314, 20–26, 1986.

Tesh RB et al., Description of Guanarito virus (Arenaviridae: Arenavirus), the etiologic agent of Venezuelan hemorrhagic fever. *Am. J. Trop. Med. Hyg.* 50, 452–459, 1994.

Weaver SC et al., Guanarito virus (Arenaviridae) isolates from endemic and outlying localities in Venezuela: sequence comparisons among and within strains isolated from Venezuelan hemorrhagic fever patients and rodents. *Virology* 266, 189–195, 2000.

1.7 Zoonoses Caused by Filoviruses

The members of the family *Filoviridae*, Marburg virus and Ebola virus, each forming a genus of its own, are known to cause hemorrhagic fevers. Hemorrhagic fever viruses belong to different virus families and are highly pathogenic, although not highly contagious. Marburg virus, the prototype virus of the family Filoviridae was discovered in 1967 in Marburg, when it caused disease in laboratory workers in Marburg and Frankfurt, Germany and in Belgrade, at that time Yugoslavia. Ebola virus is best known as an agent in hospital-associated disease outbreaks in African hospitals.

The host reservoir of filoviruses has remained undisclosed for a long time. Meanwhile, there is strong evidence that flying foxes, especially *Roussettus aegyptiacus* (s. Fig. 1.8) and other *Megachiroptera* constitute the reservoir of Filoviruses. Human infections are mostly acquired

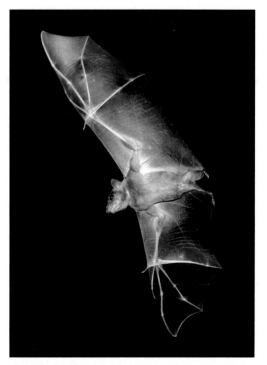

Figure 1.8 | *Roussettus aegyptiacus* (flying fox) Reservoir of filoviruses (source: Oren Peles via the PikiWiki – Israel free images collection project)

from contact with monkeys and from flying foxes that are eaten as "bushmeat." In several outbreaks in Gabon and in the Republic of Congo, the Ebola virus was transmitted to humans after contact with dead chimpanzees. The infection is as dangerous for chimpanzees and gorillas as it is for humans. The Marburg virus has been transmitted to laboratory workers in Germany and in Yugoslavia after contact with vervet monkeys (*Chrysocebus aethiops*). A third virus species in this family, Reston virus, has been imported from Southeast Asia to the United States and to Italy in Java monkeys (*Macaca fascicularis*). Animal caretakers were infected with these viruses. A seroconversion without clinical signs was diagnosed. Reston virus, therefore, is not considered to be pathogenic for humans.

Viruses in the family *Filoviridae* (L. n. *filum*, thread) are mononegavirales, which means they have an unsegmented single-stranded genome with negative polarity. Based on differences in the genetic makeup, there are three genera in this family: *Marburg virus* and *Ebola virus, and Cuevavirus*. The latter is not known to cause Human disease. Marburg virus has seven gene products. Ebola virus has an additional soluble glycoprotein (sGP) which may be connected with the regulation of its pathogenicity. The 3′ and 5′ ends of the RNA are conserved and reveal a high degree of complementarity. Both viruses have a nucleocapsid protein gene at the 3′ end of the genomic RNA. The sequence includes a phosphoprotein (VP35) connected to the capsid, a matrix protein (VP40), and the GP gene as well as VP30 and VP24. The L gene is located at the 5′ end; it codes for the RNA-dependent RNA polymerase. The product of the GP gene is cleaved proteolytically post translation into G1 and G2. Ebola virus has a mechanism of molecular editing: an additional glycosylated gene product, the sGP, is specified by the GP gene. The VP24 is associated with viral immune escape mechanisms.

Filoviruses are causes of severe outbreaks with extremely high case fatality rates. The outbreaks are characterized by human-to human-transmission with a high proportion of nosocomial transmission in the setting of African hospitals. The most severe outbreaks of Marburg virus have occurred in Angola (2004) and in Durba (1998). The cumulative number of patients is more than 560 with an overall lethality of 83% in Angola and in the Congo and 23% in Marburg in the setting of a University hospital. Ebola virus has caused more outbreaks than Marburg virus with more than fifty times as many patients. The case fatality rate was 83% (Ebola Zaire), 54% (Ebola Maridi) and 40% (Bundibugyo virus, Uganda). Reston virus, the Asian species of Ebola virus is presently not believed to be pathogenic for humans; there is only indirect evidence for clinically inapparent infections. The fourth species of Ebola virus, Ivory Coast, has been observed only in two patients. Presently (January 2014 to May 2015), the greatest outbreak is ongoing in Guinea, Sierra Leone, and in Liberia with more than 26,700 cases (>11.999 fatalities) and a case fatality rate of ca. 42%. (All these figures are preliminary).

In post mortems, extended necroses are found in parenchymatous organs, especially in liver, spleen, kidneys, and gonads. Inflammatory reactions are absent or not prominent. The spectrum of affected cell types comprises macrophages, monocytic and dendritic cells, endothelial cells, fibroblasts, hepatocytes, von Kupffer cells, and adenoid cells in the adrenals. All these cells are actively producing the virus; however, the total loss of these cells does not explain the fatal courses. The lymphopenia and the thrombopenia are most probably not caused by viral cytolysis; an increased apoptosis is discussed instead. Thrombocytopenia, of course, is a consequence of intravascular coagulation. In survivors, the counts of lymphocytes and of thrombocytes are normalized within a few days.

Hemorrhagic diathesis in some cases has caused massive intracerebral bleeding. However, in the majority of cases, loss of blood does not reach a life threatening degree and can not explain the lethal courses. Disseminated intravascular coagulation plays a role in the development of hemorrhagic diathesis. The primary cause of hemorrhage is apparently the formation of gaps in the endothelial layers of small blood vessels. These gaps are induced by TNFalpha and H_2O_2, which are secreted by virus infected monocytes/macrophages. Viral cytolysis of endothelial cells may also be a cause of gap formation.

An important factor in the pathogenesis of hemorrhagic diathesis is the dramatic loss of ionized calcium. Deposits of calcium were found in the liver and spleen of experimentally infected guinea pigs and also in organs at postmortems. Blood from infected guinea pigs did not clot on day 4 or 5 of the disease. But upon substitution with 0.01 or 0.02 m CaCl ca. 50% of the coagulation could be restored although clotting factors and platelet counts were reduced to less than 20% of normal values.

In an outbreak of Ebola Sudan strain, it was shown that the plasma concentration of ionized calcium was a prospective indicator of disease. Patients with reduced levels of Ca^{++} did not survive. Members of the family *Filoviridae* are listed in Tab. 1.3.

REFERENCES

Balter M, Emerging diseases. On the trail of Ebola and Marburg viruses. *Science* 290, 923–925, 2000.

Biot M, Tribute to Dr. Katenga Bonzali. *Trop. Med. Int. Health.* 5, 384, 2000.

Jahrling PB et al., Filoviruses and Arenaviruses. In: Murray PR et al. (eds.), *Manual of Clinical Microbiology*, 1570–1582, 8th ed. ASM Press, Washington, DC, 2003.

Kiley MP et al., Filoviridae: a taxonomic home for Marburg and Ebola viruses? *Intervirology* 18, 24–32, 1982.

Slenczka W, The Marburg Virus Outbreak of 1967 and Subsequent Episodes. In: Klenk HD (ed.), *Marburg and Ebola viruses. Current Topics Microbiol. Immunol.* 235, 49–76, 1999.

Siegert R et al., Zur Ätiologie einer unbekannten, von Affen ausgegangenen menschlichen Infektionskrankheit. *Dtsch. Med. Wschr.* 92, 2341–2343, 1967.

WHO, Marburg fever, Democratic Republic of the Congo. *Wkly. Epidemiol. Rec.* 74, 145 and 157, 1999.

WHO, Viral haemorrhagic fever/Marburg, Democratic Republic of the Congo (update). *Wkly. epidemiol Rec.* 75, 109, 2000.

Zeller H, Les leçons de l'épidémie à virus Marburg à Durba, République Démocratique du Congo (1998–2000). *Med. Trop. (Mars)* 60, 23–26, 2000.

1.7.1 MARBURG VIRUS HEMORRHAGIC FEVER

Marburg virus infection in humans produces hemorrhagic fever with a high fatality rate. Most cases in Europe occurred in laboratory personal after contact with imported *Chrysocebus (Cercopithecus) Aethiops* monkeys.

Etiology. The causative agent was isolated and identified in Marburg in 1967 and was therefore named "Marburg virus." Together with the Ebola virus, discovered in 1976, the Marburg virus constitutes the family Filoviridae, which comprises two genera, Marburg virus and Ebola virus (see Table 1.3). The name of this family

Table 1.3 | Family Filoviruses

GENUS OR SUBGENUS	TYPE SPECIES	ASSUMED SOURCE(S) OF INFECTION[1]	GEOGRAPHICAL OCCURRENCE
Genus *Marburg virus*	Marburg virus	Vervet monkeys (*Cercopithecus aethiops*)	East Africa, Angola
Genus *Ebola virus*	Ebola virus	Chimpanzees, gorillas	Equatorial Africa
	Ebola virus Zaire	Chimpanzees (*Pan troglodytes*)	Republic of Congo, Gabon
	Ebola virus	Unknown	Sudan, Uganda, Maridi
	Ebola virus	Chimpanzees	West Africa, Ivory Coast
Subgenus *Reston Virus*	Reston virus[2]	Java cynomolgus monkeys (*Macaca fascicularis*)	Southern Asia

A third genus of the family Filoviridae, cuevavirus, was found in bats in Spain. It is not known to cause human disease but might interfere with serologic techniques.
[1] Flying foxes or fruit bats (*Megachiroptera*) are now believed to be reservoir hosts of filoviruses (for details see text).
[2] Reston virus, the Asian subtype of Ebola virus, is nonpathogenic for humans.

refers to the elongated threadlike virus particles (Lat. *filum* for thread). These viruses are enveloped particles with a helical nucleocapsid that contains a single stranded RNA of negative polarity. The standard length of Marburg virus is 665 nm but there are filamentous particles with a length of ca. 1,500 to 8,000 nm. The length of these particles roughly corresponds to multiples of 665 nm, the standard length.

Occurrence. Marburg virus was first discovered in 1967, when 31 people in Belgrade, Yugoslavia, and in Frankfurt and Marburg, Germany, fell ill with a hemorrhagic fever. Laboratory personnel working in vaccine production or safety testing of vaccines were affected. The common source of infection was monkeys of the species *C. aethiops* (green guenons), which were imported to Europe from Uganda.

In the following 30 years, only three additional primary disease cases and three secondary infections have been observed in Africa were confirmed by virus isolation. Geographically, one case was associated with Zimbabwe, and two cases with the Mount Elgon region in Kenya. One of the strains isolated from patients in Kenya, Ravn, deviated from all the other strains known at that time. Humans in Africa may have antibodies against Marburg virus in the absence of an anamnestic evidence of hemorrhagic fever.

Meanwhile, there is strong evidence that flying bats, especially *Roussettus aegyptiacus* are reservoir animals of the Marburg virus. These animals are found in Sub-Saharan Africa and in Egypt, Palestine, Syria, and Cyprus. They are fructivorous bats, eating wild figs and living in caves. In Cameroon, they are found up to 1,600 mNN. Upon experimental infection, these animals do not show overt disease. Antibodies to the Marburg virus antigen were found in their serum, in some cases viral RNA was also detectable. Therefore, it is assumed that they have clinically inapparent infections.

R. aegyptiacus has a body length of 15 cm and a wingspan of 60 cm, the fur color is greyish-brown. Flying foxes are ideally suited as a virus reservoir. Monkeys, other animals, and occasionally humans, may be infected by way of bat secretions and excrements sticking on leafs and on fruits. In cages, where the bats are living in colonies, aerogenic transmissions may occur. These routes of infection are also typical for HENIPA viruses in South East Asia and in Australia. Living in cages, *R. aegyptiacus* offers a good explanation for infection of tourists visiting the Kitum cage and for the outbreak among miners in the mining region of Durba and Watsa in the Orientale province of the Democratic Republic of the Congo. In African countries, flying foxes are eaten as a delicacy. Migration of these animals might explain the epidemiology.

A large number of Marburg virus hemorrhagic fever cases occurred in 1999 and 2000 in Durba, located in the northern part of the Republic of Congo, near the border with Uganda. The case fatality rate (123/149 cases) was 82.5%. A genetic analysis revealed at least three different virus variants. Individuals working in a gold mine were primarily affected. Large numbers of bats and some rats were found in the gold mine. Secondary infections occurred after contact in families and hospitals. The search for a natural reservoir of the agent failed at that time. The greatest outbreak (up to this time) of Marburg virus fever occurred in 2004 to 2005 in Uige in Angola. In this outbreak, which happened in the region around Uige, children were mainly the victims. Most probably, the route of infection was via reused needle sticks during a vaccination campaign. There were 324 out of 388 confirmed cases; the case fatality rate was 83%.

Transmission. All primary infections occurring in Europe in 1967 could be traced to contact with monkey's blood or organs or with cell cultures prepared from monkey kidneys. Conditions were such that transmission by direct contact or aerosols was possible. Two cases in a Russian research laboratory could be traced to aerosols; one of them was fatal. Secondary infections almost always were transmitted by accidental inoculations or with patient blood through skin lesions. In one case, the virus was detected in sperm: a spouse became infected 3 months after the husband developed the disease. In the

Durba outbreak, 1999 to 2000, the primary cases were in miners and were most probably transmitted from infected bats living in the mines. In addition, there were many family infections. In the outbreak that occurred in Uige, reused needle sticks were the vehicle of transmission. The primary source of this outbreak was not identified. In addition to these modes of transmission, African funeral habits, including caressing the corpses, have contributed to the spread of the virus in most African outbreaks.

Clinical Manifestations. After the incubation period of an average of 7 days (range, 3 to 9 days), the onset of disease is sudden without a prodromal period. Patients develop high fever, severe malaise, weakness, headaches, hyperesthesia, limb pain, nausea, vomiting, abdominal pain, and diarrhea. Early signs are conjunctivitis, pharyngitis, and maculopapular rash (Fig. 1.9) spreading from the face to the body and to the proximal parts of the limbs, and an enanthem of the soft palate. Vomiting and severe diarrhea are seen in 75% of the cases. Hemorrhagic diathesis was found in less than half of the cases (Fig. 1.10).

Towards the end of the acute phase, there are signs of CNS involvement, with apathy, depression, and encephalitis. Symptoms reminiscent of a tetany with paresthesia, restless legs, sleeplessness, and the feeling of "lying on dried crumbs" were clearly described but were misinterpreted as signs of viral CNS-involvement.

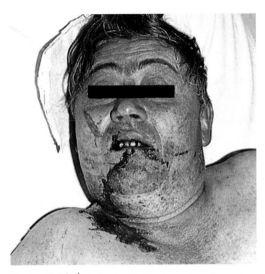

Figure 1.10 | Patient with Marburg virus disease in a prefinal stage. (Courtesy of W. Stille)

Hypocalcemia seems to be an important event in the pathogenesis. Ionized calcium apparently is the limiting factor in the development of consumption coagulopathy. In Europe, the case fatality rate of primary cases was ca. 30%. Secondary infections were less severe and not fatal. Patients with fatal courses were often admitted to the hospital in shock or with signs of a severe hemorrhagic diathesis.

Death, when it occurred, followed between days 7 and 16 after onset of the disease. The virus can be found for several months after the acute infection in immunologically privileged organs. Clinically inapparent infections have not been observed.

Clinical pathology reveals a distinct thrombocytopenia and lymphopenia with a neutrophilia in the early stage. The neutrophilic cells revealed a "pseudo-Pelger" anomaly. Transaminases are elevated, especially serum glutamine oxalacetic transaminase (SGOT). In some cases proteinuria, oliguria, and urea retention are seen. A veterinarian aged 39 years died from massive intracerebral sanguination.

Following recovery from acute disease, the Marburg virus can persist for several months in organs that are immunologically sequestered, that is, in the testes and in the anterior bulbar portion. Some of the patients may develop

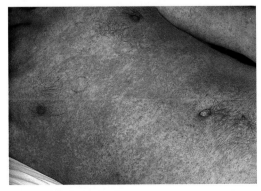

Figure 1.9 | Maculopapular exanthema at day 6 of Marburg virus disease. (Courtesy of G. Baltzer.)

uveitis in the course of their convalescent period. In such cases, the virus has been isolated from the anterior eye chamber. Relapses may occur during the convalescent phase with neurological symptoms, with orchitis or hepatitis. The clinical course of relapses was benign in the patients who were infected with Marburg virus in 1967. Retrospectively, clinically inapparent infections were found in 2 persons, who had had contact with monkeys. However, three individuals, who had had a risk of infection, developed a rather mild course of disease and were not admitted to the hospital. More than hundred healthy contact individuals were seronegative in Marburg and in Frankfurt. This, however, was not the case during the African outbreaks, where symptomatic infection of family members was often observed. Survival of the disease does not cause persisting damage of organs.

Chimpanzees and gorillas are infected under natural conditions, and, like humans, they die under the picture of hemorrhagic fever. Upon experimental transmission to laboratory animals, for example, guinea pigs and Syrian hamsters, an increased pathogenicity is observed in the course of three passages. This observation is not in accordance with clinical observation in nosocomial infections, which were made in European hospitals.

It is reported that the vervet monkeys that have introduced Marburg virus to Europe in 1967 did not show signs of overt disease. However, it is probable that some animals, convalescent of Marburg virus infection may have been in close contact with non-infected animals and that these might have infected their cage companions. Sexes were not separated in the cages. In humans, the virus may persist in immunologically privileged organs as in the testes and anterior eye chambers for up to 3 months. The same may happen in vervet monkeys, if there are any survivors in natural infections.

In experimentally infected guinea pigs and hamsters, clinical pictures and pathology are identical to the manifestations in human patients. Deposits of calcium were found in necrotic parenchyma. Laboratory studies on the pathogenesis of hemorrhagic diathesis resembled the findings in humans.

Diagnosis. The virus can be demonstrated by electron microscopy in formaldehyde-fixed blood after differential centrifugation. The structure of the virus is characteristic (665 nm elongated enveloped rods) and can only be confused with the Ebola virus, which has a length of 800 nm.

Virus isolation is possible by inoculating guinea pigs or Vero cells with blood or urine. The virus can be detected directly in EDTA-treated blood by antigen capture or by RT-PCR. Hänninen has used primers for the detection of Marburg virus aiming at a sequence from the GP gene. This test has a high sensitivity, and it can be used for all known variants of the Marburg virus genome. However, it has not yet been tested in the field. Highly conserved sequences from the N or L gene might be more convenient for the detection of variants.

It is important to avoid laboratory contamination with cDNA when evaluating the PCR. If a special strain is present in the laboratory and the PCR results have an identical sequence, it might be difficult to confirm a diagnosis.

The virus can also be detected in cell cultures prepared from kidneys of infected monkeys. Viral antigen can be seen by immunofluorescence in blood smears or in imprints from postmortem material (liver, spleen, and lymph nodes) with immunofluorescence or by IgM capture ELISA. IF and ELISA tests are useful for the detection of IgG antibodies. Virus-specific IgM antibodies are present in the second week of the disease. They can be demonstrated by IgM capture ELISA. ELISA is also useful for the detection of IgG antibodies. Recombinant antigen preparations were found satisfactory for ELISA procedures.

Differential Diagnosis. Any severe infectious disease should be considered in the differential diagnosis, especially meningococcal sepsis, typhus, cholera, yellow fever and other flavivirus infections, rickettsiosis, leptospirosis, Lassa fever, Ebola virus infection, as well as

Crimean-Congo and Korean hemorrhagic fevers. The initial clinical diagnosis would be hepatitis virus in most cases. In Africa, of course, malaria is most frequently the cause of disease with fever and malaise.

Therapy. Treatment is symptomatic, mainly to control the homeostasis and the hemorrhagic diathesis, which is believed to be the result of a disseminated intravascular coagulopathy. It has not been proven whether the acute disease phase of a patient can be improved by hemodialysis. An exchange transfusion, as has been attempted for Lassa fever, should be strictly avoided.

Regarding the finding of a hypocalcemia, substitution of ionized calcium might be advisable, at least in early cases. The risk of inducing a disseminated intravascular thrombosis might be neglectable in the presence of thrombocytopenia and deficiency in clotting factors. Hypocalcemia is most probably the explanation, why administration of clotting factors and platelet concentrates are ineffective to stop the hemorrhagic diathesis. The fact that in African populations the case fatality rate of filovirus disease is much higher as compared to European populations might in part be due to a lower efficiency of Vitamin D_3 activation in the colored skin resulting in latent hypocalcemia and inability to compensate losses of Ca^{++} in short time.

Immune serum is believed to be beneficial in some cases, but it is not available commercially and the therapeutic effect was not analyzed in clinical trials. Experimental treatment attempts with ribavirin, interferon alpha, or immunoglobulin from recovered individuals were not rewarding. Virus replication in cell culture can be stopped by lysosomotropic agents.

Transport of a patient in the acute phase to a hospital with isolation quarters is not advised, because these patients are usually in critical condition at the time of the diagnosis. Any mechanical trauma would result in extensive hematomas. A patient with hemorrhagic fever should be treated in a local hospital by personal experienced in barrier nursing techniques if such are available. High- pressure safety suits, gloves, goggles, and masks for the staff and an autoclave for disposal of infected waste are sufficient for safe barrier nursing.

Prophylaxis. Experimental vaccines have been developed. They are effective but are not clinically evaluated. Extreme caution is advisable in handling potentially infected monkeys or people and potentially infectious material. The staff should be experienced in barrier nursing techniques and appropriate equipment should be available to avoid hospital epidemics. Touching dead people with bare hands, as is common in African burial rites, can cause the spread of Marburg virus. It is mandatory, therefore, to have the cadavers cremated under controlled conditions. Convalescents are not allowed to make blood donations and should not have unprotected sexual intercourse for at least 6 months after the acute phase of the disease.

Diagnostic or experimental procedures have to be performed in BSL-4 laboratories. Safe handling of virus-infected clinical specimens in a normal clinical laboratory may present a special challenge. Whenever it is feasible, the specimens should be treated in a BSL-4 laboratory. Specimens must be inactivated by fixation or by thermal (56 °C, 30 min) or chemical treatment, before removing them from the isolation ward. The addition of detergent to a serum specimen will reduce the virus titer. Running infected specimens in a centrifuge is the most dangerous of all manipulations. Sticks with infected needles and cuts with infected knives should be avoided.

REFERENCES

Biot M, Tribute to Dr. Katenga Bonzali. *Trop. Med. Int. Health.* 5, p384, 2000.

Haenninen HM, Taï forest Ebola project: Untersuchungen von Arthropoden auf das Vorkommen von Filoviren mit der Polymerasekettenreaktion, Inauguraldissertation, Philipps-Universität Marburg, 2002.

Kiley MP et al., Filoviridae: a taxonomic home for Marburg and Ebola viruses? *Intervirology* 18, 24–32, 1982.

Siegert R et al., Zur Ätiologie einer unbekannten, von Affen ausgegangenen menschlichen *Infektionskrankheit. Dtsch. Med. Wschr.* 92, 2341–2342, 1967.

Slenczka W, The Marburg virus outbreak of 1967 and subsequent episodes. In: Klenk HD (ed.), *Marburg and Ebola Viruses. Current Topics in Microbiology and Immunology.* Vol. 235, 49–76, Springer, Berlin, Heidelberg, New York, 1999.

WHO, Marburg fever, Democratic Republic of the Congo. *Wkly. Epidemiol. Rec.* 74, 145 and 157, 1999.

WHO, Viral haemorrhagic fever/Marburg, Democratic Republic of the Congo (update). *Wkly. Epidemiol. Rec.* 75, 109, 2000.

1.7.2 EBOLA VIRUS HEMORRHAGIC FEVER

The Ebola virus has its origin in Africa. It causes hemorrhagic fever in humans with extremely high lethality rates. All known epidemics were the result of nosocomial infections with an unknown primary source of infection (index case). One case in 1994 in the Ivory Coast could be traced to an epizootic in chimpanzees with a high fatality rate. The source of three epidemics between 1996 and 2002 in Gabon, West Africa, apparently was contact with dead chimpanzees.

Etiology. The causative agent is Ebola virus. Together with Marburg virus, it forms the family *Filoviridae*. *Filoviridae* have a nonsegmented single-strand genome with minus polarity, and therefore, belong to the order *Mononegavirales*. They are closely related to the genus *Pneumovirus*. In the family of Filoviruses, Marburg virus and Ebola virus each constitute a separate genus, based on differences in their genome organization.

Maridi virus, which was isolated in 1976 during an epidemic in Sudan, is distinct from Ebola virus Zaire. Ebola virus Ivory Coast (1994) appears to represent an even more distantly related subtype. The agent of an Ebola virus epidemic in Zaire (1995), it has a close sequence homology with the agent isolated from patients in Yambuku (northern Zaire, 1976). The variation in the glycoprotein gene was only 1.2%. The primary case there apparently occurred in a forest worker who collected wood near Kikwit.

A genetically distant subtype of Ebola virus is Reston virus. The intratypic variation of the strains, which were isolated from patients in a single outbreak, is low. It is concluded that the onset of each epidemic originates from an individual index case. This is not true for the Durba outbreak of Marburg virus from 1999 to 2000.

There are remarkable differences in the pathogenicity of different subtypes of Ebola virus. Ebola Zaire has caused lethality rates of 83% or more, Ebola Sudan ca. 54%. These differences are significant, although there may be differences between outbreaks in the case definition, in data collection, and in nursing capacity.

Occurrence. Four different subtypes of the Ebola virus were isolated in Africa. The strain Maridi, originally isolated in southern Sudan in 1976 and in 1979, reappeared in Gulu, in northwest Uganda, in November 2000. In three outbreaks, the fatality rate caused by this strain has ranged between 32.5% and 65%, significantly less than the fatality rate due to the Zaire subtype. The Zaire subtype of Ebola virus, originally isolated in 1976 from a patient in Yambuku, reappeared in Kikwit in 1995. The same subtype was also isolated from patients in several outbreaks in Gabon, in the Democratic Republic of the Congo (formerly Zaire), and more recently, from outbreaks in the Republic of Congo. In these outbreaks, the fatality rate has ranged between 60% and 90%. The third African subtype, Ivory Coast, was isolated in association with an outbreak in chimpanzees in the Taï Forest in Ivory Coast. The death rate in chimpanzees was high. A scientist who had acquired the infection during an autopsy of a chimpanzee survived the disease.

The fourth subtype of Ebola virus, Reston virus, has been isolated from cynomolgus monkeys in Reston, Virginia (1989 and 1990), and in Italy (1991). The monkeys originated from the Philippines, where this subtype has also been detected. It is the first filovirus from outside of Africa. The Reston virus now has been isolated on four occasions from diseased cynomolgus monkeys that were imported from the Philippines. The latest isolate was obtained in April 1996 in Texas. Reston virus antibody was also found in swine from a Philippine pig farm. Some of the pigs died but there is no proof that they died from Ebola-Reston virus

In December 2001, Ebola virus disease appeared in the Republic of Congo and in Gabon. Thirty-two cases were diagnosed, partially by laboratory tests and by epidemiological connections. The reported fatality rate was 72%.

Monkeys were the source of human infection with the Reston virus from the Philippines. In Africa, human infections with the subtypes Zaire and Ivory Coast were associated with fatal disease in chimpanzees. Monkeys are the only known sources of filovirus infections acquired by humans. However, they can hardly be the agent reservoir because of the high filovirus pathogenicity in monkeys. The transmission cycle and reservoir of filoviruses have remained unknown in all outbreaks.

Positive serology for Ebola virus infections in humans was found in Kenya, Uganda, Liberia, and Sierra Leone (Slenczka et al. 1984). In Uganda, serologic evidence of Ebola virus infection had been obtained from human sera collected in 1992.

There is now increasing evidence that flying foxes, especially the Egyptian flying fox (*R. aegyptiacus*), may serve as the reservoir animals of the Marburg virus. These fructivorous bats may be persistently infected with filoviruses without showing overt disease. In addition, other species of Megachiroptera, such as *Hypsignathus monstrosus*, *Epomops franqueti* and *Myonycteris torquata*, may also be involved in the epidemiology. The most recent outbreak of Ebola HF in West Africa in 2014/2015 was not associated with monkeys. Instead the index case, a young boy seems to have been in contact with Megachiroptera of the species *Mops condylurus*, living in a hollow tree. The boy lived in Guinea in a village near Gueckedou and died of the disease. Slenczka et al. have published serologic data on the occurrence of Human Ebola infections in Sierra Leone in 1984 and in Liberia in 1986.

Megachiroptera live in cages and on trees eating wild figs and they contaminate the fruits with their excrements. As fruitful fig trees are also visited by a great number of other animal species, including monkeys, the fig trees may have a central position in virus transmission. The observed seasonality in filovirus outbreaks may be linked to the maturation of wild figs. Consumption of meat from monkeys and of flying foxes as "bushmeat" was in several instances identified as the primary source of outbreaks in the human population. The human-to-human spread of the virus is accelerated by family contacts and by nosocomial transmission in African hospitals with insufficient regiments of hygiene, as well as by use of non-sterile needle sticks and instruments.

The greatest Ebola outbreak, with the longest duration, and the first occurring in West Africa is presently (May 2015) going on in Guinea, Liberia and Sierra Leone, and cases were transmitted to Lagos, Nigeria, and Senegal. This outbreak became known in March 2014, some cases may have occurred earlier, and an end is not yet known. Preliminary counts of cases (26.700) and of fatalities (>11.000) are expected to be minimal estimates. The etiologic virus strain, Ebola Zaire, does not differ much from the virus that was isolated in 1976 from a case in Yambuku, Zaire. However, the epidemiologic pattern is profoundly different in a population with a high mobility and a deep distrust in Western medicine and of hospitals.

Transmission. Ebola virus epidemics have occurred predominantly during the second half of the year at the end of the rainy season. However, there is no indication of an arthropod vector. A cotton factory worker was the primary case in the Sudan epidemic. Additional cases occurred in the hospital. Almost all infections could be traced to personal contact, contact with patient blood, or accidental inoculations. Transmission by aerosol was probably not important. In the Zaire epidemic from 1976, half of the cases could be traced to inoculations with reused needle sticks in the hospital. During the latest outbreak of Ebola virus in West Africa WHO has recorded 868 cases which are believed to have resulted from nosocomial infections.

Within families, chains of up to four consecutive transmissions were found, but only 10% of contact individuals were infected and developed the disease. Burial rituals in Africa, where the deceased is touched with bare hands, has contributed significantly to the transmission of

Ebola virus in those communities. In one case, the virus was probably transmitted sexually 12 weeks after the acute disease. One infection occurred in an English high-security laboratory and could probably be explained by a defective glove used while inoculating guinea pigs. In Gabon, chimpanzees that were found dead and consumed as food gave rise to outbreaks of Ebola hemorrhagic fever on several occasions. The same route of transmission has been instrumental in the most recent outbreaks in the Republic of Congo.

An outbreak of Ebola virus disease occurred in November 2000 in Gulu, Uganda. A total of 329 disease cases were observed during a 3-month period, including 29 nurses. The case fatality rate was 32.5% (107 fatal cases). The virus isolated in Uganda was very similar to Ebola virus Maridi (1976), which may explain the low case fatality rate in comparison to outbreaks of Ebola virus Zaire. Antibodies to Ebola virus found in 1992 gave an indication that Ebola virus was present in the West Nile province of Uganda. There was probably only one primary case in the Gulu epidemic, with all additional cases being the result of human-to-human transmission. Nursing, burial rituals, and insufficient protection in the Gulu hospital were responsible.

Clinical Manifestations. The incubation period on average is 6 to 9 days, with a range of 2 to 21 days. The course of the disease is similar to that of Marburg virus disease. The onset is sudden without a prodromal period, with the following symptoms: fever, severe malaise, headaches, muscle pain, neck pain, abdominal pain, and diarrhea. In the present outbreak, it was found that a patient might lose up to 10 liters of fluid per day via the gastrointestinal tract. A hemorrhagic diathesis was found in 75% of the cases, and a maculopapular exanthema was found in 50% of the cases. During outbreaks in 1976, the case fatality rate in Sudan was 53%; in Zaire, it was 88%.

Ten percent of the diseased in Gulu, Uganda, were hospital personnel. Ebola disease was assumed in patients with fever and three additional signs: headaches (63%); nausea and vomiting (60%); anorexia; diarrhea (66%); weakness; extreme sleepiness; pain in the limbs, thorax (55%), and abdomen (48%); joint pain; discomfort in swallowing and breathing; and unexplained death. The case fatality rate in hospitalized patients was 59%; in children under 15 years of age, it was 80%. The expected dominant sign, hemorrhagic fever, was not registered in all the patients, but it signaled fatal courses, similar to the outbreak with Marburg virus in 1967.

During the latest outbreak in West Africa 868 out of 26.700 patients were classified by WHO as nosocomial infections. Several patients were treated in European and US-American hospitals and this experience has procured some additional observations. Some patients lost up to 11.000 ml of fluid per day, mainly by the enteric route. Symptoms appearing during the convalescent phase were defined as post-Ebola syndrome, which includes a state of deep exhaustion, pains in the joints and in other body regions, hearing losses, loss of vision, neurologic problems, amnesia and ataxic abasia. Intra-orbital inflammation resulted in an elevated intra-orbital pressure with refractional disturbances. As in earlier cases virus could be isolated from semen and from fluid of the anterior eye chamber. Most of these symptoms disappeared during the following weeks

Infections with a mild or clinically inapparent course have been documented in regions of endemicity. Clinically inapparent cases during an epidemic were first seen in Gabon in 1996 with an indication of virus latency. The finding might explain the occurrence of seropositive individuals who have no history of hemorrhagic fever.

A summary of Ebola virus infections up to the present—with subtype, number of cases, and percent lethality—is as follows: Zaire, 1976, 318 (88%); Zaire, 1995, 315 (81%); Ivory Coast, 1994, 2 (0%); Gabon, 1994, 44 (64%); Gabon, 1996, 37 (57%); Gabon, 1996, 60 (75%); Maridi, 1976, 284 (53%); Maridi, 1979, 34 (65%); Uganda, 2000, 329 (32.5%); Reston, 1989 and 1990, 4 (0%). There were two additional laboratory infections in England and in Russia. That makes a total of 1,430 clinical cases with 910 fatalities (64%). Filovirus infections may cause higher case fatality rates in black skinned people as compared with whites. Due to the high melanin content of their skin, black people are prone to deficiency in Vitamin D_3 and in Ca^{++} especially during the rainy season and when they are wearing western style cloths. In case of consumption coagulopathy low serum Ca^{++} seems to be the most critical factor causing hemorrhage (Egbring and Slenczka, 1971). It is not known whether or not HIV infections could have an impact on the outcome.

The outbreak of 2014/15 in West Africa (Guinea, Liberia, Sierra Leone) was caused by a virus strain resembling Ebola virus Zaire. The preliminary count of cases is >26.700, including >11.000 fatalities.

The difference in case fatality rates might be explained by a difference in pathogenicity of different virus strains. Compared with Marburg virus, Ebola virus has an additional protein, the sGP, which is believed to enhance pathogenicity by immune escape mechanisms.

Reston virus is not pathogenic for humans. Four animal caretakers became infected after contact with monkeys or by accidental inoculations. They seroconverted without clinical signs. The virus was isolated from one individual. In 2008, many pigs died on a farm on the Philippines. The cause of death was found to be a pig disease, reproductive and respiratory disease. During diagnostic work, antibodies against Ebola Reston virus were detected in the sera of some pigs, indicating that these animals had survived infections with this virus, which, however, was not the causal agent of death in the pigs.

Diagnosis. Plasma, EDTA-treated blood, urine, or liver and spleen from deceased individuals are suitable for the detection of virus by electron microscopy, isolation in cell culture (Vero cell clone E6), RT-PCR, and antigen detection with an antigen capture ELISA. These tests should only be performed by experienced personnel in special laboratories with BSL-4 precautions. Two laboratory infections with Ebola virus are known, and one of them was fatal.

Considerable sequence variations between the different African strains of Ebola virus have to be taken into account in the diagnostic RT-PCR. A highly conserved sequence from the GP gene was used by Hänninen as the target for the single-tube RT-PCR and nested PCR.

Amplification products should always be sequenced and, if possible, the diagnosis should be confirmed by the amplification of an additional sequence product from another viral gene. During a recent outbreak in the Republic of Congo (2001 to 2002), RT-PCR was proven to be useful for the diagnosis in suspected cases. During the Gulu outbreak in 2000, an antigen ELISA, an antibody ELISA, and RT-PCR were used for the diagnosis. A serological diagnosis based on IgM capture ELISA is superior to immunofluorescence towards the end of the first week of the disease. ELISA tests are used in epidemiological surveys.

Differential Diagnosis. It is important to keep in mind that hemorrhages are not seen in all the patients; they are indicators of a fatal course. Some bacterial agents may cause hemorrhagic fever more frequently than Ebola virus, for example, meningococci, leptospires, rickettsiae, salmonellae, shigellae, and EHEC. The omnipresent malaria is also to be considered. Hemorrhagic fever caused by viruses such as yellow fever and other flavivirus infections, as well as Lassa fever, Crimean-Congo hemorrhagic fever, Hantavirus, and Marburg virus infection, have to be excluded in the differential diagnosis. In children, measles has to be considered as it produces a rash and may in some cases be complicated by hemorrhagic diathesis.

Therapy. Up to 10 liters of fluid are lost per day and have to be substituted. Treatment is symptomatic predominantly to preserve homeostasis and to control the hemorrhagic diathesis and shock. Fresh blood transfusions are recommended to control the hemorrhagic diathesis under African conditions. Exchange transfusion should be strictly avoided. It has not yet been proven that hemodialysis is beneficial. Treatment with serum from recovered patients or equine hyperimmune serum is recommended but has not yet been thoroughly tested. It is presently applied in the West-African outbreak. Only limited amounts are available. Experimentally, filoviruses are susceptible to ribavirin and interferon. Replication of filoviruses in cell culture can be inhibited by lysosomotropic agents, chloroquine and quinine. An adenosine analogue, carbocyclic 3- deazadenosine, an inhibitor of the enzyme *S*- adenosylhomocysteine hydrolase, was used successfully to cure mice from an otherwise fatal Ebola virus infection. ZMapp is a preparation of monoclonal antibodies directed against the EBOV glycoprotein, which in animal experiments has prevented fatal outcome. It is only efficient against the EBOV Zaire strain.

It is not advisable to transport a patient in critical condition to a hospital with isolation wards. Patients with hemorrhagic fever should be treated in the local hospital by experienced personnel. Any mechanical trauma might result in extended hemorrhages. Pressurized safety suits for the staff and all other WHO recommended protective equipment are needed to establish safe barrier nursing techniques.

It is known that deficiency in ionized calcium is an indicator of fatal outcome in filovirus infections. Loss of calcium may be regarded as the limiting factor in the consumption coagulopathy. Maintenance of calcium homeostasis should therefore be an urgent demand, especially in fresh cases at the most early convenience. The influence of calcium substitution on the course of disease should be evaluated in animal experiments. It is very likely that the failure of transfusion, platelets and of plasma fractions to control the hemorrhagic diathesis is due to deficiency of ionized calcium. The problem of calcium substitution might be an increase of disseminated intravascular clotting as an adverse effect.

Prophylaxis. Up to this time, far more than 150 nosocomial infections have occurred in West African hospitals during the present outbreak. Two cases were transmitted in a hospital in Texas from a single patient and one case occurred in a nurse in a Madrid hospital, where two patients had been treated. In Africa, it is mandatory to have the deceased in an Ebola virus outbreak cremated by experienced personnel to prevent virus transmission by direct contact. Burial habits in which the deceased individual is touched by friends and relatives with bare hands have contributed to virus propagation in several outbreaks, not only in the Democratic Republic of Congo, but also in Uganda. People who had been in contact with the patient should be observed for 21 days, the longest known incubation period. Convalescents are not allowed to donate blood and should not have unprotected sexual intercourse for at least 6 months after the acute phase of the disease.

Extreme caution should be taken in handling infected or potentially infected individuals, as well as infected material. Experimental work has to be performed in biosafety level 4 laboratories. Safety laboratories (biosafety level 4) and experienced staff are located at the CDC in Atlanta, Georgia; Marburg, Germany (Institute for Virology); London and Sandringham, UK; Johannesburg, South Africa; Winnipeg, Canada; and Koltsovo, Russia. Safe handling of virus infected clinical specimens in a normal clinical laboratory may present a special challenge. Whenever feasible, the specimens should be treated in the level 4 lab. Specimens must be inactivated by fixation, thermal (56 °C, 30 min), or chemical treatment before they are removed from the isolation ward. Addition of detergent to a serum specimen will reduce the virus titer. Running infected specimens in a centrifuge is the most dangerous of all manipulations. Sticks with infected needles and cuts with infected knives should be avoided.

Promising candidate vaccines have been tested in animals. Protection was induced with a hybrid vaccine based on vesicular stomatitis virus recombinant for Ebola GP (VSV-Zebov GP I) vaccine. Considering the unknown epidemiology it is questionable whether there are sufficient indications for the clinical evaluation and use of such a vaccine. Improved safety regulations for hospital personnel are most important. Africans must be instructed not to use monkeys or flying foxes that are found dead for food.

REFERENCES

Baxter AG, Symptomless infection with Ebola virus. *Lancet* 355, 2178–2179, 2000.

Burton DR, Parren PW, Fighting the Ebola virus. *Nature* 408, 527–528, 2000.

CDC, Outbreak of Ebola hemorrhagic fever Uganda, August 2000–January 2001.

MMWR Morb. *Mortal Wkly. Rep.* 50, 73–74, 2001.

Haenninen HM, Taï forest Ebola Projekt: Untersuchungen von Arthropoden auf das Vorkommen von Filoviren mit der Polymerasekettenreaktion. *Inauguraldissertation*, Philipps-Universität Marburg, 2001.

Le Guenno B, Formenty P, Boesch C, Ebola virus outbreaks in the Ivory Coast and Liberia, 1994–1995. In: Klenk HD (ed.), *Marburg and Ebola viruses. Current Topics in Microbiology and Immunology*. Vol. 235, 77–84, Springer, Berlin, Heidelberg, New York, 1999.

Leroy EM et al., Human asymptomatic Ebola infection and strong inflammatory response. *Lancet* 355, 2210–2215, 2000.

MacDonald R, Ebola virus claims more lives in Uganda. *BMJ* 321, 1037, 2000.

Peters CJ, Khan AS, Filovirus diseases. In: Klenk HD (ed.), *Marburg and Ebola viruses. Current topics in microbiology and immunology*. Vol. 235, 85–96, Springer, Berlin, Heidelberg, New York, 1999.

Peters CJ, LeDuc JW, An introduction to Ebola: the virus and the disease. *J. Infect. Dis.* 179, Suppl., 9–16, 1999.

Pushko P et al., Individual and bivalent vaccines based on alphavirus replicons protect guinea pigs against infection with Lassa and Ebola viruses. *J. Virol.* 75, 11677–11685, 2001.

Slenczka, W. et al., Seroepidemiologische Untersuchungen über das Vorkommen von Antikörpern gegen Marburg- und Ebola-Virus in Afrika. *Mitt. Oesterr. Ges. Tropenmed. Parasitol.* 6, 53–60, 1984.

Sullivan NJ et al., Development of a preventive vaccine for Ebola virus infection in primates. *Nature* 408, 605–609, 2000.

Vanderzanden L et al., DNA vaccines expressing either the GP or NP genes of Ebola virus protect mice from lethal challenge. *Virology* 246, 134–144, 1998.

WHO, Ebola, Uganda (update). *Wkly Epidemiol. Rec.* 75, 369, 2000.

1.8 Zoonoses Caused by Rhabdoviruses

The family *Rhabdoviridae* includes plant viruses (two genera) and three genera of animal viruses: *Lyssavirus* (Tab. 1.4), *Vesiculovirus* (Tab. 1.5), and *Ephemerovirus*. Only lyssaviruses and some vesiculoviruses are zoonotic. The prototype of the family is rabies virus, the etiologic agent of a zoonosis with the longest known history. *Rhabdoviridae*, *Filoviridae*, and *Paramyxoviridae* are all members of the *Mononegavirales*. They have an unsegmented single-stranded RNA genome with antimessenger polarity.

The genetic program of rhabdoviruses includes only five genes: those encoding the nucleocapsid protein (N), phosphoprotein (P), matrix protein (M), receptor binding protein (G), and polymerase (L). The virus particle has the shape of a bullet with one blunt and one pointed pole. They are also called bullet-shaped

Table 1.4a | Genus *Lyssavirus*[1]

SEROTYPE	HOST	GEOGRAPHICAL OCCURRENCE
Rabies virus (lyssavirus type 1)[2]	Canids, raccoons, skunks, etc.	Worldwide
Lagos bat virus (lyssavirus type 2)	Fructivorous bats	Africa
Mokola virus (lyssavirus type 3)	Fructivorous bats	Africa
Duvenhage virus (lyssavirus type 4)	Fructivorous bats	South Africa
European bat virus type 1 (lyssavirus type 5)	Insectivorous bats	Europe
European bat virus type 2 (lyssavirus type 6)	Insectivorous bats	Europe
Australian bat virus (lyssavirus type 7)	Flying foxes (Megachiroptera)	Australia

[1] Based on molecular genetics and immunological differences, it has been proposed that two phylogroups within the seven known subtypes of rabies virus be formed. Group 1 includes the classical rabies virus (type 1) as well as bat viruses (types 4 to 7). Phylogroup 2 covers the two West African bat viruses (types 2 and 3). There are more batborne rabies viruses. Their pathogenicity is not proven in all cases.

[2] This is the most important rabies agent. It induces more than 99% of all rabies cases worldwide. Only some countries with insular or peninsular geography are free from rabies virus (e.g., New Zealand, Australia, Japan, United Kingdom, and Scandinavia).

Table 1.4b | Genus *Vesiculovirus*[1]

VIRUS	GEOGRAPHICAL OCCURRENCE	VECTOR(S)
VSV type 1 (Indiana)	USA	*Phlebotomus* sand flies VSV type 2 (New Jersey)
	USA	
VSV type 3 (Cocal)[2]	USA	
VSV type 4 (Alagoas)[2]	USA	
Chandipura virus	India	
Isfahan virus	Iran	*Phlebotomus papatasii*
Piry virus	Brazil	

[1] There are more than 20 virus types within this genus. Only five of them are known to cause human disease.
[2] Virus sometimes classified as a subtype of VSV Indiana.

viruses. The proteins N, P, and L are attached to the nucleocapsid within the virus particle. The M protein is located between the nucleocapsid and the outer membrane with the G protein as the only glycoprotein that combines the functions of receptor binding and fusion.

REFERENCES

Smith JS, Rabies virus. In: Murray PR et al. (eds.), *Manual of Clinical Microbiology*, 1544–1552, 8th ed. Vol 2. ASM Press Washington, DC, 2003.

Tsai TF, Chandler LJ, Arboviruses. In: Murray PR et al. (eds.), *Manual of Clinical Microbiology*, 1553–1569, 8th ed. Vol 2. ASM Press, Washington, DC, 2003.

Tesh R et al., Isfahan virus, a new vesiculovirus infecting humans, gerbil and sandflies in Iran. Am. *J. Trop. Med. Hyg.* 26, 299–306, 1977.

1.8.1 RABIES

Rabies is an acute, almost inevitably fatal zoonotic disease. It has a worldwide distribution. Humans and nearly all mammals are susceptible. Besides poliomyelitis and pox, rabies is one of the longest-known infectious diseases in human history.

Etiology. At least seven serotypes of rabies virus are known. Six of them are transmitted by bats. Type 1 of rabies virus is not found in insect- or fruit-eating bats worldwide. However, vampire bats in South and Central America can be infected with type 1. More recently, lyssavirus type 7 has been isolated from flying foxes (*Pteropus alecto* and *P. scapulatus*) in Australia. This virus has caused two human fatalities. Rabies had not been known to occur in Australia until that time.

Occurrence. The epidemiology of rabies is complicated. It differs from continent to continent and from country to country depending on the fauna and state of development. It is necessary to distinguish between urban and sylvan rabies (Fig. 1.11). The urban type is predominantly found in developing countries in Asia and Africa. Stray dogs transmit the disease and serve as virus reservoirs. The sylvan form of rabies is mostly seen in developed countries in the

Table 1.5a | Recommendations for treatment of animal bites

1. Immediate local treatment: wash the wound with soap and water with a detergent. If not available, use water alone. Rinse thoroughly with water and 40% to 70% alcohol, followed by tincture of iodine or a 0.1% quaternary ammonium compound.
2. Treatment by a physician: treatment of the wound as described above. Infiltration in and around the wound with rabies immunoglobulin. Rabies prophylaxis with human diploid cell culture vaccine. *No suture in the wound.* If indicated, antibiotic and tetanus prophylaxis.

Table 1.5b | Recommendations for postexposure rabies prophylaxis[1]

ANIMAL	SITUATION OF THE BITING ANIMAL	TREATMENT OF EXPOSED INDIVIDUALS
Domestic (dogs, cats)	Healthy: rabies can be ruled out for epidemiological reasons	No vaccination: observe the animal
	Healthy: rabies exposure cannot be ruled out	Active and passive vaccination
	Rabid, unknown, or stray	Active and passive vaccination
Wild (foxes, skunks, raccoons, coyotes, other carnivores, deer, bats)	Should be considered rabies positive	Active and passive vaccination
Other	Depends on epidemiological situation (consult with state veterinarian)	If needed, active and passive vaccination

[1] It is important to vaccinate within 24 h after exposure if indicated. It is life threatening to wait, for example, to observe the animal that has bitten a person. The decision to vaccinate is no longer influenced by possible side effects of the vaccine when modern vaccines are used.

Northern Hemisphere. Dogs, cats, or other domestic animals come in contact with infected sylvan or rural reservoir animals and transmit the disease. Bat rabies, which is less frequent, belongs both to the sylvan and to the urban types. Some countries with insular geography, such as Australia, New Zealand, the United Kingdom, and Japan, are free of canine rabies but may harbor bat rabies.

Rabies is most common in developing countries in Asia and Africa. Between 25,000 and 50,000 human cases are reported every year. In 1997, there were 33,000 cases in Asia, 30,000 of them in India. A total of 114 cases were seen in North and South America, four of them in the United States. Europe had 13 cases, or less than 0.1% of the total occurrence. It can be assumed that more unreported cases occurred in Asia and Africa. Rabies in developed countries is often imported. Of five cases registered in Germany since 1981, two were indigenous and three were imported from India. It is debatable whether there are rabies-free countries besides isolated islands because of the more recently discovered bat rabies problems. Island communities, such as Japan, Australia, Oceania, Great Britain, Ireland, Malta, and Cyprus, or border countries like Portugal and the countries of Scandinavia, may be free of canid (terrestrial) rabies. However, they are not free of bat rabies, as recorded in England, Australia (1998), and Denmark (1998).

Detection of lyssavirus in bats in Europe was positive in 142 bats between 1987 and 1995. The percentage of bats involved in sylvan rabies in Germany is 0.7%; in the United States it is 7.7%. Only insectivorous bats occur in the United States and Europe. Only one bat virus strain was isolated in the United States among 78 rabies virus-infected dogs and 230 rabies virus-infected cats. Occasionally, the rabies virus has been transmitted by mice (Microtinae), badgers, and martens, which seems to be of minor importance epidemiologically. Besides domestic animals (cattle, sheep, goats, horses, and pigs), the following species are involved in rabies epidemics: the arctic fox (*Alopex lagopus*); the red fox (*Vulpes vulpes*) in Canada, New York State, and Central and Western Europe; the gray fox (*Urocyon cinereoargenteus*) in focal areas in the United States; the raccoon

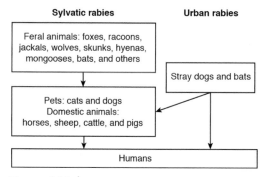

Figure 1.11 | Infection chain of rabies.

dog (*Nyctereutes procyonoides*) in Eastern Europe and Scandinavia; jackals and wild dogs (*Canis* spp.) in Asia and Africa; the striped skunk (*Mephitis mephitis*) and spotted skunk (*Spilogale putorius*) in the midwestern United States and in western Canada; raccoons (*Procyon lotor*) in the eastern United States (north to south); the yellow mongoose (*Cynictis penicillata*) in Asia and Africa; and the Indian mongoose (*Herpestris javanicus auropunctatus*) in Asia and Africa and some islands in the Caribbean. In the eastern United States, raccoon rabies spread recently from Georgia to the state of New York, introduced by imported raccoons from Florida. Rabid wolves (*Canis lupus*) are encountered in Alaska, Siberia, India, and Ethiopia.

Bat rabies occurs worldwide, including (as mentioned above) islands which are free of canid rabies. Forty species of insectivorous bats in the United States and Canada can be infected with the rabies virus. Rabies-infected bats are also present in Europe and Africa, but they are less important epidemiologically. Fruit-eating bats [flying foxes (suborder Megachiroptera, including *P. alecto* and *P. scapulatus*)] were identified in Australia as rabies carriers. They have caused two human fatalities. Vampire bats (three species, mainly *Desmodus rotundus*) are important rabies carriers that transmit the virus in the Andes from Mexico to Argentina. They live in caves and endanger tourists and researchers by biting and by transmitting rabies via aerosol. In Europe, where only insectivorous bats are known to occur, three human cases of rabies acquired from bats have been recorded since 1977. The most recent case occurred in 2002 in a British wildlife artist and bat handler who was affected in Angus, Scotland. He had refused to be vaccinated prophylactically. The bat species involved in this accident was said to have been a Daubenton's bat. This was the first human case of rabies in the United Kingdom since 1902. Nevertheless, dogs and cats (pets and stray) are the most important sources of human infections worldwide.

Transmission. The rabies virus is transmitted in saliva by the bite of an infected animal. Saliva becomes infectious by 3 to 5 days post infection. The virus travels from the site of infection along the peripheral nerves to the CNS. The salivary glands become infected via nerves from the brain. Infected saliva may contain up to 10^6 mouse ID_{50}/ml.

The virus cannot penetrate intact skin. The danger of rabies transmission by saliva-contaminated objects is small, although the virus can be found in secretions. An infection via broken skin and mucous membranes (conjunctivae) is possible. Aerosol transmission under natural conditions is rare. However, laboratory infections and infections in bat caves by aerosol are known to occur. Transmission from human-to-human is possible. This has mainly been documented in cases of corneal transplantations where rabies had not been diagnosed as the cause of death of the donor.

Close contact with infected animals enhances the chances of infection. Children playing with cats and dogs are especially endangered, even if they are not bitten. The virus can penetrate through scratch lesions. Only nine of 33 rabies cases in the United States between 1977 and 1994 could be traced to animal bites. The patients in three of the nine cases were exposed in the United States; six were exposed in other countries. In Europe (with the exception of the countries of the former USSR), there were 45 rabies cases from 1977 to 1991, 16 of which were imported.

The question of how long rabies virus remains virulent in dead animals often arises. Extreme caution should always be taken. With progressive autolysis, the virus becomes inactivated. However, during winter or under refrigeration, a cadaver may carry a live virus for 4 weeks to several months. The virus does not survive in dried secretions or blood for more than a few hours. There are no known cases of virus transmission from contaminated utensils.

One out of five individuals develops rabies after being exposed to rabies virus, if they are not protected by prophylactic or postexposure vaccination. Development of rabies in exposed individuals depends on the type and localization of the bite. Lesions on the head, neck, and arms are most dangerous. The amount of virus carried into the wound also plays a significant role; for example, when a bite has to penetrate clothing, virus in the saliva may be retained in the fabric.

The bite lesions from bats are rarely observed when they transmit rabies. Of 32 rabies cases registered in the United States since 1980, 17 were bat virus induced, but a history of a bat bite was only known in one case. One woman in Australia died from rabies exposure after being scratched by a flying fox. Bat virus has been transmitted to cave researchers by aerosol in bat caves in the Andes. There is a report from two rural communities in Peru where 636 people died in 1990 with clinical signs of rabies in the Amazon rainforest. A vampire bat virus was isolated from one patient. When 22 of the victims were questioned, 21 reported being bitten by a vampire bat.

According to reports from Asia, children are exposed to animal bites and exposure to rabies virus more frequently than adults are. Most of these bites are from dogs, but wolves are also involved.

There is little evidence for rabies infections from animal products. Several people were vaccinated in Massachusetts after they had consumed unpasteurized milk from a rabid cow. There was no evidence of virus in the milk, but its presence was considered possible.

In several instances, rabies has been transmitted with organ transplants when the donor had died from an undiagnosed rabies infection. The first cases that became known were infected with corneal transplants. Meanwhile, cases have become known from the USA and Germany in which rabies was transmitted with kidneys, liver, and lungs. All the acceptors have died from rabies. One patient who had received rabies infected lung survived. He had been vaccinated against rabies 12 years before the organ transplantation and had neutralizing antibodies.

Clinical Manifestations. The incubation period varies considerably from 10 days to 3 months and up to years. The shortest reported incubation period was 5 days, and the longest was 2 years, but 75% of patients become ill within 90 days. The closer the bite is to the CNS and the deeper it is, the shorter the incubation period is.

Pathogenic strains of rabies virus differ from attenuated variants by the marker neuroinvasiveness. Viral receptors are found in the endplates of motor neurons but not in sensory neurons. The virus migrates to the CNS by retrograde axonal transport. The incubation time is dependent on the distance from the periphery to the brain and the speed of migration. In animal experiments with "virus fixe," the speed was measured at 3 mm/h. Strains of "street virus" differ in their speed of migration. The speed is determined by mutations in the receptor binding G-protein. At the site of the bite, the virus causes only minimal inflammatory reactions. The virus blocks the type I interferon system. Structure and function of the infected neurons remain intact for some time. In the CNS, the virus is protected from humoral and cellular immune mechanisms. Virulent strains of rabies are able to block the apoptosis of infected neurons.

A prodromal period of 2 to 4 days marks the onset of the disease. The patient complains about nausea, vomiting, and headaches. Slight fever is possible. Paresthesia and pain on the side of the bite is often reported. Human rabies typically presents in two manifestations, furious and paralytic. The furious period begins with restlessness, saliva discharge, cold sweat, fear of death, rage, insomnia, convulsions, tonic-clonic spasms, and fibrillary muscle twitching: the furious rage. The patient cannot swallow; there are painful spasms of the pharynx muscles, which lead to hydrophobia. The patient is extremely sensitive to air movements (aerophobic) and noise. Death may occur during a spasm attack within days of this phase. The furious period may be followed by a paralytic stage with flaccid paralysis of the head muscles (eyes, face, tongue, and throat) and less frequently of the limbs. The patient dies in this stage after 3 or 4 days as a consequence of respiratory and heart failure. In some cases, the furious stage does not occur and the paralytic phase follows directly after the prodromal period (silent rage). In these cases, clinical diagnosis is possible only if previous animal contacts are known. The prognosis in both forms of rabies is hopeless. There are only three documented cases of unvaccinated rabies survivors.

Rabies in animals may take a variety of courses, depending on the virus strain, the age and species of the animal, and the route of infection. The disease in animals is fatal almost without exception, within 4 to 10 days of clinical signs. Change in behavior is noticed first: restlessness or apathy, enhanced or reduced excitability, aggression or daze, and finally death caused by paralysis. Wild animals hide or lose fear of humans. If touched, they respond by biting. Signs of disease can vary greatly or may even be absent. Serengeti spotted hyenas do not show symptomatic disease despite a high frequency of exposure to rabies virus. Purebred dogs are more susceptible than mixed-breed dogs.

Diagnosis. A thorough history (animal bite or contact with rabid animal) is needed to suspect rabies. An early tentative diagnosis is possible if the history includes animal bites, contact with diseased or dead animals, contact with wild animals, or a visit to countries with urban rabies or to caves in South or Central America. Cases with atypical transmission histories and atypical signs of disease are usually only diagnosed postmortem. Because corneal transplants are known to have transmitted rabies, it must be assumed that some cases may remain undiagnosed.

Pathognomonic signs, such as furious excitation, paresthesia on the side of a bite, or hydrophobia, usually appear only after uncharacteristic early signs, which may last for several days. There is a leukocytosis (20,000 to 30,000 leukocytes/mm3), a slight protein increase, and in a minority, lymphocytic pleocytosis in the CSF, as well as a slight shedding of albumin in urine.

For the detection of rabies virus in patients, only positive results are reliable. Direct immunofluorescence is a reliable test for the demonstration of viral antigen (Negri bodies) in corneal imprints, in skin biopsy specimens from the face or neck, or in brain biopsy specimens. The best areas in which to find the virus postmortem are the hippocampus, thalamus, hypothalamus, cerebellum, and brain stem. The virus can be isolated from saliva in cell culture or by intracerebral inoculation of mice. The virus can be demonstrated after 3 days in cell culture by immunofluorescence. RT-PCR can be used to detect the virus in tissue samples or in secretions.

Special reference laboratories provide the diagnosis of rabies in animals and humans. For large and small animals suspected to be infected with rabies virus, the head or the whole body, respectively, should be submitted, refrigerated but not frozen and not fixed, for analysis. For rabies diagnosis in humans and living animals, samples of saliva, conjunctival and corneal imprints, and skin biopsy specimens from the head should be examined. The samples must be refrigerated, must be protected from drying and leakage, and must be sent to the laboratory by the most expeditious route. Conjunctival and corneal imprints for immunofluorescence must be made on fat-free glass slides and air-dried. The imprint area is to be circled with a diamond point marker. The imprint must be fixed for 15 min in cold acetone (−20 °C). *Warning: fixed preparations can still be infectious!* It is best to ask the receiving laboratory for specimen requirements and the preferred manner of delivery.

The sensitivity and efficacy of the *in vivo* and postmortem diagnosis of rabies have been greatly improved by the introduction of PCR. These techniques have been successfully used for confirmation of rabies in biting animals but also for humans with suspected rabies. CSF and saliva are the best sources for the *in vivo* approach and brain tissue is used for postmortem tests. The detection of virus RNA in saliva has been shown to be considerably more sensitive than the immunohistological demonstration in skin biopsy specimens or corneal imprints. It is important to extract RNA from samples immediately, without any delay. The choice of primers depends on the anticipated rabies type. A group-specific RT-PCR targeting the N gene of rabies virus can be carried out (see the literature, end of the chapter). In addition, sequences from bat virus types 2 to 7 can be covered in a multiplex PCR, depending on the epidemiological circumstances.

Serological tests (ELISA), virus neutralization, and indirect immunofluorescence are of no use in the diagnosis because the antibody appears only late during the course of the disease, not earlier. Also, specimens from vaccinated individuals yield a positive reaction. Antibody in the CSF is diagnostic, provided it is not the result of a postvaccinal neurological reaction.

Virus detection in the brain is important for diagnostic purposes in animals that have died or have been killed. Useful tests for the detection are RT-PCR, direct immunofluorescence, and mouse inoculation.

Neutralizing antibody can be detected in people after prophylactic vaccination by means of a fluorescent focus inhibition test.

Differential Diagnosis. Tetanus, allergic postvaccinal encephalitis, poliomyelitis, Guillain-Barré syndrome, delirium tremens, and intoxication with belladonna alkaloids have to be excluded in the differential diagnosis. Acute thallium intoxication may mimic rabies in a dog. Occasionally patients were admitted to psychiatric hospitals, when symptoms of rabies were misinterpreted.

Monkey bites may transmit not only rabies virus but also herpes B virus. Coma may appear as the first sign of a herpes encephalitis. There are many other forms of encephalitis that have to be differentiated from paralytic or "dumb" rabies. Intracranial tumors and hemorrhages may cause symptoms resembling paralytic rabies. Patients with psychotic manifestations of rabies are sometimes taken to psychiatric wards. Conversely, hysterical reactions after an animal bite can produce rabies-like symptoms, which is to be suspected when a patient recovers spontaneously.

A history of traveling and animal contact is always important in the diagnosis of rabies.

Therapy. Vaccination postexposure is the only chance for potentially infected individuals. Simultaneous vaccination (active and passive) has to be applied within 24 h after exposure and can prevent the disease in humans. It is the responsibility of the physician to recognize the indication for vaccination in a person after contact with an animal known or suspected to be rabid. After exposure, bite and scratch lesions should be washed immediately with soap, water, and disinfectants. Rabies serum or, better, rabies immunoglobulin (of human origin) should be inoculated around the wounds. Postexposure vaccination should be performed as quickly as possible. Human diploid cell culture (HDC) or purified rabies cell culture vaccines are available. Six sequential injections should be made in individuals without a previous rabies vaccination. No treatment begun after symptoms have appeared has ever been successful; almost all patients die with the disease or its complications within a few weeks of onset.

Rabies is still common in Asia. Attempts are being made to reduce the number of human cases by postexposure vaccination with improved vaccines (cell culture vaccines instead of rabbit brain vaccines). Individuals at high risk for rabies will be vaccinated prophylactically. Fifteen million people annually are vaccinated postexposure. It is essential to vaccinate as soon as possible after exposure. Vaccination failures can be traced to late vaccinations. Experimentally, rats did not develop rabies if they were treated with monoclonal antibodies within 24 h after exposure.

Tab. 1.5b illustrates the WHO recommendations for postexposure rabies vaccination. If a person is bitten by a dog, it is irrelevant whether the dog was vaccinated or not. The dog can still be infectious. Contact of humans with bats that entered living quarters or that showed abnormal behavior are an indication for vaccination in the United States. Bat bites are usually not detectable.

Dogs may pick up vaccine bait for wildlife that contains modified live rabies virus. If humans come in contact with a vaccine bait, vaccination is indicated, because it is not known whether the modified virus is pathogenic for humans.

Further specific therapy for clinical rabies is not known. Although the prognosis is almost hopeless (rabies is irreversible), each person has to be treated in an intensive care setting. It is important to maintain homeostasis of fluid and electrolytes, to treat brain edema, and to sedate. Treatment with interferon alone or in combination with ribavirin can be attempted. Worldwide, three patients with overt clinical rabies recovered with intensive care therapy. A "successful cure" of a patient was reported in 2004 from the USA. She was treated with a therapeutically induced coma according to the Milwaukee protocol, and was cured with considerable neurologic defects. The Milwaukee protocol since that time has been applied several times in a modified form. It resulted in life prolongation but a cure was not achieved. In 2011, a successful cure of an 8-year-old girl was reported. Most reports on clinical cure of manifest rabies are more or less doubtful. Therefore, the diagnosis of manifest rabies still has an unfavorable prognosis.

Prophylaxis. Protective immunity can be induced by vaccination with a combination of glycoprotein and capsid protein of the rabies virus. Prophylactic vaccination with HDC or primary chick embryo culture vaccines is safe and efficacious. Both are used to vaccinate individuals who are in danger of exposure, such as veterinarians, game wardens, and farm and forest workers. People in contact with bats need prophylactic rabies vaccination, even in those countries where rabies is not known to be endemic. Three vaccinations are given at monthly intervals with booster inoculations after 1-year and again after 2 to 5 years. Protection can be monitored with an FFIT (serum neutralization test).

The annual human rabies occurrence in China has been reduced from 5,200 to 200 cases by prophylactic vaccination. There are similar reports from Thailand. The WHO supports the concept that highly endangered countries should produce their own vaccines.

The vaccination of dogs and cats is mandatory in many countries. In addition, stray animals should be euthanized to prevent the spread of rabies. Gassing of foxholes has been used to reduce the fox population. Today, vaccination of foxes and raccoons is accomplished with baits containing live virus vaccines. Three different attenuated virus vaccines and a recombinant vaccinia-rabies glycoprotein vaccine are used for wildlife vaccinations. As a result, seroconversion was found in 70% of foxes. Rabies in wild and domestic animals in Europe and rabies in feral animals has been reduced by more than 80%. Similar results were obtained with raccoons in the United States. The population of foxes in Europe has now increased considerably, creating a different potential hazard: the fox tapeworm (*Echinococcus multilocularis*) may spread and human infections might occur more frequently when more foxes are living in the vicinity of villages or in cities.

Developing countries do not have the means to control stray dogs that transmit urban rabies. Rules of religion may prevent measures being taken against stray dogs, as is the case in India. Sylvan rabies can be drastically reduced or even eliminated, as can be seen in Europe and North America. Similar concepts could be used to control urban rabies, at least in non flying carnivores. There is little experience available for the control of rabies in bats.

A specific rabies prophylaxis is usually not indicated after touching small rodents (squirrels, hamsters, guinea pigs, rabbits, rats, or mice). Children having had intensive contact with an infected pet should be vaccinated, even if they were not bitten. In the United States and many other countries, direct bat contact (bite) or even the presence of a bat in the room is an indication for rabies vaccination, including active and passive vaccination and injection of rabies hyperimmune globulin around the wound. If possible, the attacking animal should be tested for rabies virus.

Any individual with a bite or lesion caused by an animal that is rabid or suspected to be rabid should be considered to be infected (Tab. 1.5b).

It is important to notice whether any potentially infectious material (blood, saliva, or other secretions) has come in contact with open wounds or mucous membranes. The virus does not survive outside its host for extended time periods, especially when dried in secretions. Virus survival in animal cadavers depends on the outside temperature and the condition of the cadaver. When frozen, the virus can persist for weeks.

These recommendations should be followed for postexposure simultaneous vaccination of unvaccinated individuals:

1. Active immunization with a rabies vaccine, for example, Rabipur®, on days 0, 3, 7, 14, 30, and 90 postexposure. Novartis Vaccines.

2. Passive immunization once i.v. with human rabies immunoglobulin, for example, Berirab® CSL Behring.

In previously vaccinated individuals, the vaccination can be reduced to days 0 and 3 if the previous vaccination was within 1 year, or to days 0, 3, and 7 when the previous vaccination was 1 to 5 years ago.

The recommendation for prophylactic vaccination before exposure is that rabies vaccine (e.g., Rabipur or Rabivax) should be administered on days 0, 28, and 56, and again after 12 months.

REFERENCES

Badrane H et al., Evidence of two Lyssavirus phylogroups with distinct pathogenicity and immunogenicity. *J. Virol.* 75, 3268–3276, 2001.

Black EM et al., Molecular methods to distinguish between classical rabies and the rabies-related European bat lyssaviruses. *J. Virol. Methods* 87, 123–131, 2000.

Blanton JD, Rupprecht CE, Travel vaccination for rabies. *Expert Rev. Vacc.* 7, 613–620, 2008.

Bronnert J et al., Organ transplantation and rabies transmission. *J. Travel. Med.* 14, 177–180, 2007.

CDC, Human rabies prevention United States 1999 (ACIP). *Supplement to Morbidity and Mortality* Vol. 48, Jan. 1999.

CDC, Mass vaccination of humans who drank unpasteurized milk from rabid cows. *MMWR* Vol. 48, 228–229, 1999.

Crepin P et al., Intravitam diagnosis of human rabies by PCR using saliva and cerebrospinal fluid. *J. Clin. Microbiol.* 36, 1117–1121, 1998.

Echevarria JE et al., Screening of active lyssavirus infection in wild bat populations by viral RNA detection on oropharyngeal swabs. *J. Clin. Microbiol.* 39, 3678–3683, 2001.

Field H, McCall B, Barrett J, Australian bat lyssavirus infection in a captive juvenile black flying fox. *Emerg. Infect. Dis.* 5, 438–440, 1999.

Fraser GC et al., Encephalitis caused by a lyssavirus in fruit bats in *Australia. Emerg. Infect. Dis.* 2, 327–331, 1996.

Fu ZF et al., Oral vaccination of raccoons (Procyon lotor) with baculovirus-expressed rabies virus glycoprotein. *Vaccine* 11, 925–928, 1993.

Hanna JN et al., Australian bat lyssavirus infection: a second human case, with a long incubation period. *Med. J. Aust.* 172, 597–599, 2000.

Heaton PR et al., Seminested PCR assay for detection of six genotypes of rabies and rabies-related viruses. *J. Clin. Microbiol.* 35, 2762–2766, 1997.

Johnson N, Cunningham AF, Fooks AR, The immune response to rabies virus infection and vaccination. *Vaccine* 28, 3896–3901, 2010.

Johnson N et al., Human rabies due to lyssavirus infection of bat origin. *Vet. Microbiol.* 142, 151–159, 2010.

Leung AK, Davies HD, Hon KL, Rabies: epidemiology, pathogenesis, and prophylaxis. *Adv. Ther.* 24, 1340–1347, 2007.

Madsen PL, Danger from rabies-infected bats. *Lancet* 355, 934, 2000.

Moran GJ et al., Appropriateness of rabies postexposure prophylaxis treatment for animal exposures. Emergency ID Net Study Group. *JAMA* 284, 1001–1007, 2000.

Morimoto K et al., Characterization of a unique variant of bat rabies virus responsible for newly emerging human cases in North *America. Proc. Natl. Acad. Sci. USA* 93, 5653–5658, 1996.

Nel LH, Markotter W, *Lyssaviruses. Crit. Rev. Microbiol.* 33, 301–324, 2007.

Nigg AJ, Walker PL, Overview, prevention, and treatment of rabies. *Pharmacotherapy* 29, 1182–1195, 2009.

Pape WJ, Fitzsimmons TD, Hoffman RE, Risk for rabies transmission from encounters with bats, Colorado, 1977–1996. *Emerg. Infect. Dis.* 5, 433–437, 1999.

Plotkin S, Rabies: State-of-the-Art. *Clinical Picture. Clin. Inf. Dis.,* 30, 4–5, 2000.

Ruiz M, Chavez CB, Rabies in Latin America. *Neurol. Res.* 32, 272–277, 2010.

Rupprecht CE et al., Evidence for a 4-dose vaccine schedule for human rabies post-exposure prophylaxis in previously non-vaccinated individuals. *Vaccine* 27, 7141–7148, 2009.

Schnell MJ et al., The cell biology of rabies: using stealth to reach the brain. *Nat. Rev. Microbiol.* 8, 51–61, 2010.

Wacharapluesadee S, Hemachudha T, Nucleicacid sequence based amplification in the rapid diagnosis of rabies. *Lancet* 358, 892–893, 2001.

Warner CK et al., Laboratory investigation of human deaths from vampire bat rabies in Peru. Am. *J. Trop. Med. Hyg.* 60, 502–507, 1999.

Whitby JE et al., First isolation of a rabies-related virus from a Daubenton's bat in the United Kingdom. *Vet. Rec.* 147, 385–388, 2000.

Wu X et al., Reemerging rabies and lack of systemic in People's Republic of China. *Emerg. Infect. Dis.* 15, 1159–1164, 2009.

1.8.2 Vesicular Stomatitis

Vesicular stomatitis (VS) is a highly contagious infectious disease in horses, mules, cattle, and less frequently, pigs. Because of the vesicle formation in the oral mucosa and on hoofs in ruminants, it cannot be differentiated clinically from foot-and-mouth disease (FMD). A truncated VSV genome was used as a vector for a live Filovirus vaccine.

Etiology

The causative agents of VS are VS viruses (VSVs) in the genus *Vesiculovirus* of the family *Rhabdoviridae*. There are more than 20 serotypes within the genus, four of which are important as human pathogens: VSV serotype Indiana (with its subtypes Cocal virus and Alagoas virus), VSV serotype New Jersey, Chandipura virus, and Piry virus. The four virus types have a cross-reactive nucleocapsid antigen and a type-specific glycoprotein. Group-specific serological reactions exist, but there is no cross-protection see Table 1.4b). There are several other virus strains that could be considered to be subtypes or individual serotypes. Isfahan virus, for example, infects humans in Iran but it has not been associated with human disease.

Occurrence

VSV exists in North and South America, Africa, and Asia but not in Central Europe. There must be an unusually large host spectrum of VSVs, based on virus isolation and antibody detection. Host spectrum and virus reservoir may be different for the four serotypes. VSV infections have been found in humans and numerous domestic and wild mammals, but also in arthropods, especially sand flies (*Phlebotomus*). Four to 17% of inhabitants of the Amazon basin have a neutralizing antibody against the Piry virus. Antibodies against Chandipura virus are found in many animals in India.

There is a vertical (transovarial) transmission of vesiculoviruses in sand flies. VSV is often used in laboratories as an experimental model. Only on rare occasions have laboratory infections produced severe disease. Viral pseudotypes of VSV, exhibiting an envelope of an unrelated virus, can be produced with conventional virological techniques. VSV is also used as an expression vector and as a basis for recombinant vaccine viruses.

Transmission

Human infections in areas of endemicity are not unusual. Laboratory infections with VSV

have also been described. The mechanisms of transmission as well as the agent reservoir are not resolved. Transmission in cattle from animal-to-animal is probably less important than transmission via milking machines or by the hands of milkers. The sand fly (*Phlebotomus* species) appears to be most important for the transmission of VSV serotype Indiana. Other groups of diptera (Simuliidae and *Culicoides* spp.) have also been implicated.

Clinical Manifestations

Most human infections with VSV serotype Indiana or New Jersey appear to be subclinical. Human infections with Cocal virus are not known to occur. VSV virus infections in laboratories or from infected cattle may produce an influenza-like disease in humans. In one case of laboratory infection, VSV took the course of a severe hemorrhagic fever. The patient survived and recovered without sequelae.

After an incubation period of 30 h, the disease is initiated with high fever, often biphasic. Patients complain of severe malaise, headaches, myalgias, arthralgia, retrosternal pain, eye aches, and nausea. Vesicle formation in humans on the oral mucosa, lips, and nose is a rare exception; a rash does not appear. Occasionally, a disease course with hemorrhages similar to dengue has been seen. Human Piry virus infections in Brazil are associated with mild disease, lasting 3 to 4 days. Symptoms included fever, headache, myalgia, arthralgia and photophobia, and no rash. Chandipura virus was isolated from an 11-year-old girl in India suffering from encephalitic symptoms with vomiting, convulsions, and impaired consciousness. In other cases, Chandipura virus infection resembled the symptoms seen in Piry virus disease.

Vesicle formation in the oral mucosa, mouth, and snout is a typical sign of VSV infections in horses, cattle, and pigs. Fever and anorexia may be seen. The disease is not fatal, but complications due to superinfections are possible.

Diagnosis

Human disease usually appears in the context of animal disease. Human infections can be confirmed by virus isolation from throat swabs or from blood, by RT-PCR, or by serology.

In diseased animals, a rapid diagnosis is most important to exclude FMD. Virus detection in vesicle material is diagnostic. The virus can be propagated in cell cultures, for example, in Vero cells, where it grows to high titers and causes cytopathic effects. A group-specific diagnosis of the viral isolate can be made by ELISA or IFA. The neutralization test is type specific. The same tests are applicable for antibody detection in serum. A nested RT-PCR, targeting the phosphoprotein gene of VSV serotypes New Jersey and Indiana, can be used for confirmation of isolates or for direct detection of virus in the vesicle fluid.

Differential Diagnosis

Influenza-like diseases, and rarely, encephalitis and hemorrhagic fevers, should be considered in the differential diagnosis in humans, especially when vesicular disease (VD) is found in animals at the same time.

FMD and VD of pigs are first in line for the differential diagnosis in animals. Rapid serological tests and materials for antigen detection in vesicles are available. These tests have to be performed in reference laboratories.

As horses are not susceptible to FMD, only VSV and VD of pigs have to be considered if cattle, pigs, and horses are affected on a farm. When horses do not show signs of disease, FMD is the most likely diagnosis.

Therapy

There is no specific therapy. Symptomatic treatment should be addressed toward prevention of secondary infections.

Prophylaxis

Formalin-inactivated and attenuated live virus vaccines are available but of little importance. Good hygiene is sufficient to control the spread of the disease.

REFERENCES

Fu ZF et al., Stomatitis virus New Jersey serotype in clini-Oral vaccination of raccoons (Procyon lotor) cal samples by using polymerase chain reacwith baculovirus-expressed rabies virus gly-tion. *J. Clin Microbiol.* 31, 2016–2020, coprotein. *Vaccine* 11, 925–928, 1993.

Hole K, Velazques-Salinas L, Clavijo A, Improvement and optimization of a multiply real-time reverse transcription polymerase chain reaction assay for the detection and typing of vesicular stomatitis virus. *J. Vet. Diagn. Invest.* 22, 428–433, 2010.

Letchworth GJ et al., Arboviruses. In: *Mur-Vesicular stomatitis. Vet. J.* 157, 239–260.

Nunez JI et al., A RT-cal Microbiology, 1553–1569, 8th ed. Vol. *PCR assay for the differentialdiagnosis of 2.* ASM Press, Washington, DC, 2003. vesicular viral diseases of swine. *J. Virol. Methods* 72, 227–235, 1998.

Schmitt B, Vesicular stomatitis. *Vet. Clin. North Am. Food Anim. Pract.* 18, 453–459, 2002.

1.9 Zoonoses Caused by Paramyxoviruses

Several viruses in the family *Paramyxoviridae* are pathogenic for humans but not for animals, for example, mumps and measles viruses. They are not zoonotic. There are, however, pathogenic animal viruses closely related but not identical to pathogenic human paramyxoviruses. In addition, there is a small number of truly zoonotic paramyxoviruses. Most members of the *Paramyxoviridae* are capable of changing hosts, and therefore, have a wide host spectrum. Restrictions in the host range might be caused by receptor usage, by cellular transcription factors, or by immunological cross-reactivity between human and animal pathogens. For example, cross-reacting neutralizing antibodies against canine distemper virus, which is closely related to measles virus, are found in human sera. The potential of these antibodies to protect humans against infections with animal morbilliviruses has not been determined. The recently recognized human pathogens, Hendra virus and Nipah virus, are new zoonotic viruses.

Paramyxoviruses, such as rhabdoviruses and filoviruses, have a nonsegmented single-stranded RNA with negative polarity as their genome. The genome is the main constituent of the helical nucleocapsid. There is a matrix protein between the nucleocapsid and the outer membrane. Glycoproteins located in the membrane have important functions in attachment to the cell, fusion with the cellular membrane, pathogenicity, and stimulation of the immune response, as well as virus release from the cell. Viruses in this group have a common genetic structure and mechanism of gene expression. However, there are sufficient differences to allow the classification into different virus families and genera. They share the genetic organization with a gene for the nucleocapsid protein on the 5′ end and a gene for the RNA polymerase on the 3′ end. The abundance of gene expression is greatest for the 5′-end genes and least for the 3′-end genes. The gene for the matrix protein is located between both poles in addition to one or two genes for membrane glycoproteins that are responsible for receptor binding and membrane fusion. Parainfluenza viruses and rubulaviruses have a gene for neuraminidase. In addition, these viruses have a number of smaller genes for nonstructural and for structural proteins that are associated with the nucleocapsid, the matrix, or the virus membrane.

The family *Paramyxoviridae* has two subfamilies: *Paramyxovirinae* and *Pneumovirinae*. The *Paramyxovirinae* include the genera *Parainfluenzavirus* (respiroviruses), *Rubulavirus*, *Morbillivirus*, and *Henipavirus*. Respiroviruses and morbilliviruses include strictly human pathogens and related viruses pathogenic only for animals. They are not zoonotic and are not covered here. Zoonotic paramyxoviruses are listed in Tab. 1.6.

The subfamily *Pneumovirinae* contains the prototype respiratory syncytial virus, which has specific strains pathogenic for humans and others pathogenic only for animals, besides a number of other animal viruses. There is no zoonosis involved.

REFERENCES

Bowden TR et al., Molecular characterization of Menangle virus, a novel paramyxovirus which infects pigs, fruit bats, and humans. *Virology* 283, 358–373, 2001.

Chua KB et al., Tioman virus, a novel paramyxovirus isolated from fruit bats in Malaysia. *Virology* 283, 215–229, 2001.

Field HE, Mackenzie JS, Daszak P, Henipaviruses: emerging paramxyoviruses associated with fruit bats. *Curr. Top. Microbiol. Immunol.* 315, 133–159, 2007.

Halpin K, Mungall BA, Recent progress in henipavirus research. *Comp. Immunol. Microbiol. Infect. Dis.* 30, 287–307, 2007.

Harrison MS, Sakaguchi T, Schmitt AP, Paramyxoviruses assembly and budding: building particles that transmit infections. *Int. J. Biochem. Cell Biol.* 42, 1416–1429, 2010.

Mackenzie JS et al., Emerging viral diseases of Southeast Asia and the Western Pacific. *Emerg. Infect. Dis.* 7, Suppl. 3, 497–504, 2001.

Virtue ER, Marsh GA, Wang LF, Paramyxoviruses infecting humans: the old, the new and the unknown. *Future Microbiol.* 4, 537–554, 2009.

1.9.1 NEWCASTLE DISEASE

Newcastle disease, or atypical fowl plague, is a highly contagious virus infection of poultry, with respiratory, gastrointestinal, and/or CNS signs of disease. Human infection is rare and affects predominantly poultry farmers,

Table 1.6 | Zoonotic paramyxoviruses

GENUS AND VIRUS	RESERVOIR	SOURCE OF INFECTION	GEOGRAPHICAL OCCURRENCE
Rubulavirus[1]			
Newcastle disease virus	Poultry	Poultry	Worldwide
Menangle virus	*Pteropus poliocephalus*	Pigs	Australia
Henipavirus			
Hendra virus	Fruit-eating bats, flying foxes (Megachiroptera)	Horses	Australia
Nipah virus	Flying foxes (Megachiroptera)	Pigs	Malaysia

[1] An additional virus in this genus, Tioman virus, was isolated from *Pteropus hypomelanus* in Malaysia. There is at present no evidence of a zoonosis. The classification of Menangle virus and Tioman virus is preliminary.

laboratory personnel, and veterinarians. Under experimental conditions Newcastle disease virus (NDV) has been found to have oncolytic effects.

Etiology. The causative agent is NDV, in the family *Paramyxoviridae*, genus *Rubulavirus*. There are several subtypes of NDV based on pathogenetic differences, testing with monoclonal antibodies, and RNA fingerprinting. An attenuated NDV is used for vaccination of poultry. It is pathogenic for humans and frequently causes human NDV disease.

Occurrence. NDV infections of poultry occur worldwide in domestic fowl, as well as in numerous wild birds. The virus persists in the host for several weeks without signs of disease, often after an acute disease.

Transmission. Human infections occur via air or smear infection of the conjunctivae and mucosae after direct contact with infected fowl, especially chickens. Veterinarians and poultry farmers may get infected with NDV vaccine virus, which is nonpathogenic for poultry but pathogenic for humans, who may be exposed to this strain by dissolving lyophilized live virus or while using vaccine sprays. Laboratory infections occur occasionally.

Clinical Manifestations. The incubation period is 1 to 2 days, maximally 4 days. A unilateral, sometimes bilateral, follicular conjunctivitis that may turn hemorrhagic is usually seen (Fig. 1.12). The cornea is not involved. Preauricular

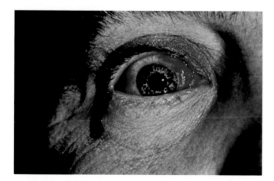

Figure 1.12 | Hemorrhagic conjunctivitis after infection with Newcastle disease virus. (Photo: J. Kösters, Institute for Poultry Diseases, University of Munich, Munich, Germany.)

lymph node swelling and pain often complicate the conjunctivitis. Less frequently, general signs with rigors, headaches, and mild fever are seen. The conjunctivitis usually lasts for 3 to 4 days. Recovery is without complications.

Disease in poultry is characterized by respiratory, gastrointestinal, and/or CNS signs. Depending on the virulence of the virus, very acute, acute, or subacute disease forms may be seen. The peracute and acute courses have a mortality of about 90%.

Diagnosis. The clinical picture of uni- or bilateral conjunctivitis with a history of contact with diseased poultry is an indication of Newcastle disease. The diagnosis can be confirmed by virus isolation or agent detection in conjunctival swabs, pharyngeal mucosa, tears, eye discharge, or throat washes. The virus can be isolated in embryonated hen's eggs or in cell culture. HI is used for serological testing.

NDV has caused great losses in chicken farms. Therefore, the rapid detection of the virus in chickens has a high economic impact. RT-PCR is used for the diagnosis in poultry. Primers for a single-tube RT-PCR targeting the fusion protein and the matrix protein are listed at the end of this section.

Human infections are always mild and secondary to poultry infections, infection with vaccine virus, or laboratory exposure. The diagnosis by RT-PCR for humans, therefore, is not needed. The HI test is useful for serodiagnosis.

Differential Diagnosis. The infection in humans has to be differentiated from other forms of virus-induced conjunctivitis, caused by adenovirus types 8 and 19 (keratoconjunctivitis epidemica), or keratoconjunctivitis haemorrhagica Apollo XI, caused by enterovirus 70. In contrast to the dispersed hemorrhages produced by these agents, hemorrhages in NDVinfection are more petechial in the inclusion body conjunctivitis caused by *Chlamydia trachomatis*.

Therapy. There is no specific therapy and treatment is symptomatic.

Prophylaxis. Prophylaxis in humans is restricted to personal hygiene and control (use of goggles and nose and mouth protection) when infected poultry or the live virus vaccine is handled.

Poultry are vaccinated on a regular basis. Vaccinated birds may shed vaccine virus, which could be a source of infection for humans, for up to 15 days.

REFERENCES

Ali A, Reynolds DL, A multiplex reverse transcription-polymerase chain reaction assay for Newcastle disease virus and avian pneumovirus (Colorado strain). *Avian Dis.* 44, 938–943, 2000.

Bukreyev A, Collins PL, Newcastle disease virus as a vector for humans. *Curr. Opin. Mol. Ther.* 10, 46–55, 2008.

Csatary LK, Csatary E, Moss RW, Scientific interest in Newcastle disease virus is reviving. *J. Natl. Cancer Inst.* 92, 493–494, 2000.

Huang HJ, Matsumoto M, Nonspecific innate immunity against Escherichia coli infection in chickens induced by vaccine strains of Newcastle disease virus. *Avian. Dis.* 44, 790–796, 2000.

Ke GM et al., Molecular characterization of Newcastle disease viruses isolated from recent outbreaks in Taiwan. *J. Virol. Methods* 97, 1–11, 2001.

Kho CL et al., Performance of an RT-nested PCR ELISA for detection of Newcastle disease virus. *J. Virol. Methods* 86, 71–83, 2000.

Lorence R et al., Phase 1 clinical experience using intravenous administration of PV701, an oncolytic Newcastle disease virus. *Curr. Cancer Drug Targets* 7, 157–167, 2007.

Miller PJ, Decanini EL, Afonso CL, Newcastle disease: evolution of genotypes and the related diagnostic challenges. *Infect. Genet. Evol.* 10, 26–35, 2010.

Seal BS, King DJ, Sellers HS, The avian response to Newcastle disease virus. *Dev. Comp. Immunol.* 24, 257–268, 2000.

Sinkovics JG, Horvath JC, Newcastle disease virus (NDV): brief history of its oncolytic strains. *J. Clin. Virol.* 16, 1–15, 2000.

Wang Z et al., Rapid detection and differentiation of Newcastle disease virus isolates by a triple one-step rtPCR. *Onderstepoort J. Vet. Res.* 68, 131–134, 2001.

Ward MD et al., Nucleotide sequence and vaccinia expression of the nucleoprotein of a highly virulent, neurotropic strain of Newcastle disease virus. *Avian. Dis.* 44, 34–44, 2000.

1.9.2 ZOONOSES CAUSED BY HENDRA VIRUS

A severe measles-like virus disease was first seen in 1994 in horses in Brisbane, Australia. A hemorrhagic fever with high lethality was seen. The virus can be transmitted to humans by close contact with infected horses and it causes a fatal infection in humans. Giant cells in vascular endothelium of capillaries and arteries mark the pathogenesis in horses and humans.

Etiology. The causative agent is Hendra virus. Hendra is a suburb of Brisbane, and the disease was first seen there. Because of the extreme length of the viral genome for paramyxoviruses, Hendra virus, together with Nipah virus, was initially classified as *megaparamyxovirus* but is now in the genus *Henipavirus* in the family *Paramyxoviridae*. Nipah virus was discovered in Malaysia in 1997. There is an antigenic relationship between Hendra virus and Nipah virus. Both viruses have a genome with more than 18,000 nucleotides. Like in other paramyxoviruses, the genetic program includes genes for N, P, C, M, fusion protein (F), receptor binding protein (H), and polymerase (L).

Occurrence. Hendra virus infections have only been observed in Australia. Fifteen horses died in two outbreaks in 1994, and one horse died in 1999. Three people became infected, and two of them died: a racehorse trainer (deceased) in Brisbane and his helper (who recovered) and a horse keeper (deceased) in Mackay.

Based on serological surveys, the virus could be traced to fruit bats or flying foxes (suborder Megachiroptera, genus *Pteropus*). The same is true of the later-discovered Nipah virus. Hendra virus has been isolated from grey-headed flying foxes (*Pteropus poliocephalus*) and from black flying foxes (*Pteropus alecto*). Thus, a new category of bat-borne zoonotic viruses, which also includes six strains of rabies virus, can be considered. Flying foxes are common in Australia, Indonesia, and Papua New Guinea, as well as on islands in the West Pacific and Indian Ocean.

Menangle virus, which causes reproductive disease in sows in Australia, and Tioman virus, recently found in Malaysia, are new viruses of the paramyxovirus family, which have a virus reservoir in flying foxes. Menangle virus is associated with *P. poliocephalus* and may cause infections of humans, Tioman virus was found in *Pteropus hypomelanus*. The classification of these viruses is preliminary, and their zoonotic potential has still to be evaluated.

Transmission. Hendra virus is probably transmitted indirectly from fruit bats to horses. Twenty percent of large fruit bats (genus *Pteropus*) have antibodies to the Hendra virus. The flying foxes stay in trees overnight. When infected, they shed infectious excrements onto pastures where horses can be exposed to the virus. Normally infected flying foxes do not show clinical manifestations. Pregnant females may infect their offspring by the vertical route without showing clinical symptoms. When infected, they shed infectious excrements onto pastures where horses can be exposed to the virus. Transmission from horse-to-horse has not been observed, and human infections were the result of close contact with infected horses (horse blood or secretions). In the years between 1994 and 2004, this was confirmed on three occasions. Two patients had been infected by contact with horses and two others during post-mortems.

Clinical Manifestations. Influenza-like disease reminiscent of *Legionella* infection was first observed in the racehorse trainer and his helper in Hendra. The helper recovered. The trainer developed acute dyspnea with increasing lung failure and signs of a hemorrhagic diathesis. He died 12 days after onset of the disease. At autopsy, a necrotizing alveolitis with giant cells, syncytium formation, and viral inclusions was found. In the second human case, the leptomeninges were infiltrated with lymphocytes and plasma cells with discrete areas of necrosis in the neocortex, basal ganglia, brain stem, and cerebellum. Viral antigen was demonstrated in the cytoplasm of some cells. A serous and hemorrhagic alveolar edema, enlarged lymph nodes, and foam in the bronchi were found. Giant cells were also found in the endothelium of lung capillaries and arteries. Similar lesions were found in the necrotic parenchyma of lymph nodes, spleen, brain, stomach, heart, and kidneys. Between 1994 and 2004, two patients died from severe meningoencephalitis. One patient was admitted after 12 days of disease

with pharyngitis, headaches, dizziness, vomiting, and stiff neck. He was demitted as a cured case but was again admitted 13 months later. He had tonic-clonic convulsions, emotional lability, and fever of low degrees. He suffered from backaches. Subsequently hemiplegia developed with inclusion of the brain stem. The patient became comatose and had to be intubated, he died after 25 days. Like other highly pathogenic paramyxoviruses, Hendra virus can block the signal cascade for interferon production.

The disease in horses was similar. Fever up to 41 °C, severe respiratory distress, and signs of hemorrhagic diathesis were dominant. Histologically, lesions similar to the ones seen in humans were found in lungs, lymph nodes, endothelium of lung capillaries and arteries, spleen, brain, stomach, heart, and kidneys. Hendra virus is highly pathogenic for pregnant mares.

As shown by immunofluorescence, sera from the diseased humans reacted with horse tissues and vice versa. Experimentally, two inoculated horses developed the disease after 6 and 10 days with high fever and severe respiratory distress. They were euthanized when moribund 2 days later.

Diagnosis. Severe disease and contact with horses on the east coast of Australia should lead to suspicion of Hendra virus infection. The diagnosis can be confirmed by virus isolation from blood and tissue extracts in Vero cell cultures, resulting in the appearance of focal syncytia usually within 3 days. IFA and the recently developed RT-PCR can be used to identify the virus and for direct demonstration.

Virus-specific antibodies can be detected by ELISA for epidemiological purposes. They are not useful for the diagnosis of acute cases.

Differential Diagnosis. Severe generalized infections with hemorrhagic diathesis and the development of ARDS—such as viral hemorrhagic fevers and hantavirus lung syndrome, as well as plague, anthrax, meningococcal sepsis, and legionellosis—are to be considered in the differential diagnosis. In less severe cases, Hendra virus disease might be reminiscent of legionellosis or influenza in their less severe courses. SARS must also be considered.

Therapy. There is no specific antiviral treatment for Hendra virus. The therapy is strictly supportive and it should address the ARDS and the hemorrhagic diathesis, as well as homeostatic maintenance. Extracorporeal elimination of carbon dioxide may be necessary.

Prophylaxis. No vaccine is available for use in horses or humans. In Australia, extreme caution is indicated in handling horses with fever, hemorrhagic diathesis, and ARDS. Gloves, goggles, and masks with respirators should be used when in contact with suspicious horses. Caution is also indicated when coming into contact with flying foxes. Excrement from these fruit bats is probably also infectious for humans. Human-to-human transmission has not yet been observed. Barrier nursing is still indicated. Experimental vaccines were developed on different bases and were successfully tested for induction of neutralizing antibodies.

REFERENCES

Aljofan M et al., Off label antiviral therapeutics for henipaviruses: new light through old windows. *J. Antivir. Antiretrovir.* 2, 1–10, 2010.

Barclay AJ, Paton DJ, Hendra (equine morbillivirus). *Vet. J.* 160, 169–176, 2000.

Bossart KN, Broder CC, Developments towards effective treatments for Nipah and Hendra virus infection. *Expert Rev. Anti. Infect. Ther.* 4, 43–55, 2006.

Daniels P, Ksiazek T, Eaton BT, Laboratory diagnosis of Nipah and Hendra virus infections. *Microbes Infect.* 3, 289–295, 2001.

Eaton BT et al., Hendra and Nipah viruses: different and dangerous. *Nat. Rev. Microbiol.* 4, 23–35, 2006.

Franke J et al., Identification and molecular characterization of 18 paramyxoviruses isolated from snakes. *Virus Res.* 80, 67–74, 2001.

Field HE et al., A fatal case of Hendra virus infection in a horse in North Queensland: clinical and epidemiological features. *Aust. Vet. J.* 78, 279–280, 2000.

Field H et al., Hendra virus outbreak with novel clinical features, *Australia. Emerg.Infect. Dis.* 16, 338–340, 2010.

Halpin K et al., Identification and molecular characterization of Hendra virus in a horse in Queensland. *Aust. Vet. J.* 78, 281–282, 2000.

Halpin K et al., Isolation of Hendra virus from pteropid bats: a natural reservoir of Hendra virus. *J. Gen. Virol.* 81, 1927–1932, 2000.

McCormack JG, Hendra, Menangle and Nipah viruses. *Aust. N. Z. J. Med.* 30, 9–10, 2000.

Smith IL et al., Development of a fluorogenic RT-PCR assay (TaqMan) for the detection of Hendra virus. *J. Virol. Methods* 98, 33–40, 2001.

Wang LF et al., The exceptionally large genome of Hendra virus: support for creation of a new genus within the family Paramyxoviridae *J. Virol.* 74, 9972–9979, 2000.

Williamson MM et al., Experimental Hendra virus infection in pregnant guinea-pigs and fruit bats (Pteropus poliocephalus). *J. Comp. Pathol.* 122, 201–204, 2000.

1.9.3 NIPAH VIRUS ENCEPHALITIS

Nipah virus may be transmitted from pigs to humans, causing a highly febrile encephalitis with a high fatality rate. Pig farmers and slaughterhouse workers are affected. The disease was first observed in Malaysia in the winter of 1998 to 1999.

Etiology. Nipah virus is a member of the family *Paramyxoviridae*, genus *Henipavirus*. The name Nipah virus is derived from the village of Sungai-Nipah in the state of Negeri Sembilan, Malaysia. The virus was isolated there for the first time from a farm worker. It is closely related structurally and antigenically to Hendra virus, which was isolated in Australia in 1994.

Menangle virus, a newly discovered paramyxovirus that causes reproductive disease with congenital malformations in sows, was isolated from *P. poliocephalus*. It resembles Nipah virus in its epidemiology and pathogenicity but is presently classified as a rubulavirus. The antibody against Menangle virus was found in piggery workers. Tioman virus, another paramyxovirus associated with Megachiroptera (*P. hypomelanus*), was isolated in Malaysia. It is not known to cause zoonotic disease.

Nipah and Hendra viruses are single stranded and have a nonsegmented genome, with negative polarity, consisting of more than 18,000 nucleotides (order *Mononegavirales*). As with other paramyxoviruses, their genetic program includes the following genes: N, P, C, V, M, F, H, and L. Because of the large size of the genome, classifying both viruses under the category of megaparamyxoviruses has been proposed.

Nipah and Hendra viruses are transmitted by flying foxes (*Pteropus vampyrus* and *P. hypomelanus*, in the suborder Megachiroptera). Together with lyssaviruses, which are transmitted by bats, these viruses form a group that could be called bat-borne viruses (viruses transmitted by bats).

Occurrence. Until now, the Nipah virus has been found only in mainland Malaysia and in Singapore. The direct source of human infection is pigs. Besides pigs and humans, serological evidence of infection has been found in horses, goats, cats, and dogs. Antibodies were also found in fruit bats [flying foxes (*Pteropus hypomelanus*)]. These animals exist in the eastern region of the Malayan peninsula and the infectious virus has been isolated from their urine. It is assumed that these bats are the reservoir and source of infection for pigs. The bats have also been identified as a reservoir of the Hendra virus in Australia.

Men aged 13 to 58 years are affected five times more frequently than women; 95.6% of the patients had contact with pigs. Human-to-human transmission or nosocomial infections have not been observed.

Porcine disease appeared first in the village of Sungai-Nipah and spread to neighboring villages. In 1999, almost all hog-raising farms were affected in the region of Bukit Pelandok in the state of Negeri Sembilan, north of the capital, Kuala Lumpur. The disease appeared in humans and dogs in direct connection with the transport of pigs. After the epidemic, 95% of pigs, 50% of dogs, 4% of cats, and 15 of 99 trapped flying foxes in the affected district were seropositive for Nipah virus. Regions with Islamic population do not have pig farming, and consequently, there are no cases with Nipah virus.

Transmission. Pigs probably become infected from the urine of bats that hang in trees at night. Evidence for transmission by arthropod vectors is lacking. Human infection is also the result of direct contact with infected pigs. Slaughterhouse workers are especially at risk.

The first cases of disease and death among hog-raising farmers and slaughterhouse workers were retroactively documented in 1997. Recognition of the new disease was initially obstructed because of the similarities between Nipah encephalitis and Japanese encephalitis, which occur in the same region.

Clinical Manifestations. In humans, subclinical, mild, and severe forms of the disease exist. The incubation period is between 1 and 3 weeks. The disease begins with fever, headache, nausea, and vomiting with variable severity. Early neurological signs are segmental myoclonus, loss of tendon reflexes, tremor, ptosis, and signs of a cerebellar inflammation. The electroencephalogram shows a slowdown of waves with bitemporal independently increased waves. Seventy-three percent of patients had inflammatory CSF changes with lymphocytosis and increased protein; 22% had convulsions; 59.3% developed drowsiness and confusion that later ended in coma, which commonly was lethal. Artificial respiration was necessary in 48%. According to official data, 259 humans became infected with Nipah virus between 1997 and 1999; 102 patients died.

Patients without disorientations survived but of those with disturbed consciousness, only 15% survived the disease. Meanwhile, clinical inapparent courses became known, and therefore, the lethality is less then was originally assumed. Most of the survivors were cured but 20% of discharged patients suffered from neurologic deficits, tetra paresis, ataxia, paralyses, and depression. Late neurologic disease became manifest in 7.5% of the patients with encephalitis and in 3.5% of the non-encephalitic courses. Relapses occurred between several months and 4 years after the acute disease. The clinical pictures of relapses resembled the picture of acute Nipah virus encephalitis. Fever, coma, meningism, segmental myoclonus were less frequent as compared to the acute disease, convulsions, and signs of cortical involvement were more frequent. In the acute phase, round or oval foci were found in the MRT. In relapses, cloudy or blot-like foci were seen, indicating massive proliferation of neuroglia. Nipah virus was not detectable in the periphery or in the cerebrospinal fluid. The relapses mostly occurred for a single time, in other cases repeated relapses occurred in a temporal distance of 6 to 7 months. Lethality was 18% in the relapses and 30% in the acute encephalitis. In postmortems, the virus was not isolated from the brain of patients with relapses.

The course of the encephalitis can be monitored by MRI. Multiple infarct-like foci are the main lesions, with asymmetric distribution in the sub-cortical and deep white matter. It is assumed that a widespread cerebral vasculopathy is the cause, with local thromboses and demyelination. The prognosis of comatose patients is usually poor. More than half of surviving patients show residual neurologic or psychopathologic signs of varying duration.

The disease in pigs has a high morbidity but low mortality. In piglets and young animals, mild to severe coughing was a typical sign. The course of the disease was less severe in these animals than in sows and boars, which expressed dyspnea, convulsions, and coma with a lethal outcome. Some animals died within a few hours. A fatal disease course was also observed in dogs. Comparable to Hendra infection of pregnant mares, Nipah virus infection is highly pathogenic during gestation.

Pathoanatomical findings in pigs and humans were pneumonic changes with consolidation, especially in the lower lung lobes, and hyperemia in the kidneys. The enteric organs appeared unremarkable. Besides some petechiae in individual cases, there were no macroscopic changes in the brain. Histologically, there was a vasculitis in small vessels of the brain and in other organs. Endothelial syncytial formation was found in the brain and in Bowman's capsule. There were cytoplasmic inclusion bodies in the brain, probably induced by the virus. Purkinje cells in the cerebellum were also infected. Primary endothelial lesions with syncytial formation, vasculitis, thrombosis, and infarcts, especially in the brain, dominate the course of the disease. In addition, there are direct lesions in infected neurons.

Diagnosis. The infectious agent can be isolated in Vero cell cultures from cerebrospinal fluid or blood. Syncytial formation can be seen within 5 days after inoculation, and viral antigen can be demonstrated in infected cells by immunofluorescence. Pleomorphic virus particles between 160 and 300 mm in diameter with the typical appearance of paramyxoviruses can be seen by electron microscopy. RT-PCR can be used for detection viral RNA in clinical specimens (blood and tissue extracts).

Differential Diagnosis. Japanese encephalitis, poliomyelitis, and other enterovirus infections, especially enterovirus 71, have to be considered. In children, the disease is expressed as acute cerebellar ataxia, an exceptional syndrome that has also been described for enteroviruses (coxsackie viruses A4, A7, A9, B3, and B4, as well as echoviruses 6, 9, and 16). Cerebellitis can also occur as a complication in varicella and infectious mononucleosis.

Therapy. There is no specific therapy for Nipah virus. Treatment is symptomatic and has to be done in multidisciplinary coordination between infectious disease experts and neurologists. The potential for infection of the attending personnel has to be considered, especially during the intensive treatment of patients in coma. Because of the thrombotic potential of the infection, all patients in the Malaysian outbreak received aspirin and pentoxifylline. Ribavirin, a nucleoside analogue, has been given to some of the patients in a nonrandomized study, because an effect against Hendra virus had been observed earlier. An analysis of the results is not yet available.

Prophylaxis. A vaccine does not exist. More than 900,000 pigs were killed in the afflicted region to stamp out the epidemic, and some human infections resulted from this activity. Because pigs are considered to be the only source of infection for humans, the contact of pigs with urine from flying foxes should be prevented.

REFERENCES

Ahmad K, Malaysia culls pigs as Nipah virus strikes again. *Lancet* 356, 230, 2000.

Bossart KN, Broder CC, Developments towards effective treatments for Nipah and Hendra virus infection. *Expert Rev. Anti. Infect. Ther.* 4, 43–55, 2006.

Bowden TR et al., Molecular characterization of Menangle virus, a novel paramyxovirus which infects pigs, fruit bats, and humans. *Virology* 283, 358–373, 2001.

CDC, Update: outbreak of Nipah virus – Malaysia and Singapore, 1999. MMWR Morb. *Mortal Wkly. Rep.* 48, 335–337, 1999.

Chadha MS et al., Nipah virus-associated encephalitis outbreak, Siliguri, *India. Emerg.Infect. Dis.* 12, 235–240, 2006.

Chew MH et al., Risk factors for Nipah virus infection among abattoir workers in Singapore. *J. Infect. Dis.* 181, 1760–1763, 2000.

Chiang CF et al., Use of monoclonal antibodies against Hendra and Nipah viruses in an antigen capture ELISA. *Virol. J.* 7, 115, 2010.

Chong HT et al., Treatment of acute Nipah encephalitis with ribavirin. *Ann. Neurol.* 49, 810–813, 2001.

Chow VT et al., Diagnosis of Nipah virus encephalitis by electron microscopy of cerebrospinal fluid. *J. Clin. Virol.* 19, 143–147, 2000.

Chua KB et al., Nipah virus: a recently emergent deadly paramyxovirus. *Science* 288, 1432–1435, 2000.

Chua KB et al., High mortality in Nipah encephalitis is associated with presence of virus in cerebrospinal fluid. *Ann. Neurol.* 48, 802–805, 2000.

Chua KB et al., Fatal encephalitis due to Nipah virus among pig-farmers in Malaysia. *Lancet.* 354, 1257–1259, 1999.

Chua KB et al., Tioman virus, a novel paramyxovirus isolated from fruit bats in Malaysia. *Virology* 283(2), 215–229, 2001.

Chua KB, Nipah virus outbreak in Malaysia. *J. Clin. Virol.* 26, 265–275, 2003.

Dimitrov DS, Wang LF, In utero transmission of Nipah virus: role played by pregnancy and vertical transmission in Henipavirus epidemiology. *J. Infect. Dis.* 196, 807–809, 2007.

Eaton BT et al., Hendra and Nipah viruses: different and dangerous. *Nat. Rev. Microbiol.* 4, 23–35, 2006.

Epstein JH et al., Nipah virus: impact, origins, and causes of emergence. *Curr. Infect. Dis. Rep.* 8, 59–65, 2006.

Goh KJ et al., Clinical features of Nipah virus encephalitis among pig farmers in Malaysia. *New Engl. J. Med.* 342, 1229–1235, 2000.

Halpin K et al., Newly discovered viruses of flying foxes. *Vet. Microbiol.* 68, 83–87, 1999.

Harcourt BH et al., Molecular characterization of Nipah virus, a newly emergent paramyxovirus. Virology 271, 334–349, 2000.

Homaira N et al., Cluster of Nipah virus infection, Kusthia District, Bangladesh, 2007. PLos One: e13570, 2010.

Homaira N et al., Nipah virus outbreak with person-to-person transmission in a district of Bangladesh, 2007. *Epidemiol. Infect.* 138, 1630–1633, 2010.

Lim CC et al., Nipah viral encephalitis or Japanese encephalitis? MR findings in a new zoonotic disease. *Am. J. Neuroradiol.* 21, 455–461, 2000.

Lo MK, Rota PA, The emergence of Nipah virus, a highly pathogenic paramyxovirus. *J. Clin. Virol.* 43, 396–400 (2008).

Luby SP et al., Foodborne transmission of Nipah virus. *Bangladesh. Emerg. Infect. Dis.* 12, 1888–1894, 2006.

NIPAH Virus Malaysia, official report Dr. Mohd Nordin Nodh Nor, Director General of Veterinary Services Ministry of Agriculture, Kuala Lumpur, 15.05.1999 ProMED-mail, 06.06.1999. http://www.healthnet.org/ programms/promed/html.

Osterholm, MT, Emerging infections – another warning. *New Engl. J. Med.* 342, 1280–1281, 2000.

Parashar UD et al., Casecontrol study of risk factors for human infection with a new zoonotic paramyxovirus, Nipahvirus, during a 1998–1999 outbreak of severe encephalitis in Malaysia. *J. Infect. Dis.* 181, 1755–1759, 2000.

Paton NI et al., Outbreak of Nipah-virus infection among abattoir workers in Singapore. *Lancet* 354, 1253–1256, 1999.

Sarji SA et al., MR imaging features of Nipah encephalitis. *Am. J. Roentgenol.* 175, 437–442, 2000.

Tan CT, Chua KB, Nipah virus encephalitis. *Curr. Infect. Dis. Rep.* 10, 315–320, 2008.

Yu F et al., Serodiagnosis using recombinant Nipah virus nucleocapsid proteins expressed in Escherichia coli. *J. Clin. Microbiol.* 44, 134–138, 2006.

Wang LF et al., The exceptionally large genome of Hendra virus: support for creation of a new genus within the family paramyxoviridae. *J. Virol.* 74, 9972–9979, 2000.

1.10 Zoonoses Caused by Orthomyxoviruses

1.10.1 INFLUENZA-VIRUSES

Besides the tick-borne Dhori and Thogoto viruses, which for a long time were believed to be nonpathogenic for humans, the family Orthomyxoviridae includes the influenza viruses. There are influenza viruses pathogenic for humans and for animals, especially birds, pigs and horses. Influenza viruses cause pandemics, epizootics, and zoonotic infections. Pigs and birds are sources of zoonotic influenza, but pandemic influenza viruses are also encountered in mammals and in birds. The relevance of these findings for the emergence of epizootics is gradually becoming clear. Based on group-specific antigens, influenza viruses are divided into A, B, and C viruses. Only viruses in the influenza A group are of zoonotic importance. Influenza B viruses have been found only in humans. Influenza C viruses have been found in humans and domestic animals, but their role as zoonotic agents is not clear.

Orthomyxoviruses, in contrast to paramyxoviruses, have a segmented genome. The genetic information in influenza A and B viruses is spread over eight segments. The three major segments code for proteins with polymerase function (PA, PB1, PB2), which are associated with the nucleocapsid in the virus particle. Additional segments code for hemagglutinin (HA), a receptor-recognizing glycoprotein, which is also involved in fusion, and a neuraminidase. Both glycoproteins are associated with the membrane in the virus particle. Three remaining segments encode the N protein (nucleocapsid), two M proteins (M1, matrix protein; M2, membrane protein), and two additional NS proteins, NS1 and NS2.

The segmented genome allows a highly efficient exchange of genes by way of genetic reassortment. Gene exchange in these viruses occurs under natural conditions. New combinations may lead to differences in immunological responses and pathogenicity. The change in antigenicity, which results from genetic reassortment, is called antigenic shift. Antigenic shift is believed to be the cause of pandemics in populations overriding the immunity to previous exposures. Besides antigenic shift, there is a continuous antigenic drift, in which the antigenicities of the receptor binding hemagglutinin and of the neuraminidase are constantly changed under the selective pressure of immune responses. The change is based on point mutation. The antigenic drift is the most important mechanism for persistence of influenza A viruses in a population.

Based on variations in the HA and neuraminidase genes, there is a binary code for influenza A viruses. Influenza viruses that are pathogenic for humans and occur in pandemics are marked as H1N1, H2N2, and H3N2. In swine influenza, H1 and H3, as well as N1 and N2, are dominant, very similar to the human pathogens. Swine influenza viruses can easily be transmitted to humans and vice versa. Among the avian influenza viruses, 14 different HA genes (H1av to H14av) and nine different neuraminidase genes (N1av to N9av) are known. Avian influenza viruses are capable of inducing catastrophic epizootics in domestic poultry and wild birds, in addition to latent infections. The avian influenza viruses can also be transmitted to mammals, especially pigs, but also to humans. Double infections with avian and mammalian viruses occur in swine and can result in genetic recombinations between influenza viruses of birds and mammals. Pigs are therefore regarded as a "melting pot" for influenza.

Influenza A viruses of horses and dogs are not of zoonotic relevance. In dogs, antibody against the actual pandemic influenza A strains are found. The infections seem to remain clinically inapparent.

During the last few years, the role of domestic cats in the spread of influenza has received considerable attention. Cats can be infected with influenza A viruses of avian as well as of human origin and can become sick with influenza. The avian H5N1 virus is especially highly pathogenic for cats. Therefore, cats, in addition to swine, could be able to play the role of a "melting pot" of influenza viruses in close neighborhood to humans. This means that swine and cats may enable genetic reassortment to occur between avian and mammalian influenza A viruses.

The pathogenicity of influenza viruses is determined by cooperation between functions of the virus and of the host organism. An important factor is the proteolysis of the hemagglutinin that is performed by cellular proteases in well-defined sites to render the virus infectious. In mammalian influenza viruses, an arginine residue marks the splitting site. Proteases, able to split on this site, are only found in the epithelial cells of the tracheobronchial tree. This is the reason why infection is restricted to the respiratory system. Avian influenza A viruses have proteolytic sites consisting of several basic amino acids. Proteases able to split on these sites are present in nearly all organs of the bird's organism, and therefore, avian influenza A is a generalized infection (Geflügelpest). Besides the host proteases bacterial proteases, for example, from *Staphylococcus aureus, S. pneumoniae, Haemophilus influenzae,* or *Klebsiella,* are able to split the hemagglutinin and activate the virus. This explains why avian influenza viruses are able to cause influenza in humans. But the capacity for epidemic spread is restricted in these cases.

A second factor restricting the host range of avian influenza A viruses is the availability of "fitting" receptors. The cellular receptor of influenza A viruses N-acetyl neuraminic acid, which is coupled to galactose in a glycosidic bond; avian influenza A viruses prefer receptors with a NANA-α-2,3 bond and these receptors are prevalent in the bird bronchial tree. Mammalian influenza A viruses infect cells, which have a NANA-α-2,6 bond, and this type is prevalent on the mucous membranes in the mammalian tracheobronchial tree. However, there are also some 2,3-receptors in mammalian lungs and these enable avian viruses to infect humans. Double infection with mammalian and avian influenza A viruses is a prerequisite for genetic reassortment!

The viral RNA polymerases in cooperation with host cell factors are determinants of the replicative speed, which is an important factor of pathogenicity in influenza. The product of the viral NS1 gene, an interferon antagonist, has a direct influence on the speed of replication.

Viral neuraminidases are important to separate virus particles from the host cell membrane and from mucin. Inhibitors of neuraminidases are used as antiviral therapeutics.

The pathogenicity of influenza viruses can be increased by immune enhancement, when protective antibodies are absent and exclusively non-protective antibodies against viral surface determinants are present. Previous infections with related viruses or ineffective vaccinations may be the cause. Up to this time there is only anecdotal but no experimental evidence and no systematic research of the occurrence of immune enhancement in influenza. There are cases in which vaccinated individuals fall ill with severe respiratory disease in the same season. Such cases are suspect of immune enhancement. In the lungs of fatal cases C4d, a marker of complement activation, is deposited in cases of immune enhancement and allows a retrospective diagnosis in case of a fatality due to vaccination failure.

Surveillance. Pandemics of influenza in the past have had a tremendous impact on human health and have paralyzed communities worldwide. Similar scenarios would have to be expected to occur in case of pandemic spread of a new influenza virus in the human population. As influenza viruses of avian or porcine origin may, by way of genetic changes, contribute to the evolution of a new pandemic variant of human influenza, it requires surveillance systems for human influenza viruses and for animal influenza. Animal influenza viruses, especially of birds and swine, have an important economic impact in addition to their zoonotic potential. Therefore, a network of influenza surveillance centers was created, with the task of tracing new virus variants, as well as estimating their epidemiological potential.

Group-specific RT-PCR techniques were established in order to detect known and unknown variants of influenza A viruses, not only in humans but also in birds, swine, and horses. Primers for a group-specific PCR for influenza A viruses, directed against the M gene, are needed for the group specific PCR.

1.10.1.1 Swine Influenza Virus H1N1

A swine influenza virus caused the influenza pandemic in 1918 to 1919, with 20 million deaths worldwide. This supposition was confirmed by serological testing and by sequencing the HA gene, which was preserved in autopsy specimens from 1919. Another outbreak occurred in 1976 in a boot camp in Fort Dix, New Jersey. Influenza A virus was isolated from five patients. This virus proved to be swine influenza virus and not the Victoria A (H3N2) virus that was prevalent in the human population at that time. One of the five patients died. The spread of this virus was expected but it did not happen, and recombinant products with H3N2 strain A Victoria, prevalent at that time, were not found.

Etiology. Swine influenza virus has the formula H1N1. A virus with this formula was first isolated from pigs in 1930. Viruses causing both the 1918 to 1919 pandemic and the cases in Fort Dix had this formula. Theoretically, it cannot be ruled out that the pandemic virus from 1918 to 1919 was originally a human influenza A virus, which in later years persisted in swine and was isolated in 1930 as a porcine influenza virus. H1N1 viruses have continued to be the prevalent pandemic strains up to the 1950s, when H1N1 was replaced by "Asiatic Influenza." In 1977, a virus closely related to the latest isolated strains of 1955 appeared in Russia. This virus infected only younger people <27 years who had no protective immunity against H1N1. This experience proves that there is a long-term immunity against influenza, which is ineffective due to the viral variability. In February 2009, a swine farm in Mexico was the origin of a new influenza A variant, which started a pandemic immediately. Most likely, this virus is a tetraparental reassortant consisting of PB2 and PA genes of North American avian viruses, a PB1 gene derived from the human H3N2 virus, the genes HA and N from the "classic" H1N1 swine virus and the NS and M genes of a "modern" H1N1 virus circulating in pigs in the Eurasian room at that time.

Occurrence. Swine influenza viruses exist worldwide. Infections in pigs are usually latent. However, outbreaks with severe losses may be seen in large pig farms.

Transmission. Influenza virus is believed to spread by aerosol. However, direct contact by handshake may also be involved. It is not known whether swine influenza virus is transmitted to humans by direct contact or by aerosol. The influenza A virus of 1918 to 1919 was very efficiently transmitted from person to person. There is no explanation as to why human-to-human transmission did not occur in the Fort Dix outbreak in 1976. There might have been a different cleavage site in the HA gene, which influenced the transmission of the virus.

Clinical Manifestations. The incubation time is 1 to 3 days. In humans, swine influenza is a febrile disease with severe malaise and head- and joint aches. Usually, the disease starts with bronchitis and seems to migrate upwards to cause rhinitis, pharyngitis, and conjunctivitis. The secretions of the mucosa are serous initially and after 2 days turn to purulent. The degree of

malaise overrates the importance of an infection that is restricted to the respiratory system.

In pigs, the influenza is a highly febrile (42 °C) disease with bronchitis, rhinitis, pharyngitis, and conjunctivitis, which can either directly, or after superinfection, cause pneumonia.

It has been hypothesized that encephalitis lethargica (von Economo), which occurred in 1922, was a late form of swine influenza. This hypothesis has never been confirmed.

Diagnosis. Serological diagnosis uses complement fixation tests, HI tests, or ELISAs. It is of limited value, as group-specific antibodies are present in most human sera. Virus-specific IgM can be detected in children but not in adults. Influenza viruses can be isolated in embryonated eggs or cell culture. Trypsin has to be added to cell culture medium to allow the proteolytic cleavage of HA. Confirmation of virus isolation and typing of the virus can be done with hemagglutination, direct immunofluorescence, or RT-PCR. Assays for typing of influenza viruses must allow detection of all currently circulating subtypes, including the influenza B virus. A set of primers for the detection and identification of viruses with the formula H1N1, H3N2, H1N2, and H3N1 are proposed by Choi et al. (see references).

Differential Diagnosis. Sporadic cases of avian or swine influenza in humans probably occur without being recognized. Human influenza A virus infections have to be considered in the differential diagnosis. In addition, all generalized infections with signs of respiratory disease up to signs of ARDS should be included. As with all zoonotic diseases, the history of professional or personal contact with diseased animals is most important. Diseases such as SARS or MERS must also be considered.

Therapy. Amantadine (100 mg of amantadine HCl, per os, twice a day; 5 mg/kg of body weight/day for children <10 years old) and rimantadine (100 mg of rimantadine per os twice a day; 5 mg/kg/day for children <10 years old; 100 mg/day for people >65 years old) prevent the maturation of viral HA. More recently, a new drug, zanamivir (Relenza) (two daily doses of 5 mg per inhalation), has become available; it inhibits the neuraminidase activity of the virus. Oseltamivir (Tamiflu) (75 mg per os twice a day for adults; for children >1 year old, dose according to weight) is another anti-influenza drug based on neuraminidase inhibition. If applied early (<48 h after onset) or prophylactically, they are effective in influenza A and B virus infections. Techniques for rapid influenza diagnosis have therefore become more important.

1.10.1.2 Avian Influenza Viruses H5N1, H7N7, H7N9, and H9N2

Avian influenza in humans was first observed in an outbreak in Hong Kong in 1997. Influenza A virus (H5N1) caused the death of six of 18 infected individuals. The genetic structure of the virus appears to prevent person-to-person transmission. Before 1997, it was believed that only swine influenza, not avian influenza, could be transmitted to humans. This virus remained prevalent in the south of China. In 2003, it started to produce zoonotic infections in people who had professional contact with livestock poultry. Since that time, it was isolated several times from farm hands, but human-to-human transmission was not observed.

Etiology. The avian influenza A virus that was responsible for the fatal human disease in Hong Kong in 1997 has the genetic formula H5N1. Meanwhile, a second avian influenza virus (H9N2) has been isolated from humans. Both viruses are genetically linked to influenza viruses found in quails. A third and a fifth avian virus, H7N7 and H7N9, can also infect humans. H7N7 was isolated during an epizootic in the Netherlands in 2003, where several people in contact with birds were infected and developed conjunctivitis. One of the patients died from pneumonia.

Other avian influenza A viruses, for example, H5N2, H7N1, and H7N3 caused epizootics with high losses of animals but zoonotic infections are neglectable. The avian strain, H9N2, has spread globally since 1980 as a pandemic strain and has produced zoonotic infections. However, it has a rather low pathogenicity for poultry.

In February 2013, a new avian influenza virus, H7N9 was isolated in China from human patients. In the course of 14 months more than 440 cases were confirmed to have H7N9, at least 155 patients have died from the disease with high fever, bronchitis, pneumonia, and dyspnea.

Occurrence. Avian influenza A viruses exist worldwide in wild and domestic birds. Infections are often latent, especially in waterfowl. The virus can be transmitted among avian species and can be carried by migrating birds. The animal trade is also an important vehicle for global distribution of avian influenza viruses. If domestic poultry on large bird farms become infected it can result in disastrous epizootics with high lethality.

Like other influenza viruses, avian influenza A viruses change by mutational events, resulting in antigenic drift, and by reassortment, resulting in antigenic shift. A molecular genome analysis of the 1997 Hong Kong isolate has shown that it might have been the product of a reassortment of a goose virus and a quail virus. Quails apparently were also the source of the H9N2 virus that was isolated from humans.

In the present epizootic, cases of H9N7 virus have occurred in many parts of China with predominance of the South Eastern provinces. Appearance of cases shows a typical seasonality in the winter season. There is no evidence of human-to-human transmission.

Transmission. The avian influenza A virus, H5N1, was transmitted to humans primarily by contact with live birds and not by contact with meat or animal products. All patients in Hong Kong were infected by direct contact with infected fowl and not by contact with infected individuals, as was demonstrated by molecular analysis of the virus isolates. However, serological surveys have shown that the virus has spread among family members and medical personnel to a lesser extent without producing clinical signs.

In the present outbreak of H9N7, no human-to human transmissions were registered. Isolated cases have occurred in the USA, in Europe, and in Malaysia in travelers returning from China but secondary spread did not occur.

Clinical Manifestations. A 3-year-old child infected with avian influenza virus H5N1 in Hong Kong in 1997 died with signs of a systemic infection and of Reye's syndrome after the child had been treated with antipyretic drugs. An additional 17 patients developed the disease in November and December of the same year with the same virus strain; six of these patients died.

Surprisingly, the autopsy did not reveal signs of a systemic infection or secondary bacterial infection as the cause of death. There was a diffuse necrosis of alveolar cells with interstitial fibrosis, necrosis of the central part of hepatic lobules, an acute tubular necrosis in the kidneys, and depletion of lymphocytes in the necrotic areas. These findings corresponded with the diagnosis of a hemophagocytic lymphohistiocytosis. Comparable to flaviviruses, a large number of influenza A viruses that exhibit extensive serologic cross-reactivity exist. Severe immunopathology may result in patients when they have a high titer of cross-reacting antibody but they are not protected against infection with a new variant.

Hemophagocytic lymphohistiocytosis (HLH) is a syndrome with fever, splenomegaly, and icterus. Hemphagocytosis is found in peripheral blood, bone marrow, and other organs: erythrocytes, leukocytes, thrombocytes, and, in bone marrow, the respective precursor cells are phagocytized by macrophages. HLH occurs in connection with neoplastic and infectious disease and with autoimmune diseases. Overstimulation of macrophages and overproduction of cytokines, including gamma interferon and tumor necrosis factor alpha, are of major pathogenetic importance. Typically, HLH can be found in cases with malignant B-cell lymphomas and in myeloic leukemia, systemic lupus erythematosus, and in graft-versus-host reactions, as well as in infections with *Leishmania, Mycobacterium tuberculosis, Brucellaceae, Campylobacter*, parvovirus B19, HIV, Epstein-Barr virus, herpesvirus hominis type 6 and other human herpesviruses, and influenza A virus.

As a rule, remissions may follow in cases with infectious diseases, when the etiologic agent can be treated successfully. In other cases, fatal courses are common.

According to the degree of pathogenicity, avian influenza A strains are divided into HP and LP strains. The presently circulating virus is a low pathogenic strain but it spreads with high efficiency.

Diagnosis. Influenza viruses can be isolated and identified relatively easily in embryonated chicken eggs or in cell culture by conventional methods. Trypsin has to be added to cell cultures for the cultivation of virus. It induces the proteolytic cleavage of the viral HA. The time-consuming virus isolation is required mainly for worldwide influenza surveillance rather than for clinical diagnosis. Group-specific serological tests or PCR can be used for preliminary identification. The PCR test is now well established for the diagnosis of influenza. At least two different gene sequences (e.g., one M protein gene and one H protein gene) should be used in a multiplex PCR because of the many types and variations of the virus. These techniques for rapidly detecting the agent become more important with better specific therapies. Primers for a group-specific RT-PCR, targeting the M gene of influenza A virus, are to be found in the literature. Primers for detection and subtyping of avian type A influenza viruses targeting the HA gene (H5 and H7) are also indicated.

Differential Diagnosis. Sporadic cases of avian or swine influenza in humans will most probably occur without being recognized. Human influenza A virus infections have to be considered in the differential diagnosis. In addition, all generalized infections with signs of respiratory disease up to signs of ARDS should be included. Hantavirus pulmonary syndrome might initially resemble influenza. As with all zoonotic diseases, the history of professional or personal contact with diseased animals is most important. SARS and MERS must also be considered. In all these cases, including zoonotic influenza A, travel history may be decisive for an early diagnosis.

Therapy. There are now four antivirals, amantadine, rimantadine, zanamivir, and oseltamivir, approved as anti-influenza drugs, which can also be used prophylactically (see discussion of swine influenza above). Techniques for rapid influenza diagnosis have therefore become more important.

Prophylaxis. In order to block widespread transmissions of the virus, all birds on poultry farms in Hong Kong were slaughtered in the 1997 outbreak of avian influenza. Vaccines are available for animals but not for humans to protect against avian and swine influenza. Human influenza vaccines do not protect against these viruses. However, vaccination is recommended to avoid superinfection of avian and human viruses. Anti-influenza drugs (see above) can also be used prophylactically. Swine should not be held in close contact with fowl, as avian influenza viruses can cross species.

In the present outbreak of H9N7 virus, the Chinese government has ordered the slaughter of chickens and ducks in poultry farms, but this did not stop the outbreak. Protection of farm hands from virus infection is the most efficient prophylactic measure.

Chicken markets are also very sensible places for virus distribution. Therefore, markets are closed. Tourists should avoid direct contact with poultry irrespective whether the animals are alive or are slaughtered.

REFERENCES

Cauthen AN et al., Continued circulation in China of highly pathogenic avian influenza viruses encoding the hemagglutinin gene associated with the 1997 H5N1 outbreak in poultry and humans. *J. Virol.* 74, 6592–6599, 2000.

CDC, Isolation of avian influenza A (H5N1) viruses from humans – Hong Kong, May– December 1997. *MMWR Morb. Mortal. Wkly. Rep.* 46, 1204–1207, 1997.

Choi YK et al., Detection and subtyping of swine influenza H1N1, H1N2 and H3N2 viruses in clinical samples using two multiplex RT-PCR assays. *J. Virol. Methods* 102, 53–59, 2002.

Cox NJ, Ziegler T, Influenza viruses. In: Murray PR et al. (eds.), *Manual of Clinical Microbiology*, 1360–1367, 8th ed. Vol. 2. ASM Press, Washington, DC, 2003.

Ellis JS, Zambon MC, Combined PCR-heteroduplex mobility assay for detection and differentiation of influenza A viruses from different animal species. *J. Clin. Microbiol.* 39, 4097–4102, 2001.

Lee MS et al., Identification and subtyping of avian influenza viruses by reverse transcription- PCR. *J. Virol. Methods* 97, 13–22, 2001.

Lin YP et al., Avian-tohuman transmission of H9N2 subtype influenza A viruses: relationship between H9N2 and H5N1 human isolates. *Proc. Natl. Acad. Sci. USA.* 97, 9654–9658, 2000.

Ku AS, Chan LT, The first case of H5N1 avian influenza infection in a human with complications of adult respiratory distress syndrome and Reye's syndrome. *J. Paediatr. Child Health* 35, 207–209, 1999.

Munch M et al., Detection and subtyping (H5 and H7) of avian type A influenza virus by reverse transcription-PCR and PCR-ELISA. *Arch. Virol.* 146, 87–97, 2001.

Saito T et al., Characterization of a human H9N2 influenza virus isolated in Hong Kong. *Vaccine* 20, 125–133, 2001.

Zhou N et al., Influenza infection in humans and pigs in southeastern *China. Arch. Virol.* 141, 649–661, 1996.

1.10.2 THOGOTOVIRUSES

Thogotoviruses, a genus in the family Orthomyxoviridae, are enveloped viruses with a segmented, minus stranded RNA-genome, consisting of 6 to 7 segments. Unlike influenza viruses the Thogotoviruses are transmitted by arthropod vectors mostly by ticks. They infect many vertebrate species, birds and also mammals. Thogotovirus, the type species infects livestock and causes disease in the animals. For several years it has been known that Thogotovirus, Dhoro virus and Bourbon virus are able to infect humans and to cause human disease. Recent case history: a patient in Eastern Kansas, USA, suffering from fever and fatigue sought medical care and gave a history of a tick bite. He had thrombocytopenia and leukopenia and was treated for suspected Lyme Borreliosis with doxycylin. But his condition did not improve. He developed exanthema of the stem, petechial bleedings and pneumonia and finally he died of multiorgan failure. Laboratory investigations, carried out at CDC in Atlanta, revealed a viral RNA sequence of a hitherto unknown Thogotovirus, which was named Bourbon virus, referring to the county, where the virus was first detected.

REFERENCE

Kosoy OI et al. Novel Thogotovirus associated with febrile illness and death, *United States, 2014. Emerg Infect Dis.* 2015 May; 21(5).

1.11 Zoonoses Caused by Picornaviruses

Many viruses pathogenic for humans are included in the large family *Picornaviridae*. However, only a few are zoonotic, and even they are of minor importance. Viruses in the family *Picornaviridae* have a cubic capsid without an envelope. The virion diameter is 28 nm. Four structural proteins make up the capsid in dodecahedral symmetry. The RNA is not segmented and has the polarity of mRNA. The genome functions as a polycistronic messenger for the translation in the cell without previous RNA synthesis. Viral proteases process the nascent poly-protein in the cell. There are six genera in the family *Picornaviridae*:

1. *Rhinovirus* (102 serotypes pathogenic for humans and three bovine rhinoviruses)

2. *Enterovirus* (eight species, including the following):

   - Enterovirus A (10 serotypes, including A2, A3, A5, A7, A10, A12, A14, A16, and enterovirus 71)

   - Enterovirus B [36 serotypes, including B1, B2, B3, B5, B6, and A9; 28 echovirus serotypes; enterovirus 69; and swine vesicular disease (SVD) virus (SVDV) (a zoonotic virus)]

   - Poliovirus (3 serotypes)

3. *Aphthovirus* [seven serotypes of foot-and-mouth disease (FMD) virus]

4. *Cardiovirus* [two serotypes of encephalomyocarditis (EMC) virus, predominantly infecting mice]

5. *Hepatovirus* (one serotype of hepatitis A virus)

6. *Parechovirus*

The following viruses in the family *Picornaviridae* are zoonotic: SVDV (with pigs as hosts), FMD virus (with cloven-hoofed animals as hosts), and EMC virus (with many species of rodents as hosts). Poliomyelitis viruses can cause outbreaks in wild monkeys; however, monkeys are not a source of human poliomyelitis.

1.11.1 SWINE VESICULAR DISEASE

SVD is an infectious disease of swine recognized since 1966. The disease is caused by an enterovirus. Clinically, the porcine disease cannot be differentiated from FMD.

Etiology. The causative agent of SVD is an enterovirus that biochemically and serologically is closely related to human Coxsackievirus B5, now classified as the human enterovirus B, serotype 5. (Porcine enterovirus types 1 to 11 are not related to human enteroviruses.) All SVDV isolates can be neutralized with immune sera against Coxsackievirus B5. However, Coxsackievirus B5 itself does not induce disease in pigs. An evolutionary connection between SVDV and Coxsackievirus B5 is assumed.

Occurrence. SVD was first observed in 1966 in Lombardy, Italy. Epizootics in numerous European and Asiatic countries followed. The disease in humans is rare. It is no longer prevalent in Europe with the exception of southern Italy, where it seems to be enzootic.

Transmission. SVD infections in humans have only been observed in individuals with close contact with infected pigs. There is no indication of human infections after eating sausage prepared from the meat of infected pigs, although the virus remains viable for months in meat products. Laboratory infections are known to occur. Human-to-human transmissions have not been observed.

Clinical Manifestations. Human infections with a clinical manifestation of vesicular formation are rare. The course of the disease is benign. Clinically inapparent infections were found in individuals with close contact with infected pigs.

The disease in pigs is not fatal. Vesicle formation with subsequent erosions on the snout, in the oral cavity, and coronary bands are typical. Occasionally, involvement of the CNS occurs.

Diagnosis. Human infection with SVDV may be suspected in individuals who have contact with infected pigs. It can be confirmed in humans as well as in swine by virus isolation or antibody detection. Serology, however, is complicated by the close relationship to Coxsackievirus B5. The diagnosis in animals is based on virus detection in vesicular material.

The fastest and safest method for the direct detection is the PCR. There is a group-specific RT-PCR technique covering all the groups of porcine enteroviruses, but it does not differentiate SVDV. Oligonucleotide primers for an SVDV-specific RT-PCR have been described previously (see the end of this section).

Differential Diagnosis. Due to the economic impact of FMD, the differential diagnosis of vesicular diseases occurring in domestic animals is most important. As the antigen content in vesicular fluids is high, a rapid diagnosis can be made with specific antisera against SVDV and FMD virus. In addition Vesicular stomatitis has to be included in the differential diagnosis.

There is a fourth vesicular disease in swine: vesicular exanthema. It was first reported in 1934 in California and it is caused by a calicivirus. The disease is considered to be extinct.

Therapy. Treatment of humans is strictly symptomatic.

Prophylaxis. Prophylaxis is by hygienic control of handling infected pigs.

REFERENCES

Callens M, de Clercq K, Highly sensitive detection of swine vesicular disease virus based on a single tube RT-PCR system and DIG-ELISA detection. *J. Virol. Methods* 77, 87–99, 1999.

Lin F, Mackay DK, Knowles NJ, The persistence of swine vesicular disease virus infection in pigs. *Epidemiol. Infect.* 121, 459–472, 1998.

Lindberg AM, Polacek C, Molecular analysis of the prototype Coxsackievirus B5 genome. *Arch. Virol.* 145, 205–221, 2000.

Nunez JI et al., A RTPCR assay for the differential diagnosis of vesicular viral diseases of swine. *J. Virol. Methods* 72, 227–235, 1998.

Oleksiewicz MB, Donaldson AI, Alexandersen S, Development of a novel real-time RTPCR assay for quantitation of foot-andmouth disease virus in diverse porcine tissues. *J. Virol. Methods* 92, 23–35, 2001.

Reid SM et al., Primary diagnosis of foot-and-mouth disease by reverse transcription polymerase chain reaction. *J. Virol. Methods* 89, 167–176, 2000.

Verstrepen WA et al., Rapid detection of enterovirus RNA in cerebrospinal fluid specimens with a novel single test-tube realtime reverse transcription PCR Assay. *J. Clin. Microbiol.* 39, 4093–4096, 2001.

Zell R et al., Detection of porcine enteroviruses by nRT-PCR: differentiation of CPE groups I–III with specific primer sets. *J. Virol. Methods* 88, 205–218, 2000.

1.11.2 FOOT-AND-MOUTH DISEASE

FMD is a highly contagious virus infection affecting almost exclusively cloven-hoofed animals (domestic and wild). Humans and animals other than those with cloven hooves are rarely affected. However, they can function as virus vectors.

Etiology. FMD virus belongs to the family *Picornaviridae*, genus *Aphthovirus*. There are seven serotypes [A, O, C, SAT 1 to SAT 3 (for South African Territories 1 to 3), and Asia 1] without serological cross-reaction. Numerous variants and subtypes exist within each serotype.

Occurrence. FMD has a worldwide distribution with the exception of Australia, New Zealand, and North America. The seven serotypes have their geographical domains: SAT 1 to SAT 3 are predominantly found in Africa. Asia 1 exists only in Asia. Types A, O, and C are found in Europe and South America. The most common type in Europe is type O.

Besides a few small episodes, Europe has been free of FMD for almost 30 years. An outbreak on one farm in Denmark in 1988 caused $60 million worth of damage. At the beginning of 2001, FMD outbreaks occurred in England, France, and in Asia. Type O was prevalent everywhere. It is possible that FMD might be introduced into FMD-free countries by bioterrorists.

The epizootic in England in February of 2001 began on a farm where restaurant scraps from a Chinese restaurant were fed to pigs. This is against legal prescriptions. The virus was then spread by sheep that had inapparent infections. When the same virus strain also appeared in continental Europe, it was suspected that the virus might have traveled by air or might have been transmitted by birds, but thorough investigations revealed that sheep had been transported from England to the European continent.

Transmission. Transmission of FMD virus is by contact or passively via vectors, by aerosol, and by contaminated water. Rodents, birds, other animals, and humans can passively spread the virus. The extended virus persistence in infected animals (6 months or more) and the high stability of the virus favor transmission under a variety of conditions. Human infections can usually be traced to direct handling of infected animals or contact during their slaughter. Laboratory infections occur. Human-to-human transmission is possible but insignificant. Insufficient hygiene favors passive transmission of FMD virus by humans, even if they do not develop disease. In 1834, three veterinarians were infected and they fell ill with FMD after having consumed raw milk from an infected cow.

During the febrile phase, the virus can be isolated from blood and organs of cattle and pigs. It is shed in milk, saliva, sweat, urine, sperm, and feces. The virus is rapidly inactivated at a pH below 5.3 and, therefore, is not found in muscle tissue of cadavers. However, it is still present in blood, bone marrow, spleen, and lymph nodes. The virus can be detected for more than 6 months in rapidly frozen meat. The infectious virus can survive at summer temperatures in the earth for 3 days, in dried feces for 14 days, and in milk at 4 °C for 6 days.

Clinical Manifestations. The course of disease in humans is biphasic. After an incubation period of 2 to 8 days, there is a general malaise, nausea, head and limb pain, and fever. The virus always enters through lesions in the skin or the oral mucous membranes. A primary vesicle

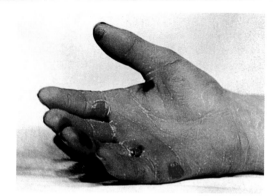

Figure 1.13 | Lesions on the hand of an animal keeper caused by foot-and-mouth disease virus infection. (Archival photo, Institute of Veterinary Hygiene and Animal Infectious Diseases, Justus Liebig University, Giessen, Germany.)

forms at the site of infection. Dissemination may follow. Mucous membranes turn red, and painful vesicles form on oral and pharyngeal mucous membranes and on fingers and toes (Fig. 1.13). Erosions remain after the vesicles dry up. Skin lesions heal in 5 to 10 days. There is no involvement of the CNS in humans.

The pathogenicity for humans of the FMD virus was proven again in England during the 2001 epizootic. Only one human case became known, with only local lesions. The patient had been in close contact with infected animals. During an epizootic of FMD in England in 1966, there also occurred only one case of FMD, in a veterinarian.

Infection with FMD virus produces clinical disease in almost all affected cloven-hoofed animals. The incubation period is 2 to 6 days. Fever and vesicle formation on oral, tongue, and pharyngeal mucous membranes are typical signs. Vesicles may form on the mouth and snout, between hooves or on the coronary band, and on teats. There is no fatality in sheep. However, secondary infections can complicate the disease, and myocarditis may develop.

The mortality rate in adult cattle is only 2% to 3%; in calves, it may be up to 50% to 70%. The mortality is lower in areas of endemicity, because calves are protected by maternal antibodies. Productivity of livestock is considerably reduced in areas of endemicity.

Diagnosis. Virus-neutralizing antibodies or a positive ELISA confirms the diagnosis of FMD in humans. Tests for viral antigens were formerly used for a rapid diagnosis in animals. These tests have now been replaced by RT-PCR.

Antigen capture ELISA uses a monoclonal antibody directed against a group-specific sequence on the amino-terminal end of capsid protein 2 (VP2).

Attempts to detect viral antigen in vesicles from infected humans are usually unsuccessful. At present, there is no generally accepted technique to differentiate between a postvaccinal and a post-infective immune response in animals. In animals, virological and serological diagnostics are done. Any isolated virus strain must be characterized to improve the vaccine design. In case of an epizootic, it may be necessary to differentiate between post-infectious and post-vaccinal immunity. Modern type FMD vaccines will only induce antibodies against structural proteins, whereas post-infectious immunity will also include antibodies against nonstructural proteins.

Differential Diagnosis. Several infectious diseases with vesicle formation should be considered in the differential diagnosis: herpesvirus infections, vesicular stomatitis, animal poxvirus infections, exsudative *erythema multiforme*, *pemphigus vulgaris,* SVD, and especially hand-foot-and-mouth disease, caused by Coxsackievirus A16 (enterovirus A). The last disease is more common in humans, especially in children, than FMD.

It is not possible to differentiate between VSV, SVD, or FMD based only on clinical manifestations. In FMD, the manifestations are graver, especially in young animals. For outbreak control, it is necessary to have a virological diagnosis in every suspected case.

Therapy. Treatment of human infections is strictly symptomatic. Antibiotics may be needed for secondary infections of extensive skin lesions. Infected calves need to be tube fed because of erosions in the mucous membranes. Adult animals may have to be slaughtered when the hoof wall becomes separated. Experimental cures are not allowed.

Prophylaxis. There is a common policy in Europe to control FMD in domestic animals. Vaccination is only allowed during outbreaks with a special permit. During an outbreak, affected herds are culled and an attempt is made to control spread of the highly contagious virus by vaccinating animals located around the infected herds.

Individual hygiene (gloves and protective clothing) suffices for human protection from infection. A formalin-inactivated vaccine against types O, A, and C was used in Europe until 1990, attended by some problems. The seroconversion was insufficient because of many variants of the virus. In some vaccine batches, the virus was not completely inactivated. In addition, it was not possible to market seropositive animals, because one could not differentiate between vaccinated and exposed animals. Administered by parenteral route vaccines may not induce sufficient mucosal immunity. It may be desirable to develop a multivalent attenuated virus vaccine that induces a good mucosal immunity. It is necessary to develop serological tests that can differentiate between seroconversion due to vaccination and those due to infection.

Ethylenimine (aziridine)-inactivated virus vaccines grown in BHK cells are currently used. Recombinant vaccines have been produced but not sufficiently tested.

REFERENCES

Bauer K, Foot-and-mouth disease as zoonosis. *Arch. Virol. Suppl. Review* 13, 95–97, 1997.

Broo K et al., Viral capsid mobility: A dynamic conduit for inactivation. *Proc. Natl. Acad. Sci. USA* 98, 2274–2277, 2001.

Garcia-Briones MM et al., Association of bovine DRB3 alleles with immune response to FMDV peptides and protection against viral challenge. *Vaccine* 19, 1167–1171, 2000.

Mayr GA et al., Immune responses and protection against foot-and-mouth disease virus (FMDV) challenge in swine vaccinated with adenovirus-FMDV constructs. *Vaccine* 19, 2152–2162, 2001.

McMinn P et al., Neurological manifestations of enterovirus 71 infection in children during an outbreak of hand, foot, and mouth disease in Western *Australia. Clin. Infect. Dis.* 32, 236–242, 2001.

Oleksiewicz MB, Donaldson AI, Alexandersen S, Development of a novel real-time RTPCR assay for quantitation of foot-andmouth disease virus in diverse porcine tissues. *J. Virol. Methods* 92, 23–35, 2001.

Pickrell J, Enserink M, Foot-and-mouth disease. U.K. outbreak is latest in global epidemic. *Science* 291, 1677, 2001.

Prempeh H, Smith R, Muller B, Foot and mouth disease: the human consequences. The health consequences are slight, the economic ones huge. *BMJ* 322, 565–566, 2001.

Reid SM et al., Primary diagnosis of foot-andmouth disease by reverse transcription polymerase chain reaction. *J. Virol. Methods* 89, 167–176, 2000.

Rodriguez-Torres JG, International approach to eradication and surveillance for footandmouth disease in the Americas. *Ann. N. Y. Acad. Sci.* 916, 194–198, 2000.

Samuel AR, Knowles NJ, Foot-and-mouth disease type O viruses exhibit genetically and geographically distinct evolutionary lineages (topotypes). *J. Gen. Virol.* 82, 609–621, 2001.

Zell R et al., Detection of porcine enteroviruses by nRT-PCR: differentiation of CPE groups I–III with specific primer sets. *J. Virol. Methods* 88, 205–218, 2000.

1.11.3 ENCEPHALOMYOCARDITIS

EMC is a virus infection of pigs and lower primates. Humans rarely develop disease and if so, only sporadically. EMC virus has been extensively used in mice as a model for myocarditis and myocardiopathy. It is still unknown whether the virus plays a role in human myocarditis.

Etiology. EMC viruses (Columbia SK and Mengovirus) belong to the family *Picornaviridae*, genus *Cardiovirus*.

Occurrence. EMC viruses exist worldwide. The human disease is seldom diagnosed, but inapparent infections have been described.

Pigs are most often affected by EMC. The lethality rate in piglets less than 2 months of age may be 10% to 100%. Several lower primates and African elephants are also highly susceptible (EMC may cause sudden death of these animals in zoos). EMC virus infections in domestic animals (horses and cattle) and in some wild rodents have also been described previously. Rats and other rodents are probably the reservoir for the EMC virus. In Sweden, EMC virus transmitted from bank voles (*Clethrionomys glareolus*) was found to have caused human myocarditis. The virus has also been isolated from birds (pheasants) and mosquitoes.

The EMC virus has only been isolated in Europe from naturally infected and diseased humans. Laboratory infections have been described. Seroepidemiological investigations revealed a wide distribution of infections in children and juveniles in North and South America, Africa, Australia, the Pacific Islands, and the Philippines. The disease has not been reported since the 1950s.

Transmission. EMC virus is shed in feces and is transmitted via feed, water, or feeding on infected cadavers. It is not known how humans become infected.

Clinical Manifestations. The rare disease in humans presents with fever, CNS disturbances (severe headaches, vomiting, stiffness of the neck, hyperactive reflexes, and delirium), and lymphocytic pleocytosis of CSF. The disease is not fatal, and there are no complications after recovery.

Myocarditis and sudden death are typical for the disease in pigs and primates. Hydrothorax, hydropericardium, and ascites may be seen. Additional signs are fever, anorexia, and progressive paralysis due to encephalomyelitis.

Diagnosis. Diseases caused by EMC virus in pigs or other domestic animals may be a hint for possible human infections. The diagnosis is confirmed by virus isolation and identification in cell culture or by serology showing increased antibody titers by virus neutralization or HI during recovery. Only a few laboratories perform serological tests for EMC.

Differential Diagnosis. Any infectious disease with CNS signs should be considered in the differential diagnosis.

Therapy. Therapy for EMC is symptomatic.

Prophylaxis. Good hygiene and cautious handling of diseased animals are sufficient for prophylaxis.

REFERENCE

Yoon JW et al., Antibody to encephalomyocarditis virus in juvenile diabetes. *New Engl. J. Med.* 297, 1235–1236, 1977.

1.12 Hepatitis E

Hepatitis E is an infectious disease, which is endemic in countries with a low standard of hygiene. In these countries, Hep E is the predominant cause of viral hepatitis. In developed countries, only sporadic cases of disease occur, which are imported or have a zoonotic origin. Compared with other forms of viral hepatitis, Hep E is characterized by high pathogenicity for pregnant women, fetuses, newborn children, and older men.

Etiology. Hepatitis E virus was detected in 1983 and it cannot be classified in any known virus family. Therefore, it is classified as the sole member in a genus Hepevirus of a new virus family named *Hepeviridae*. The genome is single stranded RNA of positive polarity. The genomic organization resembles togaviruses, and especially the rubellavirus. However, these viruses have a lipid envelope, which Hep. E has not. Reading frame 1 codes for nonstructural proteins and is translated directly. There is only one structural protein, a capsid protein, which is translated from a subgenomic RNA. Five genotypes of Hep E are known; they differ in their geographic distribution and in epidemiologic behavior.

Occurrence. Genotypes 1 and 2 are endemic in countries with low standard of hygiene, type 1 in Asia and North Africa, and type 2 in West Africa and in Middle America. These types are found only in humans and are imported to developed countries. Genotype 3, a zoonotic virus, is widely distributed in America, Europe, the Far East, and New Zealand. In Europe, Hep. E is mainly found in domestic and feral pigs, in other regions other species of feral animals, for example, in red deer. In Germany, 15% of wild boars are infected; domestic pigs are infected at the age of 2 to 4 months. In commercial pig breeding farms, 80% to 100% are seropositive. Serologic evidence of infection is also found in many other species, for example, in monkeys and rats. Genotype 4 is also a zoonotic virus. Up to this time, it was found only in Southeast Asia in humans and in pigs. Type 5 was isolated in the USA and in Australia from chickens, transmission to humans is not known to occur.

In countries, known to be endemic for types 1 or 2 of Hep.E virus, infections, are already distributed at an early age and mostly remain clinically inapparent. Children are less affected than young adults between 15 and 35 years, with males more than females. Seroprevalence in endemic regions is >60%.

In developed countries where type 3 of Hep. E virus causes zoonotic infections, sporadic cases occur only in persons with intensive animal contacts, especially with meat, blood or feces. In Germany, the reported number of cases of disease with Hep. E, type 3 rose from 51 in 2006 to 221 in 2010. The rate of imported cases, mainly that of Hep. E type 1, has in the years 2001 to 2009 amounted to an average of 25 cases per year. Mainly younger tourists (knapsack-tourists) are affected. Seroprevalence in Europe is between 3% in Spain and 13% in Sweden. In some regions, it reaches 20% to 30%. Differences in these figures may, in part, reflect methodical differences or differences in the type of antigens.

Transmission. In countries where types 1 or 2 are endemic and can cause epidemics the infection is distributed mainly by the fecal-oral route by drinking water or contaminated food. As youths, and especially male youths, are more affected than children, and male adults more than females, sexual transmission may be involved. The infection is also transmitted with blood transfusions and organ transplants.

In zoonotic infections, the route of transmission is not very well known. Contact with animal excrements, animal products or eating raw or half-raw meat, liver, or offal from domestic pigs or wild boars will play a role. Family infections are believed to be due to common risks of infection rather than human-to-human transfer.

Clinical Manifestations. Often the course is clinically inapparent. Incubation time is between 2 and 9 weeks. Symptoms such as fever, malaise, epigastric pain, vomiting, diarrhea, icterus, and dark colored urine do not differ from other forms of viral hepatitis. The severity reaches from mild courses up to a fulminant hepatitis. Viremia and virus excretion with stools ends with the cessation of clinical symptoms. The case fatality rate of Hep.E is 1% to 4%. Viral persistence may develop in patients with immunodeficiency or after organ transplantation. Reducing the immunosuppressive therapy, will, in one-third of cases, result in virus elimination. Pregnant women and their fetuses are endangered mainly in the third trimester of pregnancy, where the fatality rate is 20%. Babies and older men are also highly endangered. In patients with a chronic damage of liver parenchyma, the case fatality rate may reach 70%.

Disease in animals: chimpanzees and rhesus and cynomolgus monkeys develop hepatitis upon experimental infection. Pigs, rabbits, rats, and chickens can be infected experimentally, in pigs, the infection seems to remain inapparent.

Diagnostics. HEV is detectable by RT-PCR in stool and serum 1 week before manifestation of clinical signs and after recovery. In immunosuppressed patients, viral persistence may last for a year, often without clinical manifestations and without detectable immune answer.

Viral IgM and IgG is detectable with an ELISA test early in the course of infection. IgM is detectable up to 3 months after disease and is proof of recent infection.

Therapy. As in other forms of viral hepatitis, therapy is symptomatic; a specific antiviral therapy does not exist. In fulminant courses, liver transplantation may be needed.

Prophylaxis. A vaccine is not yet available. Antibodies against the capsid protein are protective. Vaccines containing the type 1 capsid protein in recombinant form are in phase 2 of a clinical trial. This vaccine will be of importance mainly for inhabitants of endemic countries and for travelers. In China, a vaccine is licensed under the name HEV 239.

The general prophylaxis is restricted to measures of general and personal hygiene, mainly in countries with endemic Hep. E. Animal keepers, veterinaries, butchers, and hunters have to avoid unprotected contact with animals, cadavers, animal products, blood, and excrement. Meat from wild boars and pigs should always be eaten well done. Pregnant women should especially avoid contact with meat from pigs and wild boars.

REFERENCES

Colson P et al., Pig liver sausage as a source of hepatitis E virus transmission to humans. *J Infect* 202, 825–834, 2002.

Kamar N et al., Hepatitis E-Virus and Chronic Hepatitis in Organ Transplant Recipients. *N. Engl. J. Med.* 358, 811–817, 2008.

Kamar N et al., Factors associated with chronic hepatitis in patients with hepatitis E virus infection who have received solid organ transplants. *Gastroenterology* 140, 1481–1489, 2011.

Legrand-Abravanel F et al., Characteristics of autochthonous hepatitis E virus infection in solid-organ transplant recipients in France. *J Infect Dis.* 202, 835–844, 2010.

Lul L, Hagedorn CH, Phylogenetic analysis of global hepatitis E sequences: genetic subtypes and zoonosis. *Rev. Med. Virol.* 16, 5–36, 2006.

Mushahwar JK, Hepatitis E virus: transmission, epidemiology and prevention. *Rev. Med. Virol.* 80, 645–658, 2008.

Panda SK, Thakral D, Rehmann S, Hepatitis E virus. *Rev. Med. Virol.* 17, 151–180, 2007.

Shresta MP et al., Safety and Efficacy of a Recombinant Hepatitis E-Vaccine. *N. Engl. J. Med.* 356, 895–903, 2007.

Savic B et al., Detection rates of the swine torque teno viruses (TTVs), porcine circovirus type 2 (PCV2) and hepatitis E virus (HEV) in the livers of pigs with hepatitis. *Vet Res Commun.* 34, 641–648, 2010.

Wichmann O, Koch J, Hepatitis E. Häufiger eine autochthone als ein importierte Erkrankung. *Flug-, Tropen- und Reisemedizin* 18, 74–76, 2011.

Stellungnahmen des Arbeitskreises Blut des Bundesministeriums für Gesundheit. Hepatitis E-Virus. *Bundesgesundheitsbl.-Gesundheitsforsch.- Gesundheitsschutz* 51, 90–92, 2008.

1.13 Coronaviruses

Up to 2003, no zoonotic corona virus was known. This family comprises members with a high pathogenicity for animals and humans. Host changes, a prerequisite for a zoonosis was observed in experimental conditions but not in nature. Advent of a new and hitherto unknown human disease, SARS, and isolation of the causative agent, the SARS coronavirus, has raised suspicion of a new zoonotic disease. A second zoonotic coronavirus, the MERS-CoV, was recently isolated from cases with the Middle East respiratory syndrome.

The coronaviruses are members of the nidovirus family, which comprises viruses with a special mechanism of transcription using "nested" mRNAs, *nidus* being the Latin word for nest. In negative stained preparations, coronaviruses are characterized as spherical particles of 100 to 120 nm in diameter with typical surface projections reminding of the wings of a windmill. These spikes are formed by the receptor binding S-protein. The helical nucleocapsid contains the genome, a single stranded RNA of positive polarity. With a size of 27 to 31 kb, the corona virus genome is the largest RNA genome ever found in a virus. The gene for the RNA-polymerase is located at the 5′-prime end and is translated directly from the genomic RNA immediately after infection. This results in a complimentary RNA strand, which serves as matrix for the synthesis of seven mRNA species of varying length but using a common leader sequence at the 5′-prime end, a process which is described as "nested" transcription.

The genome encodes up to 16 nonstructural proteins and five structural proteins: S, the spike protein, N, the nucleocapsid protein, a phosphoprotein, M, glycosylated membrane protein, HE, hemagglutinin/esterase glycoprotein, and E, non-glycosylated integrated membrane protein, presumed to function as an ion channel. The HE protein is found only in members of the clade ß coronaviruses; it is a functional analogue to the hemagglutinin/esterase protein of influenza C viruses.

According to their antigen relationships, the hitherto known coronaviruses are divided in clades α to γ (Tab. 1.7). The genus α comprises human pathogens (229E and NL63) as well as animal viruses infecting swine, dogs, cats, and rabbits (Tab. 1.7). A third human coronavirus (HCoV-OC43) is assigned to the genus ß together with mouse hepatitis virus, SDAV, a rat virus, HEV from swine, BCoV, a bovine virus,

and TCoV from turkeys. Infectious bursitis virus, a chicken pathogen and TCoV, a turkey virus belong to the γ-clade of corona viruses. The human coronaviruses cause respiratory and gastrointestinal disease and are held responsible for up to 30% of common colds. The pathogenic spectrum of the animal coronaviruses encompasses respiratory and gastrointestinal diseases, as well as hepatitis and ZNS disease. None of the enumerated animal pathogens has ever been incriminated in causing zoonotic disease.

Newly discovered coronaviruses, the SARS-CoV, which emerged 10 years ago in China and the MERS coronavirus, discovered in 2012 in Saudi Arabia, both causative agents of severe respiratory syndromes in humans with extremely high case/fatality rates are suspected to have a zoonotic background in chiroptera (bats). Serologic evidence of SARS-CoV was found in the large Indian civet; antibodies against MERS-CoV were detected in camels and dromedaries. Both viruses are preliminarily assigned to the clade ß of coronaviruses and they are the first examples of zoonotic pathogens in this family (Tab. 1.7).

1.13.1 SARS: SEVERE ACUTE RESPIRATORY SYNDROME

SARS was described as a new disease when clinical cases with atypical pneumonia of unusual severity were observed in Hong Kong and in Hanoi in 2002. Known causes of respiratory disease, influenza A of human or animal origin or other agents, were not found. Retrospectively, it was stated that this agent had already caused disease in November 2002 in and around Guangdong, south of China, which was not suspected to be caused by an unknown agent.

Etiology. SARS is caused by an up to that time unknown virus, the SARS associated coronavirus (SARS-CoV), which can be isolated in cell culture from throat swabs, bronchial, and fecal specimens. As a result of genetic analyses, the agent was provisionally assigned to the ß clade of coronaviruses. Concomitant infections with metapneumoviruses and chlamydiae, which

Table 1.7 | Coronaviruses and their natural hosts

VIRUS	ABBREVIATION	HOST	CLINICAL SYNDROME
Genus *Alphacoronavirus*			
Human coronavirus	HCoV-229E	Humans	Respiratory
Transmissible gastroenteritis virus	TGEV	Pigs	Respiratory and enteritis
Porcine respiratory coronavirus	PRCoV	Pigs	Respiratory and enteritis
Canine coronavirus	CCoV	Dogs	Enteritis
Feline coronavirus	FeCoV	Cats	Enteritis
Feline infectious peritonitis virus	FIPV	Cats	Respiratory, enteritis, hepatitis, central nervous system
Rabbit coronavirus	RbCoV	Rabbits	Enteritis
Genus *Betacoronavirus*			
Human Coronavirus	OC 43 HCoV-OC43	Humans	Respiratory, enteritis (?)
Human enteric coronavirus	HECoV	Humans	Enteritis
Murine hepatitis virus	MHV	Mice	Respiratory, enteritis, hepatitis, central nervous system
Sialodacryoadenitis virus	SDAV	Rats	Sialodacryoadenitis
Porcine hemagglutinating encephalitis virus	HEV	Pigs	Respiratory, enteritis, central nervous system
Bovine coronavirus	BCoV	Cows	Respiratory, enteritis
SARS coronavirus	SARS-CoV	Humans, bats, civets	Pneumonia
MERS coronavirus	MERS-CoV	Human, bats, dromedaries	Pneumonia, nephritis
Genus *Gammacoronavirus*			
Infectious bursitis virus	IBV	Chicken	Hepatitis, bursitis
Turkey coronavirus	TCoV	Turkeys	Respiratory, enteritis
Pheasant coronavirus	PCoV	Pheasants	Respiratory, enteritis

were found in some cases, seem to be irrelevant in the pathogenesis.

Occurrence. Clinical cases of SARS were first observed in Hanoi and Hong Kong; in a very short period of time, the agent was distributed by travelers throughout the world, to Taiwan, Singapore, Thailand, Canada, the USA, Ireland, France, and Germany. Originally, the virus seems to have been imported to Hong Kong by a Chinese clinician who had treated SARS patients in a Guangdong hospital. In Guangdong, several cases of pneumonia, which were retrospectively diagnosed to have suffered from SARS, had already occurred since November 2002. According to a WHO statistic, 8,098 cases of SARS were registered in 32 countries and 774 patients died of the disease, amounting to a case fatality rate of 9.56%. Seroepidemiological studies have shown that the SARS-CoV has not been present in the population before 2002/2003. The rapid pandemic spread was followed by an abrupt end of the pandemic. Since that time, 17 additional cases of SARS were registered and no case since 2004.

Transmission. In all cases, in which the source of infection could be identified, SARS-CoV was transmitted by human-to-human contact. This means that transmission from a hypothetical animal source might have been the origin of the pandemic but it was completely irrelevant for the worldwide distribution of the SARS virus. Often SARS CoV was transmitted as a nosocomial infection, 30% of the patients were members of the medical or nursery staff of hospitals, in which SARS patients were treated. These figures originated from early experience, when special protective precautions of the staff were not yet regarded to be necessary. In other cases, the virus spread had occurred in a floor of a hotel or of an apartment house. It is speculated that some "super spreaders" might have distributed the virus with an extremely high efficiency. These patients may shed 1000 times as much virus than other patients. Several clinical scientists, who had attended a congress in Hong Kong, were incubated with the infection when they traveled back to their homes and became the source of hospital outbreaks in their domestic cities.

SARS virus is excreted not only via the respiratory secretions but also via stools. There is no proof that indirect routes of transmission, for example, by contaminated meals or toilet seats might have been of significant importance for the virus spread. Enforcing principles of general and personal hygiene and the consequent application of rules of hygiene in the hospitals were sufficient to interrupt the virus transmission in hospitals. Cockroaches were suspected to have served as vectors of the virus. It is not known whether climatic factors might have influenced the virus spread. Two sporadic cases of SARS occurred during the summer of 2003 in Taipei and in Singapore. Both cases were laboratory-acquired infections due to neglect of safety precautions.

Even 10 years after the start and the end of the SARS pandemic the authentic source of the virus remains unidentified. Coronaviruses closely resembling the SARS agent but not identical with it were found in bats (*Rhinopholus sinicus)* in Guangdong and its surroundings.

Ten strains of a coronavirus resembling the SARS virus were isolated from Viverrids of the species, large Indian Civet (*Viverra zibetha*), which are prepared and consumed in China as a delicacy; but these viruses were not found to be identical to the SARS virus. A suspected case of SARS was confirmed in January 2004 in the province of Guangdong. The patient had consumed meat from a civet but no secondary cases occurred.

The closest relative of the SARS-Co virus is MERS-CoV, which was isolated in 2012 from a Saudi Arabian patient. In spite of some molecular aspects pointing to a relationship of SARS and MERS-Co viruses with avian coronaviruses, they are in the ß clade of the coronavirus family.

Clinical manifestations. The incubation time lasts 7 (4 to 12) days in the mean. The course of disease may present as a mild febrile disease with respiratory symptoms or with a range of more severe symptoms up to ARD with respiratory insufficiency. All the patients had already suffered days before hospital admission from fever to more than 38 °C and malaise more severe than in influenza. The following symptoms were stated upon hospital admission: cough (75%), myalgia (45%), respiratory distress (40%), and hypoxia. Vomiting, tendency to vomit, anorexia, and diarrhea indicating participation of the intestinal mucosa occurred in 30% of cases. Fever may last up to 3 weeks and relapses may occur; 20% of the patients complained of headaches. In the thorax X-ray, the cases with ARD showed extended signs of atypical pneumonia. At postmortem, pneumonial infiltrates, exsudate, necroses of alveolar cells, and scars were found. Infected cells were found in the lungs, the intestinal epithelium, livers, and in the kidneys. The most severe courses and the majority of fatalities occurred in patients over 40 years old and those suffering from preexisting chronic disease, for example, chronic pulmonary obstruction, diabetes, or nephritis. In children, precluding those with primary disease, severe courses were not observed. Clinical inapparent infections were not found. Between November 2002 and May 2003 more than 8,000 individuals contracted the disease, the case fatality rate was around 10%.

Some observations were published pointing to a decrease of virulence in the course of consecutive human-to-human transmissions. Some of the elderly patients had to be readmitted a few days after release from the hospital due to newly appearing health problems.

As with other coronaviruses, the angiotensin converting enzyme 2 is used by the SARS-Co virus as the cellular receptor. In analogy to chickens infected with the infectious bursitis virus, lymphocytes may be infected and lysed by the SARS virus, resulting in depletion of T- and B-cells from the lymphatic organs.

Diagnosis. Isolated cases of SARS may escape medical attention, especially when mild symptoms of disease occur during the winter season. In case of an outbreak, suspicion of SARS will be raised by a Chinese background and by the severity of some cases. The SARS virus can easily be isolated by inoculating cell cultures of human, pithecine, or murine origin, and will cause CPE within a few days after inoculation. The SARS virus can be identified by rt-PCR. Several pairs of primers re published in the internet (http://www.who.int.csr/sars.en). Indirect immunofluorescence and the western blot are preferential techniques in serodiagnostic studies.

Differential Diagnosis. In mild causes of disease, all the agents causing common colds have to be considered. In severe cases, agents causing atypical pneumonia, influenza and adenoviruses, mycoplasma, rickettsiae, and chlamydiae, as well as coxiellae and legionellae have to be excluded. Enteritis may be indicative of SARS, it may however, also occur in other respiratory infections and in cases of atypical pneumonia caused by other agents. Patients with travel anamnesis on the Arabian Peninsula may be suspected of MERS-CoV.

Therapy. A specific therapy is not available. Treatment is supportive and must be directed to control the ARDS. More than 50% of clinical cases treated for SARS need oxygen. In some severe cases, improvement was achieved with cortisol treatment.

Prophylaxis. There is no vaccine against SARS coronavirus. As the primary source of infection has not yet been identified, it is necessary to prevent familial or nosocomial transmissions. Barrier nursing techniques are needed to interrupt chains of transmission. Assuming that individuals eating zibets or bats are at risk of contracting SARS, this would place this virus in a line together with Ebola and Lassa fever, which infect people via killed animals that are prepared for meals.

1.13.2 MIDDLE EAST RESPIRATORY SYNDROME CORONAVIRUS (MERS-COV)

The MERS-coronavirus is a recently detected zoonotic coronavirus, which was identified in London in June 2012. The index case was a patient from Dschidda, Saudi Arabia, who had been transferred to a London hospital for intensive care treatment. He suffered from a respiratory infection with pneumonia and died of ARDS and acute renal failure. The postmortem confirmed the suspicion of a viral infection; however, the causal agent was not identified. Finally, amplification of a highly conserved coronavirus RNA in a PCR (Pan-Corona-PCR) proved that a novel coronavirus was involved. The PAN-corona-PCR had already been developed in 2002 in connection with the identification of the SARS associated coronavirus. In September 2012, a patient from Qatar was also transferred to a London intensive care unit and an identical coronavirus sequence was amplified. This patient had stayed in Saudi Arabia some days before onset of the first symptoms of disease. By the end of November 9, cases of this new disease had become known; all of them had lived or stayed on the Arabian Peninsula. As transmission patterns of the virus did not include human-to-human transmission and it was soon concluded that one was dealing with a zoonotic disease.

Etiology. MERS-CoV was identified as the cause of this disease. Genomically, it is related to but different from SARS-CoV, which was detected in 2002. Both viruses are now classified to the ß-clade coronaviruses.

Occurrence. All known cases of MERS-CoV syndrome can be traced back to the Arabian Peninsula. Including retrospectively diagnosed and actual cases, there is no country on the Arabian

Peninsula that has not been affected. Imported cases have occurred in the UK, in France, Italy, the Netherlands, Germany, Greece, Malaysia, Tunis, Egypt, and the USA. Recently MERS was introduced to South Korea by a tourist from Saudi Arabia. 183 cases and 33 fatalities were registered up to July 2015. Most of these cases were acquired in a hospital, probably due to problems in air conditioning.

In analogy to other coronaviruses, bats are supposed to be reservoir animals of the MERS-CoV. Genome sequences homologous to the MERS-CoV are found in stools and nasal secretions of dromedaries. Sera from dromedaries, which were taken in 2002 and had been preserved for 10 years, were reactive in tests for antibodies against MERS-CoV; 74% of presently living dromedaries are seropositive. At present, it seems that the authentic human pathogen has not yet been encountered either in bats or in dromedaries but quasispecies are found in these animals. The situation is reminiscent of the studies on SARS, where quasispecies of the SARS-CoV are found in bats as well as in civets but the authentic virus, which caused SARS in humans, has not yet found in these animals.

Transmission. Index cases can often be traced to contact with dromedaries. Human-to-human transmission seems to occur only in families or other normal social contacts but multi-sectional chains of transmission are not recorded. Most cases of human-to-human transmission are due to nosocomial infections. A high incidence of nosocomial infections occurred in Saudi Arabian hospitals, but even in France and the UK, nosocomial infections occurred at a time when the risk was not yet realized. As the virus is found in stools and in nasal mucous, it has not yet been determined which route of infection is responsible for nosocomial infections and it is not clear why the spread in hospitals seems to be more efficient than in domestic or professional settings. As high virus titers are found in nasal and in lower respiratory mucosal secretions in dromedaries, as well as in humans, it is very likely that sneezing and coughing are the predominant mechanisms of spread in inter-human, as well as zoonotic, transmissions. In

the case of SARS, it was presumed that some patients might be "super spreaders," shedding the virus with higher efficiency. It is not yet known whether the pathogenicity increases or is diminished with the number of human-to-human transmissions. The male/female ration is 3/3.1.

Clinical manifestations. According to the WHO, 636 cases of MERS are known presently, out of which, 193 were fatal. Most probably, the number of infected individuals is underestimated as mild infections, occurring in children and younger people, are not recorded. In analogy to SARS, the clinical manifestations of MERS comprise a spectrum of subclinical cases with mild respiratory symptoms up to severe courses that present with pneumonia and ARDS requiring oxygen.

Patients aged over 40 years, and especially those with comorbid conditions, such as diabetes, chronic pulmonary, cardial, or renal disease, are prone to severe courses and the majority of fatalities occur in this group, whereas mild courses are met in children and younger adults without comorbidity. Only two out of 47 hospitalized patients were previously healthy. Patients present with fever, often with chills and rigors, myalgia, cough, and shortness of breath mostly with severe hypoxemic respiratory failure. The X-ray shows signs of bronchitis and atypical pneumonia of varying intensity. Thrombocytopenia and lymphopenia are found in one-third of cases. Symptoms of hemorrhagic diathesis are not reported. Acute nephritis and shock are prognostic signs of fatal courses. In one report, 42% of the patients were alive 90 days after onset of disease.

Diagnosis. Considering the large number of agents causing respiratory disease and the uniformity of the symptoms, a tentative diagnosis in most cases will rely on epidemiological circumstances, such as a recent stay on the Arabian Peninsula or contact with dromedaries. Gastrointestinal in addition to respiratory problems may raise a suspicion but may also be present in other respiratory infections. Although virus isolation is possible, the diagnostic technique of choice is the PCR. The SARS virus can be identified by rt-PCR. Several pairs of primers are published on the internet (http://www.who.int.csr/sars.en). Serological tests are mainly important for recognition of mild and subclinical infections. Indirect immunofluorescence, ELISA, and western blot can be used for serodiagnosis.

Differential diagnosis. A large number of agents causing respiratory infections and atypical pneumonia will have to be considered. The travel anamnesis or provenience of a patient and contact with dromedaries may be helpful in these decisions.

Therapy. At present, there is no approved specific therapy against MERS-CoV syndrome. Supportive therapy will have to improve respiration that will often require oxygen respiration. As the majority of these patients have a comorbid situation, the basic disease will have to be controlled. In analogy to hepatitis C virus, a combination of ribavirin and interferon-α2b might be able to reduce the virus load. As the cellular receptor for entry of the MERS-CoV into cells is dipeptidylpeptidase 4 inhibitors or antagonists of this enzyme, for example, adenosine deaminase, might hypothetically be able to suppress the virus replication.

Prophylaxis. There is no vaccine available at present against MERS-CoV. Contact with dromedaries should be avoided, especially on the Arabian Peninsula. Pregnant women or individuals in a comorbid situation should not travel in rural regions on the Arabian Peninsula.

REFERENCES

Abdullah ASM et al., Lessons from the severe acute respiratory syndrome outbreak in Hong Kong. *Emerg. Infect. Dis.* 9, 1042–1045, 2003.

Arabi YM et al., Clinical course and outcomes of critical ill patients with Middle East respiratory syndrome coronavirus infection. *Ann. Intern. Med.* 160 (6) 389–397, 2014.

Al Tawfiq JA et al., Middle East repiratory syndrome novel corona MERS-CoV infection. Epidemiology and outcome update. *Saudi Med J* 991–994, 2013.

Assiri A et al., Epidemiological, demographic and clinical characteristics of 47 cases of Middle East respiratory syndrome coronavirus disease from Saudi Arabia, a descriptive study. *Lancet Infect Dis* 2913, 752–761.

Breiman RF et al., Role of China in the quest to define and control severe acute respiratory syndrome. *Emerg. Infect. Dis.* 9, 1037–1041, 2003.

CDC, Use of quarantine to prevent transmission of severe acute respiratory syndrome – Taiwan. *MMWR Morb. Mortal. Wkly. Rep.* 52, 680–683, 2003.

CDC, Update: Severe acute respiratory syndrome – United States, 2003. *MMWR Morb. Mortal. Wkly. Rep.* 52, 616, 2003.

Cooke FJ, Shapiro DS, Global outbreak of severe acute respiratory syndrome (SARS). *Int. J. Infect. Dis.* 7, 80–85, 2003.

Ding Y et al., The clinical pathology of severe acute respiratory syndrome (SARS): a report from China. *J. Pathol.* 200, 282–289, 2003.

Drosten C et al., Identification of a novel coronavirus in patients with severe acute respiratory syndrome. *New Engl. J. Med.* 348, 1967–1976, 2003.

Fowler RA et al., Toronto SARS Critical Care Group: Critically ill patients with severe acute respiratory syndrome. *JAMA* 290, 367–373, 2003.

Galvani AP, Lei X, Jewell NP, Severe acute respiratory syndrome: temporal stability and geographic variation in case-fatality rates and doubling times. *Emerg. Infect. Dis.* 9, 991–994, 2003.

Hartley DM, Smith DL, Uncertainty in SARS epidemiology. *Lancet* 362, 170–171, 2003.

Hsu LY et al., Severe acute respiratory syndrome in Singapore: clinical features of index patient and initial contacts. *Emerg. Infect. Dis.* 9, 713–717, 2003.

Ksiazeck TG et al., A novel coronavirus associated with severe acute respiratory syndrome. *New Engl. J. Med.* 348, 1953–1966, 2003.

Kuiken T et al., Newly discovered coronavirus as the primary cause of severe acute respiratory syndrome. *Lancet* 362, 263–270, 2003.

Lew TW et al., Acute respiratory distress syndrome in critically ill patients with severe acute respiratory syndrome. *JAMA.* 290, 374–380, 2003.

Li L, Cheng S, Gu J, SARS infection among health care workers in Beijing, China. *JAMA* 290, 2662–2663, 2003.

Loutfy MR et al., Interferon alfacon-1 plus corticosteroids in severe acute respiratory syndrome: a preliminary study. *JAMA* 290, 3222–3228, 2003.

Pang X et al., Evaluation of control measures implemented in the severe acute respiratory syndrome outbreak in Beijing, 2003. *JAMA* 290, 3215–3221, 2003.

Torpy JM, Lynm C, Glass RM, JAMA patient page. Severe acute respiratory syndrome (SARS). *JAMA* 290, 3318, 2003.

Tsui PT et al., Severe acute respiratory syndrome: clinical outcome and prognostic correlates. *Emerg. Infect. Dis.* 9, 1064–1069, 2003.

Tsui SK, Chim SS, Lo YM, Chinese University of Hong Kong Molecular SARS Research Group: Coronavirus genomic-sequence variations and the epidemiology of the severe acute respiratory syndrome. *New Engl. J. Med.* 349, 187–188, 2003.

Twu SJ et al., Control measures for severe acute respiratory syndrome (SARS) in Taiwan. *Emerg. Infect. Dis.* 9, 718–720, 2003.

Wang H et al., Fatal aspergillosis in a patient with SARS who was treated with corticosteroids. *New Engl. J. Med.* 349, 507–508, 2003.

Wong WM et al., Temporal patterns of hepatic dysfunction and disease severity in patients with SARS. *JAMA* 290, 2663–2665, 2003.

1.14 Retroviruses

This chapter is restricted on zoonotic aspects of human retrovirus infections. For an in depth discussion of the virological basis and clinical aspects, such as pathogenesis, clinical picture, diagnosis, therapy, and prophylaxis, it is recommended to consult the relevant textbooks in medical virology, immunology, internal medicine, and infectious diseases

The name "retrovirus" was coined for all the RNA viruses possessing reverse transcriptase activity, which enables them to transcribe their genome into double stranded DNA. This step is essential for the production of a so-called provirus, which can be integrated into the host cell genome. Retroviruses have a choice between two types of reproduction: production of a new generation of mature virus particles that may spread horizontally to infect new cells or remaining integrated into the host cell genome and restricting their reproductive activity to the reproduction cycle of the host cell genome. In this state, the genome is able to switch to a productive cycle resulting in a new generation of virus particles. The mature retrovirus particles are enveloped viruses of ca. 100 nm in diameter. The genome is diploid and consists of single-stranded RNA with plus-strand polarity. *Pararetroviruses* also have reverse transcriptase activity but their particles contain the genome in the form of double-stranded DNA. HepaDNA viruses and a family of plant viruses, the *caulimoviridae*, are examples of *pararetroviridae*. The reverse transcriptase does not-like other DNA-polymerases-include a proofreading mechanism; therefore, retroviruses have a high mutation rate.

Classification. The family *Retroviridae* is divided into two subfamilies, *Orthoretrovirinae* with six genera and *Spumaretrovirinae* with a single genus. The genera of *Orthoretrovirinae* are alpha- beta-, gamma-, delta-, and epsilon-retroviruses and lentivirus. An important difference between these genera is the utilization of diverse tRNA species as primers for reverse transcription. With the exception of lentiviruses and spumaviruses, the *Orthoretrovirinae* cause mostly malignant transformations of cells of the mesenchymal lines, leukemia, or sarcoma. Beta-retroviruses are transforming epithelial cells and can induce carcinomas, for example, mammary cancer in mice. The underlying mechanisms of cell transformation are different in each genus. The general principle is that cellular or viral genes, for example, oncogenes, superantigenes, or transcription activators are placed under the control of a highly active promoter of the provirus, enhancing their rate of expression and resulting in a higher concentration of the gene product. The human immunodeficiency viruses HIV I and HIV II are lentiviruses and do not induce cell transformation.

1.14.1 PRIMATE T-CELL-LYMPHOTROPIC VIRUSES: PTLV 1 AND PTLV 2 (HTLV 1 AND 2)

The human T-cell lymphotropic viruses, HTLV 1 and HTLV 2 are the only oncogenic retroviruses of humans. HTLV 1 causes adult T-cell leukemia (ATL) and HTLV-associated myelopathy (tropical spastic paraparesis). HTLV 2 is believed to be the cause of human hairy cell leukemia.

Etiology. HTLV 1 and HTLV 2 are retroviruses belonging to the genus delta-retrovirus. The term PTLV (primate T-cell leukemia virus) was coined for these viruses with regard to their close relationship with viruses occurring in monkeys. HTLV 3 and HTLV 4, viruses with a high degree of genome homology to monkey viruses of the group STLV (simian T-cell leukemia virus), were recently detected in Africans living in the south of Cameroon. The viral genomes, like all the other retroviruses, have the genes gag (capsid), pol (polymerase), and env (envelope). In addition, they have a tax gene (transcription activator) and a rex gene (splicing and regulation of intracellular transport).

Occurrence. The HTLV are mostly transmitted via human-to-human contacts; however, monkeys are believed to be the natural reservoir. In a wild caught Orangutan (*Papio hamadryas*) and a dwarf chimpanzee (*Pan paniscus*), PTLV were found having a high degree of genomic homology with HTLV 1, 2, and 3. In sera from Africans, which have contact with monkeys, PTLV sequences were found, which because of their strong divergence from HTLV 1,2, and 3 have been named HTLV 4. Correlates of these sequences have not been found up to now in simians.

HTLV 1 is endemic on some islands in the southwest of Japan, where 20% of the inhabitants are seropositive. The virus also occurs on some Caribbean islands, in central and west Africa, South Africa, Melanesia, and in India. HTLV 2 is found in i.v. drug addicts and their sex partners. Three subtypes of HTLV 2 can be differentiated: 2a in North America, 2b in Panama, Columbia, and Argentina, and 2c, which occurs in the urban populations in Brazil. In Europe, both infections are rare and are restricted to immigrants from endemic areas. HTLV 3 and 4 are at present only encountered in Cameroon inhabitants.

Transmission. PTLV are transmitted sexually, genital ulcers are predisposing factors. Transmission via blood donations is possible. Blood products are infectious only when cellular components are included. The virus content of plasma is low. The virus can be transmitted from nursing mothers via milk, 15% to 20% of the children of seropositive mothers are infected if they are breast-fed.

Clinical Manifestations. The majority of infections with HTLV 1 remain symptom-free for life, as the virus is latent in transformed cells. ATL is a lymphoproliferative disease of mature T-cells, with the markers CD^{3+}, CD^{4+}, CD^{8-}, CD^{25+}, and $HLADR^+$ having monoclonally integrated provirus in the cell genome. The latent period between infection and onset of disease is 20 to 30 years. Less than 4% of virus carriers will eventually develop ATL.

Symptoms of ATL are lymphadenopathy, lymphomas, splenomegaly, lytic bone lesions, and cutaneous foci. The patients are immune-deficient and have opportunistic infections (e.g., *Strongyloides stercoralis* in Japan).

The HTLV 1-associated (tropical) myelopathy is a demyelinating disease of the spinal cord and CNS, which is manifest in 5% of the carriers of HTLV 1. The pathogenic potential of HTLV 2 is questionable. A more detailed description of clinical pictures is found in textbooks of internal medicine and infectious diseases.

Diagnosis. Blood count, biopsy and histology are needed for the diagnosis. ELISA is used for screening of blood donors. PCR allows detection of the integrated provirus.

Therapy. ATL is treated with a protocol combining zidovudine and IFN-alpha, but long lasting remissions are only achieved in 26% of cases. Relapses occur in most cases after 12 months. There is no effective therapy against HTLV 1 associated myelopathy.

Prophylaxis. Vaccines are not available. Unprotected sexual intercourse is to be avoided. HTLV 1 infected mothers should not nurse their children. In endemic populations, donors of blood and/or organs should be tested.

REFERENCES

Balogou AA et al., Prevalence of HTLV-1 virus infection in Togo (Kozah prefecture and the University Hospital Center of Lomé). *Bull Soc Pathol Exot.* 93, 3–5, 2000.

Carles G et al., HTLV1 infection and pregnancy. *J Gynecol Obstet Biol Reprod (Paris).* 33, 14–20, 2004.

Clyti E et al., Infective dermatitis and recurrent strongyloidiasis in a child. Ann Dermatol Venerol. 131, 191–193, 2004.

Gonçalves DU et al., Epidemiology, treatment, and prevention of human T-cell leukemia virus type 1-associated diseases. *Clin Microbiol Rev.* 23, 577–589, 2010.

Grassmann R, Menschliche T-Zell-Leukämieviren (HTLV-1). In: Doerr HW, Gerlich WH (Hrsg.) *Medizinische Virologie.* 2. Aufl. Stuttgart, Georg Thieme; 2010 335–340.

Hamaad A, Davis RC, Connolly DL, Regression of HTLV1 associated intracardiac lymphoma following chemotherapy. *Heart.* 88, 621, 2002.

Hovette P et al., Pulmonary strongyloidiasis complicated by E. coli meningitis in a HIV-1 and HTLV-1 positive patient. *Presse Med.* 3, 2021–2023, 2002.

Laveaux K et al., Localized nasal cavity, sinus, and massive bilateral orbital involvement by human T cell leukemia virus 1 adult T cell lymphoma, with epidermal hypertro- phy due to mite infestation. *Rare Tumors.* 31, e59, 2010.

Mane LL et al., HTLV-1 tropism and envelope receptor Oncogene. *Sep* 5, 6016–6025, 2005.

Nicolas M, Perez JM, Carme B, Intestinal parasitosis in French West Indies: endemic evolution from 1991 to 2003 in the University Hospital of Pointe-a-Pitre, Guade-loupe. *Bull Soc Pathol Exot.* 2006 Oct; 99(4), 254–257. French.

Proietti FA et al., Global epidemiology of HTLV 1 infection and associated diseases. *Oncogene* 24, 6058–6068, 2005.

Roucoux DF, Murphy DL, The epidemiology and disease outcome of human T-lymphotropic virus type 2. *AIDS Rev.* 6, 144–154, 2004.

Yamada Y, Tomonaga M, The current status of therapy for adult T-cell leukaemia-lymphoma in Japan. *Leuk Lymphoma* 44, 611–618, 2003.

Yoshida M, Discovery of HTLV 1, the first human retrovirus, its unique regulatory mechanisms, and insights into patho-genesis. *Oncogene* 24, 5931–5937, 2005.

1.14.2 LENTIVIRUSES: HIV 1 AND HIV 2

Lentiviruses are non-transforming retroviruses, which are found in monkeys [simian immu-nodeficiency virus (SIV)], cats [feline immu-nodeficiency virus (FIV)], bovines [bovine immunodeficiency virus (BIV)], sheep [Visna virus (VV)], horses [equine infectious anemia virus (EIAV)], and goats [caprine arthritis ence-phalitis virus (CAE)]. Humans, up to that time free of lentivirus infections, became a host of the human immunodeficiency viruses, HIV 1 and HIV 2, in the mid-20th century. Since 1980, the world has seen a pandemic spread of these viruses. The human immunodefi-ciency viruses have a narrow relationship with simian immunodeficiency viruses; therefore, it is assumed that they were originally transmitted from monkeys to humans. In their primordial hosts, SIVs are not pathogenic, which provides for a further argument, that humans may not be the original hosts of HIVs. There are numer-ous examples of zoonotic viruses, which are transmitted from monkeys to humans that proves that the African habit of eating "bush meat" (monkey meat) is the route for virus pas-sage from monkeys to humans. It can be

assumed that humans are infected frequently with HIVs via bushmeat. There are many theories trying to explain why HIVs have not produced pandemic spread before the 20th cen-tury. (There is not enough space in this book to discuss this interesting problem.) Without doubt, the state of the art of the medical science would not have allowed the detection of HIVs earlier than in 1960 or 1970. If cases of AIDS had occurred before 1970, they would have been diagnosed as diseases caused by opportun-istic agents. Nobody would have been able to diagnose and to define a state of immunodefi-ciency. The first case of an HIV-infection was diagnosed retrospectively in a serum that had been taken from a patient in 1959 who was a sai-lor. All lentiviruses infect macrophages but regardless of this common feature, they produce very different clinical manifestations, for exam-ple, immunodeficiency in humans, cows, and cats, anemia in horses, encephalitis in sheep, and arthritis in goats. The reason why SIVs are nonpathogenic in their original hosts is not known.

Etiology. HIV 1, and to a smaller portion HIV 2, are the causes of the acquired human immune-deficiency syndrome (AIDS). HIV 1 originates in East Africa and stems from a chimpanzee virus (SIV^{cpz}). Three groups of HIV 1 are discernible: type M (for major) predominant with nine sub-types (A, B, C, D, E, F, G, H, J, and K), which occur in different geographic regions, and the remaining types "O" (for "outlier") and "N" (for "non M-non O"). These three types are gen-erally believed to have resulted from different events of virus transmission from chimpanzee to human. A SIV closely resembling type O of HIV was recently detected in a gorilla, thus, transmission from gorillas to humans is accepted as a possible source.

The HIV 2 epidemic originating in West Africa is most probably derived from a Mangabey monkey (*Cercocebus torquatus*). In summary, the AIDS pandemic is produced by at least four dif-ferent events of transmission from monkeys to humans. There may have been more than four events but certainly not less. Some of the viruses of group M have evolved to a greater genetic distance from the others and these are responsible for the majority of all HIV infections. Meanwhile, genetic recombinants of subtypes are found that must stem from double infections.

Occurrence. HIVs are transmitted by human-to-human contact. They are globally distributed; therefore, we are dealing with pandemic agents. Subtypes of the major type "M" differ in their geographical distribution. In Africa, all known serotypes are present with predominance of subtypes A, C, and D. In European countries and in the USA, subtype B is prevalent. Worldwide, subtype C causing 50% to 60% of all infections is the most prevalent one. HIV 2 and subtypes O and N of HIV 1 are restricted to Africa and are only rarely recognized in Europe or the USA. Subtype N was never detected outside Africa. There are constitutional factors that make people resistant against HIV. In Caucasians, 1% to 2% of the population is protected due to a deleted CCR5 gene, which encodes a chemokine receptor that serves as a co-receptor for HIV; however, only homozygotes are protected.

At present, it is estimated that there are more than 60 million people on the global scale who are infected with HIV 1. About one-third of these have succumbed to the disease. In 2007, there were 2.1 million fatalities caused by AIDS and there were 2.7 million *de novo* infections that mainly occurred in young adults aged 15 to 24 years living in developing countries; 90% of all HIV infected people (42% females) live in these countries. In the USA, the proportion of HIV-infected women increased from 7% in 1985 to 26% of newly discovered cases in 2002.

Transmission. It is generally accepted that HIV transmission from monkeys to humans is brought about by preparation and consummation of monkey meat (bush meat) that is eaten as a delicacy in most parts of Africa. Worldwide, human-to human transmission occurs in 85% of cases via heterosexual intercourse, with the exception of developed countries where homosexual transmission between men is the predominant route of transmission. In heterosexual as

well as in homosexual contacts, the risk of an insertive partner is only 10% that of the receptive partner. The probability for a successful transmission is estimated to be 0.02% to 1% per contact. In Eastern Europe, as well as in Central and Southern Asia, one-third of HIV transmissions occur in i.v. drug dependents via reused needles. A newborn child of an HIV-infected mother has a risk of 13% to 40% of being infected. The risk rises with the maternal virus load and is higher in vaginal delivery as compared to cesarean section. Breast-feeding the child increases its risk of infection. The risk of a nosocomial infection due to inadvertent needle stick injury with a blood-contaminated needle is 1:300. The probability of HIV transmission by transfusing HIV infected blood is 90%. It must be stressed that all these probabilities are arbitrary and depend on special circumstances of the case, the most critical point being the virus load.

Clinical Manifestations. As a disease, AIDS is characterized by a variable incubation period that is in the range of 1 to 4 weeks. During the incubation period, the virus load in the blood increases rapidly while antibodies are not yet produced. The risk of virus transmission is high during this period. At the end of incubation, acute disease follows with mild symptoms reminiscent of the common cold, or respecting the lymphadenopathy rather of infectious mononucleosis. There is no severe malaise, which explains that only 40% of patients would consult their practitioner. In the course of this period, 80% of memory cells have already been destroyed. The acute disease is followed by a latent period of 6 to 10 years; in HIV 2 infections, it is twice as long. The latent phase is not free of symptoms: frequent infections may raise the suspicion of immune deficiency. Virus replication causes a massive loss of CD^{4+} helper cells, which during the latent period is compensated by intensified regeneration. The patients are now highly infectious. Eventually, regeneration of helper cells can no longer compensate for cell destruction. When the count of helper cells sinks below a critical value, opportunistic diseases appear indicating the development of full-blown AIDS. Viral, bacterial, protozoan, fungal, and parasitic infections, which might be harmless for an immune competent organism, may cause life- threatening diseases. Many of these opportunistic organisms have a zoonotic background. For a more comprehensive discussion, we recommend the relevant chapters of this book and special textbooks of infectious diseases, internal medicine, and microbiology.

Diagnosis. For antibody detection (IgG and IgM), ELISA tests are available, mostly on the basis of recombinant antigens and designed to detect a broad spectrum of antibodies to HIV 1 subtypes and to HIV 2. In addition, and for confirmation of ELISA results, Western blots are used to identify false-positive results that may arise due to the very high sensitivity of the ELISA. For virus detection, the p24-ELISA is used, which is positive when there are $>10^5$/ml particles. The p24 ELISA may be combined with an ELISA detecting IgG and IgM antibodies to cover early cases in which the antibody is not present yet or the antigen is not present any more.

PCR tests are the "gold standard." Viral DNA is detected in a PCR and viral RNA in a RT-PCR. The most important diagnostic task is screening of blood donators for which ELISA tests are used throughout. Since shortly after infection, HIV-infected individuals do not yet produce antibodies and as cases with AIDS have only low antibody titers, it is necessary to include a simultaneous antigen ELISA (p24-test) in order to fill the "diagnostic gap."

To confirm a case of a suspected infection, the same techniques are used that are employed for screening of blood donors. In addition, techniques for virus detection, PCR, and RT-PCR in various modifications and measurement of the reverse transcriptase activity are available. RT-PCR and determination of the reverse transcriptase are also used to measure the virus load, so that the degree of infection, the indication for therapeutic measures, and the efficiency of antiviral therapy can be assessed. Tests for detecting resistance against antiviral drugs are also part of the diagnostic arsenal.

The uncharacteristic clinical picture of the early phase is diagnosed correctly in a minority of cases only. Specific diagnostic measures may *per se* be vulnerating and are therefore justified only in case of a suspicion with the patient's consent and accompanied by a thorough risk analysis. For this reason, infections in the early or latent phases are—as a rule—only noticed by screening blood donations or at medical checkups.

An unusual frequency of opportunistic diseases will raise the suspicion of AIDS if other explanations can be excluded. The most important clinical laboratory test in such a case is the count of $CD4^+$ cells, which can be done with an ELISA technique in combination with perfusion cytometry. Normal counts are in the range of 500 and 1500 cells/mm^3. In AIDS patients, this count declines to <250. A successful therapy should increase the $CD4^+$ count and decrease the virus load.

Therapy. The basic therapeutic concept is highly active antiretroviral therapy (HAART), which should be carried out with at least three drugs attacking three different points of action. Meanwhile, 30 different preparations are available. Points of attack are the reverse transcriptase, which may be inhibited by nucleosidic or nonnucleosidic inhibitors, protease, and integrase. Protease is responsible for processing of viral proteins and integrase accomplishes integration of the viral genome into the host cell genome. Co-receptor antagonists may interfere with virus adsorption and fusion inhibitors will prevent the virus from entering the cell. The rapid accumulation of resistant variants necessitates continuous surveillance of the therapeutic regimen. Opportunistic infections must be treated with special therapeutics (cf. the relevant chapters of this book).

Prophylaxis. Several experimental vaccines have been developed but none of these has reached maturity. The most important measure to protect the population is achieved by screening blood donors and blood donations for HIV infections. Sterile syringes and needle sticks are provided for individuals addicted to the use of i.v. drugs. The use of condoms is recommended and is propagated in cinema and TV. Unfortunately, antiviral creams for intravaginal application have not provided a sufficient protective effect. Special guidelines exist for pregnant women with HIV to prevent HIV-transmission to the fetus. To avoid nosocomial infections health professionals who have been injured with a potentially contaminated instrument will have to undergo antiviral therapy.

Prognosis. The life span of patients is prolonged by application of HAART (with relative well-being) but, after all, AIDS is, and remains, a lethal infection.

REFERENCES

Barré-Sinoussi F et al., Isolation of a T-lymphotropic retrovirus from a patient at risk of acquired immunedeficiency syndrome. *Science* 220, 868–871, 1983.

Hahn BH et al., AIDS as a zoonosis: scientific and public health implications. *Science* 28, 607–614, 2000.

Kahn JO, Walker BD, Acute human immunedeficiency virus type 1 infection. *N. Engl. J. Med.* 339, 33–39, 1998.

Letvin NL, Walker BD, Immunopathogenesis and Immunotherapy in AIDS virus infections. *Nat.Med.* 9, 861–866, 2003.

Mattapallil JJ et al., Massive infection and loss of memory CD4+ T-cells in multiple tissues during acute SIV infection. *Nature* 434, 1093–1097, 2005.

Mc Govern B, Hepatic safety and HAART. *J. Int. Assoc. Physicians AIDS Care* 3, 24–40, 2004.

Münch J et al., Semen-derived amyloid fibrils drastically enhance HIV-Infection. *Cell* 131, 1059–1071, 2007.

Plantier JC et al., A new human immune deficiency virus derived from gorillas. *Nat. Med.* 15, 871–872, 2009.

Silvestri G et al., Uderstanding the benign nature of SIV infection in natural hosts. *J. Clin. Invest.* 117, 3148–3154, 2007.

Simon V, Ho DD, Abdool Karim Q, HIV/AIDS epidemiology, pathogenesis, prevention, and treatment. *Lancet* 368, 489–504, 2006.

Van Heuverswyn F, Peeters M, Origins of HIV and implications for the global epidemic. *Curr. Inf. Dis. Rep* 9, 338–346, 2007.

Zhu T et al., An African HIV-1 sequence and implications for the origin of the epidemic. *Nature* 391, 594–597, 1998.

1.14.3 ENDOGENOUS RETROVIRUSES

Endogenous retroviruses are not transmitted under normal conditions from animals to humans. Their zoonotic potential has resulted from xenotransplantation, which means that pigs, transgenic for human transplantation antigens, are used as organ donors. The porcine endogenous retroviruses, PERV-A and PERV-B, have been shown *in vitro* to replicate in human cells. In experimental xenotransplantations (livers and pancreatic islet cells), which up to now have been carried out, no replication of PERV was recognized in the receptor organisms.

Endogenous retroviruses are not included in the above classification scheme of retroviruses as they are integrated as proviruses in the cell genome and are in their reproduction restricted to mitotic cycles of the cell genome. Integrated into the genome of the oocysts they can be propagated through generations. As proviruses are able to illegitimately integrate into the cellular genome they can fulfill the function that transposons have in the bacterial genome. As leaping genes, they are able to activate or inactivate cellular genes or cut them out of the DNA strand and translocate them.

The close relationship between exogenous and endogenous retroviruses influences the classification of the latter. Class I of ERV resembles the gamma-retroviruses, class II corresponds to alpha- and beta-retroviruses, and class III resembles the foamy agent. The differentiation criterion is the usage of different tRNA species as primers for reverse transcription.

Endogenous retroviruses guarantee a high flexibility to the host cell genomes, and therefore, they are also called the motors of evolution. While in mice and in pigs, endogenous retroviruses have retained the capability to replicate independently from the cellular genome and to produce mature virus particles; the human endogenous retroviruses have lost this ability. Thirty-one groups of human endogenous retroviruses (HERV) are known and up to 1.300 genome copies of a specific HERV are found in a single cell. The content of integrated retroviral DNA amounts to 8% of the human genome. In the placenta of humans and animals, transformation of the cytotrophoblast into the syncytiotrophoblast is brought about by retroviral fusion proteins that are encoded in the genome of endogenous retroviruses. Syncytin I is an envelope protein of HERV-W and syncytin II is a gene product of HERV-FRD.

The correct function of the syncytiotrophoblast is guaranteed by viral fusion proteins. HRVs may be looked at as slaves contributing the unique viral invention of fusion proteins to the evolution and reproduction of the *Placentalia*.

HERVs are also important in the pathogenesis of autoimmune disease. Some of these genomes have information to code for superantigens, for example, they may be transactivated by the Epstein Barr virus genome. The gene expression of HERV-K18 can be increased by an Epstein-Barr virus infection or by interferon-alpha.

REFERENCES

Bannert N, Kurth R, The evolutionary dynamics of human endogenous retroviral families. *Annu. Rv. Genomics Hum. Genet.* 7, 149–173, 2006.

Belshaw R, Dawson AL, Woolven-Allen J, Genomewide screening reveals high levels of insertional polymorphism in the human endogenous retrovirus family HERVK (HML2): implications for present-day activity. *J. Virol.* 79, 12507–12514, 2005.

Belshaw R et al., High copy number in human endogenous retrovirus families is associated with copying mechanism in addition to reinfection. *Mol. Biol. Evol.* 22, 814–817, 2005.

Choi Y, Kappler JW, Marrack P, A superantigen encoded in the open reading frame of the 3′ long terminal repeat of mouse mammary tumour virus. *Nature* 350, 203–207, 1991.

Denner J, Immunosuppression by retroviruses: implications for xenotransplantation. *Ann. NY Acad. Sci.* 862, 75–86, 1998.

Denner J, Endogene Retroviren. In: Doerr HW, Gerlich WH (eds.), *Medizinische Virologie. 2.Aufl.* Stuttgart, Georg Thieme; 341–344, 2010.

Katzourakis A, Rambaut A, Pybus OG, The evolutionary dynamics of endogenous retroviruses. *Trends Microbiol.* 13, 463–468, 2005.

Rosnett DN, Jarilina AA, Sleeping with the enemy. Endogenous superantigens in humans. *Immunity* 15, 503–506, 2001.

Ruprecht K et al., Endogenous retroviruses and cancer. *Cell Mol. Life Sci.* 65, 3366–3382, 2008.

Suttkowski N et al., Epstein-Barr virus trancactivates the human endogenous retrovirus HERV-K18 that encodes a superantigen. *Immunity* 15, 579–589, 2001.

1.15 Zoonoses Caused by Herpesviruses

The family *Herpesviridae* includes more than 100 virus species found in mammals, birds, and reptiles. These viruses are host specific,

may persist for a lifetime, and they may be reactivated. There are eight original herpesviruses pathogenic for humans, designated herpesvirus hominis type 1 (HVH-1) [also known as herpes simplex virus type 1 (HSV-1)] to HVH-8 (Kaposi sarcoma virus). There are more than 30 herpesvirus species in monkeys. Although one could expect many of these viruses to have a zoonotic potential, only one of them, herpes B virus (herpesvirus simiae), which is endemic in macaque monkeys, is highly pathogenic for humans. Conversely, human herpesviruses (HSV-1 and -2) are highly pathogenic for monkeys.

Herpesviruses are large, enveloped DNA viruses with a diameter of 120 to 300 nm and a cubic nucleocapsid composed of 162 capsomeres. The structure and size of the genome vary between virus species and genera. The genome is made of 150 to 230 kbp, which corresponds to a coding capacity of about 200 different polypeptides. At least 35 of these are present in the virus particle as structural proteins. Based on biological characteristics, the herpesviruses are divided into three subfamilies: *Alphaherpesvirinae* (e.g., herpes simplex virus), *Betaherpesvirinae* (e.g., cytomegalovirus), and *Gammaherpesvirinae* (e.g., Epstein- Barr virus).

Herpes B virus from macaques, which has zoonotic importance for humans, belongs to the subfamily *Alphaherpesvirinae*, together with HSV-1 and -2, varicella-zoster virus, and other animal herpesviruses. Viruses in this group have a short replication cycle and a relatively wide host spectrum. They cause persistent and recurrent infections of sensitive spinal and intracranial ganglia. There are several nucleoside analogues that are used as pre-drugs (inactive substances that have to be activated in the cell) in the therapy of infection. These drugs are phosphorylated only by thymidine kinases derived from the virus. Therefore, the substances (e.g., acyclovir) only block the viral DNA, but not DNA from uninfected cells.

1.15.1 HERPES B VIRUS: SIMIAN HERPES INFECTION

Among the numerous herpesviruses of monkeys, only herpes B virus is of major importance for human infections. Humans with herpes B virus infections develop ascending encephalitis and myelitis in more than 90% of cases, with a case fatality rate of 75%.

Etiology. Herpes B virus belongs to the subfamily *Alphaherpesvirinae*, genus *Simplexvirus*, and is closely related to HSV-1 and -2.

Occurrence. Human infections with herpes B virus are rare. There have been only 40 cases reported worldwide, including only one case in Europe with a clinical picture of herpes zoster.

Herpes B virus infections are almost exclusively found in *Macaca* spp. [especially *Macaca mulatta* (rhesus monkeys) and *M. fascicularis* (cynomolgus monkeys)] in different regions of Asia. Growing animals are not infected. More than 70% of monkeys in captivity and in the wild are infected. Only 2% to 3% of infected animals shed infectious virus in body secretions. Stress, immunosuppression, and pregnancy enhance virus shedding.

Monkeys from different species can become infected when kept in contact with infected macaques. Infections may become disseminated, with ascending myelitis, or they may remain latent. Infected monkeys of non-*Macaca* species can also be a source of human infections.

Modern neurological, neurophysiological, and behavioral examinations of monkeys often require close contact between humans and monkeys. The risk of exposure for humans increases with the number and intensity of these contacts. Therefore, alternative test subjects should be seriously considered if macaques are involved in research.

Transmission. Transmission of herpes B virus, like that of most herpesviruses, is by direct contact with virus-containing secretions. Indirect transmission is possible, for example, when monkeys are placed in a cage where macaques have been housed before. About 40 human infections have been known to occur since the virus was first isolated in 1933 to 1934. Only some of them have been confirmed by virus isolation. With few exceptions, infections can be traced to contact with monkeys, either in experimental work or in zoos. Half of the exposures could be traced to biting, scratching, or lesions from needles or scalpels. The source of infection of the remaining cases is unexplained. Virus in cell cultures prepared from macaques may be a source of infection. Considering the fairly frequent biting and scratching from macaques, transmission of herpes B virus to humans is an exceptional event. None of 321 individuals tested after close contact with primates, including people with lesions but without disease, had developed antibodies to the herpes B virus.

Virus transmission from an animal caretaker to his wife was observed in one case. The woman had treated herpes lesions on the hand of her husband.

Clinical Manifestations. Early local signs appear 48 h after exposure, with erythema, vesicles, ulcers, and local pain at the site of the lesion. A regional lymphadenopathy follows. Systemic signs appear 1 to 3 weeks later: paresthesia and muscle weakness up to paralysis of the infected limb, conjunctivitis, persistent hiccups, and dysphagia. Signs of progressive encephalitis are fever, headaches, nausea, vomiting, stiffness of the neck, double vision, disturbance of speech, ataxia, disturbed consciousness and respiration, spasms, ascending paralysis, and coma. Respiratory paralysis is usually the cause of death.

Recently, a case in which signs of herpes B virus appeared 10 years after the last contact with monkeys was described. The case took the form of shingles (herpes zoster oticus) and it was followed by generalized signs. This case proves the potential latency of herpes B virus in humans. It is not known whether immune responses to human alphaherpesviruses influence the course of the disease.

In contrast to other monkey species, rhesus monkeys never develop encephalitis or myelitis after herpes B virus exposure. The course of the disease in rhesus monkeys is similar to that of HSV infections in humans. In other monkey species, the herpes B virus may cause fatal disease.

Diagnosis. A tentative diagnosis can be made based on the history: contact with monkeys, their tissues, or cell cultures prepared from them. The monkeys need not be diseased. Individuals with contact with monkeys can be the source of infection. Infections by indirect contact via secretions are possible. A rapid diagnosis can be tried in cases of skin eruptions by IFA or electron microscopy or immunofluorescence with antisera to human herpesvirus 1. Therapy can be initiated before virus isolation and typing are completed.

For the isolation of the virus, epithelial cell lines from humans, monkeys, rabbits, and hamsters are suitable. The serological typing of herpes B virus is complicated by cross-reactions with other herpesviruses. Two pairs of oligonucleotide primers targeting two locations of the herpes B virus gG gene were designed and were recommended for differentiating between human herpesviruses 1 and 2 and herpes B virus. Due to the high GC content, the PCR can only run in the presence of 1 M betaine (see the end of this section).

The postmortem diagnosis in humans can be based on the history and on typical histological CNS lesions by immunofluorescence or PCR.

For research with monkeys, it is often desirable to know whether the animals are infected. Serodiagnosis is difficult. If present, antibodies to HSV-1 and -2 have to be preabsorbed with viral antigen. A competitive ELISA with monoclonal antibodies has been developed for the detection of herpes B virus antibodies. It is superior to the virus neutralization test to determine the serostatus of monkeys. A seropositive monkey can shed the virus, even if attempts to detect the virus have been negative. Any work with herpes B virus or suspicious material has to be performed in a biosafety-L4 laboratory.

Differential Diagnosis. Infections with human alphaherpesviruses and poxviruses have to be considered in the differential diagnosis. In addition, a variety of infectious and noninfectious CNS diseases should be included. The history of contact with monkeys is always important.

Therapy. In cell culture, the concentration of acyclovir has to be 10-fold higher than that for HSV-1 or -2 for a 50% blockage of herpes B virus. The minimal concentration for Ganciclovir is somewhat lower, but the toxicity is higher. Vidarabine is not recommended for herpesvirus infections today.

There are only sporadic reports available about the treatment of herpes B virus infections with acyclovir. It is too early to evaluate the results. Recommendations for treatment of encephalitis are 15 mg of acyclovir/kg i.v. every 8 h. This treatment should be continued until the virus is no longer detectable. For peripheral lesions, a dosage of 10 to 15 mg/kg of body weight three times a day is recommended.

There are insufficient data to determine the best antiherpetic nucleoside analogue for the treatment of herpes B virus infections. Therefore, trials with acyclovir alternatives (Ganciclovir, Famciclovir, and Valacyclovir) appear to be justified.

Prophylaxis. All macaques should be considered infectious unless proven otherwise. They should not be kept in contact with seronegative monkeys and should be kept separately from monkeys of other species. Even indirect contact should be avoided. If new monkeys are added to a colony, they should be tested before they are brought in contact with other animals. Attempts are being made to establish herpes B virus-free macaque colonies. By cesarean section and immediate separation of dam and offspring, the infection can be avoided in the newborn.

Strict safety measures are required when monkeys are handled. Unprotected contact with monkeys or their cages should be avoided. A face mask should be worn to avoid transmission by spitting. All contacts with potential transmission (bites or lesions) should be kept under protocol. Instructions for the treatment of bites or scratches should be readily available.

Treatment of wounds with suspected infection should proceed immediately, no later than 5 min after the bite. Deep wounds need to be drained and excised by an experienced physician. Wounds need to be rinsed for 20 min with water, or preferably with a 20% soap solution or freshly prepared 0.25% sodium hypochlorite solution, and then blotted with cotton. Conjunctivae and mucous membranes should be rinsed with physiological salt solutions.

Solutions and instruments necessary for prophylaxis must be readily available.

Before treatment, a wound swab should be taken for virus isolation. The sample should be sent refrigerated in 0.5 ml of physiological salt solution. A blood sample should be drawn for a baseline to detect a possible seroconversion later on. The serum can be stored frozen. Any material needed to take samples has to be present. A scraping of the mucous membranes from the mouth of the biting monkey should be taken and sent to a diagnostic laboratory.

The decision whether to treat prophylactically with acyclovir after a bite or not depends on the circumstances. If the bite is deep and near the head and neck, treatment should be initiated with acyclovir (10 mg/kg i.v. every 8 h to maintain a level in blood of 20 µg/ml). Low-risk lesions can be treated orally with acyclovir to reach a level in blood of 1.6 µg/ml. Because of its higher toxicity Ganciclovir is not recommended for prophylaxis.

Tetanus prophylaxis is also required after a bite. Even rabies prophylaxis has to be considered if the biting animal was caught in the wild.

REFERENCES

Artenstein AW et al., Human infection with B virus following a needlestick injury. *Rev. Infect. Dis.* 13, 288–291, 1991.

Bennet et al., Protection against herpes B virus infection in rabbits with a recombinant vaccinia virus expressing glycoprotein D. *J. Med. Virol.* 57, 47–56, 1999.

Black DH, Eberle R, Detection and differentiation of primate alpha-herpes-viruses by PCR. *J. Vet. Diagn. Invest.* 9, 225–231, 1997.

Blewett EL, Saliki JT, Eberle R, Development of a competitive ELISA for detection of primates infected with monkey B virus (Herpesvirus simiae). *J. Virol. Methods* 77, 59–67, 1999.

CDC, Fatal cercopithecine herpesvirus 1 (B virus) following a mucocutaneous exposure and interim recommendations for worker protection. *MMWR Morb. Mortal. Wkly. Rep.* 47, 1073–1076, 1998.

Hirano M et al., Rapid discrimination of monkey B virus from human herpes simplex viruses by PCR in the presence of betaine. *J. Clin. Microbiol.* 38, 1255–1257, 2000.

Holmes GP et al., Guidelines for the prevention and treatment of B-virus infections in exposed persons. The B virus working group. *Clin. Infect. Dis.* 20, 421–439, 1995.

Jerome KR, Ashley RL, Herpes simplex virus and herpes B-virus. In: Murray PR et al. (eds.), *Manual of Clinical Microbiology*, 1291–1303, 8th Ed. Vol. 2. ASM Press, Washington, DC, 2003.

Sabin AB, Wright AM, Acute ascending myelitis following a monkey bite, with the isolation of a virus capable of producing the disease. *J. Exp. Med.* 59, 115–136, 1934.

Whitley RJ, Hilliard JK, Cercopithecine Herpesvirus (B Virus). In: Knipe DP, Howley PM (eds.), *Fields Virology*, 2835–2848, 4th ed., Lippincott, Williams & Wilkins, 2006.

1.16 Zoonoses Caused by Poxviruses

Variola virus, which occurs only in humans, was the most important human poxvirus until it was eradicated in 1979. There is now a potential danger that this virus might be used as a weapon in biological warfare. Animal poxviruses had to be ruled out in the differential diagnosis while variola major existed in humans. In 1798, Edward Jenner introduced vaccinia virus, an animal poxvirus, which has been used systematically to protect against human smallpox. This vaccine made possible the worldwide eradication of smallpox in 1979. Since then, animal poxviruses have figured as potential pathogens in human medicine. There is concern that some of the orthopoxviruses could cause an epidemic in people no longer protected. Buffalopox in India and monkeypox in Africa are naturally transmitted to humans, and a serial person-to-person transmission is possible. Immunodeficient individuals in particular may be at risk.

Poxviruses are exceptional in size and structure and differ from other viruses. There is no classical geometrical capsid structure. Orthopoxviruses have an outside envelope and a second membrane underneath. Instead of a capsid, poxviruses have a nucleosome that contains DNA and it is surrounded by its own membrane. The double-stranded DNA genome of poxviruses consists of 130 to 300 kbp. These viruses have a large number of NS proteins, important for replication and pathogenesis.

Poxviruses are divided into two subfamilies: the *Chordopoxvirinae* (Tab. 1.8), with eight genera, and the *Entomopoxvirinae*, with three genera. The *Entomopoxvirinae* are arthropod viruses and have no zoonotic importance. Members of the genus *Avipoxvirus* (avian

Table 1.8 | Poxvirus subfamily *Chordopoxvirinae*

VIRUS	RESERVOIR	GEOGRAPHIC DISTRIBUTION	OTHER HOSTS AND/OR METHODS OF TRANSMISSION
Genus *Orthopoxvirus*			
Zoonotic viruses			
Monkeypox virus	Squirrels	West and Central Africa	Monkeys, person-to-person
Vaccinia virus	Unknown	Worldwide	Humans, buffaloes, rabbits, cows
Buffalopox virus[1]	Unknown	Asia	Buffaloes, person-to-person
Camelpox virus	Camels	Africa, Asia	Camels, person-to-person
Cowpox virus[2]	Rodents	Europe, Asia	Cats, cows, zoo animals, humans
Elephantpox virus	Unknown	Asia	Elephants, person-to-person
Nonzoonotic viruses			
Variola virus	Humans	Previously worldwide	Only humans
Volepox virus	Voles	Western United States	None
Ectromelia virus	Rodents	Europe	None
Raccoonpox virus	Raccoons	Eastern United States	None
Skunkpox virus	Skunks	Eastern United States	None
Uasin Gishu disease virus	Unknown	East Africa	Horses
Taterapox virus	Gerbils	West Africa	None
Genus Parapoxvirus			
Zoonotic viruses			
Bovine papular stomatitis virus	Cattle	Worldwide	Humans
Orf virus	Sheep	Worldwide	Ruminants, humans
Pseudocowpox virus (milker's nodules)	Cattle	Worldwide	Humans
Sealpox virus	Seals	Worldwide	Humans
Nonzoonotic viruses			
Auzduk disease virus	Camels	Africa, Asia	None
Parapoxvirus of red deer in New Zealand	Deer	New Zealand	None
Chamois contagious ecthyma virus	Chamois		
Genus *Yatapoxvirus*			
Tanapox virus	Rodents	East and Central Africa	Monkeys, humans
Yaba monkey tumor virus	Monkeys	West Africa	Humans

[1] Closely related to vaccinia virus.
[2] Probably identical to elephantpox virus.

poxviruses in the subfamily *Chordovirinae*) are also transmitted by arthropods among avian hosts. They also have no zoonotic importance; however, they are important for their use as expression vectors (vaccine shuttles) and less dangerous in that role than vaccinia virus.

Members of the genus *Orthopoxvirus* can be seen by light microscopy. They have a rectangular shape with dimensions of 350 by 270 nm and a genome size of around 200 kbp with a GC content of around 36%. Members of the genus *Parapoxvirus* are ovoid, with a genome of around 140 kbp and a GC content of 64%.

Only two virus species in the family *Poxviridae* are exclusively human pathogens: variola virus (smallpox virus) and molluscum contagiosum virus. In addition, numerous animal poxviruses can be transmitted to humans, especially members of the genera *Orthopoxvirus* and *Parapoxvirus* but also members of the genus *Yabapoxvirus*. Of special concern is person-to-person transmission of orthopoxviruses.

1.16.1 ZOONOSES CAUSED BY ORTHOPOXVIRUSES

Orthopoxviruses are of importance because some are closely related to variola virus and vaccinia virus and can be sequentially transmitted from person-to-person. The last case of true human smallpox (variola) was recorded in 1979. Since 1980, the world has been officially free of smallpox, but there is serious concern that smallpox virus might be used in acts of bioterrorism.

There is currently no indication that animal poxviruses might replace variola major virus as human pathogens after the discontinuation of human vaccinations. There are still diseases in animals caused by poxviruses, and there are sporadic cases of animal poxvirus infections in humans.

Etiology. Humans are susceptible to only some of the numerous animal poxviruses. The following orthopoxviruses have to be considered as zoonotic agents: monkeypox virus (only known since 1970), vaccinia virus (Jenner's smallpox vaccine virus), buffalopox virus (closely related to vaccinia virus), camelpox virus (closely related to smallpox virus), cowpox virus (not identical to vaccinia virus), and elephantpox virus (closely related to cowpox virus).

Occurrence. Animal poxvirus infections in humans occur sporadically worldwide and rarely as epidemics.

Transmission. Transmission of animal pox to humans occurs only by intensive direct or indirect contact of injured skin or small wounds with lesions of animal pox. The chances of transmission of animal pox to humans are minimal. Rarely, transmission from human-to-human might occur. It remains to be seen whether the situation remains unchanged after humans have lost their basic immunity to poxviruses.

Clinical Manifestations. The incubation period is between 7 and 14 days, when usually benign pox lesions develop. These lesions disappear without treatment, unless they are complicated by secondary bacterial infections. A generalized infection may follow, especially after vaccinia virus infections, in individuals prone to develop eczemas or with general immunosuppression. Vaccination with an incompletely inactivated recombinant vaccinia virus containing HIV gp120 produced a generalized and lethal vaccinia virus infection in individuals infected with HIV.

Diagnosis. The presence of typical pox lesions after contact with animals is diagnostic. The diagnosis can be confirmed by electron microscopy or by histology (detection of intracytoplasmic inclusion bodies in lesions and immunocytochemistry). Serology is not useful for diagnosis because there is little antibody formation at the time of disease onset.

More recently, PCR has been used to type unknown poxviruses. It is most important to recognize variola infections early, considering the potential danger of bioterrorism. Therefore, the primers for a type-specific PCR to detect the variola virus and primers for differentiation between Old World and New World orthopoxviruses are significant. For details, see the end of this chapter.

Differential Diagnosis. Before its eradication, variola virus was of primary diagnostic concern. Varicella-zoster virus and other herpesvirus infections are prominent in the differential diagnosis. In addition, molluscum contagiosum, rickettsialpox and herpetiforme dermatitis (Duhring's disease) in pregnant women, Sindbis virus, Coxsackievirus A16, and other enteroviruses can produce hand-foot-and-mouth disease, with lesions similar to cowpox.

Therapy. Specific therapy does not exist, and treatment is symptomatic. A new drug, Cidofovir [(S)-1-(3-hydroxy-2-phosphonylmethoxypropyl) cytosine) (HPMPC)], has antiviral activity against many strains of orthopoxviruses but is untried in human orthopoxvirus infections. Cidofovir resistant strains of orthopoxviruses are less pathogenic in animals than wild-type virus.

Prophylaxis. All orthopoxviruses are immunologically closely related. Vaccination with vaccinia virus or modified virus Ankara (MVA), therefore, protects not only against variola but also against other orthopoxviruses; however, it does not protect against parapoxviruses. A supply of vaccines is required for the immunization of zoo and experimental animals. If modified live virus vaccines are used, they should be harmless for humans and for animals. A highly attenuated vaccinia virus strain was developed for this purpose.

REFERENCES

Damaso CR et al., An emergent poxvirus from humans and cattle in Rio de Janeiro State: Cantagalo virus may derive from Brazilian smallpox vaccine. *Virology* 277, 439–449, 2000.

Dixon CW, Smallpox J, Churchill A., London, 1962.

Espy MJ et al., Detection of smallpox virus DNA by lightcycler PCR. *J. Clin. Microbiol.* 40, 1985–1988, 2002.

Fenner F et al., Smallpox and its eradication. Geneva: World Health Organization, 1988.

Herrlich A, *Die Pocken. 2. Aufl.*, Georg Thieme, Stuttgart, New York, 1967.

Knight JC, Massung RF, Exposito JJ, Polymerase chain reaction identification of smallpox virus. In: Becker Y, Darai G (eds.), *Diagnosis of human viruses by PCR technology*, 297–302, 2nd ed., Springer, Berlin, Heidelberg, New York, 1995.

Loparev VN et al., Detection and differentiation of Old World orthopoxviruses: restriction fragment length polymorphism of the crmB gene region. *J. Clin. Microbiol.* 39, 94–100, 2001.

Ropp SL et al., PCR strategy for identification and differentiation of smallpox and other orthopoxviruses. *J. Clin. Microbiol.* 33, 2069–2076, 1995.

Smee DF, Characterization of wild-type and cidofovir-resistant strains of camelpox, cowpox, monkeypox, and vaccinia viruses. *Antimicrob. Agents Chemother.* 46, 1329–1335, 2002.

1.16.2 INDIVIDUAL ORTHOPOXVIRUS INFECTIONS

1.16.2.1 Monkeypox

Monkeypox virus is most closely related to variola virus. The disease is seen occasionally in captive monkeys. Outbreaks in feral monkeys have not been found. Monkeypox virus causes a rare zoonosis, which has been found in humans only after the eradication of smallpox in areas of endemicity. This zoonosis occurs sporadically in tropical rainforest areas in west and central Africa, especially the Democratic Republic of Congo (formerly Zaire). It is hard to differentiate from variola. A survey conducted by the WHO in 1983 in Zaire (now Republic of Congo) found 83 cases in a population of 5 million.

Occurrence. A pox-like disease, which was transmitted from monkeys to non-vaccinated humans, was first observed in Zaire (Republic of Congo) in 1970 and 1971. Person-to-person transmission occurred in 20% to 30% of the cases, several times in a triple chain and in one case in a quadruple chain. In 1984, monkeypox was diagnosed in six non-vaccinated children in the Central African Republic. The disease was benign. Seventy-one individuals developed monkeypox in 13 townships in the Kasai Oriental region of Zaire between February and August 1996. Six cases were fatal. The rate of person-to-person transmission had increased to 71% from the earlier rate of 30%. Children and young adults, mostly those not vaccinated against variola, were affected. Another 170 individuals developed the disease in the spring of 1997 in the same region; 293 cases, including 23 fatal ones, were recognized in three locations in early 2002.

A pox-like disease caused by the monkeypox virus was seen in Gabon in four children in one family. Two of the children died with a hemorrhagic fever and involvement of internal organs. A possible person-to-person transmission was epidemiologically tested but not found.

In the United States, human disease due to the monkeypox virus was diagnosed for the first time in May 2003. The virus was transmitted by prairie dogs, which are kept as pets in some households. The virus is believed to have been introduced into the United States via Gambian giant rats – held as pets –, which were believed to have been the source of infection for the prairie dogs in captivity.

Transmission. It is not known how humans become infected with monkeypox virus. According to seroepidemiological investigations, monkeys, squirrels, porcupines, or anteaters living in the jungle could be involved in the transmission cycle. Transmission from human-to-human is rare (4% contact infection). Longer transmission chains have not been proven. It remains unclear whether monkeys are the original hosts for monkeypox virus or—like humans—only a link or a dead-end in the infection chain.

Clinical Manifestations. The disease in humans has a fatality rate of 15%. After a prodromal period of 2 days, a characteristic variola-like eruption develops over a period of 2 to 4 weeks. At the same time, lymphadenopathy becomes manifest and is more pronounced than with variola.

Diagnosis. The virus can be detected in vesicle fluid by electron microscopy and can be cultivated by inoculation of eggs or cell cultures. PCR can be used for detection of the virus and is needed for viral identification. The primers recommended for a type-specific diagnosis of monkeypox virus are to be found in the appendix.

Differential Diagnosis. The differential diagnosis has to consider all zoonotic orthopox- and parapoxvirus infections. Contact with monkeys (feral or captive) and a stay in equatorial Africa or contacts with individuals coming from Africa should raise suspicion. The possibility of a terrorist attack with smallpox virus should be kept in mind.

Therapy. See the introduction on orthopoxviruses above.

Prophylaxis. See the introduction on orthopoxviruses above.

REFERENCES

Hutin YJ et al., Outbreak of human monkeypox, Democratic Republic of Congo, 1996 to 1997. *Emerg. Infect. Dis.* 7, 434–438, 2001.

Khodakevich L et al., Orthopoxvirose simienne de l'homme en République Centrafricaine. *Bull. Soc. Pathol. Exot. Filiales.* 78, 311–315, 1985.

Meyer A et al., Première apparition au Gabon de monkeypox chez l'homme. *Med. Trop.* 51, 53–57, 1991.

Neubauer H et al., Specific detection of monkeypox virus by polymerase chain reaction. *J. Virol. Methods* 74, 201–207, 1998.

Ropp SL et al., PCR strategy for identification and differentiation of small pox and other orthopoxviruses. *J. Clin. Microbiol.* 33, 2069–2076, 1995.

Shchelkunov SN et al., Human monkeypox and smallpox viruses: genomic comparison. *FEBS Lett.* 509, 66–70, 2001.

Zaucha M et al., The pathology of experimental aerosolized monkeypox virus infection in cynomolgus monkeys (Macaca fascicularis). *Lab. Invest.* 81, 1581–1600, 2001.

1.16.2.2 Vaccinia Virus

Vaccinia (L. *vacca*, cow) is a name coined 200 years ago for a virus transmitted from cows to humans. Edward Jenner (1749 to 1823) used vesicle fluid from infected cows for "vaccination"—hence the name of the virus— of humans against smallpox.

Etiology. Vaccinia virus has been used worldwide to immunize against human smallpox. If the vaccinia virus was found in nature, it would be difficult to differentiate a wild-type virus from a vaccine virus. Buffalopox virus is very similar to vaccinia virus. It causes a disease in water buffalo in India and it can be transmitted to humans. It is debatable whether the virus, which is today classified as cowpox virus, is identical to vaccinia virus.

Occurrence. Vaccinia virus has been used to eradicate smallpox by vaccination (Fig. 1.14). A source is still not unequivocally clear. It has the widest host range of poxviruses. An old name for vaccinia virus, vaccinia officinalis, refers to the fact that this virus was used as a pharmaceutical.

Transmission. The infectious chain human-animal-human or animal-human-human has been described repeatedly. Transmission usually

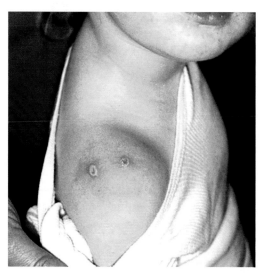

Figure 1.14 | Local pox after vaccination with vaccinia virus. (Photo: J. Pilaski.)

occurs by direct contact with infected animals or humans.

Clinical Manifestations. Contact with vaccinated humans has usually produced only localized (mammary gland) lesions in cattle, sheep, goats, and zoo animals. A generalized infection was seen occasionally. The vaccinia virus is not entirely harmless for humans. Several severe complications may result from vaccination with vaccinia virus. In highly susceptible individuals with allergies, immunosuppression, or during pregnancy, a generalized infection is a dangerous complication. Multiple pox lesions, malformation of the fetus, and abortion may be the result. Eczema vaccinatum occurs in unvaccinated adults suffering from eczema and in children suffering from milk crust. Progressive vaccinia (vaccinia necrosum) is seen in children with connatal immune defects or in adults with acquired immune deficiency. The severest complication is postvaccinal encephalitis, a demyelinating encephalitis, with a frequency of about 1/100,000 in children vaccinated for the first time at the age of >2 years. In adults, when they are vaccinated for the first time at a later age, the risk of postvaccinal encephalitis amounts to 1/10,000. In addition, there is a rare complication in small children, a

generalized infection with viremia and encephalitis. It is claimed that cessation of anti-smallpox vaccination has saved the lives of 200 children in the United States in 20 years.

An American soldier who had AIDS and was inadvertently vaccinated with vaccinia virus in 1982 developed a generalized vaccinia virus infection and died of AIDS after a year (Fig. 1.15).

Diagnosis. Vaccinia virus can be cultivated on the chorioallantoic membrane of chicken embryos or in cell cultures. As lesions of variola virus on the chorioallantoic membrane are smaller than vaccinia virus lesions, this test was used as a criterion for differentiation.

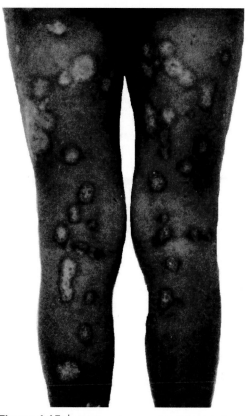

Figure 1.15 | Confluent generalized vaccinia in an American recruit, who was vaccinated without knowledge of his HIV-infection. Redield RR et al., disseminated vaccinia in a military recruit with human immunedeficiency virus (HIV) disease. New Engl. J. Med. (1987), 316, 673 – 676. (Courtesy of New Engl. J. Med.)

PCR techniques have now been developed for detection and differentiation of orthopoxviruses. Oligonucleotide primers targeting the HA open reading frame for a vaccinia virus-specific PCR have been described previously (see the end of this section).

Therapy. For therapy of vaccinia virus infections, see the introduction on orthopoxviruses above.

Prophylaxis. In the event of a smallpox outbreak, vaccination of exposed individuals with vaccinia virus is necessary, especially for those who have not been vaccinated previously. Vaccination during the incubation phase of smallpox mitigates the disease. Even pregnant women and patients suffering from an eczema must be vaccinated in such a situation, as this is their only chance to survive smallpox. There are two possibilities in avoiding complications of the vaccination. Inactivated vaccinia antigen may be injected i.m. a week before vaccination with live vaccinia virus. The other strategy is simultaneous intragluteal injection of anti-vaccinia virus hyperimmune globulin, while the vaccine is applied to the contralateral shoulder by intradermal scarification. The beneficial effect of hyperimmune globulin application on the course of vaccination is better proven than that of the vaccinia virus antigen. However, at present, the hyperimmune globulin and the inactivated vaccinia virus antigen are not available.

There is currently no licensed vaccine to be used in humans in case of a bioterrorist attack with smallpox virus (variola virus). However, the military and public health services of several countries have preserved stores of vaccine. The standards of the production of these vaccines are not in accordance with modern standards, but these vaccines were tested for safety several decades ago. They are still viable, and recently tests were conducted to determine the feasibility of using dilute vaccines in order to have more doses available for application in case of an attack. It is anticipated that 400 Americans would die from side effects of the vaccine if nationwide smallpox vaccination were necessary.

Some members of the *Poxviridae*, especially vaccinia virus, have been used as expression vectors (vaccine shuttles) because of the large size of their genome and broad host range. Replacing nonessential genes, DNA, or cDNA from different viruses can be incorporated to produce a live virus vaccine that induces immunity to five or more virus diseases. Vaccinia virus is relatively pathogenic for humans and is now even less acceptable, as smallpox has been eradicated and vaccination has been discontinued.

There is a serious problem with the use of vaccinia virus as a vector in experimental work or in recombinant vaccines. Increasingly, young scientists are exposed to poxviruses, especially vaccinia virus, which are used as vectors for other viral genes [e.g., strain WR (Western reserve), recombinant for RNA polymerase of coliphage T7]. These scientists have little or no immunity to poxviruses. One should not expect recombinant vaccinia virus strains to be nonpathogenic. A female scientist who was vaccinated against smallpox as a child and who worked in a safety hood where mouse-passaged vaccinia virus was handled previously became infected through a lesion on her hand. A pustule developed at the site of infection, followed by a significant general reaction with neurological complications (continuous dizziness). She had to be hospitalized but fortunately recovered without sequelae.

Currently, no orthopoxvirus vaccine is licensed for human use. Old-fashioned vaccinia virus vaccination would not be justified. The risk of postvaccinal encephalitis is 1:10,000, which is greater than the chance of complications after a laboratory infection. Anti-vaccinia virus hyperimmune gamma globulins are not available commercially. It is reasonable to use poxviruses (e.g., fowlpox virus) that are not human pathogenic as expression vectors. Of course, the risk of transmitting this virus to fowl has to be observed. In case of a laboratory infection with vaccinia virus, one should attempt to block the disease by use of immunoglobulin from a person with solid immunity to vaccinia virus. Cidofovir, an antiviral drug effective against orthopoxviruses, has not yet been tested in humans.

Vaccinia virus-rabies virus recombinants (vaccinia-rabies glycoprotein vaccines) have been used to immunize foxes and raccoons. Vaccinia virus–foot-and-mouth disease virus recombinants against foot-and-mouth disease or vaccinia virus-Rinderpest virus recombinants could be used in the near future. The use of these vaccinia virus recombinants could create a new zoonosis. Even if these recombinant vaccinia viruses do not initiate infectious focuses in wild or domestic animals, there is always the possibility that a recombination with cowpox viruses in rodents or with other poxviruses could create a new agent. Such an agent might be dangerous for a large group of people with immunodeficiency. As stated above, vaccination with an incompletely inactivated recombinant vaccinia virus containing HIV gp120 resulted in a generalized, lethal infection in individuals infected with HIV.

The potential danger of recombinant viruses has been documented in an experiment with mousepox (ectromelia) virus. When an interleukin-4 gene was integrated into the virus genome, it resulted in a virus that was pathogenic even for mice with genetic resistance to ectromelia virus. The recombinant virus induced a fulminant and fatal poxvirus infection. This observation exemplifies the risk of genetic experiments with human pathogenic DNA viruses.

The use of plus-strand RNA viruses, which are made replication defective and can be made recombinant for genetic material from other sources, is much more recommendable from the standpoint of biosafety, even if the maximal size of the integrated RNA were much smaller than that of poxviruses.

REFERENCES

Dixon CW, *Smallpox. J. and A. Churchill*, London, 1962.

Espy MJ et al., Detection of smallpox virus DNA by lightcycler PCR. *J. Clin. Microbiol.* 40, 1985–1988, 2002.

Fenner F et al., *Smallpox and its eradication*. Geneva: World Health Organization, 1988.

Herrlich A, *Die Pocken. 2. Aufl.*, Georg Thieme, Stuttgart, New York, 1967.

Moss B, Poxviridae: The viruses and their replication. In: Knipe DM, Howley PM, Griffin DE (eds.), *Fields Virology*, 2849–2885, 4th ed., Raven Press, New York, 2001.

Redfield RR et al., Disseminated vaccinia in a military recruit with human immunodeficiency virus (HIV) disease. *New Engl. J. Med.* 316, 673–676, 1987.

Ropp SL et al., Poxviruses infecting humans. In: Murray PR et al. (eds.), *Manual of Clinical Microbiology*, 1137–1144, 7th ed. American Society of Microbiology, Washington, 1999.

1.16.2.3 Buffalopox

Buffalopox has been known to only occur in India. It was characterized there in 1971. Buffalopox virus was transmitted to humans and it induced a disease in young adults in the state of Maharashtra between 1992 and 1996. Buffalopox virus is markedly different from cowpox virus.

Etiology. Buffalopox virus is more closely related to vaccinia virus than to cowpox virus. The question remains open whether buffalopox virus is vaccinia virus adapted to buffaloes or the original virus and precursor of vaccinia virus. There appears to be great variation in virus strains isolated from different outbreaks.

Clinical Manifestations. Local skin eruptions on the udder are the only lesions produced in buffaloes and cows. The infection produced poxlike skin eruptions especially on hands of young adult individuals who had not been vaccinated against smallpox. A total of 22 buffalopox virus strains have been isolated from humans and animals. Disseminated pox lesions on the face, arms, and buttocks were seen in children who did not have contact with cattle. It must be assumed that person-to-person transmission infected the children.

Neutralizing antibodies against buffalopox virus was found not only in individuals recovering from the disease but also in contact individuals without clinical signs. It can be assumed that subclinical infections are common.

As had been expected, animal poxvirus infections in humans have increased since smallpox vaccinations were discontinued. The transmission of buffalopox and monkeypox viruses to humans confirms the expectation.

1.16.2.4 Camelpox

Camelpox virus is classified as an orthopoxvirus. The disease caused by camelpox virus exists in Africa and Asia, especially in camels and dromedaries in the Sahara, in Somalia, in the Asiatic part of the former USSR, and in India. Among the zoonotic orthopoxviruses, camelpox virus is most closely related to smallpox virus (variola virus).

The camelpox virus can be transmitted to humans by milking, resulting in benign eruptions on hands and arms. After consumption of infected camel milk, lesions may be seen in the mouth. Transmission of camelpox from human-to-human has recently been observed in India. For diagnosis of camelpox virus by PCR, see the end of this section.

1.16.2.5 Cowpox
Etiology. Cowpox virus is not as closely related to vaccinia virus as buffalopox virus is. The disease produced by cowpox virus was frequently seen in the United States and in Central Europe in earlier times. Today, cowpox in cattle and consequently in humans is rarely seen.

Occurrence. In milking cows, the udder and teats are predominantly affected. A generalized disease with pustular exanthema may be seen occasionally.

Cowpox infections in humans cannot always be traced to diseased cattle. The epidemiology of cowpox is largely unresolved. Occasionally, cowpox infections have been seen in domestic cats (Fig. 1.16), in large cats in zoos, and in other zoo animals (rhinos and okapis). The

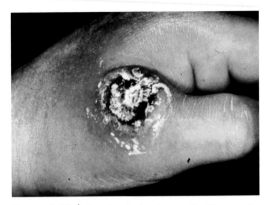

Figure 1.17 | Poxvirus lesion transmitted from a diseased cat. (Photo: T. Nasemann.)

natural reservoir of cowpox virus may be small rodents. Cattle and humans may constitute a dead-end link in the chain of transmission.

Of 11 cowpox virus infections seen in humans between 1965 and 1991, cats were the source of the infection in four cases (Fig. 1.17), rodents were the source in three cases, and a cow was the source in only one case. Antibodies to cowpox virus have been detected in more than 60% of domestic cats and in feral rodents of different species. There is a report of a lethal cowpox virus infection in a patient with eczema.

Cowpox virus was isolated from a 4-year-old child in Russia with signs of pox disease. The child had been in contact with a mole. Cowpox virus was identified in several studies in rodents, especially *Clethrionomys glareolus* and *Apodemus sylvaticus*.

Transmission. Milkers who come into contact with pox on teats develop the disease on the hands, arms, and face. Besides local pox lesions, there may be a febrile lymphangitis, severe conjunctivitis, and meningoencephalitis.

Diagnosis. For diagnosis of cowpox by PCR, see the end of this section.

1.16.2.6 Elephantpox
Elephantpox virus is closely related to cowpox virus. Based on DNA analysis, the agent is assumed to be a separate orthopoxvirus.

The disease caused by elephantpox virus has repeatedly been seen in circus or zoo elephants, sometimes with a lethal outcome. Contact with

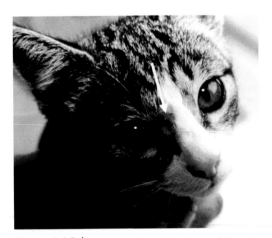

Figure 1.16 | Facial poxvirus lesion (arrow) in a cat. (Photo: D. von Bomhard.)

diseased or dead animals has produced the disease in animal caretakers, veterinarians, and technicians involved in necropsies. The reservoir for elephantpox virus is not known. Rodents may be the reservoir, as is suspected for cowpox virus. Transmission occurs by contact with pox lesions or infected material.

Elephants can be vaccinated against the disease with a live attenuated virus based on vaccinia virus. An "emergency" vaccination can be tried in healthy animals at the beginning of an outbreak.

REFERENCES

Anonymus, Don't underestimate the enemy. *Nature* 409, 269, 2001.

Baxby D, Hill BJ, Characteristics of a new poxvirus isolated from Indian buffaloes. *Arch. Gesamte Virusforsch.* 35, 70–79, 1971.

Dixon CW, *Smallpox. J. and A. Churchill*, London, 1962.

Espy MJ et al., Detection of smallpox virus DNA by lightcycler PCR. *J. Clin. Microbiol.* 40, 1985–1988, 2002.

Fenner F et al., *Smallpox and its eradication*. Geneva: World Health Organization, 1988.

Gubser C, Smith GL, The sequence of camelpox virus shows it is most closely related to variola virus, the cause of smallpox. *J. Gen. Virol.* 83, 855–872, 2002.

Herrlich A, *Die Pocken. 2. Aufl.*, Georg Thieme, Stuttgart, New York, 1967.

Jackson RJ et al., Expression of mouse interleukin-4 by a recombinant ectromelia virus suppresses cytolytic lymphocyte responses and overcomes genetic resistance to mousepox. *J. Virol.* 75, 1205–1210, 2001.

Kolhapure RM et al., Investigation of buffalopox outbreaks in Maharashtra State during 1992–1996. *Indian J. Med. Res.* 106, 441–446, 1997.

Lal SM, Singh IP, Buffalopox – a review. *Trop. Anim. Health Prod.* 9, 107–112, 1977.

Marennikova SS et al., The biotype and genetic characteristics of an isolate of the cowpox virus causing infection in a child. *Zh. Microbiol. Epidemiol. Immunobiol.* (4), 6–10, in Russisch, 1996.

Pfeffer M et al., Fatal form of camelpox virus infection. *Vet. J.* 155, 107–109, 1998.

Pfeffer M et al., Comparison of camelpox viruses isolated in Dubai. *Vet. Microbiol.* 49, 135–146, 1996.

Ropp SL et al., PCR strategy for identification and differentiation of smallpox and other orthopoxviruses. *J. Clin. Microbiol.* 33, 2069–2076, 1995.

1.16.3 PARAPOXVIRUS INFECTIONS

Parapoxviruses include the Orf virus of sheep and the viruses causing "milker's nodules" and papular stomatitis of cattle. Parapoxviruses are poxviruses that differ from other poxviruses in morphology and other biological characteristics. Disease and lesions produced by parapoxviruses are similar to those induced by other poxviruses. Apart from a common precipitating antigen, the parapoxviruses are antigenically different from other poxviruses.

Diagnosis. Parapoxviruses are closely related, and type-specific diagnosis is not easily performed. Virus detection by a group-specific PCR is available for confirmation of isolates and in clinical specimens. Oligonucleotide primers for the detection of parapoxviruses by a seminested two-step PCR are to be found in the appendix.

1.16.3.1 Contagious Ecthyma of Sheep (Orf)
Lambs become infected with Orf virus from asymptomatic mothers. They develop an ulcerative inflammation on the lips and mouth (Fig. 1.18), on the vulva (genital form), or around

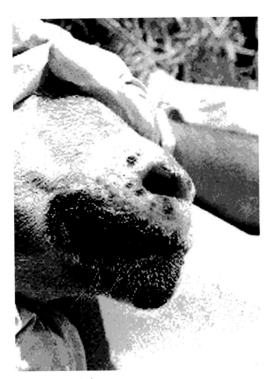

Figure 1.18 | Contagious ecthyma of sheep. (Photo: J. Pilaski.)

the margins of a hoof (pedal form). More severe forms have been seen in sheep in recent years. Cauliflower-like tumors of the mouth mucous membrane, deep ulcerative stomatitis, pharyngitis, esophagitis, and frequently loss of the hoof have been observed with a high mortality. Endemic infections in herds of sheep are common. Contact with diseased sheep leads to infection through small skin lesions in shepherds, farmers, slaughterhouse workers, and veterinarians. After an incubation period of 3 to 7 days, lesions develop on the hands and/or arms: papulovesicular (Fig. 1.19) or granulomatous eruptions similar to milker's nodules, which are not painful. Axillary lymphadenitis may develop. A generalized form is occasionally seen with lesions on the entire body. Healing takes several weeks, unless secondary infections cause complications. Contact transmission from human-to-human is possible.

Orf lesions in humans may create special diagnostic problems when they look like a malignant melanoma. If a malignant melanoma is suspected, histology of a pox section reveals a benign inflammatory skin eruption. The etiology of the disease becomes apparent with the anamnesis (contact with diseased sheep). A rapid diagnosis by electron microscopy reveals parapoxvirus. Once the diagnosis is made, surgical removal of pox lesions should not be performed, as generalization of the disease might be a consequence.

If a secondary infection is established, it is not always easy to differentiate the lesion from

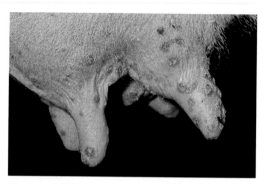

Figure 1.20 | Pseudocowpox infection on the udder of a cow (udder pox).

ulcerative pyodermitis. If crusts have formed, differentiation from impetigo contagiosa or telangiectatic granuloma becomes difficult. A precise anamnestic report usually leads to a proper diagnosis.

1.16.3.2 Milker's Nodules (Pseudocowpox)
Pseudocowpox virus causes pox lesions on the udder of cows (Fig. 1.20). They cannot be differentiated from lesions produced by cowpox virus or vaccinia virus.

The disease has been known in Europe and the United States for many years. Milkers become infected from pox lesions on the udder of milking cows. They develop vesicles and papules together with an inflammation of axillary lymph nodes. One or several pox lesions on one hand are usually seen. The lesions may extend towards the arms and body (Fig. 1.21). Occasionally, urticaria may develop. Without secondary infections, the lesions disappear within several weeks without scars.

Vaccination with vaccinia virus does not induce protection against milker's nodules, and a history of milker's nodules does not result in protection against smallpox.

1.16.3.3 Papular Stomatitis
Papular stomatitis occurs in Europe, the United States, Australia, and East Africa. An erosive or proliferative stomatitis is seen in young cattle, usually without a generalized disease. In exceptional cases, fever, salivation, and diarrhea may be seen.

The disease is transmissible to humans by contact, for example, by examination of the

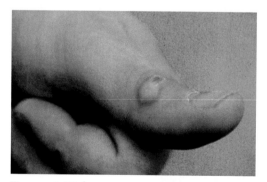

Figure 1.19 | Human infection with orf virus. (Photo: Dr. Valder, Bundesministerium für Ernährung, Land- wirtschaft und Forster, Bonn, Germany.)

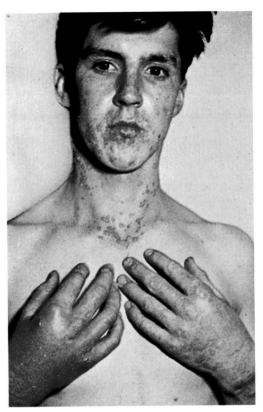

Figure 1.21 | Generalized pseudocowpox virus infection in a human. (Photo: J. Pilaski.)

oral cavity of infected animals. The virus enters through small skin lesions. The clinical manifestation is the same as that for pseudocowpox. Veterinarians and veterinary students are mostly affected. Three to 6 days after contact with infected cattle, vesicles and later circumscribed wart-like nodules develop on the hands, which disappear after 3 to 4 weeks. Recurrent lesions may develop several months after the primary infection. This infection has to be kept in mind if papules, pustules, and vesicles appear on the hands of individuals handling cattle.

1.16.4 ZOONOSES CAUSED BY YABAPOXVIRUSES

1.16.4.1 Tanapox Virus

Tanapox virus and yaba monkey tumor virus constitute a separate genus of poxviruses with a linear genome. Primates in Africa and monkeys in experimental stations may be affected. Enzootic infections in monkeys and illness in humans have been observed in the Tana River region in Kenya and in animal caretakers in primate centers in the United States.

Human disease is characterized by pox lesions on the hands and arms, sometimes together with fever, headache, and malaise. Infected monkeys do not show signs of a generalized infection. They develop only one or more pox vesicles on the face or limbs.

1.16.4.2 Yaba Monkey Tumor Virus

Yaba monkey tumor virus was discovered from subcutaneous tumors that appeared in a colony of Asian rhesus monkeys kept in Nigeria. The disease can be transmitted to humans but has never been observed in the field in monkeys or humans.

REFERENCES

Damon IK, Esposito JJ, Poxviruses that infect humans. In: Murray PR et al. (eds.), *Manual of Clinical Microbiology,* 1583–1591, 8th ed. Vol. 2. ASM Press, Washington, DC.

Inoshima Y, Morooka A, Sentsui H, Detection and diagnosis of parapoxvirus by the polymerase chain reaction. *J. Virol. Methods* 84, 201–208, 2000.

Mercer A et al., Molecular genetic analyses of parapoxviruses pathogenic for humans. *Arch. Virol. Suppl.* 13, 25–34, 1997.

Redfield RR et al., Disseminated vaccinia in a military recruit with human immunodeficiency virus (HIV) disease. *New Engl. J. Med.* 316, 673–676, 1987.

Ropp SL et al., Poxviruses infecting humans. In: Murray PR et al. (eds.), *Manual of Clinical Microbiology,* 1137–1144, 7th ed. American Society of Microbiology, Washington, DC, 1999.

1.17 Zoonoses Associated with Prions

A group of CNS diseases with extremely long incubation periods (several years) are designated "transmissible spongiform encephalopathies" (Tab. 1.9). They occur in humans and animals and are always fatal after a subacute course of the disease. These diseases have histological markers in common, which are expressed as spongiform vacuolization and an impressive

Table 1.9 | Transmissible encephalopathies in animals and humans

DISEASE	NATURAL HOST	ADDITIONAL HOST(S)	EXPERIMENTAL TRANSMISSION	COMMENT
Scrapie	Sheep	Goats, cattle?	Hamsters, mice, etc.	6 different strains
TME	Mink			Similar to scrapie
CWD	Elk, mule deer			Similar to scrapie
CJD	Humans	Unknown	Chimpanzees, gorillas	Sporadic (alimentary?), iatrogenic (cornea, dura, pituitary hormone), and familial
GSS	Humans	Unknown		Familial (vertically transmitted)
Kuru	Humans	Unknown	Chimpanzees	Only in New Guinea (Fore people)
BSE	Cattle	Cats, zoo animals, humans	Mice, hamsters, etc.	Alimentary transmission

TME, transmissible mink encephalopathy; CWD, chronic wasting disease; CJD, Creutzfeldt-Jakob disease; GSS, Gerstmann-Sträussler-Scheinker syndrome; BSE, bovine spongiform encephalopathy.

ballooning of neurons and of their processes, with a deposit of amyloid plaques. Inflammatory changes are entirely missing. Infectious agents in the classical sense are not detectable in this disease group. Besides horizontal transmission of some of these diseases, a vertical transmission might occur in others.

The transmissibility is marked by the presence of so-called prions (proteinaceous infectious particles), which apparently consist only of protein. They do not have a genome themselves but are encoded by a host gene, the prion protein (PrP) gene. Different types of the original agent and their host specificity are determined by the base sequence in the PrP gene of the host. Numerous alleles of the PrP gene exist in humans and animals. Resistance and susceptibility to the disease, as well as the predisposition to the familial forms, are always predetermined by certain alleles.

The physiological gene product of the cellular PrP gene is a glycoprotein of 27 to 31 kDa. It has a potential transmembrane domain and is connected with a glycolipid anchor in the membrane. This globular protein is transported via the Golgi apparatus to the cytoplasmic membrane. It has a half-life of hours and it is degraded by proteinases. The function of this protein is unclear. It might participate in signal transduction and come in contact with a structural protein, caveolin, after external stimulation. Caveolin phosphorylates FYN, which is a soluble tyrosine kinase. Experiments with knockout mice have shown that the physiological PrP gene product is not essential. Recently, it has been shown that in the mouse genome, a second copy of the PrP gene, "double," exists in close vicinity to the known PrP gene. Knockout of both genes resulted in infertility of male mice. Sperm was made at a normal rate but were unable to invade the egg, while the zona pellucida was intact.

Antibodies to cellular PrP do not induce recognizable damage when applied *in vivo*. However, mutation of this gene causes severe disease. There is a familial human disease, familial fatal insomnia, which may lead to depression and suicide because of insomnia. This disease is connected with a characteristic mutation of the PrP gene without the formation of a prion.

The transmissible spongiform encephalopathies have in common a characteristic mutation of the PrP gene, which leads to the incorporation of false amino acids into the protein. The altered amino acid sequence renders the protein post-translationally into an insoluble and proteinase-resistant isoform, the prion. This process can be stimulated spontaneously or may be triggered by the presence of added prions.

Prions have abnormal folded structures of pleated sheets, have a half-life of days, accumulate in intracellular vesicles that increase into large vacuoles, and can be deposited as so-called "florid plaques" (focal amyloid deposits surrounded by vacuolated cells). The accumulation of prion protein in the brain may be explained solely by the extended half-life in comparison to the half-life of the physiological gene product. An increased gene expression does not appear to be involved.

It is assumed that the prions that are present in the brain in extremely high titers (10^{12} ID_{50} per g of tissue) are also the infectious form of the causative agent. This has not yet been proven in the sense of the Henle-Koch postulate. It has not yet been possible to reproduce the disease experimentally by inoculating purified prions or recombinant prions into new hosts. Moreover, under controlled experimental conditions no causal link between oral uptake of prion material and transmission of bovine spongiform encephalopathy (BSE) has been shown. The epidemiological evidence, however, seems to be conclusive. The mechanism of disease transmission and multiplication of the agent in the host cannot be called an infection in the conventional sense.

After exposure of a susceptible host to prion containing material, there is initially an extended period of reproduction in lymphatic organs: the spleen and tonsils may contain infectious material. Mature B lymphocytes are essential for the migration into the CNS and possibly for extraneural replication.

BSE has not yet been found in cattle in the United States. However, other prion diseases [scrapie of sheep and chronic wasting disease (CWD) of cervids] are present in North America. At this time, there is no convincing evidence that scrapie or CWD could be pathogenic for humans. However, there is some concern about three cases of Creutzfeldt-Jakob disease (CJD) that occurred in individuals who had participated in wild game feasts in Wisconsin. CWD was first detected in free-ranging cervids in northeastern Colorado, southeastern Wyoming,

and the adjacent parts of Nebraska. In Nebraska, 24 of 62 deer were found to be infected. Farmed elks in Colorado, Montana, Nebraska, Oklahoma, Kansas, South Dakota, and Saskatchewan (Canada) were found to be positive for CWD prions.

1.17.1 BOVINE SPONGIFORM ENCEPHALOPATHY AND THE NEW VARIANT OF CREUTZFELDT - JAKOB DISEASE

BSE was described for the first time in 1985. Since that time, 2,000,000 cattle have died from it or have been slaughtered in Brittany, and approximately 1,500 cattle have died of BSE in other European countries. In the UK, the name "mad cow disease" has been introduced. The incubation period in cattle is 3 to 6 years. The disease is marked by behavioral disturbances and ataxia, followed by wasting and paralysis. The fear that the disease could cross species barriers became obvious early in the epidemic. Identical clinical signs were seen in cats and zoo animals and in experimentally infected mice. Meanwhile the suspicion that humans are susceptible to the disease has been confirmed. Since 1995, 128 human cases of BSE have been diagnosed in the UK, three have been diagnosed in France, two have been diagnosed in Ireland, and one has been diagnosed in Italy. The diagnosis has been confirmed in more than 117 cases. BSE, therefore, has to be considered a zoonosis. The course of the disease in humans has been falsely labeled "new variant of CJD" (nvCJD). This name does not point out important differences and disguises the fact that we are dealing with a zoonosis. It would be better and more honest to call it a human variant of BSE.

BSE is one of the transmissible encephalopathies. It is also called a transmissible subacute dementia. This group of diseases has in common a special form of spongiform changes in the cortex of the cerebrum and cerebellum. Inflammatory changes are missing. It appears, therefore, as a degenerative rather than an inflammatory disease. Infectious agents of conventional nature cannot be found. Transmission is dependent on the presence of so-called prions. Transmission occurs in connection with acts of cannibalism as well as with organ and tissue transplantations.

The longest-known and best-researched transmissible spongiform encephalopathy is scrapie in sheep. Diseases resembling scrapie are known to occur in mink (transmissible mink encephalopathy) and in deer and elk in North America (CWD). There are now six different forms of transmissible subacute dementias known in humans since the appearance of BSE. CJD, which was first described in 1920, is now known in three different forms: a sporadically occurring form, an iatrogenic form, and a hereditary transmitted form. A familial occurrence also exists in Gerstmann-Sträussler-Scheinker syndrome. Kuru is an encephalopathy in the Fore people of New Guinea, which is believed to be transmitted by cannibalism and cannibalism-like practices. The disease disappeared after the population was informed about the mode of transmission and it ceased these practices.

Etiology. Prions, the insoluble isoform of the PrP gene product, are thought to be the causative agent of BSE. There is no agreement about the question whether BSE is a disease *sui generis* or is derived from scrapie of sheep. As BSE could not be reproduced in cattle by feeding them scrapie-infected meat, the scrapie hypothesis has been discarded. As an alternative, it is assumed that BSE has existed in cattle earlier and that it has increased due to enforced cannibalism. However, Prusiner points out the fact that scrapie exists in six different types with different biological characteristics.

Theories about the prime cause of the appearance of BSE produce long lists with pros and cons. It is of interest that 17,000 cattle became diseased in Northern Ireland while only 300 diseased cattle were found in the Republic of Ireland. Perhaps the British feed was not used in the Republic of Ireland. Northern Ireland has British regulations in veterinary medicine. Nothing is known about genetic differences between cattle in Northern Ireland and the Republic of Ireland.

Occurrence. The alimentary route appears to be the most important route of infection for cattle. Cannibalism was previously forced on cattle, as they were fed animal offal (cadavers, meat of inferior quality, and slaughterhouse scraps). As long as this feed was heated to 130 °C, mainly to inactivate anthrax spores, the prions, as well as the spores, were inactivated. Because of the energy crisis in the 1970s, the production formula in the UK was changed and the temperature for the process was lowered. This has led to the widely accepted theory that prions were no longer inactivated and the disease, therefore, began to spread. The incriminated animal feed was still produced even after its connection with the disease was established.

After it was banned in the UK, it was exported to other countries, which proved to be fatal because of the resulting spread of BSE. Cattle and calves were also exported. Initially, it was assumed that vertical transmission is possible because animals, which were probably infected shortly after birth, developed the disease. Meanwhile, it became obvious that these animals were fed a milk replacement that contained cadaver feed produced in the conventional manner. Prions have been detected in this feed. There is no indication for a transmission by artificial insemination, where thawed semen is directly deposited on the stimulated uterine mucous membrane. Larvae of meat flies can pick up prion-containing material. This material remains infectious for hamsters after the larvae pupate and even after the larvae die.

The disease of cattle exists in England (in 2003 there were 228.24 new cases per 1 million bovines per year), Portugal (107.8 cases), Ireland (88.39 cases), Spain (37.95 cases), Switzerland (27.93 cases), Belgium (25.75 cases), France (20.96 cases), Slovakia (18.73 cases), Germany (17.02 cases), and Luxemburg (14.54 cases). In Germany, in total, 413 infected cows were found, and in 2009, there were two animals. Based on export analyses, it is expected that up to 100 additional countries could be affected In the province of Alberta, Canada, the first BSE case on the American continent was detected in May 2003 in a Black Angus cow. In December 2003, BSE was found in the USA in a Holstein cow. A total of four BSE cases were detected in the USA, the last was found in 2012 in a dairy cow.

Between 1 January and 31 May 2002, a total of 427 new cases of BSE were detected in British cattle, most of them born after the ban on offal powder. In 2001, a total of 8,516,227 bovine animals were tested for BSE, and 2,153 were found positive. In 2002, about 40 animals per month were found positive for BSE, the youngest having been born in 1997. Among the members of the European Union, only Luxembourg and Sweden have not yet had cases of BSE. Besides cattle, zoo animals, pets, pigs, chickens, and farmed fish have been exposed to prion-containing feed. Some zoo animals and pets have acquired the disease. The feeding of pigs did not produce disease. It is possible to induce a spongiform encephalopathy in pigs after intra-cerebral inoculation of the brain from BSE-diseased cattle. As has been seen with experimental exposure of rodents, one cannot rule out the possibility that pig organs replicate prions after feeding without producing disease in the pigs. Sheep and goats develop disease after feeding with BSE material.

The summit of BSE cases was reached in 1992 with 37,000 cases worldwide of which more than 36,000 were registered in the UK. The annual number of cases began to decrease in 2003 and this was bisected year by year. In 2005, 474 cases were found, and in 2011, only 29 BSE cases occurred worldwide.

The human disease of BSE (nvCJD) represents a new form of transmissible encephalopathy in Europe. It is similar to kuru, which previously existed only in the Fore people of New Guinea and which has been eradicated. As of July 2002, more than 130 cases of nvCJD have been reported since 1995: at least 128 cases in England, three in France, two in Ireland, and one in Italy. From present data, a total number of >220 cases of nvCJD were diagnosed worldwide of which 177 occurred in the UK and 27 in France. Four cases were found in the USA and it was found that all of them had a travel history in European countries, where BSE cases had occurred. The latest case of nvCJD was confirmed in June 2014 in Texas according to CDC news. NvCJD has not been diagnosed in individuals who had never stayed in a country known to have BSE cases. Out of 1,592 cases of spongiform encephalitis that were diagnosed in the United Kingdom in a 10-year period since 1990 ca. 7.5% were confirmed to be nvCJD.

The age of patients who died of nvCJD in the years 1995 to 2003 ranged between 19 and 40 years with a maximum at 25 years. In "classic" CJD, the age distribution was 35 to 90 years with a maximum of 70 years at the time of death.

Transmission. Transmission to humans appears to be predominantly by the alimentary route. There is, however, no proof for this generally accepted theory. Contrary to what could be expected, contact with BSE-infected cows does not seem to have created an occupational risk for nvCJD in individuals known to be exposed to cattle diseases. In cattle, the prions can be found mainly in the brain but also in extracerebral neural tissues and in lymphatic organs. Initially after infection, prions are amplified in peripheral organs, mainly in the spleen and lymphatic tissues. B cells are needed for the invasion of the brain. Muscles are free of infectious agents. In experimentally infected mice, prions were also detected in the muscles. The use of brain, lymphatic tissues, and offal as food for humans or animals should be strictly avoided. With the exception of colostrum, milk does not appear to be infectious. Cattle blood, serum albumin, and products from cattle, such as gelatin and casings, could be potentially infectious and should not be used.

The possibility of an iatrogenic transmission from human-to-human by medical or dental instruments or by transplantations and blood transfusions cannot be ruled out. So-called clusters of the disease in several people in the same village might be explained by human-to-human transmission, for example, by manipulations by dentists or otolaryngologists. In analogy with CJD, one can assume that BSE can be transmitted by corneal grafts, dura mater, or pituitary extracts. Scrapie in sheep has been transmitted by blood transfusion.

Genetic disposition. The susceptibility of humans for BSE appears to be genetically determined. Codon 129 of the PrP gene codes in both alleles for the amino acid methionine (Met/Met) in 100% of the patients with BSE disease, but only for 39% of the population in general. In contrast to CJD, and in contrast to BSE in humans, a genetic predisposition and a primary resistance are not known for BSE in cattle. It has been maintained by some that the decrease in the rate of BSE cases might not have occurred due to the ban of offal feeding but it was brought about instead by killing of all the animals susceptible to the disease.

Clinical Manifestations. The clinical disease of BSE (nvCJD) in humans becomes apparent after an incubation period of more than 16 years. It presents with neurological and psychomotor deficits. Leading symptoms are typical cerebellar syndromes with unsteady walking and inability to stand on one leg. In addition, emotional disturbances develop, ranging from a state of annoyance up to fits of rage and depression. With progressing disease, cortical signs appear, with loss of memory, dementia, and myoclonus. The Babinski reflex remains negative. The Achilles tendon and patellar reflexes become pathologic in most cases. These symptoms correspond with pathoanatomical changes, with vacuole formation in neurons of the cerebellum with astrogliosis and then of the brain stem, and only later with the involvement of the cortex. Amyloid plaques are rare in CJD but common in BSE of humans. In contrast to CJD, there are so-called florid plaques in human BSE (nvCJD). Similar plaques are found in kuru, a spongiform encephalopathy that existed in the Fore people in New Guinea but it has never been seen in Europe, and not in BSE of cattle. In respect to its clinical picture and neuropathology BSE in humans is rather corresponding to kuru.

Diagnosis. Besides a histopathological diagnosis, a diagnosis based on antigen detection is possible. Antibodies against the PrP protein, which also detect prions, are used. A pretreatment of the test material with proteases causes only protease-resistant prions to react. Antibodies against prions cannot be found in infected animals. Tests for the detection of prion disease in living animals and people are being developed but are not yet reliable for general application. Tab. 1.10 lists criteria for diagnosis of human BSE (nvCJD).

Differential Diagnosis. It is important to differentiate the picture of human BSE (nvCJD) from that of CJD (Tab. 1.11). In CJD symptoms like loss of memory and progressive dementia, as well as motor deficits (pyramidal tract), are predominant. Vacuolization and astrogliosis in the cortex, cerebellum, and brain stem neuron are less pronounced in CJD and appear only late in the disease and to a lesser extent. In CJD, amyloid plaques are rare. Alzheimer's disease and dementia of old age need to be differentiated diagnostically from CJD and human BSE. In some cases, the autopsy confirms spongiform encephalopathy, whereas the clinical diagnosis varied from brain tumor to stroke. Conversely, only 50% of cases with an anticipated diagnosis of CJD can be confirmed by pathoanatomy. Every clinical diagnosis of human BSE (nvCJD) and CJD, therefore, has to be confirmed by an autopsy.

Therapy. There is no specific therapy for BSE.

Prophylaxis. Slaughtered animals older than 2 years must be tested before release for consumption. If a positive animal is found on one farm, the entire herd must be slaughtered and burned, a practice that has been criticized emphatically. Tests to demonstrate prions become positive not before 24 months. Risky material, such as nervous and lymphatic tissues, therefore, should be carefully removed and should not be eaten or fed to animals. Risky material includes most of all the offal. However, prions were also detected in muscle tissue. Risky products from cattle, for example, gelatin, serum albumin, guts, and catgut, are not to be used for the production of drugs and vaccines or for food products. Some countries do not allow blood donation from donors who come from countries, or who have been to such countries, where BSE is present

Table 1.10 | Criteria for diagnosis of human bovine spongiform encephalopathy (nvCJD)[1]

I. A.	Progressive neuropsychiatric disturbance in a young patient [mean age for nvCJD (years), late 20s; mean age for classical Creutzfeldt-Jakob disease (years), late 60s]
B.	6-month duration of disease
C.	No indication of another diagnosis by routine testing
D.	No previous treatment (transfusion, transplantation, brain surgery)
II. A.	Early psychiatric symptoms (depression, anxiety, apathy, denial, delusions)
B.	Persistent hyperesthesia (very painful) and dysesthesia
C.	Ataxia
D.	Myoclonus or chorea or dystony
E.	Dementia
III. A.	An electroencephalogram does not show the generalized periodical triphasic complexes (1/s) typical of Creutzfeldt-Jakob disease
B.	High pulvinal signal on both sides in magnetic resonance imaging scans
IV. A.	Tonsillar biopsy positive for prions
V.	Neuropathologic results. Spongiform changes and extensive PrP depositions in florid plaques in the brain and cerebellum. (Florid plaques are amyloid plaques, which are surrounded by vacuoles in rosette formation.) Only these findings confirm the diagnosis. Codon 129 of the patient's PrP gene being homozygous for Met/Met seems to be essential for the diagnosis but does not prove it.

[1]Roman.

because of the possible transmission of prions by blood products.

For surgical operations, for example, tonsillectomy, it is recommended to use disposable instruments. Prion-contaminated material should be burned. The following conditions are recommended for steam sterilization: 2 h of running steam at 132 °C. Disinfection of prions can be accomplished by treatment with 5.25% sodium hypochlorite or 2 M NaOH. Formic acid and disinfectants containing phenol reduce the infectivity significantly. The flaming of previously mechanically cleaned instruments, such as scissors and forceps, with alcohol is a

Table 1.11 | Differential diagnosis of Creutzfeldt-Jakob disease (CJD) and human bovine spongiform encephalopathy (nvCJD)[1]

FINDING	HUMAN BSE (NVCJD)	CJD (SPORADIC)
Median age at death (range)	29 years (19 to 41 years)	65 years
Median duration of disease (range)	12 months (8 to 23 months)	4 months
Initial symptom(s)	Abnormal behavior, dysesthesia	Dementia
Late symptoms	Dementia, ataxia, myoclonus	Ataxia, myoclonus
Periodic complexes in electroencephalogram	Not present	Usually present
Codon 129 Met/Met	100% of human cases	83% of human cases
Histopathology	Vacuolization, loss of neurons, astrogliosis, amyloid plaques (100% of patients)	Vacuolization, loss of neurons, astrogliosis, amyloid plaques (1% to 15% of patients)
% of patients with florid plaques[2]	100	0
Glycosylation products of PrP	Similar to BSE	Never like BSE

[1] Modified from Will RG et al., A new variant of Creutzfeldt-Jakob disease in the UK. *Lancet* 347, 921–925, 1996.
[2] Florid plaques are amyloid plaques surrounded by vacuoles in rosette formation.

fire hazard but may reduce the risk of transmitting prions. Unfortunately, convincing data for the reduction in risk of transmission do not exist.

REFERENCES

Appel TR et al., Heat stability of prion rods and recombinant prion protein in water, lipid and lipid-water mixtures. *J. Gen. Virol.* 82, 465–473, 2001.

Asher DM, Transmissible spongiform encephalopathies. In: Murray PR et al. (eds.), *Manual of Clinical Microbiology*, 1125–1136, 7th ed. American Society of Microbiology, Washington, DC, 1999.

Baron TG, Biacabe AG, Molecular analysis of the abnormal prion protein during coinfection of mice by bovine spongiform encephalopathy and a scrapie agent. *J. Virol.* 75, 107–114, 2001.

Chesebro B, Fields B, Transmissible spongiform encephalopathies: A brief introduction. In: Fields BA et al. (eds.), *Virology*, 2845–2850, 3rd ed., Raven Press, New York, 1996.

Foster J et al., Partial dissociation of PrP(Sc) deposition and vacuolation in the brains of scrapie and BSE experimentally affected goats. *J. Gen. Virol.* 82, 267–273, 2001.

Fraser H, Phillips report and the origin of BSE. *Vet. Rec.* 147, 724, 2000.

Gajdusek DC, Infectious amyloids: subacute spongiform encephalopathies as transmissible cerebral amyloidoses. In: Fields BA et al. (eds.), *Virology*, 2851–2900, 3rd ed., Raven Press, New York, 1996.

Haltia M, Human prion diseases. *Ann. Med.* 32(7), 493–500, 2000.

Laffling AJ et al., A monoclonal antibody that enables specific immunohistological detection of prion protein in bovine spongiform encephalopathy cases. *Neurosci. Lett.* 300, 99–102, 2001.

Prusiner SB, Prions. In: Fields BA et al. (eds.), *Virology*. 3rd ed., 2901–2949, Raven Press, New York, 1996.

Shaked GM et al., Protease-resistant and detergent-insoluble prion protein is not necessarily associated with prion infectivity. *J. Biol. Chem.* 274, 17981–17982, 1999.

Shaked GM et al., Reconstitution of prion infectivity from solubilized protease-resistant PrP and nonprotein components of prion rods. *J. Biol. Chem.* 276, 2001.

Van Keulen LJ et al., Diagnosis of bovine spongiform encephalopathy: a review. *Vet. Q.* 22, 197–200, 2000.

Weissmann C, Aguzzi A, PrP's double causes trouble. *Science* 286, 914–915, 1999.

Wrathall AE et al., Studies of embryo transfer from cattle clinically affected by bovine spongiform encephalopathy (BSE). *Vet. Rec.* 150, 365–378, 2002.

Bacterial Zoonoses | 2

2.1 Introduction

Beside the "classical" bacterial zoonoses, this chapter covers infectious diseases such as listeriosis, in which the causative agents are frequently found in animals and that are traditionally regarded as zoonoses. However, since these agents may also be found in the environment and are not necessarily transmitted directly from animals to humans, diseases caused by them have also been termed "sapronoses," "geonoses," or "saprozoonoses."

2.2 Anthrax

Anthrax, already described by Greek and Roman writers, is primarily an acute infection of herbivores that can be transmitted to humans. In humans, three manifestations are seen: cutaneous, pulmonary, and intestinal anthrax.

Etiology. *Bacillus anthracis* is a nonmotile, sporeforming, aerobic Gram-positive rod. The vegetative (propagating) form is found in the host. Outside the host, it forms an endospore ("spore") that is resistant to environmental changes, such as desiccation, heat, cold, and ultraviolet light, and may remain infectious in

soil for decades. Virulence factors are the capsule and the plasmid-encoded exotoxins: protective, lethal, and edema toxin.

Occurrence. Anthrax occurs worldwide. In countries with insufficient veterinary services, above all, in Central and South America, Southern and Eastern Europe, Asia, Africa, the Caribbean, and the Middle East, the disease is either sporadic or epidemic.

Spores arise under natural conditions, primarily through putrefaction of carcasses or their breakup by scavengers, less often through the secretions of diseased animals. Susceptible animals maintain the circulation in endemic areas. Contaminated effluent from factories handling animal products (skin, hides, furs, hair, wool, bones) can spread the disease as well (Fig. 2.1) and imported animal products may introduce spores from endemic areas.

Animals become infected mostly by intake of spores during grazing. Under normal conditions, cattle, sheep, goats, equines, buffalo, camels, reindeer, and mink are most often affected, pigs and carnivores rarely, and birds practically never, with the exception of ostriches, ducks, and birds of prey. As the European Union has banned the feeding of animal parts to ruminants, pigs, and horses, contaminated bone-,

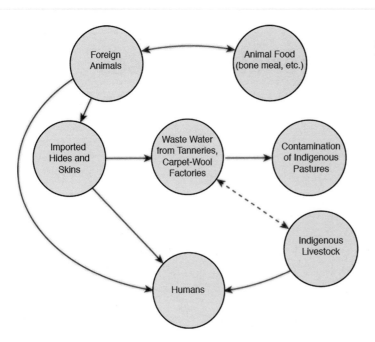

Figure 2.1 | Important transmission chains and avenues for contamination of *Bacillus anthracis*.

blood- and other meals have disappeared as sources of anthrax spores.

At particular risk are people in contact with susceptible animals, their products and carcasses, for example, those working with furs, horsehair, wool, carpets, brushes, paintbrushes, yarns, rags, and those employed in the production of glue from bone meal. Furthermore, veterinarians, animal dealers, farmers, butchers, knackers, and workers in the transportation industry can come into contact.

B. anthracis spores are potential bioweapons. In one famous episode in 2001 ("Amerithrax"), letters contaminated with anthrax spores were sent to politicians and journalists in the USA. Twenty-two people contracted anthrax and five of them died.

Transmission. Humans are primarily infected through contact with animals and their products. Transmission from human to human is possible but remains without epidemiological significance. The most frequent portals of entry are skin abrasions, injuries, and small blemishes. Transmission by arthropods cannot be ruled out yet. Airborne infection through sheep shearing or work in tanneries is particularly dangerous.

Consumption of meat or milk from infected animals may also lead to infection and severe illness. Even contaminated hides on exotic drums have been the source of infection.

Clinical Manifestations. Depending on the portal of entry, anthrax may take on several forms. Approximately 95% of all cases represent cutaneous anthrax. The incubation period is 2 to 5 (0.5 to 17) days. At the portal of entry, the first symptom is redness, followed by formation of a small papule and, after 12 to 24 h, a blister containing serosanguinous or seropurulent fluid. At the end of the first week, the central area ulcerates and develops a dark blue-red crust that later enlargens, blackens, and becomes dry and tough (Fig. 2.2). The surrounding tissue may become edematous ("malignant pustule"). Several carbuncles may develop simultaneously. The lesions are painless unless associated with lymphangitis or lymphadenitis. Depending on the severity of the illness, general symptoms such as fever, malaise, vomiting, and hypotension may develop. Drug addicts in Europe who inadvertently injected heroin contaminated with anthrax spores developed subcutaneous anthrax with massive edematous areas on the

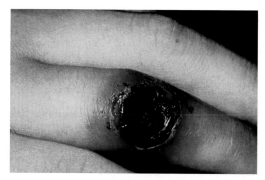

Figure 2.2 | Anthrax carbuncle. Eschar with black, adherent crust (courtesy of Klinische Visite Bildtafeln Thomae No. 114, Bildarchiv für Medizin GmbH, Munich, Germany).

extremities but without the typical anthrax skin lesions. Fever, compartmental syndromes, and shock have been reported.

Pulmonary anthrax [minimum infective dose 8000 to 50 000 spores; incubation period 9 to 10 (1 to 43) days] begins with nonspecific symptoms such as a sore throat, dry cough, and moderately high fever after which tachycardia, dyspnea, wheezing, high fever, sweats, tachypnea, hematemesis, bloody diarrhea, meningitis and, eventually, shock and coma will set in.

Intestinal anthrax (incubation period 1 to 7 days) starts with anorexia, nausea, and vomiting; later, abdominal pain, hematemesis, bloody diarrhea, and shock will develop. On autopsy, ulcers and necrotic areas in the intestinal tract, areas of bleeding in the mesenterium, and, frequently, extensive hemorrhagic lymphadenitis are found.

Oropharyngeal anthrax, also following oral uptake of spores, is characterized by sore throat, pain on swallowing, painful lymphadenopathy, and, occasionally, massive edema of the neck. The mucous membranes of the mouth and throat show 2 to 3 cm large foci of inflammation that may ulcerate and become covered with a grayish-white pseudomembrane.

Anthrax is always a life-threatening infection. Untreated cutaneous anthrax has a case-fatality rate of 10 to 40% (the latter if septicemia or meningitis develop). The prognosis is poor if the portal of entry is on either head or neck. The case-fatality rate of pulmonary, intestinal, and meningeal anthrax without early treatment approaches 90 to 100%.

In animals, anthrax is a peracute to chronic generalized infection. Herbivores are particularly prone to a severe illness. Sudden death, extensive edema, shock, colicky pain, and oral/nasal/intestinal hemorrhages are suspicious. High fever, dyspnea, cyanosis, difficulty swallowing, and diarrhea may be present in acute cases. In dead animals, rigidity may be missing but splenomegaly and hemorrhagic infiltrates of subcutaneous and subserous tissues should point to the diagnosis. In less susceptible animals, for example, pigs, mild, chronic, and localized forms (throat or mesenterial anthrax) may be seen.

Diagnosis. Cutaneous anthrax can be diagnosed clinically by a rapid development of an indolent carbuncle. The diagnosis of pulmonary and intestinal anthrax is more difficult; however, the patient's history may provide a hint. In cases of cutaneous anthrax, vesicular exudate is obtained by swab or by aspiration with a capillary tube below the edge of the eschar; the sample is then submitted for microscopy (Gram, Foth or McFadyean stain) and culture. Skin biopsy should be done under antibiotic coverage to prevent dissemination; the sample may also be used for immunohistochemical analysis.

Pulmonary anthrax is diagnosed by the characteristic radiological finding of symmetric mediastinal widening (indicating hemorrhagic mediastinitis) or by computer tomography showing abnormally large hilar lymphnodes and fluid accumulation in the respiratory tract. Confirmation is by microscopy and culture of sputum. When intestinal anthrax is suspected, feces, vomitus, secretions from nose, mouth, or anus, peritoneal fluid, and/or mesenterial lymphnodes may be cultured.

Bacteremia occurs in most cases of pulmonary and intestinal anthrax and is detected by blood culture. In meningitis, the spinal fluid is bloody and contains numerous bacilli. *B. anthracis* grows well and often sporulates at 37 °C. For contaminated samples, polymyxin-lysozyme-EDTA-thallous acetate agar has been recommended as a selective medium. PCR methods that amplify plasmid encoded virulence factors have been developed. Antibody titers against virulence factors can be measured by enzyme linked immunosorbent assay (ELISA) or indirect hemagglutination assay (IHA) techniques. These tests have not been standardized for routine use.

In the countries of the former USSR, positive results of an anthracin skin test, using a subcutaneous injection of an extract from an attenuated strain of B. anthracis, were used to indicate cell-mediated immunity against B.anthracis. The test was said to be positive in 81% of the cases within 3 days and in 97% within 2 to 3 weeks following infection.

In animals, the diagnosis is based on culture, with a direct stain used for orientation. In extracts of animal products, B. anthracis antigen can be detected by thermoprecipitation (Ascoli and Valenti) but this test lacks specificity and is of no use for environmental samples.

Differential Diagnosis. For cutaneous anthrax: erysipelas, insect bites, glanders, tularemia; for pulmonary anthrax: ornithosis; for intestinal anthrax: salmonellosis, cholera, mushroom, mercury, and arsenic poisoning; for septicemia cerebral malaria should be considered.

Therapy. Cutaneous anthrax with penicillin-susceptible strains: penicillin G 4 mio. IE every 4 h intravenously (i.v.), or amoxicillin 3 × 500 mg/day orally (p.o.) for 7 to 10 days; alternatively, doxycycline 2 × 100 mg/day p.o. (in the setting of bioterrorism, for 60 days). If susceptibility is unknown: ciprofloxacin 2 × 500 mg/day p.o., or levofloxacin 500 mg/day i.v. or p.o. for 60 days, or doxycycline 2 × 100 mg/day p.o. for 60 days. Bed rest, compresses, fluid and electrolyte substitution are necessary. Surgery is contraindicated. Pulmonary and intestinal anthrax, septicemia, and meningitis: ciprofloxacin 400 mg i.v. every 12 h, or levofloxacin 500 mg i.v. every 12 h, or doxycycline 100 mg i.v. every 12 h plus clindamycin 900 mg every 8 h and/or rifampicin 300 mg i.v. every 12 h. Intensive care is necessary. Children require lower doses.

Prophylaxis. The most important prophylactic measure to be taken is the control of anthrax in animals. This includes early recognition of B. anthracis infection followed by segregation, closure of stables or entire farms, killing of infected animals and of those suspected to have an infection, removal of animal products, and disinfection of suspicious items with 10% aqueous solution of sodium hypochlorite, soap or detergents, followed by exposure to chlorine, ethylene oxide, vaporized hydrogen peroxide, or a gas plasma system (Abtox or Sterrad). Spores will be killed by exposure to 60 Cobalt (20 to 30 kGy).

In cases of exposure, p.o. prophylaxis with ciprofloxacin (2 × 500 mg/day) or doxycycline (2 × 100 mg/day) for 10 days, in the setting of bioterrorism with presumed spore exposure for 60 days, are necessary. A different protocol follows the combination of immediate vaccination with an antibiotic treatment for 6 weeks. Live vaccines from spores of attenuated B. anthracis strains without capsule have been developed in Russia and China and they were used on humans and animals. In the USA and UK, two vaccines have been approved, they are called anthrax vaccine adsorbed (AVA) and anthrax vaccine precipitated. Both are produced from culture filtrates of toxigenic B. anthracis strains and both contain the protective antigen as primary immunogen. AVA may be injected (i) subcutaneous (s.c.) on days 1, 14, and 28, with boosters after 6, 12, and 18 months; or (ii) intramuscular (i.m.) on days 1 and 28 and after 6, 12, and 18 months.

For both, boosters are then recommended for every year. The use of vaccines is restricted to persons at high risk, for example, laboratory or military personnel. For work with B. anthracis or potentially contaminated specimens, Biosafety level (BSL) 3 practices should be followed.

Reporting. Anthrax is a notifiable disease in the USA and in Canada.

REFERENCES

Baggett HC et al., No evidence of a mild form of inhalational Bacillus anthracis infection during a bioterrorism-related inhalational anthrax outbreak in Washington, D.C., in 2001. *Clin. Infect. Dis.* 41, 991–997, 2005.

Bales ME et al., Epidemiologic response to anthrax outbreaks: field investigations, 1950–2001. *Emerg. Infect. Dis.* 8, 1163–1174, 2002.

Bartlett JG, Inglesby TV, Borio L Jr, Management of anthrax. *Clin. Infect. Dis.* 35, 851–858, 2002.

Bell DM, Kozarsky PE, Stephens DS., Clinical issues in the prophylaxis, diagnosis, and treatment of anthrax. *Emerg. Infect. Dis.* 8, 222–225, 2002.

Centers for: Disease Control and Prevention (CDC). Advisory Committee on Immunization Practices. Use of anthrax vaccine in the United States. MMWR Recomm. Rep. 49(RR15), 1–20, 2000.

Cieslak TJ, Eitzen EM Jr, Clinical and epidemiologic principles of anthrax. *Emerg. Infect. Dis.* 5, 552–555, 1999.

Dixon TC et al. Anthrax. *N. Engl. J. Med.* 341, 815–826, 1999.

Doganay M, Metan G, Alp EL. A review of cutaneous anthrax and its outcome. J. Infect. *Public Health* 3, 98–105, 2010.

Friedlander AM, Little SF, Advances in the development of next-generation anthrax vaccines. *Vaccine.* 27 (Suppl 4), D28–32, 2009.

Gombe NT et al., Risk factors for contracting anthrax in Kuwirirana ward, Gokwe North, Zimbabwe. *Afr. Health Sci.* 10, 159–164, 2010.

Hendricks KA et al., Centers for disease control and prevention expert panel meetings on prevention and treatment of anthrax in adults. *Emerg. Infect. Dis.* 20(2), e130687, 2014.

Hicks CW et al., An overview of anthrax infection including the recently identified form of disease in injection drug users. *Intensive Care Med* 38, 1092–1094, 2012.

Hugh-Jones ME, de Vos V, Anthrax and wildlife. *Rev. Sci. Tech.* 21, 359–383, 2002.

Inglesby TV, Anthrax as a biological weapon: medical and public health management. Working Group on Civilian Biodefense. *JAMA* 281, 1735–1745, 1999.

Jernigan JA et al., Bioterrorism-related inhalational anthrax: the first 10 cases reported in the United States. *Emerg. Infect. Dis.* 7, 933–944, 2001.

Knox D et al., Subcutaneous anthrax in three intravenous drug users: a new clinical diagnosis. *J. Bone Joint Surg. Br.* 93, 414–417, 2011.

McGovern TW, Norton SA, Recognition and management of anthrax. *N. Engl. J. Med.* 346, 943–945, 2002.

Patra G et al., Molecular characterization of Bacillus strains involved in outbreaks of anthrax in France in 1997. *J. Clin. Microbiol.* 36, 3412–3414, 1998.

Penn CC, Klotz SA, Anthrax pneumonia. *Semin.Respir. Infect.* 12, 28–30, 1997.

Rao SS, Mohan KV, Atreya CD, Detection technologies for Bacillus anthracis: prospects and challenges. *J. Microbiol. Methods* 82, 1–10, 2010.

Shlyakhov E, Rubinstein E, Evaluation of the anthraxin skin test for diagnosis of acute and past human anthrax. *Eur. J. Clin. Microbiol. Infect. Dis.* 15, 242–245, 1996.

Singh BB, Gajadhar AA, Role of India's wildlife in the emergence and re-emergence of zoonotic pathogens, risk factors and public health implications. *Acta Trop* 138C, 67–77, 2014.

Sirisanthana T, Brown AE, Anthrax of the gastrointestinal tract. *Emerg. Infect. Dis.* 8, 649–651, 2002.

Swartz MN, Recognition and management of anthrax – an update. *N. Engl. J. Med.* 345, 1621–1626, 2001.

Weiss S et al., Antibiotics cure anthrax in animal models. *Antimicrob. Agents Chemother.* 55, 1533–1542, 2011.

Turnbull P, *Anthrax in Humans and Animals.* World Health Organization, Food and Agriculture Organization of the United Nations, World Organisation for Animal Health, Geneva, 2008.

2.3 Bartonelloses

A wide spectrum of infections with various *Bartonella* spp. is known in humans and animals. These include Carrion's disease (Oroya fever or verruca peruana), bacillary angiomatosis, bacillary peliosis (peliosis hepatis, peliosis lienalis), cat scratch disease, chronic bacteremia, endocarditis, and neurological disease, the latter particularly in HIV-infected patients.

Etiology. Until 1993, the genus *Bartonella* consisted of one species only: *B. bacilliformis*. Later, 16SrRNA sequence analysis showed that the former genera *Rochalimaea* and *Grahamella* belong to the genus *Bartonella*.

With *B. henselae*, a "non-culturable" agent was, for the first time, identified by molecular techniques as a distinct species causing a particular disease, that is, bacillary angiomatosis. Subsequently, the genus has expanded and now comprises approximately 35 species, at least 13 of which are considered human pathogens (www.bacterio.net).

Bartonella spp. belong to the class alpha-2-proteobacteria and are phylogenetically related to *Brucella* spp. They are small (0.3 to 0.5 by 1.0 to 1.7 μm), slightly curved, oxidase-negative, microaerophilic fastidious Gram-negative rods that can be cultured on media containing blood or hemin in a moist 5 to 10% CO_2 atmosphere. Growth may require 9 to 40 days. Some species (*B. bacilliformis*, *B. clarridgeiae*) are motile with flagella; others have pili only or show twitching motility. Pili (fimbriae) allow the bacteria to adhere to eukaryotic cells and to transport them into red blood and endothelial cells. While *B. bacilliformis* is located within and outside such cells, *B. quintana* is an exclusively epicellular bacterium. With the help of a protease-sensitive angiogenic factor, bartonellae (e.g., *B. bacilliformis, B. quintana, B. henselae*) induce proliferation of endothelial cells.

Occurrence. The reservoir of potentially infected animals is large and comprises cats (*B. henselae, B. clarridgeiae, B. koehlerae, B. elizabethae, B. weissii*), dogs, coyote (*B. vinsonii* subsp. *berkhoffii*), wild rabbits (*B. alsatica*), rats (*B. tribocorum*), mice (*B. vinsonii* subspp. *vinsonii* and *arupensis*) and other rodents (*B. washoensis*), other mammals, birds, and fish (*B. grahamii, B. talpae, B. peromysci, B. taylori, B. doshiae*) and bats (Candidatus B. mayotimonensis). Cats and rodents may be infected by several species at the same time. In a few animals, depending on the type of placentation, transplacentar transmission is possible. Some animals are asymptomatic, others (e.g., dogs) show symptoms of disease. Human infections are frequent: healthy blood donors have shown prevalence rates of 5 to 30%.

Transmission. Transmission depends on the species of *Bartonella* and on the hosts (animal or human), some of whom show a high preference for certain vectors. Sandflies (*Lutzomyia* spp.) for *B. bacilliformis*, body lice (*Pediculus humanus* var. *corporis*) for *B. quintana*, cat fleas (*Ctenocephalides felis*) for *B. henselae*, mites (*Trombicula microti*) for *B. vinsonii* subsp. *vinsonii*, ticks (*Ixodes scapularis*) for *B. vinsonii* subspp. *berkhoffii* and *arupensis*. *Amblyomma americanum* in the southeastern USA and *Ixodes ricinus* in the Czech Republic carry bartonellae in 0.4% and 1.2%, respectively. However, the potential for a *Bartonella* infection after tick bites is still being discussed. Human pathogens are mainly *B. bacilliformis* and *B. quintana*, which are transmitted from human to human only (anthroponoses) by the vectors mentioned. Among the zoonotic agents, *B. henselae* is by far the most important one. Others are listed in Tab. 2.1.

2.3.1 CAT SCRATCH DISEASE

Etiology. The most important agents of cat scratch disease (CSD) is *B. henselae* (formerly *Rochalimaea henselae*); more rarely, other species, such as *B. clarridgeiae, B. doshiae*, and *B. koehlerae*, may be involved. *Afipia felis*, described in 1988 as a further agent, may have a minor role, if any.

Occurrence. CSD occurs only in humans, particularly in children and in adolescents, and hardly, if ever, in domestic animals. It is more frequent in temperate climates during fall and winter. Sporadic cases, family outbreaks, and miniepidemics have been reported. The incidence in the USA is approximately 25 000 cases per year. The reservoir for *B. henselae* is domestic cats who do not become symptomatic but can be bacteremic for long periods. The rate of feline infections is highest in moist and warm regions (up to 70%) and lower in northern areas (0% in Norway!). *B. henselae* has also been detected in fleas of infected cats. These fleas are probably host-specific and transmit the organism from cat to cat. It is assumed that dried infected flea feces can be transmitted to humans through the claws of mostly young cats by scratching.

Transmission. In >90% of cases, a history of scratch or bite wounds from cats or contact with mostly young cats, rarely with dogs, can be elicited. Direct human-to-human transmission is extremely unlikely.

Clinical Manifestations. Following a 3 to 10 day incubation period, a primary lesion appears as an erythematous papule. After 1 to 2 weeks, a subacute regional lymphadenitis will develop which may lead in 10 to 15% of all cases to a purulent secretion (Fig. 2.3). Axillar, cervical, or inguinal nodes are most often affected and they remain enlarged from several weeks to months until recovery sets in. In individual cases, fever, chills, anorexia, malaise, and a generalized exanthema may be seen. Systemic

Table 2.1 | Human pathogenic *Bartonella* spp.

SPECIES	VECTOR	RESERVOIR	DISEASE	OCCURRENCE
Human-specific				
B. bacilliformis	*Lutzomyia* spp.	Humans	Oroya fever	S. America
B. quintana	*Pediculus humanus vestimenti*	Humans bacteremia, endocarditis	Trench fever	S. America, USA, Europe, Africa
Zoonotic				
B. henselae	*Ctenocephalides felis*, ticks	Cats, (dogs)	Cat scratch disease, bacteremia, endocarditis, bacill. angiomatosis, peliosis	Europe, USA, S. America, Asia, Africa
B. koehlerae	Fleas?	Cats	Cat scratch disease	USA
B. clarridgeiae	*Ctenocephalides Felis*	Cats, (dogs)	Cat scratch disease, endocarditis	Europe, USA, Asia
B. vinsonii subsp. *berkhoffii*	Ticks?	Dogs	Fever, myocarditis	Europe, USA
B. elisabethae	*Xenopsylla cheopis*	Rats, (dogs)	Bacteremia, endocarditis	Europe, USA
B. rochalimae	Sand flies?	Rats	Bacteremia	
B. grahamii	*Ctenophthalmus nobilis*	Mice, voles	Neuroretinitis	Europe, Asia, Canada
B. vinsonii subsp. *arupensis*	?	Mice	Fever, bacteremia	Europe, USA
B. vinsonii subsp. *vinsonii*	Fleas? Mites?	Mice	Fever, bacteremia	Europe, USA
B. doshiae	Fleas	Rodents	Cat scratch disease	Europe
B. washoensis	*Ixodes* spp.?	Ground squirrels	Myocarditis	USA
B. alsatica	?	Rabbits	Bacteremia, endocarditis	Europe
B. tamiae	?	?	Fever	Thailand
Candidatus B. mayotimonensis	?	Bats, mice?	Endocarditis	USA

Modified from Kempf V, Autenrieth I. *Bartonella* spp. and *Afipia* spp. In: Neumeister B.: Mikrobiologische Diagnostik, Thieme, Stuttgart, Germany, 2009.

infection can manifest itself in a long-lasting bacteremia with rapidly increasing intermittent or persisting fever, with local symptoms being mostly absent. Rare complications are meningitis and endocarditis. In approximately 6% of all cases, CSD manifests itself as Parinaud's oculoglandular syndrome. Severe complications are encephalopathies (2%) with long-lasting fever, coma, convulsions, and (reversible) blindness due to optic neuritis. Granulomatous hepatitis (0.3%), arthritis/arthralgia, osteomyelitis (0.3%), and pneumonia (0.2%) are rare. The general outlook is favorable.

Diagnosis. CSD may be suspected from the typical clinical picture (primary lesion, regional lymphadenopathy) and a history of contact with cats, occasionally with dogs through licking, biting, or scratching. The laboratory diagnosis is primarily a serological one, mostly by use of an immunofluorescence test using *B. henselae* antigen from Vero cell cultures. A variety of commercial tests are available. Antibodies can usually be detected when lymphadenopathy has developed; however, low titers are difficult to interpret because of high seroprevalence (e.g., in 6 to 10% of the German population) and cross-reactions.

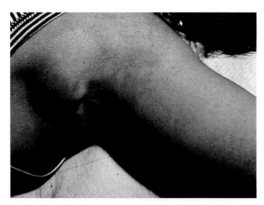

Figure 2.3 | Clinical presentation of cat scratch disease with adenopathy of the axillar lymphnode (Dr. A. Sander, Freiburg, Germany).

Bartonellae can be detected directly from lymph node biopsies by PCR. Histologically, nonspecific granulomatous inflammation with necrotic centers surrounded by epithelioid cells, eosinophils, and giant cells can be seen. A Warthin-Starry stain may show bartonellae but lacks specificity. Positive cultures are rare.

Differential Diagnosis. Infectious mononucleosis, mycobacterial infections, lymphogranuloma venereum, lues, Hodgkin's and other lymphomas and tumors, tularemia, brucellosis, toxoplasmosis, and histoplasmosis.

Treatment. Generally, CSD is benign, self-limited and does not require antimicrobial treatment. Therapy essentially consists of analgesics and antipyretics. A persisting primary lesion should be treated with warm moist compresses and it will heal in 2 to 3 months. Incision of purulent lymph nodes may sometimes be necessary and should provide samples for histological and microbiological analysis. In immunosuppressed individuals, and in severe cases, oral azithromycin (500 mg on day 1 and 250 mg from day 2 to day 5) is recommended. In cases of optical neuritis, oral doxycycline 2×100 mg/day plus rifampicin 2×300 mg/day for 4 to 6 weeks is recommended.

Prophylaxis. Immunocompromised individuals carry a high risk and should avoid contact with wild or stray cats, with those that are flea-infested, and with kittens <12 months. Scratches are particularly dangerous.

2.3.2 ENDOCARDITIS DUE TO *BARTONELLA* SPECIES

Trench fever, which is caused by *B. quintana*, has become a rarity. This bacterium, as well as *B. henselae* and other *Bartonella* spp., have become known as important causes of long-lasting bacteremia and culture-negative endocarditis. While *B. quintana* infections occur particularly in homeless persons, patients with preexisting valve lesions are at risk for *B. henselae* endocarditis.

Diagnosis. Serology may reveal high IF titers (>6400). PCR on heart valve biopsies is the preferred method for a direct demonstration of the agent. Cultures in cell lines or blood cultures are rarely positive.

Therapy. Ceftriaxone 2 g/day i.v. for 6 weeks plus gentamicin 3 mg/kg/day i.v. for 2 weeks plus doxycycline 2×100 mg/day p.o. for 6 weeks. Infected valves should be surgically removed.

2.3.3 *BARTONELLA* INFECTIONS IN IMMUNOCOMPROMISED PATIENTS

Etiology. The most frequent agents are *B. henselae* and *B. quintana*; other species (*B. elisabethae*, *B. vinsonii* subspp. *berkoffii* and *arupensis*, *B. washoensis*) have rarely been implicated. Patients with cellular immune defects (e.g., HIV infection) may show particular pathologies, that is, bacillary angiomatosis and peliosis hepatis, as well as osteomyelitis and endocarditis. In HIV+ patients, the disease begins slowly with general malaise, diffuse pains, tiredness, headache, weight loss, hepatomegaly, and extended febrile periods with occasional high temperatures.

In bacillary angiomatosis, bartonellae propagate in endothelial cells and induce angiogenesis in the skin and subcutis, more rarely in mucous membranes, and in intestinal organs, such as liver, spleen, brain, lung, and intestine, as well as in bones. Skin and subcutaneous tissues show single or multiple (>100) skin-colored or light/dark red nodules that may ulcerate, secrete serous or bloody fluid, or form crusts. Regional lymph nodes are enlarged. Lesions may bleed profusely if injured. Bacillary peliosis is characterized by microscopic to millimeter-size blood-filled cysts in the liver, more rarely in spleen and lymph nodes, which may bleed profusely. Part of the neuropsychiatric problems in HIV+ patients, such as chronic or acute meningoencephalitis and progressive dementia, may be due to *Bartonella* infection.

Diagnosis. Serological diagnosis is unreliable in immunocompromised patients, the direct visualization of the agents in tissues with Warthin-Starry stain nonspecific and difficult to interpret. The best method in cases of bacillary angiomatosis and peliosis hepatis is PCR from tissue, with a sensitivity of 50 to almost 100%. Culture of tissue homogenates on solid media, possibly cocultured with cell lines, requires long incubation periods (7 to 10 days) and is often negative.

Differential Diagnosis. The differential diagnosis includes endocarditis of other etiology (e.g., *Coxiella burnetii*), and other encephalopathies (HIV, *Cryptococcus neoformans*, *Toxoplasma gondii*).

Therapy. Recommended are oral clarithromycin 2 × 500 mg/day or azithromycin 250 mg/day or ciprofloxacin 500 to 700 mg/day or doxycycline 2 × 100 mg/day; in severe cases, doxycycline 2 × 100 mg/day p.o. plus rifampicin 2 × 300 mg/day, each for 8 weeks.

REFERENCES

Angelakis E et al., Potential for tick-borne Bartonelloses. *Emerg. Infect. Dis.* 16, 385–391, 2010.

Breitschwerdt EB, Kordick DL, Bartonella infection in animals: carriership, reservoir potential, pathogenicity, and zoonotic potential for human infection. *Clin. Microbiol. Rev.* 13, 428–438, 2000.

Breitschwerdt EB et al., Bartonellosis: an emerging infectious disease of zoonotic importance to animals and human beings. *J. Vet. Emerg. Crit. Care (San Antonio)* 20, 8–30, 2010.

Buffet JP, Kosoy M, Vayssier-Taussat M., Natural history of Bartonella-infecting rodents in light of new knowledge on genomics, diversity and evolution. *Future Microbiol* 8, 1117–1128, 2013.

Chomel BB et al., Bartonella spp. in pets and effect on human health. *Emerg. Infect. Dis.* 12, 389–394, 2006.

Chomel BB, Kasten RW, Bartonellosis, an increasingly recognized zoonosis. *J. Appl. Microbiol.* 109, 743–750, 2010.

Guphill L, Bartonellosis. *Vet. Microbiol.* 27, 347–359, 2010.

Kaiser PO et al., Bartonella spp.: throwing light on uncommon human infections. *Int. J. Med. Microbiol.* 30, 7–15, 2011.

Maggi RG et al., Bartonella. In: Versalovic J et al., (eds.): *Manual of Clinical Microbiology*, 10th ed., 786–798, American Society for Microbiology, Washington D.C., 2011.

Molin Y et al., Migratory birds, ticks, and Bartonella. *Infect Ecol Epidemiol* 1, 2011 (Epub Feb. 11).

Mühldorfer K, Bats and bacterial pathogens: a review. *Zoonoses Public Health* 60, 93–103, 2013.

Regnery R, Tappero J, Unraveling mysteries associated with cat-scratch disease, bacillary angiomatosis, and related syndromes. *Emerg. Infect. Dis.* 1, 16–21, 1995.

2.4 Borrelioses

Of prime importance for humans are Lyme borreliosis and relapsing fever. Several *Borrelia* species occurring in animals have thus far not been decribed as infectious agents in humans, for example, *B. anserina* (worldwide in geese, ducks, chickens, turkeys), *B. coriaceae* (cause of stillbirths in North American cattle), *B. latyschewii* (in reptiles in Iran and Central Asia), and *B. theileri* (agent of bovine and equine borreliosis in South Africa and Australia).

2.4.1 LYME BORRELIOSIS

Lyme borreliosis, an infectious disease caused by B. *burgdorferi sensu lato*, manifests itself in humans and animals with a multitude of dermatological, rheumatological, neurological, and cardiac symptoms. It was named after the town of Lyme in Connecticut, where it was first observed in the 1970s in the form of joint diseases in adolescents, which were initially diagnosed as juvenile rheumatoid arthritis. The etiological agent was identified by Willy Burgdorfer in 1982.

Etiology. Spirochetes isolated from the main vector, that is, hard ticks (*Ixodes* spp.) and from patients with Lyme borreliosis belong to the genus *Borrelia*. They are Gram-negative and have a typical spirochetal structure with a protoplasmic cylinder surrounded by an internal membrane and a peptidoglycan wall. The protoplasma contains a linear chromosome and many linear and circular plasmids. Flagella in variable numbers (7 to 11 in *B.burgdorferi*; 15 to 30 in *B. recurrentis*) originate at the ends of the protoplasmic cylinder and they are enveloped by the outer membrane. Thus, they are endoflagella that cause the spiral shape as well as the screw-like motility. The outer membrane contains immunogenic proteins used in diagnostic tests.

The Lyme borreliosis spirochetes form a complex (*B.burgdorferi s.l.*) that by now contains 37 named genospecies (see www.bacterio.net). Within this complex, *B. burgdorferi sensu stricto*, *B. garinii*, and *B. afzelii* are the most important human pathogens. All US isolates belong to *B. burgdorferi s.s.*, while in Europe, all three species have been isolated, although most of them belong to the latter two species. These epidemiological differences may account for regional differences in clinical symptomatology. Whether borreliae other than those mentioned in Tab. 2.2a and b may infect humans has not been established.

Occurrence. Lyme borreliosis has been found in the entire Northern Hemisphere. The incidence in Central Europe is estimated at 60 to 130 cases per 100 000 inhabitants per year,

that is, 40 000 to 90 000 new cases per year in Germany. The early stage (erythema migrans) is seen most often during summer, with a peak in June/July. Weeks to months later, with a peak in October, neurological and cardiac symptoms will appear. The late stage with chronic skin and joint disease and neurological symptoms become manifest 2 to 3 years after infection.

The most important reservoirs are wild rodents, particularly wood and yellow necked mice, bank voles, and hedgehogs whose complement does not affect borreliae (by contrast, the complement of domestic animals and deer is able to lyse borreliae). The main vectors of *B. burgdorferi s.l.* are various hard ticks that feed over several days: in Europe, *I. ricinus*; in the USA, *I.scapularis* (syn. *I. dammini*), and *I. pacificus*; in Asia, primarily *I. persulcatus*. In Central Europe, the rate of infestation of *I. ricinus* with *B.burgdorferi s.l.* may be as high as 42%, and all stages (1% of larvae, 10% of nymphs, and 20% of adults) may be infested. For *I. hexagonus*, the hedgehog tick, rates of up to 12% have been found. In Connecticut, 10 to 50% of nymphal and adult *I. scapularis* are infested. The risk of borreliae being transmitted to humans in the western USA is much lower (1 to 3%) as only a small part of the tick parasitize rodents, with their main intermediate host being lizards, which are not susceptible to infection. The tick may nevertheless contribute to the spread of the disease as it can be found in many wild and domestic animals, including birds. The

Table 2.2a | *Borrelia* spp. of medical and veterinarian significance occurring in North America

SPECIES	VECTOR	RESERVOIR	OCCURRENCE	DISEASE	HOSTS
B.burgdorferi s.s.***	*Ixodes scapularis*, *I. pacificus*	Mice, small rodents, hare	North America	Lyme borreliosis	Human, dog, cat (horse, cattle)
B. andersonii	*I. dentatus*, *I. scapularis*	Unknown	North America	unknown	(Human)
B. bissettii	*I. spinipalpus*, *I. pacificus*	Mice, birds, rabbit	North America	Lyme borreliosis (erythema migrans, lymphocytoma)	Human

*** s.s., sensu stricto

Modified from Straubinger RK. Genus Borrelia. In: Selbitz JJ, U Truyen, P Valentin-Weigand (eds.): Tiermedizinische Mikrobiologie, Infektions-und Seuchenlehre; Enke, Stuttgart, 2011; and Stanek G. Borreliosen. In: H Aspöck (ed.): Krank durch Arthropoden, 605–624, Denisia 30, Linz, 2011.

Table 2.2b | *Borrelia* spp. of medical and veterinarian significance occurring in Europe and Asia

SPECIES	VECTOR	RESERVOIR	OCCURRENCE	DISEASE	HOST
B. burgdorferi s.s.****	*I. ricinus*, *I. persulcatus*	Mice, other rodents, lagomorphs	Europe, Japan	Lyme borreliosis	Human, dog, cat (horse, cattle)
B. garinii	*I. ricinus*, *I. persulcatus*	Mice, small mammals, birds	Europe, Asia	Lyme borreliosis	Human (dog, cattle, cat, horse)
B. afzelii	*I. ricinus*, *I. persulcatus*	Mice, small mammals, lagomorphs	Europe, Asia Europe, Asia	Lyme borreliosis	Human (dog, cattle, cat, horse)
B. valaisiana	*I. ricinus* *I. persulcatus*	Mice, small mammals, lagomorphs, birds	Europe, Asia	Lyme borreliosis (?)	Human
B. spielmanii	*I. ricinus*	Dormouse, hedgehog	Europe, Asia	Skin lesions (?), vasculitis (?)	Human
B. lusitaniae	*I. ricinus*, *I. columnae*	Mice, lizards	Europe, Japan	Skin lesions (?),	Human
B. bissettii	*I. ricinus*	Mice, birds, rabbits	Europe (Slovenia)	Lyme borreliosis (erythema migans, lymphocytoma)	Human
B. japonica	*I. ovatus*, *I. persulcatus*	Mice, birds	Japan	Unknown	Human, dog
B. tanukii	*I. tanuki*, *I. ovatus*	Unknown	Europe, Asia (Japan)	Unknown	Dog, cat
B. turdi	*I. turdus*	Unknown	Asia (Japan)	Unknown	Dog, cat
B. sinica	*I. ovatus*	Unknown	Asia (China)	Unknown	Unknown

**** s.s., sensu stricto
Modified from Straubinger RK, Genus Borrelia. In: Selbitz JJ, Truyen U, Valentin-Weigand P (eds.): Tiermedizinische Mikrobiologie, Infektions-und Seuchenlehre; Enke, Stuttgart, 2011; and Stanek G. Borreliosen. In: Aspöck H (ed.): Krank durch Arthropoden, 605–624, Denisia 30, Linz, 2011.
The recently described *B. miyamotoi* is genetically closer to the relapsing fever borreliae but is transmitted by the same ticks as *B. burgdorferi s.s.* and has its reservoir in rodents.

occurrence of Lyme borreliosis in humans is closely associated with tick infestation. Ticks prefer moist areas: lightly grown deciduous forests, meadows adjacent to rivers, parks, and gardens. At special risk are forest workers, tourists sleeping in tents, and walkers.

Transmission. *B. burgdorferi s.l.* residing in the midgut of a tick expresses outer surface protein A (OspA) that mediates binding to the midgut epithelium of the tick. When the tick starts feeding on a host, most borreliae cease to express OspA at the higher temperature and begin to express OspC. These processes enable the borreliae to exit from the midgut, to spread via the hemolymph and to invade the salivary gland.

They then manage to enter the bite wound via the infected saliva. During the first hours of tick attachment, the risk of infection is minimal but increases after 36 h. Prospective studies have estimated the risk of infection after any tick bite to be 4 to 8%. The risk after the bite of a tick infected with borreliae is, however, 23%. Whether other blood-sucking insects such as deer flies (*Stomoxys calcitrans*) or horse flies (*Tabanidae*) may transmit borreliae has not been elucidated but is would probably be of minor epidemiological importance. Simultaneous infections with *Babesia* spp. or *Ehrlichia* spp. are possible and should be taken into account.

Clinical Manifestations. In analogy to infection with *Treponema pallidum*, the clinical course of Lyme borreliosis has been subdivided into three stages. Stage 1 the early-localized infection; Stage 2, the dissemination; and stage 3 the persistent infection (Tab. 2.3).

Stage 1: following the bite of an infected tick, *B. burgdorferi* spreads centrifugally in the skin which, after an incubation period of a few days to >1 month, reacts in 60 to 80% of the patients with a typical erythema migrans (Fig. 2.4), occasionally accompanied by fever and regional lymphadenopathy. Usually, the erythema develops slowly from a small red papule and spreads within days to weeks over larger areas while fading centrally. Fading may not always occur, however, and cockade forms are occasionally seen. Much rarer is lymphocytoma, a painless, blue-red nodule or plaque, which in children is mostly on the earlobes or scrotum, and in the nipple area in adults.

Stage 2: 3 to 5 weeks following the tick bite, borreliae disseminate via the bloodstream and, perhaps, via peripheral nerves, as suggested by ipsilateral erythema migrans and central or peripheral neuropathies. Manifestations of dissemination include:

- Signs of generalized infection, such as malaise, fatigue, weakness, myalgias, arthralgias;

- Fever (rare) and night sweats;
- Multiple erythema migrans lesions or disseminated lymphocytomas (rare in Europe, more frequent in America);
- Intermittent joint, tendon, muscle or bone pain lasting for a few hours;
- Signs of early neuroborreliosis in approximately 5% of symptomatic infections. Following an incubation period of 4 to 7 weeks, children will develop mild aseptic meningitis and/or peripheral neuritis of cranial nerves, mostly of the nervus facialis. In adults, meningoradiculoneuritis (Bannwarth) and/or paresis of cranial nerves are typical. Symptoms start with burning, piercing radicular pain attacks that react poorly to analgesics. One to 4 weeks later most patients experience motor or sensory deficits, particularly of the cranial nerves;
- Cardiopathy. If the conduction system is affected, tachyarrhythmias and 2nd or 3rd degree atrioventricular (AV) blocks may occur. Cardiomyopathies have also been described.

Stage 3: this stage is characterized by the presence of borreliae in organs, primarily in the collagenous connective tissue of skin and joints.

Acrodermatitis chronica atrophicans (ACA): this is a chronic progressive fibrosing skin disease, generally occurring several years after the primary infection. Hands and feet become swollen with a blue-red discoloration, particularly

Table 2.3 | Clinical stages of Lyme borrelioses

STAGE	INFECTION	CLINICAL MANIFESTATION
Stage 1	Early localized	Erythema chronicum migrans Lymphadenosis cutis (solitary lymphocytoma)
Stage 2	Disseminated	Multiple erythema migrans Disseminated lymphocytoma Systemic infection with general malaise, myalgias, arthralgias Early Lyme borreliosis (aseptic meningitis, neuritis, meningoradiculitis Bannwarth) Carditis (tachyarrhyhmias, a-v block)
Stage 3	Chronic	Acrodermatitis chronica atrophicans Arthritis Peripheral neuropathies, progressive encephalomyelitis (very rare)

Modified from Stanek G, Borreliosen. In: Aspöck H (ed.): Krank durch Arthropoden, 605–624, Denisia 30, Linz, 2010.

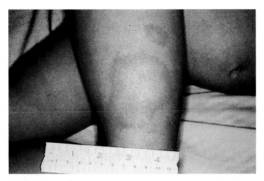

Figure 2.4 | Erythema migrans following tick bite on the right thigh (Prof. R.C. Johnson, Minneapolis, MN, USA).

over the extensor surfaces of the joints. Later, the skin becomes atrophic, paper-thin, and almost transparent. Persisting signs are often combined with polyneuropathy.

Classical Lyme arthritis: joint symptoms start years after the primary infection. They manifest themselves as mono- or oligoarthritis of the large joints (hip, knee, ankles). Inflammation may "jump" from joint to joint, with effusions forming within a few hours. Arthritis may recede spontaneously; in other cases, IL-1 and prostaglandins induce synovial proliferation and activate collagenases, leading to irreversible damage to the cartilage. Such patients have histocompatibility antigens Human Leukocyte Antigen (HLA) DR2 and HLA DR4 ci. three times more often than healthy individuals.

Chronic Lyme borreliosis: axonal degeneration of peripheral nerves leads to a painful neuropathy and sensory loss. In Europe, polyneuropathy is generally associated with acrodermatitis; in the USA, it may occur without ACA.

Chronic progressive Lyme encephalomyelitis: rare and associated with central nervous symptoms. Depending on the localization of the affected parts of the brain, chronic progressive encephalomyelitis, cerebellitis, spastic paraspareses, ataxia, transverse myelopathy, cranial nerve palsies, and mental disturbance (rarely, dementia) may result. Borreliae may persist in the central nervous system (CNS) in spite of antibiotic treatment. Symptoms may resemble those of multiple sclerosis or neurosyphilis but it can be differentiated from them by the presence of specific intrathecal antibodies.

Occasional reports of transplacentar infections with damage to the fetus have been met with skepticism. While rodents and wild animals seem to only have inapparent infections dogs, possibly also horses and cattle may have overt borreliosis. In dogs, recurrent mono- or oligoarthritis, fever and malaise have been observed, and renal disease such as glomerulonephritis and kidney failure were seen in Bernese mountain dogs and in retrievers. Neurological and cardiac manifestations are rare. After an incubation period of 2 to 4 months, one to five exacerbations will generally take place, each lasting from 2 to 5 days. Recovery occurs after 6 to 8 weeks, although the organisms may persist in various tissues. Horses may also show a multitude of symptoms, mostly recurrent arthritis, neuropathy, and ulcerative keratitis. They have been interpreted as signs of borreliosis as diagnostic tests were positive but could not be reproduced in controlled experiments. In cattle, arthritis, myocarditis, pneumonia, and stillbirth were seen and interpreted as signs of borreliosis.

Diagnosis. While a history of tick bite may provide a valuable clue, the diagnosis must be based on clinical and serological findings.

The Centers for Disease Control (CDC) and the German Society for Hygiene and Microbiology quality standards recommend a step-by-step diagnosis. The first test is an ELISA with purified or recombinant antigens. If it is positive, a confirmatory test, generally an immunoblot differentiating between IgM and IgG is required. In *B. burgdorferi s.l.* infections, many immunologically relevant proteins can be found which are located at the surface (Osp) and in the cell itself. A few weeks after infection IgM antibodies against cross-reacting flagellin and against the specific OspC can be detected. In stage 2, antibodies against other proteins, for example, VlsE or BmpA, expressed *in vivo*, can be found. In Stage 3, antibodies against p83/100 are characteristic. Immunoblot bands should be interpreted according to official recommendations. The sensitivity of antibody tests in stage 1 is ci. 20 to 50%, in stage 2, 70 to 90% (IgM); in stage 3, almost 100% (IgG). The diagnosis of a florid Lyme borreliosis, however, can only be made in connection with clinical symptoms. If treatment has been successful, the serological response will decrease but may take years. The proof of neuroborreliosis rests with the finding of intrathecal antibodies. A positive cerebrospinal fluid (CSF)/serum index could remain even after successful treatment.

Isolation of the organism on selective media such as Barbour-Stoenner-Kelly medium at 30 to 35 °C is difficult and time-consuming. Isolation from blood is quite unusual; from CSF, it succeeds in 10 to 30% of all cases. Optimal are skin biopsies (60 to 80% positivity rate). PCR has been successful in a number of cases, with the best sensitivity in joint fluid (50 to 70%). It may remain positive in spite of successful treatment but does not necessarily mean that borreliae are viable.

Differential Diagnosis. The differential diagnosis of erythema migrans must consider erythema annulare centrifugum (associated with rheumatic fever), erysipelas (which develops faster and spreads within days), erysipeloid (associated with a professional history, e.g., in butchers), and erythema exsudativum multiforme. Arthritis also occurs in primary chronic polyarthritis and as para- or postinfectious complication of infections with yersiniae, salmonellae, *Campylobacter*, and chlamydiae.

Therapy. Therapy depends on stage and localization. Stage 1: doxycycline 2×100 mg/day p.o., or amoxicillin 3×500 mg/day p.o., or cefuroxime acetil 2 to 3×500 mg/day p.o. for 2 to 3 weeks; or oral azithromycin 500 mg/day for 10 days. Success rate >90%. Cardiopathy: 1st degree AV block: p.o. treatment as for stage 1; 2nd and 3rd degree AV block: Ceftriaxone 2 g/day i.v. or penicillin G 4 to 5 mio. IE/day i.v. for 2 to 3 weeks. Arthritis: doxycycline or amoxicillin as above or ceftriaxone or penicillin G as above but for 2 to 3 months. Acrodermatitis: doxycycline as above for 1 to 2 months. Meningitis and encephalitis: ceftriaxone as above or penicillin as above for 2 to 4 weeks

Prophylaxis. A vaccine against *B.burgdorferi s.s.* developed in the USA that prevented adhesion of borreliae in the tick with OspA antibodies is not being produced any more. Individual prophylaxis, therefore, has to focus on exposition,that is, wearing protective clothing, rubber boots, etc. Long trousers should be tucked into socks. Spraying of permethrin on clothing and of repellents on wrists will improve protection. Wearing of light-colored clothing will facilitate the discovery of ticks. The risk of disease is low at 24 to 36 h after the bite. After walking through infested areas, the search for ticks should start right away, and at the latest, 24 h later. When trying to remove a tick, turn it with a tick tweezers at the mouth parts. Most tick forceps are not fine enough and they will crush the tick. Better are tick cards that are pushed underneath the tick (do not use oil or glue). If an area is known for a high degree of infestation and if the time of the bite is known, prophylactic oral doxycycline 1×200 mg should be considered. Elimination of ticks from their natural environment has so far not met with success. The use of fungal blastospores and of nematodes is in an experimental stage.

Reporting. Lyme disease is a notifiable disease in the USA and in Canada.

REFERENCES

Aguero-Rosenfeld ME et al., Diagnosis of Lyme borreliosis. *Clin Microbiol Rev* 18, 484–509, 2005.

Blanc F et al., Relevance of the antibody index to diagnose Lyme neuroborreliosis among seropositive patients. *Neurology* 69, 953–958, 2007.

Chan K, Marras SA, Parveen N., Sensitive multiplex PCR assay to differentiate Lyme spirochetes and emerging pathogens Anaplasma phagocytophilum and Babesia microti. *BMC Microbiol* 13, 295, 2013.

Gern L, Humair PF., Ecology of Borrelia burgdorferi sensu lato in Europe. In: Gray JS et al. (eds.), *Lyme-Borreliosis Biology, Epidemiology and Control.* CABI Publishing, UK, 149–174, 2002.

Hassler D et al., Disappearance of specific immune response after treatment of chronic Lyme borreliosis. *Int. J. Med. Microbiol.* 293(Suppl 37), 161–164, 2004.

Hubalek Z, Epidemiology of Lyme borreliosis. *Curr. Probl. Dermatol.* 37, 31–50, 2009.

Kalish RA et al., Evaluation of study patients with Lyme disease, 10–20-year follow-up. *J. Infect. Dis.* 183, 453–460, 2001.

Kalish RA et al. Persistence of immunoglobulin M or immunoglobulin G antibody responses to Borrelia burgdorferi 10–20 years after active Lyme disease. *Clin. Infect. Dis.* 33, 780–785, 2001.

Kurtenbach K et al., Borrelia burgdorferi sensu lato in vertebrate hosts. In: Gray JS et al. (eds.): *Lyme-Borreliosis Biology, Epidemiology and Control*, 117–128, CABI Publishing, UK, 2002.

Nadelman RB et al., Prophylaxis with single-dose doxycycline for the prevention of Lyme disease after an Ixodes scapularis tick bite. *New Engl. J. Med.* 345, 79–84, 2001.

Petersen LR et al., Epidemiological and clinical features of 1149 persons with Lyme disease identified by laboratory based-surveillance in Connecticut. *Yale J. Biol Med* 62, 253–262, 1989.

Pfister HW, Rupprecht TA, Clinical aspects of neuroborreliosis and post-Lyme disease syndrome in adult patients. *Int J. Med. Microbiol.* 296(Suppl. 40), 11–16, 2006.

Reed KD, Laboratory testing for Lyme disease: possibilities and practicalities. *J. Clin. Microbiol.* 40, 319–324, 2002.

Schwan TG, Piesman J, Vector interactions and molecular adaptations of Lyme disease and relapsing fever spirochetes associated with transmission by ticks. *Emerg. Infect. Dis.* 8, 115–121, 2002.

Seriburi V et al., High frequency of false positive IgM immunoblots for Borrelia burgdorferi in clinical practice. *Clin Microbiol Infect* 18, 1236–1240, 2012.

Shapiro ED, Clinical practice. Lyme disease. *New Engl J Med* 370, 1724–1731, 2014.

Skuballa J et al., Occurrence of different Borrelia burgdorferi sensu lato genospecies including B. afzelii, B. bavariensis, and B. spielmanii in hedgehogs (Erinaceus spp.) in Europe. *Ticks Tick Borne Dis.* 3, 8–13, 2012.

Stanek G et al., Lyme borreliosis. *Lancet* 379, 461–473, 2012.

Stanek G, Reiter M, The expanding Lyme borrelia complex – clinical significance of genomic species? *Clin Microbiol Infect* 17, 487–493,2011.

Steere A et al., Prospective study of serologic tests for Lyme disease. *Clin Infect Dis* 47, 188–195, 2008.

2.4.2 RELAPSING FEVER

Relapsing fever is an acute infectious disease caused by borreliae that are transmitted to humans by arthropods, which has the characteristic of periodic bouts of fever. For epidemiological reasons, two forms can be distinguished: the epidemic, louse-borne and the endemic, tick-borne form.

Etiology. The causative agent of the epidemic form is *Borrelia recurrentis*, while the endemic form is primarily caused by *B. duttonii* and rarely by *B. persica, B. hermsii, B. venezuelensis, B. mazzottii,* and *B. hispanica* (Tab. 2.4). The morphologically indistinguishable borreliae are motile Gram-negative bacteria with a typical spirochetal structure (see above).

Relapsing fever borreliae are able to evade immunological defenses through antigenic variation within the host. A single cell can give rise to ci. 30 antigenic variants, each of which is expressing a unique variable major protein (Vmp) that occurs in two classes: a large one (Vlps) of 36 KDa and a small one (Vsps) of ci. 20 KDa. In each phase of spirochetemia, a population composed almost entirely of one type prevails. During relapse, the population is dominated by a type different from the preceding one.

Occurrence. Relapsing fever occurs worldwide. The louse-borne variety is transmitted by head and body lice that carry the borreliae in their hemolymph. There is no mammal reservoir. Humans in endemic areas (northeast Africa, Bolivia, and Peru) are at particular risk if they are in close contact under conditions of war and deprivation. The tick-borne variety is endemic in central, eastern, and southern Africa where it is caused by *B. duttonii* and other borreliae, while in the western US, *B. hermsii* is the main agent. The infected ticks transmit the bacteria mainly transovarially to the offspring. Reservoirs are wild rodents (mice, rats, hamsters, weasels, chipmunks) and domestic animals (horses, cattle, pigs). At special risk are tourists who camp and trek in areas of endemicity at any time during the entire year.

Transmission. Human infection with *B. recurrentis* does not occur through the bite of the louse but rather through infected hemolymph, which is released on crushing the louse, or through rubbing of louse feces into the skin that the borreliae actively penetrate. *B. duttonii,* however, is transmitted by fast (15 to 90 min) blood-sucking soft ticks (*Ornithodoros* spp.) that carry the organism in their saliva or coxal fluid. Direct transmission of *B. duttonii* from human to human is rare.

Table 2.4 | Relapsing fever *Borrelia* spp. of medical and veterinary significance

SPECIES	VECTOR	RESERVOIR	OCCURRENCE	DISEASE, RELAPSING FEVER	HOST(S)
B. recurrentis	*Pediculus humanus*	Human	Worldwide[1]	Louse-borne	Human
B. duttonii	*O.*[2] *moubata*	Mice, small mammals	East Africa	Tick-borne	Human
B. crocidurae	*O. erraticus*	Mammals	N./E. Africa, Near East, S.E. Europe	Tick-borne	Human
B. persica	*O. thozolani*	Mice, small mammals	Asia	Tick-borne	Human, cat (?)
B. hispanica	*O. erraticus*	Mice, small mammals	Spain	Tick-borne	Human
B. hermsii	*O. hermsii*	Small mammals, birds	N. America	Tick-borne	Human
B. turicatae	*O. turicata*	Mice, small mammals	N. America	Tick-borne	Human
B. parkeri	*O. parkeri*	Mice, small mammals	N. America	Tick-borne	Human
B. coriaceae	*O. coriaceus*	Cattle, black-tailed deer, small mammals	N. America (S.E.)	Tick-borne, abortion in cattle	Human, cattle
B. lonestari	*Amblyomma americanum*	Black-tailed deer, cattle	N. America	STARI[3]	Human
B. anserina	*Argas persicus*	Birds	Worldwide	Avian	Turkey, chicken, geese
B. theileri	*Rhipicephalus* spp., *Boophilus* spp.	Ruminants, horses	Africa, Australia	Tick spirochetosis	Ruminants, horses

Modified from Straubinger RK, Genus Borrelia. In: Selbitz HJ, U Truyen, P Valentin-Weigand (eds.): Tiermedizinische Mikrobiologie, Infektions-und Seuchenlehre, Enke, Stuttgart, 2011; and Stanek G, Borreliosen, In: Aspöck H (ed.): Krank durch Arthropoden, 605–624, Denisa 30, Linz, 2011
[1] At present, Sudan and Ethiopia
[2] O, *Ornithodoros*
[3] STARI, erythema, fatigue, headache, muscle ache

Clinical Manifestations. The epidemic form is clinically more severe than the endemic one. After an incubation period of 2 to 12 (mostly 5 to 8) days, the disease begins suddenly without prodromi with fever (39 to 41 °C) and chills. The spirochetemia may reach a density of 10 000 or 100 000 000 per ml of blood in the louse- and tick-borne varieties, respectively. Temperature will turn to normal after 5 to 7 and 3 to 4 days for each form. During the afebrile intervals, the patient feels normal, and febrile intervals will become shorter and less intense with time with head and muscle aches, loss of appetite, dizziness, nausea, vomiting, and tachycardia. Hepatosplenomegaly may already be present after the second day of illness. The conjunctivae are infected or may show a yellowish hue. Signs of bleeding, such as petechiae and ecchymoses, may be present on the skin. Complications include bronchitis, bronchopneumonia, myocarditis with arrhythmia, hepatitis, arthritis, nephritis, iridocyclitis, and CNS involvement (cranial nerve deficits, hemiplegia, and coma). Abortion may occur. In less severe cases, spontaneous resolution will set in after several febrile episodes. Prognosis is generally good but without treatment, the case fatality may be as high as 50% due to cerebral hemorrhage or liver failure. There is a short-lived immunity that extends only to the homologous *Borrelia* species.

Diagnosis. The diagnosis is confirmed by microscopy of a stained blood smear taken during a febrile episode. Actively motile borreliae may already be seen in an unstained drop of blood with the use of phase contrast or darkfield microscopy or fluorescence microhematocrit enrichment (QBC enrichment as used in the diagnosis of malaria) with acridine orange staining. Permanent preparations are best obtained by methanol fixation of blood smears or thick drops stained with Giemsa (Fig. 2.5) or acridine orange. PCR is done in specialized laboratories. Isolation of borreliae on modified Kelly medium has been successful for some species but, like animal inoculation and xenodiagnosis, is of no importance today. Serological test are not routine. The usual treponemal tests show cross reactions with borreliae. If they are negative 2 weeks after the infection, relapsing fever can be ruled out. The blood shows leukocytosis (15 000 to 30 000 per microliter), with an occasional anemia.

Differential Diagnosis. Typhoid fever, typhus, trench fever, malaria, leptospirosis, brucellosis, yellow fever, and other hemorrhagic fevers.

Therapy. Doxycycline 2 × 100 mg/day p.o. or erythromycin 4 × 500 mg/day p.o. for 7 to 10 days. In patients with CNS symptoms,

ceftriaxone 2 g/day i.v. for at least 2 weeks. The frequent occurrence of a Jarisch-Herxheimer reaction calls for hospitalization during treatment. For the louse-borne form, delousing is essential.

Prophylaxis. The most important measures are control of lice and ticks and protection from these arthropods. In endemic areas, emphasis must be on hygienic conditions in homes, especially with regard to clothing.

REFERENCES

Assous MV, Willamamowski A, Relapsing fever borreliosis in Eurasia- forgotten but certainly not gone. *Clin. Microbiol. Infect* 15, 407–414, 2009.

Barbour AG, Restrepo BI., Antigenic variation in vector-borne pathogens. *Emerg. Infect. Dis.* 6, 449–457, 2000.

Bunikis J et al., Typing of Borrelia relapsing fever group strains. *Emerg. Infect. Dis.* 10, 1661–1664, 2004.

Cadavid D, Barbour AG, Neuroborreliosis during relapsing fever: review of the clinical manifestations, pathology, and treatment of infections of humans and experimental animals. *Clin. Infect. Dis.* 26, 151–164, 1998.

Cutler SJ, Possibilities for relapsing fever reemergence. *Emerg. Infect. Dis.* 12, 369–374, 2006.

Cutler SJ, Abdissa M, Trape JF, New concepts for the old challenge of African relapsing fever borreliosis. *Clin. Microbiol. Infect.*, 15, 400–406, 2009.

Dworkin MS et al., Tick borne relapsing fever. *Infect. Dis. Clin. North. Am.* 22, 449–468, 2008.

Elbir H, Raoult D, Drancourt M, Relapsing fever borreliae in Africa. *Am J Trop Med Hyg.* 89, 288–292, 2013.

Krause PJ et al., Human Borrelia miyamotoi infection in the United States. *N Engl J Med* 368, 291–293, 2013.

Larsson C et al., Persistent brain infection and disease reactivation in relapsing fever borreliosis. *Microbes Infect.* 8, 2213–2219, 2006.

Larsson C, Andersson M, Bergström S, Current issues in relapsing fever. *Curr. Opin. Infect. Dis.* 22, 443–449, 2009.

Schwan TG, Piesman J, Vector interactions and molecular adaptations of Lyme disease and relapsing fever spirochetes associated with transmission by ticks. *Emerg. Infect. Dis.* 8, 115–121, 2002.

Schwan TG et al., Diversity and distribution of Borrelia hermsii. *Emerg. Infect. Dis.* 13, 436–442, 2007.

Scott JC. Typing: African relapsing fever spirochetes. *Emerg. Infect. Dis.* 11, 1722–1729, 2005.

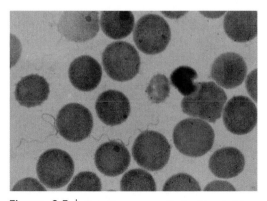

Figure 2.5 | *Borrelia recurrentis* in blood (May-Grünwald-Giemsa stain).

2.5 Brucelloses

Brucelloses are acute or chronic infectious diseases of humans and animals caused by Gram-negative bacteria of the genus *Brucella*. They may affect single or all organ systems. Human infections have also been called Bang's disease (caused by *B. abortus*) and Maltese fever (caused by *B. melitensis*). From a taxonomic point of view based on DNA-DNA hybridization and sequence homology of 16SrRNA gene sequences, *Brucella* has been considered a monospecific genus and the "species" mere biovars of *B. melitensis*. This chapter, however, will follow the 1980 Approved List of Bacterial Names (www.bacterio.net).

Etiology. Brucellae are Gram-negative coccoid to short rods, nonmotile, obligately parasitic, with a moderate ability to survive outside the host. Agents infecting humans are *B. abortus* (main host, cattle), *B. melitensis* (sheep, goats, camels), *B. suis* (pig, reindeer, wild boar, hare; in South America, also cattle), and occasionally, *B. canis* (dog). Brucellae infecting marine mammals *B. ceti* (whales), *B. pinnipedialis* (seals, dolphins) may be transmitted to humans and cause disease. *B. neotomae* (desert rat), *B. ovis* (sheep), and *B. microti* (field mouse) have not been isolated from humans. The newly discovered *B. inopinata* has so far only been isolated from one human case.

Occurrence. Brucellosis in humans is closely associated with occurrence and spread of *Brucella* spp. in animals, particularly in farm animals. The incidence has decreased after many sources of animal brucellae were cleared. In Europe, animal brucellosis is still seen in Mediterranean and Balkan countries (Portugal, Spain, Italy, Malta, Bosnia-Herzegovina, Croatia, Greece, Cyprus, Turkey, Macedonia, and Serbia). Outside of this area, countries in Africa (Algeria), Asia (Syria, Iran), and Latin America (particularly Brazil and Mexico) show a relatively high incidence in farm animals. Dog brucellosis has been sporadic in Europe since 1973. In several European countries including Germany, field hares and wild boars are epidemiologically relevant reservoirs for *B. suis*.

At particular risk are people in contact with the main hosts, such as veterinarians, farmers, animal care personnel, milkers, those handling artificial insemination, abattoir and slaughterhouse personnel, hunters and, above all, those working in endemic areas where there is also a danger of infection from insufficiently heated or raw milk. Laboratory infections show that microbiologists are also at risk. Brucellae are considered potential bioweapons.

Transmission. Infection in humans occurs by direct contact with secretions and excreta of infected animals (e.g., lochia during delivery or abortion), via the mouth, conjunctivae, or small skin lesions. Another pathway is oral uptake of raw or insufficiently heated milk or milk products, for example, cheese prepared from nonpasteurized sheep or goat milk. Infected mothers may excrete brucellae with their milk, thereby infecting the infant. Aerogenic transmission is also possible, for example, through infectious aerosols or dust particles in abattoirs or in the laboratory. The infectious dose for humans is very small (below 100 organisms). Venereal transmission is possible but plays a major role only in animals (Fig. 2.6).

Clinical Manifestations. The exact incubation period in humans is unknown; it may range from 1 to 3 weeks (for *B. melitensis*) to 3 months. Monocytes and macrophages are target cells for brucellae. They are taken up in phagosomes, remain viable by suppressing phagosome-lysosome fusion, and inhibit apoptosis of host cells. They multiply in vacuoles within the endoplasmic reticulum and from there spread to various organs, particularly into the cells of the reticuloendothelial system, liver, spleen, skeletal muscle, and urogenital tract where they give rise to granulocytic inflammation with or without necrosis or caseation.

The clinical symptoms of brucellosis are manifold and depend, among other items, on the species. The most severe infections are due to *B. melitensis*, followed by *B. suis* and *B. abortus*. *B. canis* is the least virulent agent. Prodromes, often vague and scant, are headache, backache, depression, fever (in >90%), sweats, anorexia, lymphadenopathy (10 to 20%), and hepatosplenomegaly (20 to 30%). As the diseases progresses, gastrointestinal symptoms such as abdominal pain, nausea, vomiting,

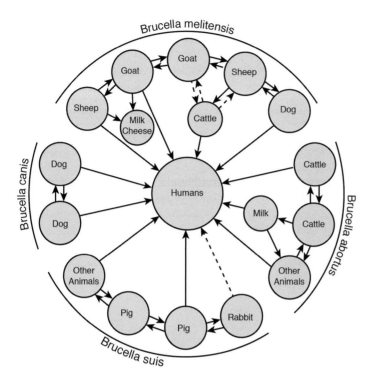

Figure 2.6 | The most important transmission chains of *Brucella*.

hepatitis, diarrhea, or constipation become conspicuous. The musculoskeletal system is affected in 20 to 60% with spondylitis, arthritis (particularly sacroiliitis), and osteomyelitis, the CNS in 5% with meningoencephalitis and radiculoneuritis, the heart in 2% with endo- or pericarditis, the respiratory system with bronchopneumonia and pleural effusions, and the urogenital tract with epididymitis and orchitis, rarely with abortion. Patients may present with anemia, leukopenia, and thrombocytopenia that are due to hemophagocytic lymphohistiocytosis. Iridocyclitis, chorioiditis, thyreoiditis, and neuritis are other manifestations. Infections with *B. melitensis* and *B. suis* may be accompanied by undulating fever, that is, episodes of fever lasting for 1 to 3 days, alternating with afebrile periods of several days.

In animals, brucellosis can be latent for several years. In females, it manifests itself as abortion, neonatal weakness, retention of the placenta, and, rarely, mastitis. In males, orchitis and epididymitis, with subsequent infertility. In cattle and other animals, polyarthirits, tendovaginitis, and bursitis have been observed.

Diagnosis. Brucellosis is best proven by blood culture that is most likely positive in the acute stage and during a febrile episode. Prolonged incubation (up to 14 days in a 5% CO_2 atmosphere) of blood culture systems seems to be optimal (sensitivity in acute cases, 80 to 90%; 30 to 70% in chronic ones). Bone marrow and joint fluid, spinal fluid, urine, excised lymph nodes, and biopsy material from liver or spleen may also be cultured. PCR allows for a fast diagnosis and appropriate protocols have been established. Initial routine diagnostic biochemical tests may confuse *Brucella* with other urease-positive Gram-negative rods such as *Moraxella phenylpyruvica*. Species differentiation, not done in routine laboratories, has used dye inhibition, biochemical and molecular tests, and reactions in monospecific antisera. Serology includes agglutination (e.g., Rose Bengal test with *B. abortus* 99 Weybridge strain for screening) and Coombs tests. IgM and IgG are determined by ELISA. At least two serum samples should be taken 8 to 10 days apart. Only significant changes in titer (3 to 4 dilutions) are significant. Western blots have been used to distinguish between active, past, and subclinical infection. The antigens of the three main human species are closely related and may be cross-reacting with those of *Yersinia enterocolitica* serovar 09, *Escherichia coli* O157, *E. hermannii, Francisella tularensis, Stenotrophomonas maltophilia, Afipia clevelandensis, Salmonella* Group 030 (e.g., *S. Urbana, S. Godesberg*) and *Vibrio cholerae* O1. Persons vaccinated against cholera may show false-positive *Brucella* reactions. If *B. canis* infection is suspected, serological tests should use *B. canis* antigen, which does not show cross-reactivity with other *Brucella* antigens except *B. ovis*.

In animals, the diagnosis is made by culture of aborted fetuses, placenta, vaginal secretions, milk or udder secretion, testicular tissue, semen, preputial, joint, bursa fluid or lymph node aspirates. Direct microscopy with Köster stain (which uses the alkali resistance of brucellae) provides for a rapid orientation. Internationally recognized are Rose Bengal and complement fixation (CF) tests and, in pigs and cattle, agglutination, ELISA (also for milk samples) and fluorescence polarization tests. *Brucella*-specific cell-mediated immune reactions can be shown by positive brucellin or gamma interferon tests. Brucellae belong to the biosafety 3 organisms.

Differential Diagnosis. In the acute stage, influenza, ornithosis, Q fever, typhoid and paratyphoid fever, malaria, military tuberculosis, Kala-azar, and infectious mononucleosis must be ruled out. In chronic brucellosis, viral meningoencephalitis, rheumatic fever, endocarditis, collagenoses, Hodgkin's disease, ankylosing spondylarthritis, tuberculosis of the spine, and even hepatitis have to be taken into consideration.

Therapy. Antimicrobials used for brucellosis must be effective intracellularly. The high frequency of relapse with monotherapy requires at least two antibiotics. For adults and children >8 years doxycycline 2 × 100 mg/day p.o. for 6 weeks plus gentamicin 5 mg/kg/day i.m. or i.v. for 7 to 10 days have been recommended. The regimen proposed by the World Health

Organization (WHO) with doxycycline (as above) plus rifampicin 600 to 900 mg/day p.o. for 6 weeks has led to more frequent relapses (10 to 20% vs. 5 to 10%). For children <8 years trimethoprim-sulfamethoxazole 2 × 5 mg/kg/day p.o. for 6 weeks plus gentamicin 3 × 2 mg/kg/day i.v. or i.m. for 2 weeks are recommended. Pregnant women should receive double-strength trimethoprim-sulfamethoxazole 2 × 1 to 2 tablets/day plus rifampicin 1 × 600 to 900 mg/day p.o. for 6 weeks. Patients with neurobrucellosis or osteomyelitis have to be treated for 3 to 6 months, those with endocarditis for at least 6 months with doxycycline plus an aminoglycoside and rifampicin, possibly also with ceftriaxone and/or a fluoroquinolone. Controls should extend over 2 years. In Europe, therapeutic trials with infected cattle, sheep, goats, and pigs are prohibited.

Prophylaxis. Unpasteurized milk and milk products, for example, sheep and goat cheeses from endemic areas should be avoided. Individuals exposed to potential sources of *Brucella* should wear gloves and facemasks when working with animals, for example, those in labor. Infected mothers should not breast feed and milk must be heated before feeding.

Vaccination with attenuated *Brucella* strains (19BA and 104M) has not proven to be reliable and they will interfere with the results of serological assays. One of the most effective measures is the systematic eradication of brucellosis in domestic animals. Many countries run surveillance programs for farm animals using serological controls. In positive cases, the stables will be closed and the animals killed (not slaughtered!).

Reporting. Brucellosis is a notifiable disease in the USA and in Canada

REFERENCES

Al Dahouk S, Sprague LD, Neubauer H, New developments in the diagnostic procedures for zoonotic brucellosis in humans. *Rev Sci Tech* 32, 177–188, 2013.

Araj GF, Update on laboratory diagnosis of human brucellosis. *Int. J. Antimicrob. Agents* 36 (Suppl 1), S12–17, 2010.

Baldi P et al., Serological follow-up of human brucellosis by measuring IgG antibodies to lipopolysaccharide and cytoplasmic proteins of Brucella species. *Clin. Infect. Dis.* 22, 446–455, 1996.

Batchelor BI et al., Biochemical mis-identification of Brucella melitensis and subsequent laboratory-acquired infections. *J. Hosp. Infect.* 22, 159–162, 1992.

Blasco JM, Molina-Flores B, Control and eradication of Brucella melitensis infection in sheep and goats. *Vet. Clin. North Am. Food Anim. Pract.* 27, 95–104, 2011.

Buzgan T et al., Clinical manifestations and complications in 1028 cases of brucellosis: a retrospective evaluation and review of the literature. *Int. J. Infect. Dis.* 14, e469–478, 2010.

Carvalho Neta AV et al., Pathogenesis of bovine brucellosis. *Vet. J.* 184, 146–155, 2010.

Corbel MJ, *Brucellosis in Humans and Animals*. World Health Organization, Geneva, 2006.

Drancourt M, Brouqui P, Raoult D, Afipia clevelandensis antibodies and cross-reactivity with Brucella spp. and Yersinia enterocolitica O:9. *Clin. Diagn. Lab. Immunol.* 4, 748–752, 1997.

Ferreira L et al., Identification of Brucella by MALDI-TOF mass spectrometry. Fast and reliable identification from agar plates and blood cultures. *PLoS ONE.* 5, e14235, 2010.

Foster G et al., Brucella ceti sp. nov. and Brucella pinnipedialis sp. nov. for Brucella strains with cetaceans and seals as their preferred hosts. *Int. J. Syst. Evol. Microbiol.* 57, 2688–2693, 2007.

Martin-Mazuelos E et al., Outbreak of Brucella melitensis among microbiology laboratory workers. *J. Clin. Microbiol.* 32, 2035–2036, 1994.

Marzetti S et al., Recent trends in human Brucella canis infection. *Comp.Immunol. Microbiol Infect Dis* 36, 55–61, 2013.

Mayer-Scholl A et al., Advancement of a multiplex PCR for the differentiation of all currently described Brucella species. *J. Microbiol. Methods* 80, 112–114, 2010.

Meng XJ, Lindsay DS, Sriranganathan N, Wild boars as sources for infectious diseases in livestock and humans. *Philos Trans R Soc Lond B Biol Sci* 364, 2697–2707, 2009.

Nielsen K et al., Salmonella enterica serotype Urbana interference with brucellosis serology. *J. Immunoassay Immunochem.* 28, 289–296, 2007.

Palanduz A et al., Brucellosis in a mother and her young infant: probable transmission by breast milk. *Int. J. Infect. Dis.* 4, 55–56, 2000.

Pappas G, The changing Brucella ecology: novel reservoirs, new threats. *Int. J. Antimicrob. Agents* 36(Suppl 1), S8–11, 2010.

Pappas G et al., Brucellosis. *N. Engl. J. Med.* 352, 2325–2336, 2005.

Scholz HC et al., Brucella microti sp. nov., isolated from the common vole Microtus arvalis. *Int. J. Syst. Evol. Microbiol.* 58, 375–382, 2008.

Scholz H et al., Brucella inopinata sp. nov., isolated from a breast implant infection. *Int. J. Syst. Evol. Microbiol.* 60, 801–808, 2010.

Solera J, Update on brucellosis: therapeutic challenges. *Int. J. Antimicrob. Agents 36, Suppl 1, S18–20, 2010.

Solera J et al., Brucellar spondylitis: review of 35 cases and literature survey. *Clin. Infect. Dis.* 29, 1440–1449, 1999.

Traxler RM et al., A literature review of laboratory-acquired brucellosis. *J. Clin. Microbiol.* 51, 3055–3062, 2013.

Whatmore AM et al., Marine mammal Brucella genotype associated with zoonotic infection. *Emerg. Infect. Dis.* 14, 517–518, 2008.

Yagupsky P, Detection of brucellae in blood cultures. *J. Clin. Microbiol* 37, 3437–3442, 1999.

2.6 Campylobacterioses

Campylobacterioses are acute to chronic infections of humans and animals caused by several species of the genus *Campylobacter* (formerly *Vibrio*). Direct or indirect transmission from vertebrates to humans has been established for *C. jejuni, C. coli, C. lari, C. upsaliensis,* and *C. hyointestinalis*. In humans, these species cause mild to severe diarrhea with or without metastatic infections or generalization. *Arcobacter* spp., aerotolerant Gram-negative bacteria morphologically resembling *Campylobacter*, have been isolated from farm animals and from humans with diarrhea but transmission between them has not been proven.

Etiology. *Campylobacter* spp. are motile, slender, comma-like or spiral Gram-negative rods that grow best in an atmosphere of 5% O_2, 10% CO_2, and 85% N_2. They can be separated by cultural and biochemical characteristics. The zoonotic agents, *C. jejuni* subsp. *jejuni, C. coli, C. lari* and *C. upsaliensis*, grow even at 42 °C and are called thermophilic. They are obligately parasitic inhabitants of mucous membranes in vertebrates. Outside of their hosts, they remain infectious only for a few weeks.

C. fetus subsp. *venerealis* is highly adapted to cattle and causes enzootic abortion while *C. fetus* subsp. *fetus* has a wider range of animal hosts. It causes enzootic abortion in sheep and occasionally in goats, pigs and cattle. As these two species are mainly isolated from animals (in whom they are obligate pathogens), the infrequent human cases, mostly septicemia and extraintestinal infections in immunocopromised persons, are regarded as zoonotic. However, direct or indirect transmission from animals to humans has not been unequivocally demonstrated either by serology or by culture. In addition, both species have not been isolated more frequently from humans in close contact with animals or their products than from others.

Occurrence. Infections with *Campylobacter* spp. in humans have increased worldwide and are, in many European countries, more frequent than salmonellae as agents of enteric disease. In the European Union, *C. jejuni* subsp. *jejuni* causes >80% of all campylobacterioses in which agents have been speciated. *C. coli* takes approximately 5 to 10% while *C. lari* and *C. upsaliensis* are still rare. All infections occur during the year; however, they are more frequent during summer.

The natural habitat of the zoonotic species is the gastrointestinal tract of various animals, with prevalence rates and relative frequency of the different *Campylobacter* spp. varying between animal species. The main reservoir for *C. jejuni* subsp. *jejuni* are wild birds and poultry. The high frequency in chickens can be explained by problems in rearing and slaughtering. Pet birds can also be carriers. *C. coli* occurs mainly in pigs: >90% of *Campylobacter* spp. isolated from pigs belong to this species. Feces of cattle, calves, sheep, and zoo animals often carry zoonotic *Campylobacter* spp. *C. jejuni* and *C. coli* are also found in dogs, cats, hamsters, guinea pigs, and mice. *C. lari* is most frequent in seagulls and is more rarely found in other birds and domestic animals. The main host for *C. upsaliensis* is the dog.

While people of any age and sex may be affected, the disease shows a peak in small children up to 5 years of age and a smaller one in young adults between 20 and 29 years. At high risk are individuals who are in frequent contact with animals.

Transmission. Infection in humans occurs primarily by ingestion of contaminated food, that is, raw or undercooked poultry, pork or milk. As the minimal infective dose is approximately 500 bacteria, multiplication of *C. jejuni* in such foods is not necessary to cause infection, which is also possible via contaminated drinking or surface water, moist soil, contact with animal excreta, or directly from human to human (Fig. 2.7).

Clinical Manifestations. *C. jejuni* in humans: after an incubation period of 3 to 5 days (range, 1.5 to 11 days), acute enteritis develops in most cases. Regular prodromes are fever up to 40 °C, chills, headache, muscle aches, nausea, and lassitude. Abdominal symptoms may lead to laparotomy or appendectomy. From 12 to 24 weeks to 2 days after the onset of prodromes, diarrhea follows with stools of soft, later liquid to watery consistency with a putrid odor.

Beginning on day 2 or 3, the stool may contain blood, bile, pus, or mucus. Colicky abdominal pain and vomiting, as well as colitis and proctitis, are possible, and fever may reach 40 °C. Radiologically, there is a Crohn-like terminal ileitis. Individual cases of meningitis, peritonitis, urinary tract infection, and septicemia, particularly in immunocompromised patients, have been reported. The prognosis is good and a fatal outcome rare. Relapses (5 to 10% of untreated cases), however, are not as infrequent as in other diarrheal diseases.

Within 1 to 5 weeks following enteritis, symptoms of reactive arthritis may arise. Twenty to 40% of all cases of Guillain-Barré syndrome and its Miller-Fisher variant, presenting as acute, and frequently severe, polyradiculopathy, are preceded within 1 to 3 weeks by infection with *C. jejuni*. Certain serovars of *C. jejuni*, particularly O19 and O41, have oligosaccharides containing neuraminic acid in the outer core polysaccharides that are identical to the terminal oligosaccharides present in complex gangliosides of peripheral nervous tissue. Antibodies induced by *C. jejuni* are probably cross-reacting with nerve receptors and induce an antibody-mediated demyelinization and axonal degeneration.

C. fetus in humans: *C. fetus* subsp. *fetus* may cause septicemia in immunocompromised patients with diabetes, liver disease, or tumors. Spread manifests itself in endovascular infections, septic arthritis, endo- or pericarditis, cellulitis, peritonitis, and meningitis. In pregnancy, abortion and premature contractions as well as neonatal septicemia and meningitis have also been reported.

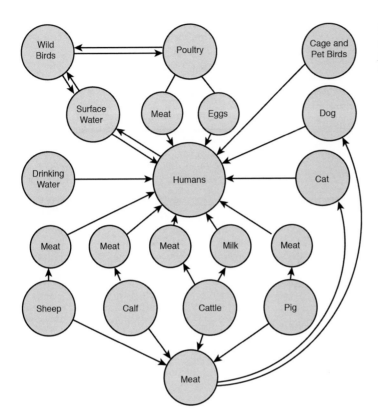

Figure 2.7 | Possible transmission chains of *Campylobacter jejuni* subsp. *jejuni* and *Campylobacter coli*.

Campylobacter in animals: most cases in animals remain inapparent except in some younger ones who may show diarrhea. In cattle, sheep, goats, pigs, dogs, ferrets, and mink, *C. jejuni* (in pigs also *C. coli*) may cause sporadic abortion. Mastitis in cattle is rare. In some birds, hepatitis has been observed ("avian Vibrio hepatitis"). *C. fetus* subsp. *fetus* is a commensal in the intestine of sheep and cattle. *C. fetus* subsp. *venerealis* causes bovine venereal campylobacteriosis (enzootic abortion) and infertility.

Diagnosis. Proof of the disease and its complications is obtained by culture of fresh material, with optimal samples being liquid stools or rectal swabs.

In cases of unexplained fever or septicemia, if prior enteric symptoms are present, blood cultures should be obtained. Various PCR methods have also been developed for different species. Results of serological tests have not been satisfactory as there are over 50 different serovars of *C. jejuni*. At best, these tests may be useful for epidemiological purposes. Patients with *C. jejuni* enteritis may yield false-positive results for *Legionella pneumophila*. In animals, the diagnosis is by culture from stool, milk, or material from abortion.

Differential Diagnosis. *Campylobacter* enteritis cannot be distinguished from infection with *Salmonella*, *Shigella*, *Yersinia* and *Clostridium difficile* by clinical symptoms alone.

Therapy. Replacement of fluid and electrolytes is of prime importance. Antibiotics should be used only if there are long-lasting diarrhea (>1 week), high fever, or signs of septicemia. Recommended are azithromycin 500 mg (in children, 10 mg/kg)/day p.o. for 3 days or ciprofloxacin (up to 30% resistant strains!) 2 × 500 mg/day p.o. for 5 to 7 days. *C. fetus* infections are treated with gentamicin 5 to 7 mg/kg/day i.m. or i.v., or aminopenicillin 4 × 25 mg/kg/day i.v., or imipenem 4 × 500 mg/day i.v. in immunocompetent patients for two weeks and in immunocompromised patients for 4 weeks.

Prophylaxis. Food hygiene is of prime importance. This includes cooking or frying of pork and poultry, extreme care when working at the same time with raw and heated meat, avoidance of unpasteurized milk, and proper hygiene of drinking water. General rules of hygiene should be observed when there has been contact with animals, that is, immediate handwashing with soap and disinfection if animals suffer from diarrhea.

Reporting. Campylobacteriosis is a notifiable disease in Canada

REFERENCES

Altekruse SF et al., Campylobacter jejuni – an emerging foodborne pathogen. *Emerg. Infect. Dis.* 5, 28–35, 1999.

Bell JA, Manning DD, Reproductive failure in mink and ferrets after intravenous or oral inoculation of Campylobacter jejuni. *Can. J. Vet. Res.* 54, 432–437, 1990.

Bessède E, et al., New methods for detection of campylobacters in stool samples in comparison to culture. *J Clin Microbiol* 49, 941–944, 2011.

Coker AO et al., Human campylobacteriosis in developing countries. *Emerg. Infect. Dis.* 8, 237–244, 2002.

Cone LA et al., Cellulitis and septic arthritis caused by Campylobacter fetus and Campylobacter jejuni: report of 2 cases and review of the literature. *J. Clin. Rheumatol.* 9, 362–369, 2003.

Debruyne L, Gevers D, Vandamme P, Taxonomy of the family Campylobacteriaceae. In: Nachamkin I, Szymanski CM, Blaser M: *Campylobacter.* ASM Press, Washington DC, USA, 2008.

Debruyne L et al., Comparative performance of different PCR assays for the identification of Campylobacter jejuni and Campylobacter coli. *Res Microbiol* 159, 88–93, 2008.

Drenthen J et al., Guillain-Barre syndrome subtypes related to Campylobacter infection. *J. Neurol. Neurosurg. Psychiatry* 82, 300–305, 2011.

EFSA, European Food Safety Authority. Control: the European Union Summary Report on Trends and Sources of Zoonoses, Zoonotic Agents and Food-borne Outbreaks in 2009. *EFSA J.* 9, 2090, 2011.

Endtz HP et al., Molecular characterization of Campylobacter jejuni from patients with Guillain-Barre and Miller-Fisher syndromes. *J. Clin. Microbiol.* 38, 2297–2301, 2000.

Engberg J et al., Quinolone and macrolide resistance in Campylobacter jejuni and C. coli: resistance mechanisms and trends in human isolates. *Emerg. Infect. Dis.* 7, 24–34, 2001.

Fujihara N et al., A case of perinatal sepsis by: Campylobacter fetus subsp. fetus infection successfully treated with carbapenem – case report and literature review. *J. Infect.* 53, e199–202, 2006.

Gorkiewicz G et al., Transmission of Campylobacter hyointestinalis from a pig to a human. *J. Clin. Microbiol.* 40, 2601–2605, 2002.

Gorkiewicz G et al., A genomic island defines subspecies-specific virulence features of the host-adapted pathogen: Campylobacter fetus subsp. venerealis. *J. Bacteriol.* 192, 502–517, 2010.

Hara-Kudo Y, Takatori K, Contamination level and ingestion dose of foodborne pathogens associated with infections. *Epidemiol. Infect.* 139, 1505–1510, 2011.

Kuschner RA, Thomas et al., Use of azithromycin for the treatment of Campylobacter enteritis in travelers to Thailand, an area where ciprofloxacin resistance is prevalent. *Clin. Infect. Dis.* 21, 536–541, 1995.

McGoldrick A et al., Real time PCR to detect and differentiate Campylobacter fetus subspecies fetus from Campylobacter fetus subspecies venerealis. *J Microbiol Methods* 94, 199–204, 2013.

Nachamkin I, Allos BM, Ho T, Campylobacter species and Guillain-Barre syndrome. *Clin. Microbiol. Rev.* 11, 555–567, 1998.

Odendaal MW et al., First isolation of Campylobacter jejuni from the vaginal discharge of three bitches after abortion in South Africa. *Onderstepoort J. Vet. Res.* 61, 193–195, 1994.

Pope J et al., Campylobacter reactive arthritis: a systematic review. *Semin. Arthritis Rheum.* 37, 48–55, 2007.

Robinson DA, Infective dose of Campylobacter jejuni in milk. *Br. Med. J. (Clin. Res. Ed.)* 282, 1584, 1981.

Scanlon KA et al., Occurrence and characteristics of fastidious Campylobacteraceae species in porcine samples. *Int J Food Microbiol* 163, 6–13, 2013.

Scallan E et al., Foodborne illness acquired in the United States – major pathogens. *Emerg. Infect. Dis.* 17, 7–15, 2011.

Stuart TL et al., Campylobacteriosis outbreak associated with ingestion of mud during a mountain bike race. *Epidemiol. Infect.* 138, 1695–1703, 2010.

2.7 Chlamydioses

Etiology. Chlamydiae are nonmotile, very small, obligately intracellular bacteria. Their cell wall resembles that of Gram-negative bacteria but contains only traces of peptidoglycan. They undergo a characteristic developmental cycle. Extracellular round to oval, highly infectious elementary bodies with diameters of 0.2 to 0.6 µm are taken up into cell vacuoles by endocytosis. There, they develop into vegetative, noninfectious pleomorphic reticulate bodies (diameter, 0.5 to 1.5 µm) that divide by binary fission and are metabolically active. Eventually, the vacuole fills up with >1000 intracytoplasmic inclusions but does not fuse with the cellular lysosomes due to an inhibitory mechanism produced by the chlamydiae. This vacuole is a characteristic morphological sign of infected cells and can be used for the microscopic diagnosis. The reticulate bodies then differentiate via intermediate condensing forms into mature infectious elementary bodies that are released when their membranes and those of the host cells burst, thereby initiating a new cycle.

There are now four families in the order *Chlamydiales*: *Chlamydiaceae, Parachlamydiaceae, Simkaniaceae, and Waddliaceae*. In the family *Chlamydiaceae*, two genera have been described: *Chlamydia* and *Chlamydophila*. Zoonotic agents belong to the latter genus. More recent sequence homology data of the 16S and 23S rRNA genes suggest, however, that there may actually be only one genus; therefore, the division into *Chlamydia* and *Chlamydophila* has not been universally accepted (in www.bacterio.net, several species are listed with both genera).

C. psittaci (in birds), *C. abortus* (in ruminants), and *C. felis* (in cats) are found in animals. The main host for *C. pneumoniae* are humans but sporadic cases have been reported in coala bear, bandicoots, horses, snakes, turtles, iguanas, chameleons, and frogs. These isolates, however, have proven to be animal-specific biovars; therefore, *C. pneumoniae* has not been regarded as a zoonotic bacterium.

2.7.1 PSITTACOSIS/ORNITHOSIS

C. psittaci has six serovars (A to F) that correspond to six OmpA genotypes. Three more OmpA genotypes (EB, WC, and M56) are known. Avian chlamydiae are of particular significance for humans because they are able to cause severe disease, generally referred to as ornithosis. Psittacosis refers to disease in psittacine birds transmitted to humans. Clinical symptoms include fever, chills, headache, photophobia, interstitial pneumonia, cough, and myalgias (see below).

Occurrence. *C. psittaci* is distributed worldwide. Natural hosts are birds. Thus far, infection in more than 460 avian species has been described, with parrots and pigeons being most frequently affected. Occasionally, *C. psittaci* is isolated from healthy or diseased mammals, such as cattle, sheep, pigs, and dogs.

In the past 10 years, 70 to 200 annual outbreaks of psittacosis in psittacines and approximately 10 to >100 cases of psittacosis/ornithosis have been officially registered. Psittacine strains are particularly virulent in humans but strains from other birds may cause severe disease as well, for example, in pigeon breeders or employees of the poultry industry. At high risk are people in contact with birds and their excreta, that is, veterinarians, bird breeders and dealers, animal caretakers, slaughterhouse employees (poultry!), microbiologists, and people working with bird feathers. *C. psittaci* is a potential bioterrorism (and biosafety level 3) agent.

Transmission. Transmission to humans occurs by inhalation of contaminated dust or through contact with the excreta of infected animals. Asymptomatic birds, particularly psittacines and pigeons, are the most important sources of infection (Figs 2.8 and 2.9). Transmission from human to human seems possible but is probably rare.

Clinical Manifestations. The clinical picture of psittacosis/ornithosis is quite variable, from inapparent infections detected by chance to slight respiratory symptoms to severe life-threatening atypical pneumonias with high fever, severe headache, and multiorgan failure. The incubation period is 7 to 21 days but may extend to 3 months. Disease begins either suddenly with chills, fever up to 40 °C, and relative bradycardia, or slowly with malaise, cough, and a rise in temperature. Variable symptoms are headache, myalgias, persistent nonproductive cough, occasional dyspnea and cyanosis, as well as mental symptoms, such as lethargy, confusion, stupor, and coma. While physical signs may be discrete, chest radiographs are abnormal in 50 to 90% of patients. Extensive, rarely spotty, infiltrates with a ground-glass appearance are pathognomonic of interstitial pneumonia. Rare manifestations are monosymptomatic peri- or myocarditis and thromboembolic

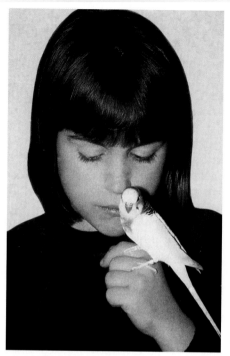

Figure 2.8 | Possible danger in transmitting chlamydiae when kissing birds (courtesy of Archiv Bayerisches Landesamt für Gesundheit und Lebensmittelsicherheit, Erlangen, Germany).

complications requiring surgical intervention. Erythema nodosum has also been recorded. Peracute courses may involve pancreatitis. Less severe cases last from 10 to 14 days, severe cases from 3 to 7 weeks. Without treatment, the case-

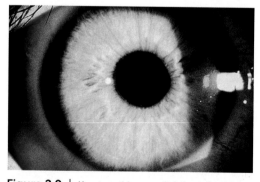

Figure 2.9 | Keratopathia superficialis and epithelial and subepithelial infiltrations across the entire cornea, caused by human chlamydiae. The source was a chlamydia-infected cat that suffered from a upper respiratory infection (Prof. G. J. Jahn, Erlangen, Germany).

fatality rate may reach 20% in the latter group; with appropriate treatment, it is close to 1%.

Inapparent infection is most frequent in mammals and birds. Disease may be limited to local symptoms, such as bilateral conjunctivitis in pigeons, but may also be an acute or chronic generalized infection. Sick birds lose appetite, show ruffled feathers, serous or purulent nasal discharge, tachypnea, diarrhea, and bloody stools. Pneumonia, tracheitis, conjunctivitis, polyserositis, pericarditis, arthritis, splenomegaly, and encephalitis may follow. Simultaneous affection of respiratory and intestinal tracts is not infrequent. Epidemics in domestic poultry (turkey, ducks, and geese), pigeons, and pet birds may lead to substantial economic losses.

Diagnosis. Private or professional contact with birds provide initial hints for a clinical diagnosis. A positive culture from sputum or blood from the febrile phase using cell cultures [McCoy or BGM cells, sometimes, specific pathogen free (SPF) chick embryos] is diagnostic. Visualization is by Giménez, immunoperoxidase or immunofluorescent staining. These methods, however, are labor intensive and carry the risk of a laboratory infection. Work with *C. psittaci* is, therefore, limited to BSL level 3 laboratories. A highly sensitive test is provided by PCR. Species identification is possible if suitable primers are available. In some reference laboratories, microarray assays are available.

In diseased birds, direct microscopic proof of inclusion (reticulate) or extracellular elementary bodies may be attempted, for example, from nasal secretions. An alternative would be the demonstration of antigens by ELISA or immunofluorescence assay (IFA). In humans, the diagnosis can also be made by antibody assays using micro-IFA or ELISA. Both are able to demonstrate IgM in the early and IgG in subsequent stages. These antibodies are only genus- and not species-specific, neither are those assayed with CF tests (which are not in use any more). Species-specific antibodies are produced against mitochondrial outer membrane protein.

Differential Diagnosis. Atypical pneumonias due to *M. pneumoniae, C. burnetii, Legionella* spp., and viruses.

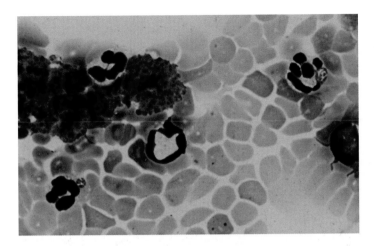

Figure 2.10 | Granulocytic anaplasmosis caused by *A. phagocytophilum* Within the two granulocytes (left lower corner) morulae, that is, the reproductive stages of the organism can be seen. Hamster blood (Dr. B. Munderloh, Minneapolis, MN, USA).

Therapy. The antibiotic of first choice is doxycycline 2 × 100 mg/day p.o. or tetracycline 4 × 500 mg/day p.o. for 2 to 3 weeks. An alternative in pregnancy and for children would be azithromycin (first 500 mg, then 250 mg/day p.o. for 2 to 3 weeks; in children <8 years, 10 mg/kg/day).

Prophylaxis. People at risk (see above) should be made aware of the possibility of infections and they should take appropriate preventive measures, such as use of protective clothing and facemasks. Infected birds should be treated with tetracycline through their feeds for 45 days. The United States Department of Agriculture requires that imported birds be quarantined for 30 days, primarily to prevent introduction of Newcastle disease. A bird's beak should not be held close to the human mouth (Fig. 2.8). Pet birds should only be bought from a dealer who carries a permit to sell them.

Reporting. Psittacosis/ornithosis are notifiable diseases in the USA and in Canada.

2.7.2 CHLAMYDIOSES TRANSMITTED FROM MAMMALS

Chlamydioses have been reported to occur in at least 32 mammal species, including ruminants, horses, cats, dogs, pigs, and guinea pigs. Human infections occur sporadically as a consequence of contact with infected animals and their excreta.

C. abortus is the frequent agent of chlamydial abortion in sheep and goats, causing fertility problems, abortion, and offspring with diminished life expectancy. Transmission occurs most often via abortions, lochia, or chorions/amnions of infected animals. In humans, a variety of diseases have been reported: influenza-like syndromes with thrombopenia and coagulopathies, conjunctivitis, chronic upper genital tract infections, septicemia with dysfunction of lung, liver, and kidneys. In pregnancy, miscarriage and fetal death may occur; therefore, pregnant women who are close to delivery should avoid contact with sheep and goats.

C. felis occurs mainly in cats in whom it causes inflammation of the conjunctivae and the mucous membranes of mouth, throat, and nose. Humans may become infected through contact with an infected cat and they may acquire mono- or bilateral follicular acute or chronic conjunctivitis. Cases of atypical pneumonia and endocarditis have also been reported. *Parachlamydia acanthamoebae* in humans has mainly been reported as agent of lower respiratory infections but zoonotic transmission between animals (ruminants) and humans remains to be proven.

REFERENCES

Borel N et al., Parachlamydia acanthamoebae and its zoonotic risk. *Clin. Microbiol. Newsletter* 32, 185–195, 2010.

Centers for: Disease Control and Prevention. (CDC). Compendium of measures to control Chlamydia psittaci infection among humans (psittacosis) and pet birds (avian chlamydiosis). MMWR Morbid. Mortal. Wkl. Rep. 49(RR8), 2000.

Cotton MM, Partridge MR, Infection with feline Chlamydia psittaci. *Thorax* 53, 75–76, 1998.

Dickx V, Vanrompay D, Zoonotic transmission of Chlamydia psittaci in a chicken and turkey hatchery. *J. Med. Microbiol.* 60, 775–779, 2011.

Everett KD, Bush RM, Andersen AA, Emended description of the order Chlamydiales, proposal of Parachlamydiaceae fam. nov. and Simkaniaceae fam. nov., each containing one monotypic genus, revised taxonomy of the family Chlamydiaceae, including a new genus and five new species, and standards for the identification of organisms. *Int. J. Syst. Bacteriol.* 49 (Pt 2), 415–440, 1999.

Fraeyman A et al., Atypical pneumonia due to Chlamydophila psittaci: 3 case reports and review of literature. *Acta Clin. Belg.* 65, 192–196, 2010.

Geens T, Sequencing of the Chlamydophila psittaci ompA gene reveals a new genotype, E/B, and the need for a rapid discriminatory genotyping method. *J. Clin. Microbiol.* 43, 2456–2461, 2005.

Greub G, International committee on systematics of Prokaryotes. Subcommittee on the taxonomy of the Chlamydiae. *Int. J. Syst. Evol. Microbiol.* 60, 2694, 2010.

Hadley K et al., Ovine chlamydiosis in an abattoir worker. *J. Infect.* 25(Suppl 1), 105–109, 1992.

Horn H, Phylum XXIV: Chlamydiae Garrity and Holt 2001. In: Krieg NR et al. (eds.): *Bergey's Manual of Systematic Bacteriology*. Springer, New York, Dordrecht, Heidelberg, London, 2011.

Hughes C et al., Possible nosocomial transmission of psittacosis. *Infect. Control Hosp. Epidemiol.* 18, 165–168, 1997.

Ito I et al., Familial cases of psittacosis: possible person-to-person transmission. *Intern. Med.* 41, 580–583, 2002.

Kaleta EF, Taday EM, Avian host range of Chlamydophila spp. based on isolation, antigen detection and serology. *Avian Pathol.* 32, 435–461, 2003.

Messmer TO et al., Application of a nested multiplex PCR to psittacosis outbreaks. *J. Clin. Microbiol.* 35, 2043–2046, 1997.

Mitchell CM et al., Chlamydia pneumoniae is genetically diverse in animals and appears to have crossed the host barrier to humans on (at least) two occasions. *PLoS Pathog.* 6, e1000903, 2010.

Pantchev A et al., New real-time PCR tests for species-specific detection of Chlamydophila psittaci and Chlamydophila abortus from tissue samples. *Vet. J.* 181, 145–150, 2009.

Pantchev A et al., Detection of all Chlamydophila and Chlamydia spp. of veterinary interest using species-specific real-time PCR assays. *Comp. Immunol. Microbiol. Infect. Dis.* 33, 473–484, 2010.

Pospischil A et al., Abortion in woman caused by caprine Chlamydophila abortus (Chlamydia psittaci serovar 1). *Swiss Med. Wkly.* 132, 64–66, 2002.

Senn L, Hammerschlag MR, Greub G, Therapeutic approaches to Chlamydia infections. *Expert Opin. Pharmacother.* 6, 2281–2290, 2005.

Sprague LD et al., The detection of Chlamydophila psittaci genotype C infection in dogs. *Vet. J.* 181, 274–279, 2009.

Teankum K et al., Prevalence of chlamydiae in semen and genital tracts of bulls, rams and bucks. *Theriogenology* 67, 303–310, 2007.

Vanrompay D, Ducatelle R, Haesebrouck F, Chlamydia psittaci infections: a review with emphasis on avian chlamydiosis. *Vet. Microbiol.* 45, 93–119, 1995.

Vanrompay D et al., Chlamydophila psittaci transmission from pet birds to humans. *Emerg. Infect. Dis.* 13, 1108–1110, 2007.

Verweij PE et al., Severe human psittacosis requiring artificial ventilation: case report and review. *Clin. Infect. Dis.* 20, 440–442, 1995.

Walder G et al., An unusual cause of sepsis during pregnancy: recognizing infection with Chlamydophila abortus. *Obstet. Gynecol.* 106, 1215–1217, 2005.

Walder G et al., Chlamydophila abortus pelvic inflammatory disease. *Emerg. Infect. Dis.* 9, 1642–1644, 2003.

2.8 Ehrlichioses/Anaplasmosis

Human ehrlichioses and anaplasmosis are caused by various *Ehrlichia* spp. and *Anaplasma phagocytophilum*. Most cases are acute but occasional chronic febrile systemic infections are characterized by headache, myalgia, arthralgia, nausea, vomiting, pancytopenia, and liver or kidney damage. Some of these are lethal, particularly if complicated by secondary infections.

Etiology. Ehrlichiae and anaplasmata are pleomorphic, nonmotile Gram-negative intracellular bacteria that parasitize monocytes and granulocytes. Species pathogenic for animals may also attack lymphocytes and megakaryocytes. Multiplication by fission inside cytoplasmic vacuoles (initial bodies) leads to elementary bodies that divide in the phagosome, forming a "morula" 2 to 5 µm in size and containing ci. 100 elementary bodies. Cell lysis releases the bacteria that can infect other cells.

The most recent systematic distinguishes in the order *Rickettsiales* are these families: *Bartonellaceae* (genus *Bartonella*), *Anaplasmataceae* (genera: *Anaplasma, Ehrlichia, Neorickettsia, Wolbachia*), and *Rickettsiaceae* (genera: *Rickettsia, Orientia*) (Fig. 2.11). Human pathogens

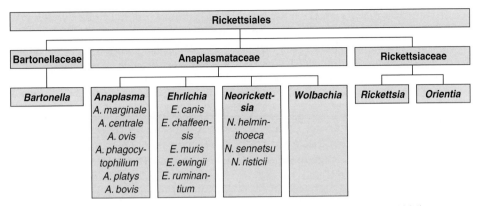

Figure 2.11 | Systematics of the Order Rickettsiales (Dumler S 2001, modified Hartelt K 2004).

are *Anaplasma phagocytophilum* and *Ehrlichia chaffeensis, E. ewingii,* and possibly *E. canis* (Tab. 2.5). Ehrlichiae have been known as animal pathogens for over 100 years but their pathogenicity for humans has only been described at the end of the last century.

Occurrence. The epidemiology of *Ehrlichia* spp. is insufficiently known. Vectors are various species of ticks. Disease due to *E. chaffeensis* is most frequently found in the US, particularly in Missouri, Tennessee, Oklahoma, Texas, Arkansas, Virginia, Georgia, California, Oregon, and Washington; 5500 cases have been reported through 2009. This pattern resembles that of Rocky Mountain spotted fever (RMSF) as the

vector for both is the tick *Amblyomma americanum*. In Oklahoma, ehrlichiosis occurs with a frequency equal to RMSF; in Georgia, it is even more frequent than RMSF. Clusters were observed following camping in tick-infested areas. Seroepidemiological studies have shown high antibody prevalence in white-tailed deer (54%), foxes (83%), raccoons (60%), and rabbits (16%). These animals are probably the main reservoir. Wild boars, dogs and horses are also assumed to be hosts. Sporadic cases have also been reported from Latin America, Africa, Europe, and Asia.

A. phagocytophilum is endemic in Wisconsin, Minnesota, Connecticut, and Massachusetts. As of 2009, >6200 cases had been reported in the

Table 2.5 | *Anaplasma* and *Ehrlichia* spp. pathogenic for humans

SPECIES	HOSTS	VECTORS	DISEASE
Anaplasma phagocytophilum	Ruminants, horse, dog, human	*Ixodes ricinus, I. persulcatus, I. scapularis*	Equine/canine human granulocytic anaplasmosis (HGA)
Ehrlichia chaffeensis	White-tailed deer, dog	*Amblyomma americanum*	Canine/human monocytic ehrlichiosis (HME)
Ehrlichia ewingii	Dog, human	*Amblyomma americanum*	Human *E. ewingii* ehrlichiosis (HEE)
Ehrlichia canis	Dog (human)	*Rhipicephalus sanguineus, Dermacentor variabilis*	Canine/(human) monocytic ehrlichiosis
Neorickettsia sennetsu	Human	Trematodes(?), *Stellantchasmus falcatus*	Sennetsu fever
Candidatus Neoehrlichia mikurensis	Human, Rodents	Ixodes spp.	Nonspecific symptoms

Modified from Straubinger RK, Rickettsiales and *Coxiella burnetii*. In: Selbitz HJ, Truyen U, Valentin-Weigand P (eds.): Tiermedizinische Mikrobiologie, Infektions- und Seuchenlehre. Enke, Stuttgart, 2011.

US. Vectors are ticks (*Ixodes* spp.); hosts are small rodents, particularly white-footed mice, chipmunks and voles but also horses, red deer, ruminants, dogs, and horses. Infested *I. ricinus* have been found in Germany, France, the UK, Italy, the Netherlands, Switzerland, and Slovenia. Rates for nymphs were between 0.5% (Switzerland) and 25% (Italy), for adults in Southern Germany 0.2 to 1.2%. Hosts are primarily bank voles, with an average *Anaplasma* carriage rate of 10.3% as detected by PCR. True mice are infected only sporadically. Thus, there seem to be locally variable natural foci that can serve as infectious sources for humans. Woodworkers in Southern Germany showed seroprevalence rates of up to 16% (average, 10%) but none of them have reported signs of disease. This may mean that certain strains are not particularly virulent as seems to be the case in other European countries as well. The few human cases reported from Sweden and Slovenia were slight, transient febrile infections with minimal thrombocytopenia and leukopenia.

Neorickettsia sunnetsu had already been found in 1954 in Japan in patients with a mononucleosis-like disease. Later, similar infections were seen in Thailand and Malaysia. The source has been uncooked fish, with the neorickettsiae most likely parasites of fish trematodes

Various ticks are known or suspected vectors for ehrlichiae: in the US, for *E. chaffeensis,* they are *Amblyomma americanum* and *Dermacentor variabilis*; (in other countries, probably other tick species) for *A. phagocytophilum* it is *Ixodes scapularis* in the Eastern and *I. pacificus* in the western states of the US, and *I. ricinus* in Europe. These ticks also transmit *Borrelia burgdorferi* and *Babesia microti*. *E. canis* is transmitted by the brown dog tick, *Rhipicephalus sanguineus,* and by various *Ixodes* spp., *E. ewingii* by *Amblyomma americanum*, and Candidatus Neoehrlichia mikurensis by various *Ixodes* spp. Tick bites can be elicited in the histories of 73% of patients with ehrlichiosis and anaplasmosis; the rest of these patients live in tick-infested areas. More than 90% acquire the disease during the months of highest tick activity, that is, from April to October, with a peak during June/July. For work with both *Ehrlichia* and *Anaplasma,* biosafety 3 level laboratories are required.

Clinical Manifestations. Target cells of both bacterial genera are leukocytes: for *E. chaffeensis* and *E. canis*, monocytes and macrophages and, more rarely, lymphocytes, for *A. phagocytophilum*, granulocytes. Hence the distinction between human monocytic ehrlichiosis (HME) and human granulocytic anaplasmosis (HGA or HGE). HME and HGA resemble each other clinically but there may be differences in severity and frequency of certain symptoms. Approximately 60% of the infections are asymptomatic or present as a nonspecific viral syndrome; 15% of Wisconsin's population have antibodies against the agent of HGA but have never been manifestly ill. Hospitalization was necessary for 30 to 50% of HGA patients and for >60% of HME patients. Men are affected 2 to 4 times more frequently than women.

After a median incubation period of 1 week, the disease starts as a generalized febrile infection with marked malaise, chills, severe headache, myalgia, and more rarely, arthralgias, loss of appetite and weight, nausea, and vomiting. In approximately 30% of HME patients, a maculo-papular, occasionally petechial, skin rash is noted. Severe and often fatal courses are seen in older individuals and in patients with severe underlying diseases or immunosuppression. Frequent complications are acute respiratory distress syndrome (ARDS), shock, and severe opportunistic infections.

Complications of HME may be meningitis or meningoencephalitis, and in HGA, long-lasting nephropathy. Moderate anemia and marked granulo/lympho/thrombocytopenia as well as elevated transaminase levels are characteristic. Unless treated, the disease lasts for 10 to 14 days, occasionally even for 1 to 2 months. The case-fatality rate is 2 to 5% in patients with HME and 7 to 10% in those with HGA, depending on age, immune status, timely start of antibiotic treatment, and presence of opportunistic infections. The latter occur particularly in HGA, with esophagitis due to *Candida* or herpesviruses, and pneumonia due to *Cryptococcus neoformans* or *Aspergillus* spp. Six to 21% of HGA patients show antibodies against *B. burgdorferi sensu lato* and *Babesia microti*. Double infections of HGA with *B. burgdorferi s.l.* have been reported but their effects on severity, duration and complications of HGA are unknown.

E. ewingii was identified in 1999 as a new agent of granulocytic ehrlichiosis that runs a mild, HME-like course and occurs mainly in immunocompromised individuals.

N. sennetsu causes Hyuganetsu (Kagama) fever in Japan, Malaysia, and Laos, a mononucleosis-like disease with fever, chills, severe headache, myalgias, loss of appetite and later, retroauricular and cervical lymphadenopathy and, in half of the patients, hepatosplenomegaly. Leukopenia followed by lymphocytosis and moderately elevated transaminase levels are characteristic.

Ehrlichiae and anaplasmata are also of importance in veterinary medicine. In dogs, *E. platys* causes infectious cyclic thrombocytopenia and *E. canis* causes monocytic ehrlichiosis (tropical canine panleukopenia). Initially, nonspecific symptoms, such as high fever, anorexia, lassitude, nasal and ocular discharge, and pallor of the mucous membranes prevail. In the following chronic phase, thrombocytopenia is most conspicuous, leading to hemorrhages and anemia. *E. canis* is transmitted by *Rhipicephalus sanguineus* (see above) and it mainly occurs in Mediterranean countries. *E. ewingii* and *A. phagocytophilum* are also pathogenic for dogs. The former, in the US, causes canine granulocytic ehrlichiosis with a course similar to, but milder, than *E. canis* infection. *A. phagocytophilicum* has also been found in dogs in Germany, with a seroprevalence of 20 to 30%. Canine granulocytic anaplasmosis shows few specific symptoms: fever, anorexia, weight loss, dyspnea, lethargy, lymphadenopathy, and polyarthritis.

N. helminthoeca is the agent of salmon poisoning disease that is transmitted by trematodes. *N. risticii* causes equine monocytic neorickettsiosis (Potomac horse fever); vectors are cercariae. In ruminants, ehrlichioses have been known for some time, that is, *E. (Cowdria) ruminantium*

in cattle leading to heartwater disease, and *A. phagocytophilum* to gall sickness.

Diagnosis. Ehrlichioses should be suspected from the history of tick bites, the clinical picture and the epidemiological situation, that is, occurrence in endemic tick-infested areas from April to October. A generalized infection with lymphadenopathy following ingestion of raw fish in endemic areas should raise the suspicion of Sennetsu fever.

In the first week, morulae may be detected in blood smears or buffy coats by Giemsa stains, either in monocytes (HME, <10%) or in granulocytes (HGA, 25 to 75%). *E, chaffeensis, E. canis, N. risticii,* and *N. sennetsu* may be cultured by inoculation of peripheral blood leukocytes into cell cultures of macrophages from dogs or mice. *A. phagocytophilum* can be cultured in a promyelocytic cell line. Cell culture, however, is not a routine diagnostic method because it requires several weeks of incubation. Routine serological methods are IFA and ELISA; ehrlichial antigens being available mostly from public health and research laboratories. A fourfold increase in antibody titers is generally obtained after 2 weeks so that the diagnosis mostly becomes retrospective. As persistent titers, high seroprevalence, and cross-reactions have to be taken into account, PCR in the first week has become the gold standard and it can also be used for a species diagnosis.

Differential Diagnosis. Primarily, RMSF, tularemia, Lyme borreliosis, infectious mononucleosis. Double infections are possible (see above). Depending on the combination of symptoms, murine typhus, typhoid fever, viral infections, and toxic shock syndrome have to be ruled out as well.

Therapy. In view of the possibly lethal outcome, suspicion of HME or HGA justifies an immediate onset of treatment. The drug of choice is doxycycline 2 × 100 mg/day p.o. for 7 to 14 days. In pregnancy or in children <8 years rifampicin (2 × 300 mg/day p.o.; 10 mg/kg) can be attempted.

Prophylaxis. Contact with ticks should be minimized (appropriate clothing and insect repellents). As infection occurs only after a tick bite that lasts for several hours, frequent checks for ticks are advised in areas of heavy infestation.

Reporting. Ehrlichiosis and Anaplasmosis are notifiable diseases in the USA and in Canada

REFERENCES

Bakken JS et al., The serological response of patients infected with the agent of human granulocytic ehrlichiosis. *Clin. Infect. Dis.* 34, 22–27, 1978.

Bakken JS, Dumler S, Clinical diagnosis and treatment of human granulocytotropic anaplasmosis. *Ann. N.Y. Acad. Sci.* 1078, 236–247, 2006.

Bakken JS, Dumler S, Human granulocytic anaplasmosis. *Infect. Dis. Clin. North. Am.* 22, 433–448, 1978.

Buller RS et al., Ehrlichia ewingii, a newly recognized agent of human ehrlichiosis. *New Engl. J. Med.* 341, 148–155, 1999.

Doudier B et al., Factors contributing to emergence of Ehrlichia and Anaplasma spp. as human pathogens. *Vet. Parasitol.* 167, 149–154, 2010.

Dumler JS et al., Reorganization of genera in the families Rickettsiaceae and Anaplasmataceae in the order Rickettsiales: unification of some species of Ehrlichia with Anaplasma, Cowdria with Ehrlichia and Ehrlichia with Neorickettsia, descriptions of six new species combinations and designation of Ehrlichia equi and „HGE agent" as subjective synonyms of Ehrlichia phagocytophila. *Int. J. Syst. Evol. Microbiol.* 51, 2145–2165, 2001.

Dumler JS et al., Ehrlichioses in humans: epidemiology, clinical presentation, diagnosis and treatment. *Clin. Infect. Dis.* 15 (Suppl. 1), 45–51, 2007.

Horowitz HW et al., Antimicrobial susceptibility of Ehrlichia phagocytophila. *Antimicrob. Agents Chemother.* 45, 786–788, 2001.

Horowitz HW et al., Lyme disease and human granulocytic anaplasmosis coinfection: impact of case definition on coinfection rates and illness severity. *Clin Infect Dis* 56, 93–99, 2013.

Ismail N, Bloch KC, McBride JW, Human ehrlichiosis and anaplasmosis. *Clin. Lab. Med.* 30, 261–292, 2010.

Paddock CD et al., Infections with Ehrlichia chaffeensis and Ehrlichia ewingii in persons coinfected with human immunodeficiency virus. *Clin. Infect. Dis.* 33, 1586–1594, 2001.

Paddock CD, Childs JE, Ehrlichia chaffeensis: a prototypical emerging pathogen. *Clin. Microbiol. Rev.* 16, 37–64, 2003.

Ramsey AH et al., Outcomes of treated human granulocytic ehrlichiosis cases. *Emerg. Infect. Dis.* 8, 398–401, 2002.

Standaert SM et al., Primary isolation of Ehrlichia chaffeensis from patients with febrile illnesses: clinical and molecular characteristics. *J. Infect. Dis.* 181, 1082–1088, 2000.

Strle F, Human granulocytic ehrlichiosis in Europe. *Int.J. Med. Microbiol.* 293(Suppl. 37), 27–35, 2004.

Unver A et al., Western blot analysis of sera reactive to human monocytic ehrlichiosis and human granulocytic ehrlichiosis agents. *J. Clin. Microbiol.* 39, 3982–3986, 2001.

Walker DH and the: Task Force on Consensus Approach for Ehrlichiosis, Diagnosing human ehrlichioses: current status and recommendations. *ASM News* 66, 287–290, 2000.

2.9 Enterohemorrhagic *Escherichia coli* (EHEC) Infections

EHEC strains cause intestinal infections in humans that cover a spectrum from uncomplicated diarrhea to severe hemorrhagic colitis. Life-threatening complications occur in 5 to 20% of these patients; that is, hemolytic-uremic syndrome (HUS), mostly in children <10 years, and thrombotic-thrombocytopenic purpura (TTP), mostly in adults. Most cases of EHEC infection are zoonotic.

Etiology. *Escherichia coli* strains causing intestinal diseases are grouped according to virulence factors (adhesins, exotoxins) and diseases (pathovars; see Tab. 2.6). EHEC are a subgroup of Shiga toxin producing *Escherichia coli* (STEC), the strains producing one or more Shiga toxins (Stx) that cause bloody diarrhea in humans. Many of them also have the ability to cause attachment and effacement (A/E) lesions, primarily in the cecum and the colon. These lesions are characterized by adhesion (attachment) of the bacteria to the intestinal epithelium with subsequent cellular changes consisting of loss of microvilli and effacement at the adhesion site.

Shiga toxins are a family of very potent cytotoxins (verotoxins) to which belong Stx produced by *Shigella dysenteriae* serotype 1, as well as some strains of *Citrobacter freundii*, *Enterobacter cloacae*, and *S. flexneri*. Within the Stx family, two types based on structural features can be distinguished: Stx 1(including Stx) and Stx2 as well as several subtypes (Stx 1a, 1b, 1c, 1d, 2a, 2b, 2c, 2d, 2e, 2f, and 2g). Bloody diarrhea and HUS are particularly associated with EHEC forming Stx 2a, 2c, and/or 2d. The structural genes for Stx are in the genome of lysogenic lambda-like bacteriophages that are integrated into the *E. coli* chromosome.

Table 2.6 | Classification of diarrheagenic *Escherichia coli*

E. COLI PATHOVAR	VIRULENCE FACTORS			DIARRHEA	
	ADHESINS	TOXINS	INVASINS	HUMANS	DOMESTIC ANIMALS
Enteropathogenic *E. coli* (EPEC)	Intimin, BFP, Paa, Lpf	(EAST-1)	−	Infants, small children	+
Enterotoxic *E. coli* (ETEC)	CFAs, Tia, F4, F5, F6, F17, F18, F41, F42 (Paa)	ST and/or LT (EAST -1)	−	Cholera-like, travel-associated	Newborn and young animals
Enteroinvasive *E. coli* (EIEC)	−	−	Ipa A, B, C, D	Like shigellosis	−
Enterohemorrhagic *E.coli* (EHEC)[1]	Intimin, Efa1 (Paa, Saa, Lpf)	Stx, Hly$_{EHEC}$ (EAST-1, CDTs)	−	HC, HUS/TTP	+, HC
Diffusely adherent *E. coli* (EAEC)	F1845, AIDA-1	(ShET1)	−	+	?
Enteroaggregative *E. coli*	AAFs, HdaA	EAST-1, Pet (EAEC)	−	+	−

AAF, aggregative adherence factors; AIDA, antigen involved in diffuse adherence; BFP, bundle-forming pili; CDTs, cytolethal distending toxins; CFAs, colonization factor antigens; EAST, heat-labile enterotoxin of EAEC; Efa1, *E.coli* adherence factor 1; F, fimbrial antigen; HC, hemorrhagic colitis; Hda, HUS-associated diffuse adherence; Hly$_{EHEC}$, EHEC hemolysin; HUS, hemolytic-uremic syndrome; Ipa, invasion plasmid antigen; Lpf, long polar fimbriae; LT, heat-labile *E.coli* enterotoxin; Paa, porcine attaching-and-effacing associated; Pet, plasmid-encoded toxin; Saa, STEC autoagglutinating adhesin; Shet1, *Shigella* enterotoxin; Stx, Shiga toxins; ST, heat-stable *E.coli* enterotoxin; Tia, enterotoxigenic invasion locus a; Tib, enterotoxigenic invasion locus b; TTP, thrombotic thrombocytopenic purpura
[1] The only proven zoonotic agent

Shiga toxins are hetero-hexameric protein molecules with an AB5 structure. The A subunit has N-glycosidase activity and catalyzes the hydrolytic cleavage of adenine in the nucleoproteid position 4324 of the 28S rRNA of the target cell. This discrete molecular lesion inhibits cellular protein synthesis and leads to the death of the target cells; that is, the small endothelial cells in the small blood vessels of the kidney, the intestine, and the brain ("vasculotoxin").

Intimin (*eae* gene) is a well characterized EHEC adhesin. Its gene *eae* lies on a ci. 35 kbp segment of the EHEC chromosome [locus of enterocyte effacement (LEE)], which represents a pathogenicity island. LEE also contains other genes whose products participate in creating the A/E lesions, for example, a gene cluster encoding a type III protein secretion system. This system, resembling an injection needle, translocates in EHEC and enteropathogenic *Escherichia coli* (who also possess an LEE) several effector proteins from the bacterial cytoplasm into the target cell cytoplasm. One of these effector proteins is the translocated intimin receptor (Tir), which is incorporated by the target cell into its cytoplasmic membrane. Tir binds to intimin and is a receptor of high affinity for the intimin-carrying bacterium. Together with other effector proteins such as Map, EspF, EspH, EspJ, NleA, NleB, and NleC EHEC manipulate cellular signal cascades and thereby rearrange the cytoskeleton and damage function and structure of the intestinal epithelium.

Many other factors that are expressed by different EHEC strains in different combinations determine their putative virulence: Saa, Iha, Sfp fimbriae, long polar fimbriae (Lpf), EHEC adherence factor 1 (Efa1), and hemorrhagic coli pilus as (putative) adherence factors, as well as subtilase cytotoxin, cytolethal distending toxins, EHEC hemolysin ("enterohemolysin"), urease, the serine protease EspP, and a bifunctional catalase/peroxidase (KatP).

Today, one assumes that EHEC arose from "harmless, normal" *E. coli* by horizontal gene transfer (e.g., through transduction and/or conjugation) that provided the bacteria with genes for a parasitic/pathogenic existence in the host.

EHEC and potential EHEC strains (see below) belong to many serovars: by now, >200 of them have been detected worldwide. In most countries, the sorbitol-negative serovar O157:H7, more rarely O157:H-, is the dominating one and the cause of 70 to 80% of all HUS and of 40 to 50% of all EHEC enteritis cases. Other serovars, however, are being isolated from hemorrhagic colitis, particularly in Europe: a sorbitol-fermenting, nonmotile serovar O157: NM and serovars O26:H11/H-, O91:H14/H21, O103:H2, O104:H4, O111:H2/H8/NM, O118: H16/NM, O121:H19, O145:H25/H28/NM, and O146:H21/H28. These serovars are called non-O157:H7 EHEC.

Occurrence. Disease caused by EHEC was first described in 1982/83 in the USA. Since then, sporadic cases and smaller epidemics with several hundred cases have been reported from the Americas, Europe, Asia, and Africa, with a peak incidence between June and September. Although incidence data are not always reliable, the EU reported in the year 2000 approximately 0.75 confirmed new cases per 100 000 inhabitants, with differences between countries ranging from 0.0 to 5.33 (Ireland). Germany reported an incidence of 800 to 1300 new cases, that is, 1 per 100 000 inhabitants, with 40 to 120 cases of HUS. Approximately 50% of the EHEC infections occurred in children <5 years of age. In the US, there are reportedly eight cases per 100 000 inhabitants per year, which would translate into 20 000 cases and 250 fatalities. In some states, EHEC O157:H7 is the second or third most frequent enteropathogen and is more frequent than yersiniae or shigellae. It is the most frequent agent of bloody diarrhea, taking 40% of those cases.

Domestic and wild ruminants, particularly cattle, sheep, and goats are carriers and excrete STEC strains, but not all STEC seem to be EHEC. Conversely, every STEC strain should be regarded as a potential EHEC as diagnostic laboratories are unable to differentiate between the two. STEC is found in >50% of all cattle and can

also be found in pigs, horses, dogs, cats, fowl, and wild birds. The reservoir of some serovars, however, is not known, for example, that of O157: NM and of the enteroaggregative O104:H4.

Transmission. EHEC are transmitted by the fecal-oral route. The minimal infective dose is small and resembles that of shigellae (10 to 100 bacteria for EHEC O157:H7) as the bacteria are relatively resistant to stomach acid. Human infections are primarily due to consumption of fecally contaminated, uncooked or insufficiently heated foodstuffs. Examples are hamburgers, raw sausage spreads, raw milk, and milk products. EHEC may also contaminate potatoes, spinach, salad dressings, apple sauce and apple cider from fallen fruit, unchlorinated drinking water, and surface waters. Large epidemics in Japan (1996) and Germany (2011) with several thousand cases each could be traced to EHEC-contaminated sprouts of radish and fenugreek, respectively. In some instances, EHEC were transmitted by direct contact with infected animals (cattle, sheep, goats, horses) and their excreta, for example, in petting zoos. Human-to-human transmission, mostly by direct contact, is not rare in infant wards, kindergartens, nursing homes, and families.

Clinical Manifestations. Asymptomatic infections are known to occur but very few data have been published. The following symptoms appear after an incubation period of 3 to 4 days (range, 1 to 8 days) in 80 to 90% of the patients: severe abdominal pain accompanied by initially nonbloody watery diarrhea, nausea and vomiting. Fever is rare. After 1 to 4 days, diarrhea becomes bloody in most patients; in approximately 10%, it remains nonbloody. In the residual 10 to 20% (frequently small children), a severe hemorrhagic colitis will develop, accompanied by colicky pain, a diarrhea that is "all blood and no stool," and sometimes fever. The abdomen is exquisitely tender, resembling an "acute abdomen." Symptoms last for 4 to 10 days. No protective immunity will develop.

HUS and TTP will complicate the disease in ci. 5 to 20% of the patients 4 to 13 days after diarrhea has set in but preceding gastrointestinal symptoms may be absent. These complications can often not be distinguished easily, as in both, microangiopathic hemolytic anemia with thrombocytopenia occur, with renal failure in HUS and CNS involvement in TTP most conspicuous. Both are caused by spillover of Shiga toxin into the bloodstream and its stereospecific binding to globotriasylceramide (Gb3), the glycosphingolipoid receptor located on endothelial and renal cortical cells, intestinal epithelium, and red blood cells. The damage to endothelial cells, probably augmented by lipopolysaccharide (LPS), leads to release of coagulation factors and initially increases but later inhibits prostacyclin synthesis. As a consequence, platelet aggregation, thrombotic obstruction of glomerular capillaries, microinfarcts, reduced glomerular filtration, and hypertension will ensue. Endothelial damage and platelet aggregates are found in other organs as well. Red cell damage in the partially obstructed small vessels leads to anemia, hemoglobinuria, and formation of fragmentocytes.

HUS generally starts out as an acute disease in children <10 years of age with pallor, oliguria to anuria, hypertension, edema, heart failure, coma, convulsions, and focal CNS symptoms to hemiplegia. Laboratory findings include anemia, hemolysis with elevated bilirubin and reticulocyte counts, thrombocytopenia, coagulopathy, and fragmentocytes. Signs of renal failure are increased serum potassium, urea and creatinine, metabolic acidosis, hematuria, hemoglobinuria, and proteinuria. Ultrasound shows enlargement of the kidneys. The case-fatality rate is 3 to 5%; approximately 10% of the patients will develop renal failure. In adults with TTP, fever, hemolysis, renal insufficiency, and CNS symptoms are generally more pronounced than in children.

In animals, EHEC infections are generally asymptomatic. In experiments, human EHEC strains were able to cause diarrhea in calves and severe hemorrhagic colitis in rabbits. In greyhounds, an EHEC infection is known that resembles human disease in pathogenesis and symptomatology, that is, cutaneous and renal glomerular vasculopathy (CRVG, Alabama rot). Acutely ill dogs show subcutaneous edema,

multifocal cutaneous necroses and venous thromboses. Severe infections with the hematological and renal disorders described above are mostly fatal. The so-called "coli enterotoxemia" in pigs is caused by STEC strains exclusively adapted to these animals.

Diagnosis. Patients with bloody stools, HUS, and TTP, or a history of bloody diarrhea as well as children <6 years hospitalized for diarrhea or those with acute renal failure should be evaluated for EHEC. It should also be kept in mind that these organisms may induce nonbloody, watery diarrhea and a clinically mild course. There have even been suggestions to examine every diarrhoic stool for EHEC.

The multitude of EHEC serovars, the small number of bacteria and the short period of excretion (13 to 21; range 2 to 124 days) create problems for the microbiological diagnosis. Therefore, a combination of cultural, immunological, and molecular tests would be optimal. Most important, however, is the proof of Shiga toxin or its genes directly from stool or, better yet, from a culture. The presence of toxin can be proven in enzyme immunoassay (EIA) from cultures or by Vero cell toxicity tests while the genes are best demonstrated by PCR or DNA-DNA hybridization. O157 EHEC can also be detected directly in stools by use of fluorescein-marked O157-specific antibodies but non-O157 will not be detected by this method. It also requires a large number of bacteria. Immunomagnetic separation has also been used for isolation of O157 EHEC from stool and food samples; the detection of non-O157 strains by this method has so far been limited to specialized laboratories.

Enrichment media, for example, trypticase soy broth with or without novobiocin and cefsulodin, may be used for culture. Differential media serve for isolation and presumptive recognition, for example, Sorbitol-MacConkey agar (SMAC) for O157 strains that cannot metabolize sorbitol (NSF; in contrast to 95% of all other *E. coli* strains). Addition of tellurite and cefixime increases the selectivity of SMAC. As O157 EHEC do not produce beta-glucuronidase, newer media contain chromogenic or fluorogenic substrate of this enzyme. Colonies of NSF EHEC O157:H7/NM remain colorless or do not fluoresce on these media.

Also, almost all O157 EHEC and >80% of the non-O157 ones express the EHEC-characteristic hemolysin. A special medium containing washed sheep erythrocytes, antibiotics, and calcium ions (WSBA-Ca) in a Columbia agar base can detect the enterohemolysin. Finally, antibody assays against the LPS of EHEC O157 may be helpful.

Differential Diagnosis. Diseases that caused acute abdominal symptoms, such as acute cholecystitis, appendicitis, diverticulitis, intussusception, ulcerative colitis, and ileus, must be included in the differential diagnosis, as must be infections due to *C. jejuni, C. difficile, Salmonella* spp., *Shigella* spp., *Yersinia enterocolitica*, and *Entamoeba histolytica*.

Therapy. Fluid and electrolyte replacement is of prime importance in order to keep up kidney perfusion and to prevent HUS and TTP. Treatment against the underlying condition is, at present, impossible. Antimicrobial treatment is contraindicated as it contributes to increased verotoxin production and release, prolongs EHEC excretion, and thus, increases the risk for HUS and TTP. Motility-inhibiting drugs are also contraindicated as they lead to retention of EHEC, and thereby increase the risk of toxin absorption.

Patients with HUS/TTP must be treated in intensive care units as early dialysis, control of electrolytes and treatment of hypertension, blood transfusion, and plasmapheresis, may be necessary. Improved clinical management and dialysis have reduced the case-fatality rate to <10%. However, approximately 30% of the survivors will suffer from permanent disabilities, such as chronic renal insufficiency, hypertension, and neurological deficits. Some patients will have to be permanently maintained on dialysis.

Prophylaxis. The risk of EHEC infection can be minimized by general hygienic measures: handwashing with water and soap before meals and after contact with animals (particularly ruminants) and items in contact with them. Children must be supervised accordingly. Proper hygiene in food processing and in preparation of meals, especially separation of meat from other foodstuffs, are the most important steps. Uncooked foods should always be kept at refrigerator temperature, and heating should always take place at least at 70 °C (158 F) for 10 min.

Of items bought on the market, unpasteurized milk should be boiled before consumption. Meat, especially hamburgers, should be heated so that the entire patty is exposed to 70 °C (158F); the same applies to vegetable sprouts. Raw vegetables must be peeled or thoroughly washed. Patients and convalescent individuals with stools positive for EHEC (possible for up to 8 weeks after infection) should not be employed in the food-processing industry or in establishments caring for people at risk, for example, kindergartens, schools, and nursing homes.

Reporting. Disease due to EHEC is notifiable in the USA and in Canada; HUS following diarrhea also in the USA.

REFERENCES

Besser RE et al., An outbreak of diarrhea and hemolytic uremic syndrome from Escherichia coli O157:H7 in fresh-pressed apple cider. *JAMA* 269, 2217–2220, 1993.

Beutin L et al., Characterization of Shiga toxin-producing Escherichia coli strains isolated from human patients in Germany over a 3-year period. *J. Clin. Microbiol.* 42, 1099–1108, 2004.

Brzuszkiewicz E, et al., Genome sequence analyses of two isolates from the recent Escherichia coli outbreak in Germany reveal the emergence of a new pathotype: Entero-Aggregative-Haemorrhagic Escherichia coli (EAHEC). *Arch Microbiol* 193, 883–891, 2011.

Chapman PA, Cornell J, Green C, Infection with verocytotoxin-producing Escherichia coli O157 during a visit to an inner city open farm. *Epidemiol. Infect.* 125, 531–536, 2000.

Cowan LA et al., Clinical and clinicopathologic abnormalities in greyhounds with cutaneous and renal glomerular vasculopathy: 18 cases (1992–1994). *J. Am. Vet. Med. Assoc.* 210, 789–793, 1997.

Croxen MA, Finlay BB, Molecular mechanisms of Escherichia coli pathogenicity. *Nat. Rev. Microbiol.* 8, 26–38, 2010.

Dundas S et al., The central Scotland Escherichia coli O157:H7 outbreak: risk factors for the hemolytic uremic syndrome and death among hospitalized patients. *Clin. Infect. Dis.* 33, 923–931, 2001.

EFSA, European Food Safety Authority. Control: the European Union Summary Report on Trends and Sources of Zoonoses, Zoonotic Agents and Food-borne Outbreaks in 2009. *EFSA J.* 9, 2090, 2011.

Fratamico P et al., Prevalence and characterization of shiga toxin-producing Escherichia coli in swine feces recovered in the National Animal Health Monitoring System's Swine 2000 study. *Appl. Environ. Microbiol.* 70, 7173–7178, 2004.

Garcia A et al., A naturally occurring rabbit model of enterohemorrhagic, Escherichia coli-induced disease. *J. Infect. Dis.* 186, 1682–1686, 2002.

Kaper JB, Nataro JP, Mobley HL, Pathogenic Escherichia coli. *Nat. Rev. Microbiol.* 2, 123–140, 2004.

Karch H, Mellmann A, Bielaszewska M, Epidemiology and pathogenesis of enterohaemorrhagic Escherichia coli. *Berl. Munch. Tierarztl. Wochenschr.* 122, 417–424, 2009.

Karch H, Mellmann A, Bielaszewska M, Epidemiology and pathogenesis of enterohaemorrhagic Escherichia coli. *Berl. Munch. Tierarztl. Wochenschr.* 122, 417–424, 2009.

Mellmann A et al., Analysis of collection of hemolytic uremic syndrome-associated enterohemorrhagic Escherichia coli. *Emerg. Infect. Dis.* 14, 1287–1290, 2008.

O'Brien SJ, Adak GK, Gilham C, Contact with farming environment as a major risk factor for Shiga toxin (Vero cytotoxin)-producing Escherichia coli O157 infection in humans. *Emerg. Infect. Dis.* 7, 1049–1051, 2001.

Orth D et al., Cytolethal distending toxins in Shiga toxin-producing Escherichia coli: alleles, serotype distribution and biological effects. *J. Med. Microbiol.* 55, 1487–1492, 2006.

Page AV, Liles WC, Enterohemorrhagic Escherichia coli infections and the hemolytic-uremic syndrome. *Med Clin North Am* 97, 681–695, 2013.

Paton AW, Paton JC, Escherichia coli subtilase cytotoxin. *Toxins (Basel)* 2, 215–228, 2010.

Persson S et al., Subtyping method for Escherichia coli shiga toxin (verocytotoxin) 2 variants and correlations to clinical manifestations. *J. Clin. Microbiol.* 45, 2020–2024, 2007.

Salvadori M, Bertoni E, Update on hemolytic uremic syndrome: diagnostic and therapeutic recommendations. *World J Nephrol* 2, 56–76, 2013.

Schmidt MA, LEEways: tales of EPEC, ATEC and EHEC. *Cell. Microbiol.* 12, 1544–1552, 2010.

Tarr PI, Gordon CA, Chandler WL, Shiga-toxin-producing Escherichia coli and haemolytic uraemic syndrome. *Lancet* 365, 1073–1086, 2005.

Yukioka H, Kurita S, Escherichia coli O157 infection disaster in Japan, 1996. *Eur. J. Emerg. Med.* 4, 165, 1997.

Erickson MC, Doyle MP, Food as a vehicle for transmission of Shiga toxin-producing Escherichia coli. *J. Food Prot.* 70, 2426–2449, 2007.

2.10 Erysipeloid

Erysipeloid is a mostly acute infection, particularly of pigs, but also of other animals and even of humans. The causative agent is *Erysipelothrix rhusiopathiae*. In humans, the disease is characterized by a localized or diffuse cutaneous inflammation.

E. rhusiopathiae is a nonmotile, slender, straight or slightly curved Gram-positive rod, is nonfastidious, and grows between 5 and 42 °C. The genus shows 26 serovars and an N (nonreactive) group that do not parallel the subdivision into species (*E. rhusiopathiae*, *E. tonsillarum*, and *E. inopinata*). Seventy-five to 80% of all pig isolates belong to serovars 1 and 2. There are distinct differences in the virulence of individual strains, an important factor being the heat-labile anionic polysaccharide capsule that protects *E. rhusiopathiae* from phagocytosis. The significance of the adhesive surface proteins RspA and RspB and of the hemolysin have not been elucidated.

The other two species have not been identified as being zoonotic. *E. tonsillarum* has been found in the tonsils of healthy pigs, in heart valves of dogs with endocarditis, and in surface waters. *E. inopinata* was found in a peptone broth prepared from plant material.

Occurrence. *E. rhusiopathiae* occurs worldwide. Under natural conditions, it is probably able to multiply only in a host. That spectrum is wide and encompasses many mammals (including marine ones), birds, reptiles, and fish, but also cephalopods, crustaceans, and arthropods. Outside of such hosts, *E. rhusiopathiae* is frequently found on decaying substrates, in moist soil, and in sewage, which offer optimal survival conditions (up to 9 months).

Human disease is closely associated with the occurrence in pigs, poultry (particularly turkey and ducks), as well as fresh and salt water fish. Other birds and mammals, such as lambs, horses, cattle, dogs, mice, rats, and fur-bearing animals, are rare as sources. Human erysipeloid is primarily a professional disease. At risk are butchers, veterinarians, farmers, animal care personnel, fisher, fish vendors, knackers, personnel in the fish, meat, and poultry industry, cooks and people in contact with sewage from slaughterhouses. In them, erysipeloid is a sporadic infection. Group disease and smaller epidemics with dozens of cases have been reported.

Transmission. In animals, *E. rhusiopathiae* is frequently found on tonsils and in the throat. Infected animals excrete the organism in urine, feces, saliva, and nasal secretions. Infection in humans is established through skin lesions in contact with infectious animal organs and secretions, for example, mucus from fish or through contaminated instruments. Even dog bites may lead to infection. Foodborne infections could occur but seem to be rare.

Clinical Manifestations. Three manifestations can be discerned: a localized cutaneous infection (erysipeloid), a diffuse skin infections, and septicemia.

In the localized infection, a sharply demarcated, centrifugal redness develops at the portal of entry after an incubation period of 2 to 5 days (Fig. 2.12). Initially, the erythema is bluish, later blue-red, and then fades centrally. Sometimes, a small blister or an ulcer will develop at this site. There is no pus but the site and its surroundings are edematous. Edema, itching, and pain can be so intense that there will be limitation of motion in the adjacent joints. Occasionally, erysipeloid is accompanied by fever, lymphangitis, and regional lymphadenitis. Painful arthritis of the adjacent joints is rare. The symptoms tend to disappear within 1 to 3 weeks.

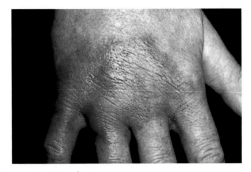

Figure 2.12 | Erysipeloid. Progressive erythema with edema and hemorrhagic areas (courtesy of Klinische Visite Bildtafeln Thomae, No. 114, Bildarchiv für Medizin GmbH, Munich, Germany).

The diffuse/generalized form is rare. Starting from the primary lesion, inflammatory foci show at several distant sites. A protracted course is the rule, and patients often complain of fever, joint and muscle pain. There may be relapses.

Septicemia is rare (<1%) but frequently leads to endocarditis, particularly on already damaged valves. The case-fatality rate can reach 38%. Chronic arthritis, encephalitis, meningitis, nephritis with renal failure, and peritonitis are further rare complications.

Pigs are frequently infected with *E. rhusiopathiae* but develop disease, that is, chronic to peracute septicemia, only if other diseases are present or the animals are poorly kept. Acutely and subacutely ill animals show fever and edematous red areas looking like maps or rectangles. Pregnant sows may abort. A peracute course quickly leads to septicemia without cutaneous symptoms (white erysipeloid). Chronic erysipeloid leads to stunting, mostly accompanied by dermatitis, arthritis, endocarditis, and spondylitis. Erysipeloid in pigs is a widespread, frequent, and economically important disease.

In sheep, particularly in lambs from the second to the third month of life, eysipeloid manifests itself mostly as chronic polyarthritis, less frequently as septicemia. In poultry, especially in turkeys and ducks, and in zoo- and wild birds, erysipeloid appears as a septicemia with fever, lassitude, dyspnea, cyanosis, diarrhea, arthritis, and hemorrhages. The case-fatality rate may be up to 40%. Erysipeloid in other animals (cattle, horse, dog, rodents, fur-bearing zoo- and wild animals) is sporadic, mostly in young ones, but, similar to pigs, acute septicemic and chronic cases may occur.

Diagnosis. The diagnosis can be secured by culture of a biopsy specimen from the edge of the lesion, which should extend to the subcutis. *E. rhusiopathiae* grows well aerobically at 37 °C within 1 to 3 days. Many strains prefer a 5 to 10% CO_2 atmosphere. Dissociation into S and R forms with characteristic cellular and colonial morphology develops particularly following repeated passages. Speciation is based on morphological and biochemical characteristics. Various (multiplex) PCR methods have been designed for genus and species recognition. Serological tests are without merit. In pigs, the characteristic skin changes allow for a tentative diagnosis, which will be confirmed by culture of various organs, including skin.

Differential Diagnosis. Because of its characteristic aspect, the typical localization (hand, finger) and history (profession, injury), erysipeloid is easily distinguished from streptococcal erysipelas and from erythema chronicum migrans. Erysipelas shows a stronger redness, a tendency to spread over large areas, fever, and general symptoms. Erythema chronicum migrans is rare on the hands, is not painful, is often ring or double ring-like, and enlarges more slowly.

Therapy. Keeping the affected extremity in a resting position plus moist compresses may suffice. Penicillin V 1 to 2 mio. IU/day p.o. for 5 to 10 days may shorten the duration. For septicemia, 10 to 20 mio. IU penicillin/day should be used for 4 to 6 weeks. Patients with penicillin allergy may receive a cephalosporin or a fluoroquinolone although in a few instances resistance against the latter has been reported. Vancomycin, trimethoprim-sulfamethoxazole and aminoglycosides are ineffective.

Acute diseases in animals are treated with penicillin, formerly in combination with an erysipeloid antiserum. Chronic arthritis and spondylitis do not react to these therapies.

Prophylaxis. Contact with infected animals or contaminated material (carcasses, furs, bones, fish bones) requires wearing of gloves. Instruments, tabletops, and hands are to be cleaned and disinfected. Wounds should be cleaned and disinfected. Injuries showing signs of inflammation must be treated immediately. In pigs and turkeys, whole cell inactivated and live vaccines have been used.

REFERENCES

Brooke CJ, Riley TV, Erysipelothrix rhusiopathiae, bacteriology, epidemiology and clinical manifestations of an occupational pathogen. *J. Med. Microbiol.* 48, 789–799, 1999.

Eamens GJ et al., Evaluation of Erysipelothrix rhusiopathiae vaccines in pigs by intradermal challenge and immune responses. *Vet. Microbiol.* 116, 138–148, 2006.

Fidalgo SG, Longbottom CJ, Rjley TV, Susceptibility of Erysipelothrix rhusiopathiae to antimicrobial agents and home disinfectants. *Pathology (Phila.)* 34, 462–465, 2002.

Gorby GL, Peacock JEJr, Erysipelothrix rhusiopathiae endocarditis: microbiologic, epidemiologic, and clinical features of an occupational disease. *Rev. Infect. Dis.* 10, 317–325, 1988.

Hocqueloux L et al., Septic arthritis caused by Erysipelothrix rhusiopathiae in a prosthetic knee joint. *J. Clin. Microbiol.* 48, 333–335, 2010.

Imada Y et al., Serotyping of 800 strains of Erysipelothrix isolated from pigs affected with erysipelas and discrimination of attenuated live vaccine strain by genotyping. *J. Clin. Microbiol.* 42, 2121–2126, 2004.

Kanai Y et al., Occurrence of zoonotic bacteria in retail game meat in Japan with special reference to Erysipelothrix. *J Food Prot.* 60, 328–331, 1997.

Ko SB et al., A case of multiple brain infarctions associated with Erysipelothrix rhusiopathiae endocarditis. *Arch. Neurol.* 60, 434–436, 2003.

Neumann EJ et al., Safety of a live attenuated Erysipelothrix rhusiopathiae vaccine for swine. *Vet. Microbiol.* 135, 297–303, 2009.

Ogawa Y et al., The genome of Erysipelothrix rhusiopathiae, the causative agent of swine erysipelas, reveals new insights into the evolution of firmicutes and the organism's intracellular adaptations. *J. Bacteriol.* 193, 2959–2971, 2011.

Pal N, Bender JS, Opriessnig T, Rapid detection and differentiation of Erysipelothrix spp. by a novel multiplex real-time PCR assay. *J. Appl. Microbiol.* 108, 1083–1093, 2010.

Reboli AC, Farrar WE, Erysipelothrix rhusiopathiae: an occupational pathogen. *Clin. Microbiol. Rev.* 2, 354–359, 1989.

Romney M, Cheung S, Montessori V, Erysipelothrix rhusiopathiae endocarditis and presumed osteomyelitis. *Can J Infect Dis* 12, 254–256, 2001.

Rosskopf-Streicher U et al., Quality control of inactivated erysipelas vaccines: results of an international collaborative study to establish a new regulatory test. *Vaccine* 19, 1477–1483, 2001.

Ruiz ME et al., Erysipelothrix rhusiopathiae septic arthritis. *Arthritis Rheum.* 48, 1156–1157, 2003.

Schuster MG, Brennan PJ, Edelstein P, Persistent bacteremia with Erysipelothrix rhusiopathiae in a hospitalized patient. *Clin. Infect. Dis.* 17, 783–784, 1993.

Shimoji Y, Pathogenicity of Erysipelothrix rhusiopathiae: virulence factors and protective immunity. *Microbes Infect.* 2, 965–972, 2000.

Stenström IM et al., Occurrence of different serotypes of Erysipelothrix rhusiopathiae in retail pork and fish. *Acta Vet. Scand.* 33, 169–173, 1992.

Tlougan BE, Podjasek JO, Adams BB, Aquatic sports dermatoses: Part 3. On the water. *Int. J. Dermatol.* 49, 1111–1120, 2010.

Umana E, Erysipelothrix rhusiopathiae: an unusual pathogen of infective endocarditis. *Int. J. Cardiol.* 88, 297–299, 2003.

Veraldi S et al., Erysipeloid: a review. *Clin. Exp. Dermatol.* 34, 859–862, 2009.

Wang Q, Chang BJ, Riley TV, Erysipelothrix rhusiopathiae. *Vet. Microbiol.* 140, 405–417, 2010.

2.11 Glanders

Malleus (glanders, farcy) is an acute to chronic bacterial infection primarily of horses and other ungulates, characterized by pustular skin lesions, multiple abscesses, necrotic processes in the respiratory tract, pneumonia, and septicemia. It is occasionally transmitted to humans, resulting in a mostly fatal disease.

Etiology. Glanders is caused by *Burkholderia mallei*, a nonfermenting Gram-negative coccoid to pleomorphic, nonmotile, aerobic rod. In contrast to other *Burkholderia* species, *B. mallei* is obligately parasitic, multiplying intracellularly in epithelial cells and phagocytes. Virulence factors are the polysaccharide capsule and type III and VI protein secretion systems.

Occurrence. Horses, donkeys, and mules are the animals most susceptible to *B. mallei*. Important reservoirs are infected horses, sheep, goats, dogs, and large cats, for example, lions, tigers, etc. Public health programs have eliminated glanders in many countries; the last cases in Germany were seen several years ago. At present, the disease is still seen in Mongolia, China, India, Pakistan, Indonesia, the Philippines, Iraq, Iran, the United Arab Emirates, Eritrea, Ethiopia, and Brazil. Single cases have also been reported from Turkey. The first case in the US, after more than 50 years of absence, was reported in a military microbiologist.

At particular risk are animal caretakers, veterinarians, horse dealers, butchers, abattoir workers, knackers, and laboratory personnel. *B. mallei* is considered a potential bioweapon, with work restricted to biosafety level 3 laboratories.

Transmission. Transmission occurs mainly through contact with infected animals or indirectly through fomites, such as food, litter, cleaning tools, troughs, and water containers. All excreta from infected animals, particularly nasal discharge, secretions and pus, are potential sources. Portals of entry are the mucous membranes of the mouth, throat, nose, and eyes, or small skin lesions arising from animal dissections. Aerogenic transmission through inhalation is particularly dangerous. Rare cases of human-to-human transmission have been reported under conditions of patient care and sexual contact.

Clinical Manifestations. The incubation period lasts from 1 to 5 days in acute and possibly longer in chronic infections. Prodromes are nonspecific. The portal of entry at first shows an indolent soft swelling that later ulcerates and eventually becomes gangrenous with involvement of regional lymph channels and nodes. Within a few days, septicemia will develop with high fever, chills, myalgias, and widespread involvement of internal organs (lung, liver, spleen, meninges, brain). During the second week, the temperature may rise further and a maculopapular exanthema may be seen, which becomes pustulous and finally exulcerates. In some cases, the patient dies within 7 to 10 days.

Chronic suppurative glanders may take a course lasting for several months and even years. It is characterized by multiple subcutaneous and intramuscular abscesses and ulcers with regional lymphadenitis (Fig. 2.13), which will have to be drained surgically. The disease may be limited to the nose and mouth but may also develop into the acute, generalized form with a lethal outcome.

Nasal glanders is a special form characterized by bloody and/or purulent inflammation of the mucosa and surrounding tissues. Bony and cartilaginous structures of the nose may break down. Extension to pharynx and upper respiratory tract is possible. The case-fatality rate of untreated glanders is close to 100%; in chronic cases, it approaches 50%.

In ungulates, malleus is often a chronic disease with formation of exudative/necrotizing and proliferative areas, pustules and nodules in skin, nose, lung, and, occasionally, other organs

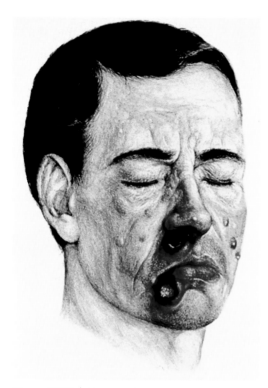

Figure 2.13 | Glanders: Multiple eschars.

(e.g., testes). The draining lymph nodes are swollen, painful and may become purulent. In donkeys and mules, an acute/subacute form with high fever will develop; in horses, the disease is frequently chronic or latent. Both lead to excretion of *B. mallei* that is epidemiologically significant but often overlooked.

Diagnosis. A definite diagnosis can only be made by isolation of *B. mallei* from pustules, pus, or sputum. The organism grows well on routine laboratory media. Speciation is accomplished by biochemical tests or by PCR. CF tests and ELISA are positive from the 10th day of illness. Agglutination titers of 1:>400 are suspicious. In ungulates, CF and agglutination, as well as intradermal mallein tests, are internationally accepted. Culture and PCR can also be used but should only be performed in safety level 3 laboratories.

Differential Diagnosis. Melioidosis, tuberculosis, anthrax, erysipelas, smallpox, and syphilis have to be considered.

Therapy. Ceftazidime or imipenem i.v. for 2 to 4 weeks or until clinical improvement has set in, then doxycycline or trimethoprim-sulfamethoxazole for another 20 weeks. Susceptibility tests should be performed as there may be resistance to multiple antibiotics. Treatment of diseased or possibly infected animals is prohibited in many countries.

Prophylaxis. No vaccines or antisera are available. Postexposition prophylaxis may be undertaken with trimethoprim-sulfamethoxazole or doxycycline plus ampicillin-clavulanic acid for 3 weeks. The most effective means is veterinary control of animals, particularly of those imported from endemic areas. If an epidemic is suspected, diseased animals are killed, with appropriate protection for humans. Fomites have to be destroyed or thoroughly cleaned and disinfected.

REFERENCES

Anonymous, *Glanders*. The Center for Food Security and Public Health, Iowa State University. http://www.cfsph.iastate.edu/Factsheets/pdfs/glanders.pdf. 2007.

Anonymous, *Glanders and Meliodosis, Guidelines for Action in the Event of Deliberate Release*. http://www.hpa.org.uk/web/HPAwebFile/HPAweb_C/1194947412449. Health Protection Agency, 2008.

Bondi SK, Goldberg JB, Strategies toward vaccines against Burkholderia mallei and Burkholderia pseudomallei. *Expert Rev. Vaccines*, 7, 1357–1365, 2008.

Centers for: Disease Control and Prevention(CDC). Laboratory-acquired human glanders—Maryland, May, 2000. MMWR Morb Mortal Wkly Rep. 49, 532–535, 2000.

Elschner M et al., Use of a Western blot technique for the serodiagnosis of glanders. *BMC Vet. Res.* 7, 4, 2011.

Estes D et al., Present and future therapeutic strategies for melioidosis and glanders. *Expert Rev. Anti Infect. Ther.* 8, 325–338, 2010.

Galyov EE, Brett PJ, DeShazer D, Molecular insights into Burkholderia pseudomallei and Burkholderia mallei pathogenesis. *Annu. Rev. Microbiol.* 64, 495–517, 2010.

Kenny DJ et al., In vitro susceptibilities of Burkholderia mallei in comparison to those of other pathogenic Burkholderia spp. Antimicrob. *Agents Chemother.* 43, 2773–2775, 1999.

Mohammad TJ, Sawa MI, Yousif YA, Orchitis in Arab stallion due to Pseudomonas mallei. *Indian J. Vet. Med.* 9, 15–17, 1989.

Rowland CA et al., Protective cellular responses to Burkholderia mallei infection. *Microbes Infect.* 12, 846–853, 2010.

Schmoock G et al., DNA microarray-based detection and identification of: Burkholderia mallei, Burkholderia pseudomallei and Burkholderia spp. *Mol. Cell. Probes* 23, 178–187, 2009.

Srinivasan A et al., Glanders in a military research microbiologist. *N. Engl. J. Med.* 345, 256–258, 2001.

Van Zandt KE, Greer MT, Gelhaus HC., Glanders: an overview of infections in humans. *Orphanet. J. Rare. Dis.* 8, 131, 2013.

Verma RD et al., Development of an avidin-biotin dot enzyme-linked immunosorbent assay and its comparison with other serological tests for diagnosis of glanders in equines. *Vet. Microbiol.* 25, 77–85, 1990.

Whitlock GC, Estes DM, Torres AG, Glanders: off to the races with Burkholderia mallei. *FEMS Microbiol. Lett.* 277, 115–122, 2007.

2.12 Leptospiroses

Leptospiroses are acute systemic infections of humans and animals caused by various serovars of the genus *Leptospira*. For names of the diseases, see Tab. 2.7. The most serious infection is Weil's disease, with fever, hemorrhagic complications, and renal failure.

Etiology. Leptospirae are spiral-shaped, motile bacteria measuring 6 to 20×0.1 µm, with both ends bent hook-like in the same direction. The cellular structure is that of a Gram-negative bacterium but staining results in a Gram-labile appearance. Culture is difficult and requires long-chain fatty acids as sources for carbon and energy. Optimal are liquid or semisolid media containing serum, that is, Tween 80/BSA-, Fletcher-, Ellinghausen-McCullough-Johnson-Harris (EMJH) or Korthof medium with rabbit serum incubated at 28 to 30 °C. Visualization is by darkfield microscopy.

Molecular genetic research has led to a revision of the genus. The former subdivision in to two species, *L. interrogans* (pathogenic) and *L. biflexa* (saprophytic, environmental, nonpathogenic) has been abandoned in favor of 21 genomospecies (www.bacterio.net), with 25 serogroups and >200 serovars. Both pathogenic and nonpathogenic serovars may occur within one species, and some serovars belong to multiple species. The former *L. interrogans* and *L. biflexa* are now genospecies *sensu stricto*.

Occurrence. The pathogenic leptospires have a wide spectrum of hosts including humans. Each serovar is adapted to one or a few animal species in which it is maintained and serves as a reservoir. Hosts can remain infected for years or life-long as permanent excretors even without symptoms. The relevant serovars for humans and their hosts are listed in Tab. 2.7.

Carriers of pathogenic leptospires have a worldwide distribution in >180 animal species, particularly in tropical and subtropical countries and mainly in farm animals (pigs, cattle, horses) and pets (dogs). Infections have also been

Table 2.7 | Most important agents of leptospirosis in humans

LEPTOSPIRA SEROVAR(S)	MAIN AND PERSISTENT HOST(S)	COMMON NAMES OF HUMAN DISEASE
Australis	Hedgehogs, rats	Field fever, canefield fever, canecutter fever, pea pickers' disease
Autumnalis	Mice	Fort Bragg fever
Bataviae, sejro	Mice, rats	Harvest fever, rice field fever
Canicola	Dogs, jackals	Canicola fever
Grippotyphosa	Mice, hamsters, raccoons	Mud fever, field fever, pea pickers' disease
Hardjo	Cattle, sheep	Dairy farm fever
Ictero-haemorrhagiae, copenhageni	Rats	Weil's disease, rice field fever
Pomona	Pigs, cattle, sheep	Swine herd disease
Tarassovi	Pigs, mice	Swine herd disease

observed in wild animals, such as wild boar, foxes, hares, hedgehogs, bats, and marsupials.

In human populations, leptospires occur throughout the year with a peak in summer and fall. The yearly incidence in moderate climates is ci. 0.1 to 1.0 and in tropical and subtropical countries 1.0 to 10 per 100 000 inhabitants. At risk are farm workers, veterinarians, breeders and animal caretakers, slaughterhouse personnel, butchers, workers in meat processing plants, abattoirs and sewage systems, hunters in general but especially rat and mouse hunters, animal trappers, and cooks. Leptospiroses are also more frequent in people living in inundated areas, those engaged in water sports, and adventure tourists traversing swamps and primeval forests. In industrialized countries, individual cases or small epidemics may occur, whereas in developing countries, one may figure with epidemics comprising several thousand infections and possibly hundreds of fatal cases.

Transmission. Leptospires have a particular affinity for the urogenital tract, especially the kidneys. Infected animals excrete large numbers with urine, amniotic fluid, and materials from abortion. The tenacity of leptospires is generally low but they are able to remain infectious for several months in moist environments with a slightly alkaline pH.

Transmission to humans is mostly indirect via items contaminated with sources such as moist soil and surface waters. The usual portals of entry are skin lesions due to professional exposure, swimming, or barefoot walking. In infections following bites by rats, mice, or hamsters, animal urine voided at the time of the bite is the most likely source of infection. Lesions in the mucous membranes of nose, mouth, and eyes may also become portals of entry, for example, after drinking from brooks or swimming and diving in contaminated (e.g., canal) water. Infection via contaminated foodstuffs is rare.

Clinical Manifestations. Leptospires are able to invade any organ system. They cause damage to endothelial cells by means of a cytotoxic glycoprotein and induce vasculitides with bleeding or ischemic lesions.

Most infections follow a subclinical course. The incubation period in symptomatic cases is 5 to 14 days (range, 2 to 26 days). All leptospiroses follow a similar diphasic course. The first bacteremic phase (4 to 7 days) lacks prodromes and starts out with a sudden bout of fever up to 40 °C, chills, malaise, headache, signs of meningeal irritation, a nonproductive cough, myalgias (particularly in the calf and lumbar areas), conjunctival hyperemia, and hemorrhages. Hepatomegaly, mild jaundice, abdominal pain, loss of appetite, nausea, vomiting, and diarrhea may also be observed. During this phase, leptospires can be detected in blood and CSF. After specific antibodies have been formed, fever and clinical symptoms will abate for 1 to 5 days but leptospires can still be found in the kidney, CSF, and urine.

In approximately 50% of cases, the disease will go into a second, "immune" phase that may last up to 3 months and in which leptospires are still excreted in the urine. Then, fever will return and, depending on the serovar, certain organ systems will be affected with various degrees of severity: aseptic meningitis, iridocyclitis, jaundice, renal failure (azotemia, oligo- or anuria), anemia, thrombocytopenia, hemorrhages (petechiae to severe bleeding in skin, lung, kidneys, intestine), hemorrhagic pneumonia with ARDS, interstitial myocarditis with arrhythmia, and circulatory collapse. Leptospires may also cause fetal death and abortion. Late sequelae in 25% of patients with severe disease are myalgias, lassitude, headache, tinnitus, and psychoses. The worldwide case-fatality rate is, on average, ci. 10%; however, in severe cases it may reach 40%, mostly due to renal and liver failure.

In animals, particularly in reservoir hosts, leptospiral infections are mostly inapparent. Leptospiroses may yet occur in domestic animals, manifesting themselves, similar to disease in humans, as acute or chronic systemic infections with nonspecific symptoms (fever, loss of appetite and energy) and anemia, bloody urine, hemorrhages (sclerae), vomiting, convulsions, nephritis, and hepatitis with jaundice. Depending on the infecting serovar, animal species and the immune status, fatal outcome may be possible. In farm animals, leptospirae may cause agalactia, stillbirths, abortion, neonatal weakness, and infertility. Recurrent equine uveitis (periodic eye inflammation, moon blindness) is perhaps an immunopathological sequel of acute leptospirosis.

Diagnosis. A thorough history of the patient is important, including a review of occupational and recreational activities, animal contacts, and occurrence of sudden or recurrent fever. Proof of the diagnosis is provided by microbiological and serological testing. During the first 10 days of illness, an attempt can be made to visualize leptospirae in blood or urine by darkfield examination (low sensitivity!) or immunofluorescence. Urine will contain few organisms, generally beginning with the second week.

Cultures have to be incubated for up to 13 weeks and examined weekly by microscopy. PCR is possible but has limitations (low number of organisms, inhibitory substances or contamination of the sample), although sensitivity is higher than that of culture (which is up to 50%). The microagglutination test (MAT) is the method of choice for detection of antibodies and will yield positive results at the earliest on the 5th to 9th day of illness. It should be followed up by repeat testing within 8 to 10 days, with a fourfold increase in titer being diagnostic. Depending on the choice of antigens used, the serogroup can be diagnosed but cross-reactivity will account for problems with the serovar identification. ELISA, in particular, dot-ELISA and dipstick-ELISA, which measure IgM, will be positive earlier than MAT. IgM antibodies can persist over months and they should not be interpreted as signs of a persistent infection. Positive results should be checked with MAT. Cross reactions are said to occur in patients with *Borrelia* or *Treponema* infections. Early treatment may suppress antibody formation. In animals, MAT is the test of choice.

Differential Diagnosis. During the first week, influenza, rheumatic fever, streptococcal tonsillitis, salmonellosis, brucellosis, septicemia of various etiologies, and, in areas of endemicity, malaria, dengue, and typhus should be considered. During the second week, all forms of hepatitis, tuberculous meningitis, acute glomerulonephritis, EHEC infections as well as hantavirus infection, and in the tropics, yellow fever should be included in the differential diagnosis.

Therapy. Penicillin G 4 × 1.5 mio IE/day i.v.; or ceftriaxone 1 × 1 g/day i.v.; or doxycycline 2 × 100 mg/day i.v. or p.o.; or ampicillin 4 × 0.5 to 1.0 gm/day i.v. for 7 days; or azithromycin (first day, 1 g; 2nd and 3rd day 500 mg each p.o.). A Jarisch-Herxheimer reaction is possible. Severe cases have to be hospitalized. In cases of renal failure, dialysis will increase the chance of survival. Diseased animals are treated with tetracycline or streptomycin.

Prophylaxis. Chains of transmission between infected animals and humans must be broken, especially by rat and mouse control as well as cleansing and disinfection of items contaminated with urine or stool. People exposed through professional or recreational activities (see above) should wear protective clothing, such as watertight boots, gloves, and goggles, and should cover blemishes with tightly fitting compresses. Barefoot walking and swimming in stagnant waters should be avoided in endemic areas. Chemoprophylaxis with doxycycline 1 × 200 mg p.o. per week seems to be efficacious in >95% of exposed people.

Active immunoprophylaxis has been reported from China, Cuba, France, and Russia. Immunity was serovar-specific and lasted for a few months. For cattle, pigs, and dogs, vaccination has been approved in many countries. Its protection is also serovar-specific but has led to a reduction in the numbers of leptospirae excreted, thereby contributing to the protection of contacts.

Reporting. Leptospirosis is a notifiable disease in the U.S.

REFERENCES

Agampodi S, Peacock SJ, Thevanesam V, The potential emergence of leptospirosis in Sri Lanka. *Lancet Infect. Dis.* 9, 524–526, 2009.

Ahmed A et al., Development and validation of a real-time PCR for detection of pathogenic Leptospira species in clinical materials. *PLoS ONE* 4, e7093, 2009.

Anonymous, *Human Leptospirosis: Guidance for Diagnosis, Surveillance and Control*. World Health Organization, Geneva, 2003.

Anonymous, *Leptospirosis*. World Organization for Animal Health, Paris, 2008.

Bharti AR et al., Leptospirosis: a zoonotic disease of global importance. *Lancet Infect. Dis.* 3, 757–771, 2003.

Bolin CA, Koellner P, Human-to-human transmission of Leptospira interrogans by milk. *J. Infect. Dis.* 158, 246–247, 1988.

Bovet P et al., Factors associated with clinical leptospirosis: a population-based case-control study in the Seychelles (Indian Ocean). *Int. J. Epidemiol.* 28, 583–590, 1999.

Centers for: Disease Control and Prevention (CDC). Update: outbreak of acute febrile illness among athletes participating in Eco-Challenge-Sabah 2000-Borneo, Malaysia, 2000. MMWR Morb. Mortal. Wkly. Rep. 50, 21–24, 2001.

Chappel RJ et al., Impact of proficiency testing on results of the microscopic agglutination test for diagnosis of leptospirosis. *J. Clin. Microbiol.* 42, 5484–5488, 2004.

Dupont H et al., Leptospirosis: prognostic factors associated with mortality. *Clin. Infect. Dis.* 25, 720–724, 1997.

Emmanouilides CE, Kohn OF, Garibaldi R, Leptospirosis complicated by a Jarisch-Herxheimer reaction and adult respiratory distress syndrome: case report. *Clin. Infect. Dis.* 18, 1004–1006, 1994.

Faine S et al., Fatal congenital human leptospirosis. *Zentralbl. Bakteriol. Mikrobiol. Hyg.* A 257, 548, 1984.

Guerra MA, Leptospirosis: public health perspectives. *Biologicals* 41, 295–297, 2013.

Hartskeerl RA, Collares-Pereira M, Ellis WA, Emergence, control and re-emerging leptospirosis: dynamics of infection in the changing world. *Clin. Microbiol. Infect.* 17, 494–501, 2011.

Heron LG et al., Leptospirosis presenting as a haemorrhagic fever in a traveller from Africa. *Med. J. Aust.* 167, 477–479, 1997.

Jansen A et al., Leptospirosis in Germany, 1962–2003. *Emerg. Infect. Dis.* 11, 1048–1054, 2005.

Katz AR et al., Assessment of the clinical presentation and treatment of 353 cases of laboratory-confirmed leptospirosis in Hawaii, 1974–1998. *Clin. Infect. Dis.* 33, 1834–1841, 2001.

Koizumi N et al., Serological and genetic analysis of leptospirosis in patients with acute febrile illness in Kandy, Sri Lanka. *Jpn. J. Infect. Dis.* 62, 474–475, 2009.

Levett PN et al., Leptospirosis. *Clin. Microbiol. Rev.* 14, 296–326, 2001.

Nardone A et al., Risk factors for leptospirosis in metropolitan France: results of a national case-control study, 1999–2000. *Clin. Infect. Dis.* 39, 751–753, 2004.

Seijo A et al., Lethal leptospiral pulmonary hemorrhage: an emerging disease in Buenos Aires, Argentina. *Emerg. Infect. Dis.* 8, 1004–1005, 2002.

Sejvar J et al., Leptospirosis in "Eco-Challenge" athletes, Malaysian Borneo, 2000. *Emerg. Infect. Dis.* 9, 702–707, 2003.

Smythe LD, Leptospirosis worldwide, 1999. *Wkly. Epidemiol. Rec.* 74, 237–242, 1999.

Svan Crevel R et al., Leptospirosis in travelers. *Clin. Infect. Dis.* 19, 132–134, 1994.

2.13 Listeriosis

Listeriosis is an infectious disease in animals and humans that manifests itself in a large variety of forms. Recent research has shown that it is primarily a foodborne disease, with animals being occasional sources for the bacterium (Fig. 2.14).

Etiology. *Listeria monocytogenes* is a Gram-positive, facultatively anaerobic, motile, non-sporeforming coccoid rod. On the basis of O and H antigens, 13 serovars can be distinguished, with ser 1/2a, 1/2b, and 4b the most frequent agents of disease. *L. monocytogenes* is not fastidious and is able to multiply at temperatures from 0° to 45 °C; therefore, it is regarded as psychrotolerant. It lives as a facultatively intracellular bacterium in vertebrates and is able to penetrate various host cells by a zipper mechanism, thereby transgressing epithelial barriers. Its parasitic lifestyle rests on a coordinated expression of several virulence factors, the most important ones being internalin InlA and InlB, listeriolysin O (LLO) and the actin-assembly inducing protein ActA. *L. ivanovii* subspp. *ivanovii* and *londoniensis*, *L. seeligeri*, and *L. innocua* have only rarely been reported as human pathogens. *L. murrayi, L. grayi, L. marthii, L. rocourtiae,* and *L. welshimeri* are not regarded as human pathogens.

Occurrence. *L. monocytogenes* is geophilic and ubiquitous in nature (soil, plants, surface waters). Material from soil and low quality, poorly ripened silage of corn, grass, oats, and legumes (pH >4.5), but not silage of beet leaves, play an important role as reservoirs. Listeriae have also been isolated from the intestine of farm animals (cattle, sheep, pigs), various pets (dogs, cats) and roebuck; zoo-, fur-, and laboratory animals, birds, cold blooded animals, and even from insects. In the stools of clinically healthy humans, listeriae have been found from 0.5 up to 70% (on repeat cultures); at

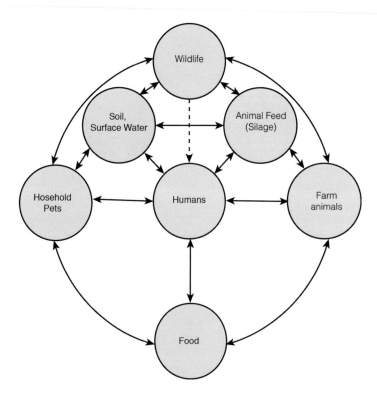

Figure 2.14 | Possible transmission chains for *Listeria monocytogenes*.

any time, 5 to 10% seem to be carriers. As the organism is excreted in the stool of humans and animals it can, via manure or sewage, contaminate plants and water sources.

Listeriosis occurs worldwide in humans and animals. In humans, it is more frequent in summer and fall than in winter; in animals, there is a peak between February and April. The incidence of human listeriosis in Germany is ci. 0.4 new infections per 100 000 inhabitants. It is one of the more frequent causes of newborn meningitis. Professional risk is highest in veterinarians, farm personnel, animal caretakers, slaughterhouse workers, and butchers.

Transmission. Epidemics and most individual cases are caused by consumption of contaminated foodstuffs. Among the latter, raw milk and soft cheeses (Brie, Camembert, Vacherin, Feta), meat and meat products such as sausages (raw ones and those heated during processing), tongue in aspic, raw smoked fish (e.g., vacuum packed smoked salmon), mussels, vegetables, sprouts, and salads. Pasteurized milk has been reported to contain listeriae if the bacterial load is very high but it seems possible that post-pasteurization played a role in these cases. Contamination with soil, dust, or feces is due to insufficient hygiene in handling food. Milk may also be contaminated through *Listeria* mastitis in cows or sheep due to hematogenous dissemination or direct ascending infection of the udder, with clinical symptoms of mastitis present or absent.

The initial number of listeriae in the food in question may be low but under storage conditions it may become high enough to cause disease (the minimum infectious dose is unknown but probably depends on host susceptibility and differences in virulence of individual strains). Enrichment at refrigerator temperature is possible because of the psychrotolerance of *Listeria*.

During pregnancy, *L. monocytogenes* may be transmitted *in utero* or colonize the infant at the time of delivery. Horizontal transmission in obstetrical wards is also possible, which increases the risk for healthy infants, physicians, midwives, and nurses.

Direct contact with diseased, for example, aborting, animals is another risk factor. Healthy carriers may transmit the organism via the conjunctivae of contacts. Airborne infections occurring after inhalation of dust during stable cleaning have also been described.

Clinical Manifestations. Certain factors predispose individuals to infection with *Listeria*: pregnancy, a compromised immune status, leukemia, Hodgkin's disease, diabetes, cytostatic treatment, but rarely HIV infection. Approximately two-thirds of all cases occur in people >60 years of age. The incubation period is uncertain but may range from 1 to 4 weeks. Symptoms have already been observed 3 to 4 days after ingestion of contaminated food. The following types of infection are known:

- Listeriosis in pregnancy. Mostly during the third trimester, an influenza-like illness with fever, chills, malaise, myalgias, arthralgias, back pain, and occasional diarrhea may occur. In many cases, however, the infection is subclinical or inapparent. Intrauterine infection may lead to miscarriage or premature delivery. Newborn disease is either early-onset (1 to 5 days p.p.) and occurs mostly in premature infants due to intrauterine infection, with signs of pneumonia, ARDS, and widespread abscesses ("granulomatosis infantiseptica"), or late-onset (>5 days p.p.), occurring mostly in infants apparently healthy at birth, due to colonization at birth, with signs of meningitis;
- Listeriosis of the CNS. Manifested as either meningitis or encephalitis, or meningoencephalitis. It may occur during *Listeria* septicemia or as a disease in itself. Mortality is between 40 and 50% even with treatment;
- Glandular listeriosis. It resembles infectious mononucleosis with swelling of the salivary glands and the nuchal lymph nodes. The oculoglandular type (Parinaud's syndrome) is characterized by local conjunctivitis with swelling of the regional lymph nodes;
- Localized form. Papulous and pustulous skin lesions on hands, arms, thorax. and face are prominent and are accompanied by fever;
- Typhoid form. Characterized by high fever and occurrence in immunocompromised individuals;

- Noninvasive febrile gastroenteritis. It occurs typically in immunocompetent individuals 6 to 10 days after ingestion of large inocula of *L. monocytogenes* and lasts for 1 to 3 days;
- Atypical cases: endocarditis, purulent pleuritis, pneumonia;
- Liver abscesses, arthritis, etc.

Listeriosis in animals may manifest itself in several forms occurring in all domestic animals. Cerebral listeriosis, characterized by loss of orientation, cranial nerve paresis, ataxia, occasional opisthotonus and coma, is most frequent in young sheep. In cattle, sheep, and pigs abortion, premature delivery, newborn weakness, and placentar retention are signs of genital listeriosis. In young animals (lambs, calves, piglets, foals), in rodents and poultry, septicemia is of particular concern because of its high mortality. Cases of mastitis, gastroenteritis, and ocular infection have been reported as well. Many animals are asymptomatically infected.

Diagnosis. The mainstay of the diagnosis is culture. Blood, CSF, pus, amniotic fluid, menstrual blood, lochia, and meconium are appropriate specimens for culture. In epidemics, stool culture may also be indicated. For sources containing mixed flora, for example, stool and selective media have been designed. These include lithium chloride-phenylethanol-moxalactam (LPM) agar, Oxford medium (Columbia agar with esculin, ferric ammonium citrate, lithium chloride, cycloheximide, colistin, acriflavin, cefotetan, and fosfomycin), and polymyxin B-acriflavin-lithium chloride-ceftazidime-esculin-mannitol (PALCAM) agar. Cold enrichment is less sensitive and tedious. Species identification is accomplished by biochemical tests and, recently, by MALDI-TOF mass spectrometry. Because of the high incidence of a few serovars, their determination for epidemiological purposes is not helpful. Molecular typing methods, such as multilocus enzmyme electrophoresis and DNA macrorestriction analysis (PFGE), are more useful. Antibody tests against listeriolysin O have not been standardized.

In live animals, the organism can be cultured from blood, CSF, feces or placenta. In dead animals, culture from brain, liver, or stomach contants of aborted fetuses may be attempted.

Differential Diagnosis.

- Newborn listeriosis: toxoplasmosis, cytome-galovirus disease, newborn septicemia and meningitis due to B streptococci or *Escherichia coli*;
- Glandular form: infectious mononucleosis, toxoplasmosis, yersiniosis;
- CNS listeriosis: meningoencephalitis due to *Streptococcus pneumoniae, Neisseria meningitidis, Haemophilus influenzae*;
- Other bacteria or viruses (e.g., adeno- or enteroviruses);
- Cutaneous form: dermatitis due to streptococci, staphylococci, Candida, and cercariae;
- *Candida* and cercariae;
- Typhoid form: septicemias due to other bacteria;
- Gastrointestinal form: gastrointestinal infections due to other bacteria.

Therapy. Ampicillin 6 × 2 g/day i.v. plus gentamicin 5 mg/kg/day i.v. or i.m. Equally effective is trimethoprim-sulfamethoxazole 3 to 4 × 15 to 20 mg/day i.v. Duration: in bacteremia, 2 weeks; in meningitis, 3 weeks; in other CNS infections, 6 to 8 weeks; in newborn listeriosis (early onset), >2 weeks. Listeriae are resistant to cephalosporins and the bactericidal effect of fluorochinolones against intracellular bacteria is diminished.

Prophylaxis. General hygienic measures should be observed, particularly in patients at high risk: peeling or thorough washing of raw vegetables, keeping uncooked separate from cooked food, and thorough cooking of raw food from animal sources. Pregnant women and immunocompromised individuals should avoid raw meat and vegetables, soft cheeses, and raw or marinated seafood.

Reporting. Leptospirosis is a notifiable disease in the U.S. and in Canada; in the latter, however, only the invasive forms.

REFERENCES

Allerberger F, Wagner M, Listeriosis: a resurgent food-borne infection. *Clin. Microbiol. Infect.* 16, 16–23, 2010.

Barbuddhe SB et al., Rapid identification and typing of Listeria species by matrix-assisted laser desorption ionization-time of flight mass spectrometry. *Appl. Environ. Microbiol.* 74, 5402–5407, 2008.

Centers for: Disease Control and Prevention (CDC). Vital signs: Listeria illnesses, deaths, and outbreaks – United States, 2009–2011. MMWR Morb Mortal Wkly Rep 62, 448–452, 2013.

Chakraborty T, The molecular mechanisms of actin-based intracellular motility by Listeria monocytogenes. *Microbiologia* 12, 237–244, 1996.

Drevets DA, Bronze MS, Listeria monocytogenes: epidemiology, human disease, and mechanisms of brain invasion. *FEMS Immunol. Med. Microbiol.* 53, 151–165, 2008.

Dussurget O, Pizarro-Cerda J, Cossart P, Molecular determinants of Listeria monocytogenes virulence. *Annu. Rev. Microbiol.* 58, 587–610, 2004.

Freitag NE, Port GC, Miner MD, Listeria monocytogenes - from saprophyte to intracellular pathogen. *Nat. Rev. Microbiol.* 7, 623–628, 2009.

Fretz R et al., Update: multinational listeriosis outbreak due to 'Quargel', a sour milk curd cheese, caused by two different L. monocytogenes serotype 1/2a strains, 2009–2010. *Euro Surveill.* 15, pii19543, 2010.

Gasanov U, Hughes D, Hansbro PM, Methods for the isolation and identification of Listeria spp. and Listeria monocytogenes: a review. *FEMS Microbiol. Rev.* 29, 851–875, 2005.

Hof H, An update on the medical management of listeriosis. *Expert Opin. Pharmacother.* 5, 1727–1735, 2004.

Jackson Br et al., Outbreak-associated Salmonella enterica serotypes and food commodities, United States, 1998–2008. *Emerg Infect Dis* 19, 1239–1244, 2013.

Johnsen BO et al., A large outbreak of: Listeria monocytogenes infection with short incubation period in a tertiary care hospital. *J. Infect.* 61, 465–470, 2010.

Koch J et al., Large listeriosis outbreak linked to cheese made from pasteurized milk, Germany, 2006–2007. *Foodborne Pathog. Dis.* 7, 1581–1584, 2010.

Koch J, Stark L, Significant increase of listeriosis in Germany – epidemiological patterns 2001–2005. *Euro Surveill.* 11, 85–88, 2006.

Lamont RF et al., Listeriosis in human pregnancy: a systematic review. *J. Perinat. Med.* 39, 227–236, 2011.

Lianou A, Sofos JN, A review of the incidence and transmission of: Listeria monocytogenes in ready-to-eat products in retail and food service environments. *J. Food Prot.* 70, 2172–2198, 2007.

McCollum JT et al., Multistate outbreak of listeriosis associated with cantaloupe. *N Engl J Med* 369, 944–953, 2013.

Orndorff PE et al., Host and bacterial factors in listeriosis pathogenesis. *Vet. Microbiol.* 114, 1–15, 2006.

Orsi RH, den Bakker HC, Wiedmann M, Listeria monocytogenes lineages: genomics, evolution, ecology, and phenotypic characteristics. *Int. J. Med. Microbiol.* 301, 79–96, 2010.

Perrin M, Bemer M, Delamare C, Fatal case of Listeria innocua bacteremia. *J. Clin. Microbiol.* 41, 5308–5309, 2003.

Rocourt J et al., Quantitative risk assessment of Listeria monocytogenes in ready-to-eat foods: the FAO/WHO approach. *FEMS Immunol. Med. Microbiol.* 35, 263–267, 2003.

Silk BJ et al., Invasive listeriosis in the Foodborne Diseases Active Surveillance Network (FoodNet), 2004–2009: Further targeted prevention needed for higher-.risk groups. *Clin Infect Dis* 54(Suppl 5), S396–404, 2012.

Thévenot D, Dernburg A, Vernozy-Rozand C, An updated review of Listeria monocytogenes in the pork meat industry and its products. *J. Appl. Microbiol.* 101, 7–17, 2006.

Vazquez-Boland J, Listeria pathogenesis and molecular virulence determinants. *Clin. Microbiol. Rev.* 14, 584–640, 2001.

Winter P et al., Clinical and histopathological aspects of naturally occurring mastitis caused by Listeria monocytogenes in cattle and ewes. *J. Vet. Med. B Infect. Dis. Vet. Public Health* 51, 176–179, 2004.

2.14 Mycobacterioses

2.14.1 INFECTIONS WITH THE *MYCOBACTERIUM TUBERCULOSIS* COMPLEX

Tuberculosis is a chronic disease of humans and animals caused by several pathogenic species of the genus *Mycobacterium*. Almost all of them can be transmitted between humans and animals.Tuberculosis, malaria, and AIDS belong to the three most frequent infectious diseases in humans. According to WHO statistics, 30% of the world's population is infected with tuberculosis, approximately 9 million people per year acquire the disease, and 1.7 million die. The large majority of human infections is due to transmission from other humans; only a small part (<10%) has its origin in animals.

Etiology. Mycobacteria are acid-fast rods that can be differentiated by cultural, biochemical, and molecular characteristics into more than 100 species and subspecies (www.bacterio.net). Important characteristics are aerobiosis, growth on special media, lack of motility, and a high content of lipids and mycolic acids in the cell wall. This special cell wall structure enables mycobacteria to resist chemical (disinfectants) and physical (heat) factors and to survive, even in the obligately parasitic species, for several months outside the host, for example, in dust or desiccated secretions.

Worldwide, the most frequent agent of human tuberculosis is *M. tuberculosis*, followed by *M. africanum* (mostly in western and central Africa), *M. bovis*, and *M. caprae*. Disease due to *M. microti*, *M. pinnipedii*, and *M. canettii* are sporadic. These species form the "*M. tuberculosis* complex." The most important agent of zoonotic tuberculosis is *M. bovis*, the agent of tuberculosis in cattle. *M. microti* was regarded as a commensal in humans until it was observed as an agent of human pulmonary tuberculosis in the Netherlands, France, and Germany. In some patients, contact with mice could be elicited but zoonotic chains of infection have not been fully elucidated.

Occurrence. Tuberculosis occurs worldwide in humans, as well as in wild and domesticated or captive mammals. All species of the *M.tuberculosis* complex have a wide spectrum of hosts including humans.

The main reservoir of *M. tuberculosis* and *M. africanum* are humans. Both species can be transmitted from infected individuals to animals. While infection in cattle does not cause disease, it can become symptomatic in parrots, wild and zoo animals, and may occasionally be transmitted to other animals or humans. *M. africanum*, frequent in tropical Africa, has also been sporadically observed in cattle, pigs, and zoo animals (rock hyraxes) in Europe but chains of transmission are still unclear.

The most important source for human *M. bovis* infections are cattle, although the risk of transmission has substantially declined because of successful control of disease in these animals. Actually, older people, or those coming from areas of endemic cattle tuberculosis and with open tuberculosis, are now endangering cattle. In 2008, the incidence of *M. bovis* tuberculosis in the European Union was 0.02 per 100 000 inhabitants. In Germany, only 1.9% of all cases of tuberculosis that were diagnosed by species were caused by *M. bovis* and 97.3% by *M. tuberculosis*.

The reduction in cattle tuberculosis has also led to a reduction in tuberculosis of pigs, horses, sheep, goats, dogs, and cats. The rare cases of the disease in dogs or cats are mostly caused by contact with human excretors of *M. tuberculosis* or *M. bovis*. Tuberculosis is still relatively frequent in large cats, cattle, antilopes, elephants, and primates in zoos, parks, and animal stores. In some countries, *M. bovis* has established itself in wild animals, which has rendered elimination of cattle tuberculosis more difficult. Examples are badgers (in the UK), wild boar (Spain), common brushtail possum (New Zealand), water buffalo (South Africa), white-tailed deer (USA), wood bison, and red deer (Canada).

M. caprae was originally detected in goats (Spain) but has since been found as an agent of tuberculosis in other European countries and other animal species, as well as in humans. *M. microti* causes naturally acquired generalized tuberculosis in mice ("vole bacillus" in wood mice and shrews) but has also been found in rock (Cape) hyraxes, llamas, badgers, ferrets, cattle, pigs, and cats. *M. pinnipedii* causes tuberculosis in seals. It can be transmitted to humans and, at a minimum, to camels and tapirs.

At particular risk for tuberculosis are people in contact with tuberculous animals, their secretions, and organs: veterinarians, farmers, milkers, abattoir workers, meat inspectors, autopsy personnel, animal keepers (also in zoos) and dealers, laboratory personnel, and owners of potentially infected pets (e.g., monkeys).

Transmission. Infected animals excrete tubercle bacteria with bronchial secretions, milk, urine, vaginal mucus, semen, or feces. Humans may acquire the disease through droplets or inhalation of infected dust, by the oral route (insufficiently heated milk or meat) or through direct injury to skin or mucous membranes (Fig. 2.15). Work with *M. tuberculosis* complex and *M. avium* requires biosafety 3 laboratories.

Clinical Manifestations. *M. tuberculosis* and *M. bovis* cause similar symptoms and pathologies. The incubation period is between 4 and 6 weeks. Symptoms may be manifold.

Primary tuberculosis is generally symptomless and recognizable only by conversion of tuberculin tests. Following inhalation of bacteria, a primary pulmonary focus develops that

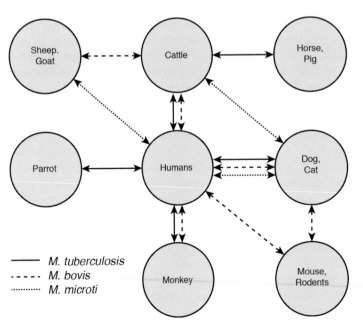

Figure 2.15 | Possible transmission chains for the *Mycobacterium tuberculosis* complex.

will become necrotic and is walled off. The regional lymph nodes are affected as well, forming the "primary complex" together with the primary pulmonary focus. Both will eventually heal. If the bacteria enter the gastrointestinal tract, the primary complex will form there.

Symptoms of progression are subfebrile temperatures, night sweats, lymph node swellings, cough, and possibly hemoptysis, fatigue, anorexia, and erythema nodosum on the extremities. If a pulmonary lymph node breaks down and discharges into a bronchus, caseating pneumonia or "galloping phthisis" will develop. Primary pulmonary tuberculosis may not only show proliferative or cavernous lesions but also an exudative course with pleural effusion. This begins with a sudden high fever, chest pain, cough, and notable differences in the depths of respiration between the two sides. The exudate is yellowish green, clear, or turbid.

Extrapulmonary tuberculosis may affect virtually every organ system, in particular, lymph nodes, the gastrointestinal, genitourinary and skeletal system, the meninges, and the peritoneum. Particularly dangerous is the hematogenous dissemination of mycobacteria. Depending on the immune system of the host, it may lead to a number of different syndromes.

Miliary tuberculosis may take an acute, subchronic, or chronic course. The most conspicuous symptoms are high and sustained fever, night sweats, dry cough, malaise, splenomegaly, and occasional skin lesions. Chest X-ray shows multiple minute nodules. Without treatment, tuberculous meningitis will develop in ci. 50% of the cases, with a high case-fatality rate. The main symptoms are fever, headache, cranial nerve deficits, and mental changes. In addition, tuberculous peritonitis may develop with fever, ascites, and subsequent increase in abdominal girth.

Bone and joint tuberculosis becomes manifest mainly in hip and knees, with pain, swelling, and limitation of motion. Destruction of vertebrae with damage to the spinal cord are typical sequelae of spinal tuberculosis (Pott's disease: kyphosis, abscess, paraplegia).

The clinical picture of skin tuberculosis (lupus vulgaris) is highly variable. Patients may show maculopapular, nodular, ulcerative or sometimes hemorrhagic skin lesions that either may spread superficially or extend to deeper skin layers.

In animals, tuberculosis is a chronic generalized disease that resembles human tuberculosis in pathogenesis, course, and symptoms. Primary complexes are mostly localized in lung or intestine. The clinical picture develops slowly with nonspecific symptoms, such as anorexia, emaciation, lassitude, and reduced capacity for work. Later, organ-specific symptoms will show up, such as fever, cough, dyspnea, diarrhea, loss of milk production, pareses, skin ulcers and fistulas, and lymph node abscesses. Early and late generalizations are manifested in severe, acutely febrile disease and are mostly lethal. Suspicious findings on slaughtering or dissection are caseous or calcified granulomas in internal organs and lymph nodes, or numerous miliary nodules in internal organs, lymph nodes, or in the serous cavities.

Diagnosis. Clinical symptoms, for example, chronic cough lasting >2 weeks, subfebrile temperatures, night sweats, and anorexia may arouse the suspicion of tuberculosis, particularly in high risk patients, for example, homeless or alcoholic persons, immunosuppressed patients, elderly, nursing home residents, patients suffering from lymphomas or diabetes, and immigrants from countries with a high prevalence of tuberculosis.

No chest X-ray can be considered pathognomonic as virtually any pattern may be seen: patchy or nodular infiltrates or, more typically, upper lobe infiltrates with or without cavities and with or without pleural effusion. The presence of mycobacteria in a specimen can be proven by microscopy, culture and/or molecular methods. Animal inoculation is obsolete. Suitable samples are sputum, bronchial secretions, gastric juice, spinal fluid, other body fluids, biopsy material from skin, mucous membranes, and bone.

Microscopy (Ziehl-Neelsen or auramin/rhodamin stains) allows detection of acid-fast rods only. Smear-positivity indicates 5×10^3 to 10^4 bacteria per ml. While *M. tuberculosis*, *M. avium-intracellulare* and other species can be diagnosed today directly by molecular biological techniques, for other species, culture is mandatory but may take 6 to 8 weeks. Media are egg-based (Lowenstein-Jensen) or agar-based (Middlebrook 7H10 or 7H11). Addition of antimicrobials is helpful for elimination of contaminants. Nonradiometric systems (Mycobacteria Growth Indicator Tube; Becton-Dickinson, Franklin Lakes, NJ, USA) or MB Bact/Alert (bio-Mérieux, Marcy l'Etoile. France) may be used. DNA amplification (e.g., PCR) techniques allow direct identification of the *M.tuberculosis* complex and are able to detect <10 bacteria per specimen. Compared to culture, their sensitivity is 95%, but in smear-negative cases, only 50 to 60%. This is why today's amplification techniques cannot obviate culture, which is necessary in any case for testing antimicrobial susceptibilities (recently, however, molecular tests for susceptibility testing have also come into use). *M. microti* infections are diagnosed by DNA amplification as culture of this species presents considerable difficulties.

IS6110 fingerprinting, spoligo- and mycobacterial interspersed repetitive (MIRU-VNTR) typing are used for typing of *M. tuberculosis* complex isolates with the aim of resolving etiological and epidemiological problems, for example, chains of infection, reservoirs, geographical, and animal distribution of dominant strain types.

In the tuberculin skin test, patients are tested for delayed hypersensitivity to antigens of the *M. tuberculosis* complex. A positive result indicates earlier or actual exposure to species of the *M.tuberculosis* complex. These tests are partially cross-reactive with nontuberculous mycobacteria and do not indicate degree of activity, severity of disease, or the causative species. Severe cases, for example, miliary tuberculosis, may lead to an anergic reaction; and vaccination with the Bacille Calmette-Guérin (BCG) vaccine to a positive result. The preferred format is the intradermal Mendel-Mantoux test (MMT): Five units of Purified Protein Derivative in 0.1 ml solution are injected intracutaneously on the volar side of the forearm. The result is read after 48 to 72 h and the diameter of the reaction is recorded. Based on the sensitivity

and specificity of the test, and the prevalence of tuberculosis in various groups of patients, three cutoff levels have been recommended for defining a positive result. People with the highest risk for tuberculosis, that is, immunosuppressed patients (due to HIV infection, organ transplantation, or immunosuppressive treatment), people with recent contact to tuberculous patients, and people with a suspicious X-ray picture are deemed positive at a diameter of <5 mm. A reaction of >10 mm would be called positive in immunocompetent people with a higher likelihood of a recent infection, for example, immigrants from countries with a high tuberculosis prevalence, immunocompetent drug addicts, prisoners and prison employees, people in nursing homes and homeless shelters, and laboratory personnel. For people without any known risk factors, a positive result would read >15 mm.

The interferon gamma release assay is an indirect test that uses whole blood and appropriate test antigens for *M.tuberculosis* complex-specific T cells. As this test is more specific than the skin test, it is recommended for confirmation of MMT-positive results. The diagnosis on live animals is done with an intracutaneous tuberculin test. In slaughtered or killed animals, it is made by using the results of pathology, histology, culture, or molecular biology.

Differential Diagnosis. Depending on the localization of the lesion(s), a large number of diseases must be included in the differential diagnosis: nonspecific lymphadenopathies, lymphomas, tularemia, pulmonary diseases, such as chronic bronchitis, viral pneumonias, pulmonary mycoses (aspergillosis, cryptococcosis, histoplasmosis), actinomycosis, silicosis, sarcoidosis, bronchial carcinoma, pleuritis of other origin, and gastrointestinal diseases, such as peritonitis, Crohn's disease, diverticulitis, small bowel, and colorectal cancer.

Mycobacterioses due to nontuberculous mycobacteria may mimic tuberculosis. These mycobacteria (*M. kansasii, M.avium, M.intracellulare, M. malmoense, M. haemophilum, M. simiae,* and *M. xenopi*, and rapid growers such as *M. fortuitum* and *M. chelonae*) are ubiquitous in the environment and cause disease mainly in immunocompromised hosts.

Therapy. Therapy nowadays must take into consideration the increasing spread of *M. tuberculosis* strains with multiple resistance (MDR; at least against rifampicin and isoniacid) and those with extensive resistance (XDR; multi-resistance plus resistance against second line drugs such as fluoroquinolones, amikacin, capreomycin, kanamycin).

During the initial phase, newly discovered, smear- or culture-positive patients are treated with peroral rifampicin (RMP) 10 mg/kg/day (maximally 600 mg/day) plus isoniacid (INH) 5 mg/kg/day (max. 300 mg/day) plus pyrazinamide (PZA) 15 to 30 mg/kg/day (max. 2 g/day), plus ethambutol (ETB) 15 to 25 mg/kg/day, all for 2 months (bactericidal phase). If the strain turns out to be fully susceptible in subsequent susceptibility tests, ETB may be omitted. Following the bactericidal phase, the patient should be treated with RMP plus INH for 4 months. Alternative regimens that allow all drugs to be given intermittently 2 or 3 times per week have been developed. This kind of treatment especially calls for directly observed therapy.

M. bovis is PZA-resistant. Therapy with INH plus RMP plus ETB should be prolonged for 9 to 12 months. According to drug susceptibility testing in liquid media, *M. microti* is susceptible to conventional antituberculous therapy including RMP, INH, and PZA. However, pulmonary infiltrates of HIV-infected patients have disappeared only if a six-drug regimen including clarithromycin, ETB, and ofloxacin was followed. Antituberculous therapy can have adverse effects, such as hepatitis, peripheral neuropathy, optic neuritis, encephalopathy, hyperuricemia, and arthralgia.

Tuberculous cattle, or those suspected to have tuberculosis, should not be treated at all, and treatment of other domestic animals should not be attempted because of doubtful prognosis and the danger of spread.

Prophylaxis. Biosafety level 3 facilities are required for laboratories performing cultures, identification, and susceptibility testing of the *M. tuberculosis* complex.

The BCG vaccination is effective in children and prevents dissemination but not infection or reactivation of latent pulmonary tuberculosis. If tuberculin-negative people encounter humans or animals suffering from open tuberculosis, they should take prophylactic INH (5 mg/kg/day). If conversion takes place, INH, perhaps in combination with RMP, should be taken for 3 to 6 months. Sputum smear-positive patients should be isolated, initially for 2 weeks, during which time they, and their care personnel, should wear facemasks.

The most important measure to prevent human infection with *M. bovis* is control of cattle tuberculosis. This is generally accomplished by regular control measures, such as meat inspection, tuberculin tests, shutting of suspicious stables, killing of diseased animals, or of those suspected to have tuberculosis, prohibition of treatment, vaccination, and slaughtering. Disinfectants used must have been tested for effectiveness against *M. tuberculosis* complex.

Reporting. Tuberculosis is a notifiable disease in the USA and in Canada

REFERENCES

Alfredsen S, Saxegaard F, An outbreak of tuberculosis in pigs and cattle caused by Mycobacterium africanum. *Vet. Rec.* 131, 51–53, 1992.

Aranaz A et al., Elevation of Mycobacterium tuberculosis subsp. caprae Aranaz et al. 1999 to species rank as Mycobacterium caprae comb. nov., sp. nov. *Int. J. Syst. Evol. Microbiol.* 53, 1785–1789, 2003.

Caminero JA et al., Best drug treatment for multidrug-resistant and extensively drug-resistant tuberculosis. *Lancet Infect. Dis.* 10, 621–629, 2010.

Cosivi O et al., Zoonotic tuberculosis due to Mycobacterium bovis in developing countries. *Emerg. Infect. Dis.* 4, 59–70, 1998.

Cousins DV et al., Tuberculosis in seals caused by a novel member of the Mycobacterium tuberculosis complex: Mycobacterium pinnipedii sp. nov. *Int. J. Syst. Evol. Microbiol.* 53, 1305–1314, 2003.

Dalovisio JR, Stetter M, Mikota-Wells S, Rhinoceros' rhinorrhea: cause of an outbreak of infection due to airborne Mycobacterium bovis in zookeepers. *Clin. Infect. Dis.* 15, 598–600, 1992.

De Vos V et al., The epidemiology of tuberculosis in free-ranging African buffalo (Syncerus caffer) in the Kruger National Park, South Africa. *Onderstepoort J. Vet. Res.* 68, 119–130, 2001.

Delahay RJ et al., The status of Mycobacterium bovis infection in UK wild mammals: a review. *Vet. J.* 164, 90–105, 2002.

Dheda K et al., Extensively drug-resistant tuberculosis: epidemiology and management challenges. *Infect. Dis. Clin. North Am.* 24, 705–725, 2010.

Eker B et al., Multidrug- and extensively drug-resistant tuberculosis, Germany. *Emerg. Infect. Dis.* 14, 1700–1706, 2008.

Frank W et al., Mycobacterium microti–pulmonary tuberculosis in an immunocompetent patient. *Wien. Klin. Wochenschr.* 121, 282–286, 2009.

Ghodbane R, Drancourt M, Non-human sources of Mycobacterium tuberculosis. *Tuberculosis* 93, 589–595, 2013.

Huard R et al., PCR-based method to differentiate the subspecies of the: Mycobacterium tuberculosis complex on the basis of genomic deletions. *J. Clin. Microbiol.* 41, 1637–1650, 2003.

Kiers A et al., Transmission of Mycobacterium pinnipedii to humans in a zoo with marine mammals. *Int. J. Tuberc. Lung Dis.* 12, 1469–1473, 2008.

Kubica T, Rüsch-Gerdes S, Niemann S, Mycobacterium bovis subsp. caprae caused one-third of human M. bovis-associated tuberculosis cases reported in Germany between 1999 and 2001. *J. Clin. Microbiol.* 41, 3070–3077, 2003.

Michalak K et al., Mycobacterium tuberculosis infection as a zoonotic disease: transmission between humans and elephants. *Emerg. Infect. Dis.* 4, 283–287, 1998.

Michel AL et al., Mycobacterium tuberculosis at the human/wildlife interface in a high TB burden country. *Transbound Emerg Dis* 60, 46–52, 2013.

Miltgen J et al., Two cases of pulmonary tuberculosis caused by Mycobacterium tuberculosis subsp canetti. *Emerg. Infect. Dis.* 8, 1350–1352, 2002.

Montali RJ, Mikota SK, Cheng LI, Mycobacterium tuberculosis in zoo and wildlife species. *Rev. Sci. Tech.* 20, 291–303, 2001.

Nishi JS, Shury T, Elkin BZ, Wildlife reservoirs for bovine tuberculosis (Mycobacterium bovis) in Canada: strategies for management and research. *Vet. Microbiol.* 112, 325–338, 2006.

Oh P et al., Human exposure following Mycobacterium tuberculosis infection of multiple animal species in a metropolitan Zoo. *Emerg. Infect. Dis.* 8, 1290–1293, 2002.

Reddington K et al., A novel multiplex real-time PCR for the identification of mycobacteria associated with zoonotic tuberculosis. *PLoS One* 6, e23481, 2011.

Sougakoff W, Molecular epidemiology of multidrug-resistant strains of Mycobacterium tuberculosis. *Clin. Microbiol. Infect.* 17, 800–805, 2011.

WHO, Global tuberculosis control. WHO report 2010. World Health Organization, Geneva, 2010.

2.14.2 INFECTIONS WITH *MYCOBACTERIUM MARINUM*

M. marinum infections mainly affect the skin and they are called swimming pool granuloma, fish tank granuloma, or fish tuberculosis.

Etiology. The main agent is *M. marinum* but in individual cases, *M. fortuitum* or *M. chelonae* have been isolated. All of them belong to the non-tuberculous mycobacteria (NTM; see 2.14.3)

Occurrence. On a worldwide scale, *M. marinum* infection is one of the most frequent infections of pet fish. The host spectrum of *M. marinum* is extensive and includes many fresh water and salt water fish. The bacterium is able to survive for months in aquatic habitats. At particular risk for infection are people exposed to contaminated fish tanks.

Transmission. The organisms invade the human skin through minor lesions that occur when a contaminated aquarium is cleaned, or through contact with salt water fish. There has been no human-to-human transmission.

Clinical Manifestations. Following an incubation period of 2 to 3 (1 to 8, occasionally up to 36) weeks small erythematous papules arise on the hand and upper arms that develop into granulomas, abscesses, or ulcers persisting for months, but occasionally healing spontaneously, forming a scar. Rare complications are tenosynovitis, arthritis, bursitis, and osteomyelitis. In immunocompromised patients, dissemination of granulomas may lead to a lethal outcome.

The clinical picture in fish is acute or chronic. Diseased fish avoid contact with others, become anorexic, lethargic, and lose weight. Nodules, ulcers, depigmentation, bloating, exophthalmos, and deformations may be seen. In some cases, disseminated granulomatous foci become obvious only at autopsy.

Diagnosis. The clinical picture and the patient's history (recreational or occupational contact with aquariums or salt water fish) should arouse suspicion. Histology of early lesions reveals acid-fast bacteria, polymorphonuclear leukocytes, and histiocytes, whereas older lesions consist of lymphocytes, epithelioid cells, and some Langhans giant cells, usually without caseation. Proof is provided by culture. Growth (aerobic for 2 to 3 weeks) is better at 28° to 30 °C than at 37 °C. The final diagnosis rests with molecular tests.

Differential Diagnosis. Noninfectious granulomas (cutaneous sarcoidosis, granuloma annulare, lymphomas) and infections due to streptococci, staphylococci, other mycobacteria (*M. tuberculosis* complex), fungi (*Candida* spp., *Cryptococcus neoformans, Sporothrix schenckii, Trichophyton* spp.), cutaneous leishmaniosis, nocardiosis, cowpox, and infections with papilloma viruses.

Therapy. *M. marinum* is IHN- and PZA-resistant. The recommended treatment is with peroral doxycycline (2 × 100 mg/day), or clarithromycin (2 × 500 mg/day), or trimethoprim-sulfamethoxazole double strength (2 × 1 tablet/day),or RMP 600 mg/d plus ETB 15 mg/kg/day for at least 12 weeks (attention: hepatitis and optical neuritis!). Deep lesions have to be treated surgically.

Prophylaxis. Wearing gloves when cleaning aquariums or handling fish, particularly if skin blemishes are present. Swimming pool water should be adequately treated with chlorine.

REFERENCES

Cheung JP et al., Review article: mycobacterium marinum infection of the hand and wrist. *J. Orthop. Surg. (Hong Kong)* 18, 98–103, 2010.

Gray SF et al., Fish tank granuloma. *BMJ* 300, 1069–1070, 1990.

Jacobs JM et al., A review of mycobacteriosis in marine fish. *J: Fish Dis* 32, 119–130, 2009.

Jernigan JA, Farr BM, Incubation period and sources of exposure for cutaneous Mycobacterium marinum infection: case report and review of the literature. *Clin. Infect. Dis.* 31, 439–443, 2000.

Lacaille F et al., Persistent Mycobacterium marinum infection in a child with probable visceral involvement. *Pediatr. Infect. Dis. J.* 9, 58–60, 1990.

Macek P et al., Mycobacterium marinum epididymoorchitis: case report and literature review. *Urol. Int.* 87, 120–124, 2011.

Rallis E, Koumantaki-Mathioudaki E, Treatment of Mycobacterium marinum cutaneous infections. *Expert Opin. Pharmacother.* 8, 2965–2978, 2007.

Streit M et al., Disseminated Mycobacterium marinum infection with extensive cutaneous eruption and bacteremia in an immunocompromised patient. *Eur. J. Dermatol.* 16, 79–83, 2006.

2.14.3 POSSIBLE ZOONOTIC MYCOBACTERIOSES

There are several pathogenic mycobacterial species beside the *M. tuberculosis* complex that are included in a group called nontuberculous mycobacteria (NTM). Some of them are opportunists, primarily infecting humans and animals with generally or locally weakened defense mechanisms. Risk factors in humans are HIV infection, tumors, immunosuppressive therapy, chronic obstructive pulmonary disease, cystic fibrosis, and alcoholism. In industrial countries, NTM infection was, up to the introduction of highly active retroviral treatment (HAART) in the mid-1990s, one of the most frequent AIDS-defining diseases. Besides *M. marinum*, the species *M. fortuitum, M. abscessus,* and *M. chelonae* (see also 2.15.2), which have also been isolated from cats, wild boars, and pigs, belong to the NTM.

Some other NTM, particularly of the *M. avium-intracellulare* (MAI) complex, have been suspected of being zoonotic agents. The MAI complex includes the four *M. avium* subspp. *avium, silvaticum, paratuberculosis,* and *hominissuis,* and the species *M. intracellulare.* They are frequently found in mammals and birds as obligate or facultatively pathogenic agents.

REFERENCES

Bercovier H, Vincent V, Mycobacterial infections in domestic and wild animals due to Mycobacterium marinum, M. fortuitum, M. chelonae, M. porcinum, M. farcinogenes, M. smegmatis, M. scrofulaceum, M. xenopi, M. kansasii, M. simiae and M. genavense. *Rev. Sci. Tech.* 20, 265–290, 2001.

Cadmus SI et al., Mycobacterium fortuitum from lesions of slaughtered pigs in Ibadan, Nigeria. *Rev Sci Tech* 29, 706–711, 2010.

Esteban J, Ortiz-Pérez A, Current treatment of atypical mycobacteriosis. *Expert Opin. Pharmacother.* 10, 2787–2799, 2009.

Falkinham JO, Epidemiology of infection by nontuberculous mycobacteria. *Clin. Microbiol. Rev.* 9, 177–215, 1996.

Falkinham JO, Ecology of nontuberculous mycobacteria – where do human infections come from? *Semin Respir Crit Care Med* 34, 95–102, 2013.

Garcia-Jimenez WL et al., Non-tuberculous mycobacteria in wild boar (Sus scrofa) from southern Spain: epidemiological, clinical and diagnostic concerns. *Transbound Emerg Dis*, 62, 72–80, 2015.

Griffith DE et al., An official ATS/IDSA statement: diagnosis, treatment, and prevention of non-tuberculous mycobacterial disease. *Am J Respir Crit Care Med* 175, 367–416, 2007.

Malik R et al., Infection of the subcutis and skin of cats with rapidly growing mycobacteria: a review of microbiological and clinical findings. *J Feline Med Surg* 2, 35–48, 2000.

Tortoli E et al., Impact of genotypic studies on mycobacterial taxonomy: the new mycobacteria of the 1990s. *Clin Microbiol Rev* 16, 319–354, 2003.

2.14.3.1 Infections with M. avium subsp. avium

This species [*Mycobacterium avium* subsp. *Avium* (MAA), MAI serotypes 1,2, and 3] is the agent of fowl tuberculosis, a generalized chronic granulomatous disease of birds with a progressive loss of weight, frequently leading to death. It has a worldwide distribution and affects most often older animals. Nowadays, it has lost significance for intensive poultry farming but can still be isolated from pet birds and zoos. MAA has also been found sporadically in association with tuberculous foci in mammals and humans, although restriction fragment length polymorphism profiles (and even techniques with higher resolution) of human and avian isolates did not match. As MAA and other agents of the MAI complex seem to occur ubiquitously in our environment water and soil may be the common source for birds and humans, and not birds the source for human infections.

REFERENCES

Anonymous, *Mycobacteriosis (Fact sheet)*. Center for Food Security and Public Health, Iowa, USA, 2006.

Biet F et al., Zoonotic aspects of Mycobacterium bovis and Mycobacterium avium-intracellulare complex (MAC). *Vet. Res.* 36, 411–436, 2005.

Komijn RE et al., Prevalence of Mycobacterium avium in slaughter pigs in the Netherlands and comparison of IS1245 restriction fragment length polymorphism patterns of porcine and human isolates. *J. Clin. Microbiol.* 37, 1254–1259, 1999.

Oloya J et al., Mycobacteria causing human cervical lymphadenitis in pastoral communities in the Karamoja region of Uganda. *Epidemiol. Infect.* 136, 636–643, 2008.

Thorel MF, Huchzermeyer HF, Michel AL, Mycobacterium avium and Mycobacterium intracellulare infection in mammals. *Rev. Sci. Tech.* 20, 204–218, 2001.

Tirkkonen T et al., High genetic relatedness among Mycobacterium avium strains isolated from pigs and humans revealed by comparative IS1245 RFLP analysis. *Vet. Microbiol.* 125, 175–181, 2007.

Tran QT, Han XY. Subspecies identification and significance of 257 clinical strains of *Mycobacterium avium*. *J Clin Microbiol.* 52, 1201–1206, 2014.

Turenne CY, Wallace R, Behr MA, Mycobacterium avium in the postgenomic era. *Clin. Microbiol. Rev.* 20, 205–229, 2007.

Von Reyn CF et al., Persistent colonisation of potable water as a source of Mycobacterium avium infection in AIDS. *Lancet* 343, 1137–1141, 1994.

Yajko DM et al., Mycobacterium avium complex in water, food, and soil samples collected from the environment of HIV-infected individuals. *J. Acquir. Immune Defic. Syndr. Hum. Retrovirol.* 9, 176–182, 1995.

2.14.3.2 Infections with M. avium subsp. hominissuis

M. avium subsp. *hominissuis* (MAH) is the most frequently found mycobacterium of the MAI complex in mammals, humans, and in the environment. The finding of tuberculous foci in lymph nodes and organs during inspection of pork has become rare following control of cattle tuberculosis (in Germany, <1% of pigs). Positive cases most often show tuberculous changes in submandibular and mesenteric lymph nodes. More than 90% of these pigs have infections with the MAI complex, mostly with MAH.

Molecular analyses have shown that MAH is genetically more diverse than the other MAI species and subspecies. There are, however, no associations between MAH genotypes and animal species. Rather, some human isolates resembled those from pigs, some even in every detail. This observation, however, cannot be taken as proof of transmission from pigs to humans as MAH and other MAI subspecies occur naturally in water and soil, which could be the common source.

Infection via contaminated food, for example, insufficiently heated pork, has not been documented thus far, and neither has transmission through contact with infected animals.

REFERENCES

Bruijnesteijn van Coppenraet L. E. et al., Lymphadenitis in children is caused by Mycobacterium avium hominissuis and not related to "bird tuberculosis". *Eur. J. Clin. Microbiol. Infect. Dis.* 27, 293–299, 2008.

Kaevska M et al., "Mycobacterium avium subsp. hominissuis" in neck lymph nodes of children and their environment examined by culture and triplex quantitative real-time PCR. *J. Clin. Microbiol.* 49, 167–172, 2011.

Mijs W et al., Molecular evidence to support a proposal to reserve the designation Mycobacterium avium subsp. avium for bird-type isolates and "M. avium subsp. hominissuis" for the human/porcine type of M. avium. *Int. J. Syst. Evol. Microbiol.* 52, 1505–1518, 2002.

Möbius P et al., Macrorestriction and RFLP analysis of Mycobacterium avium subsp. avium and Mycobacterium avium subsp. hominissuis isolates from man, pig, and cattle. *Vet. Microbiol.* 117, 284–291, 2006.

Moravkova M, et al., High incidence of Mycobacterium avium subspecies hominissuis infection in a zoo population of bongo antilopes (Tragelaphuis eurycerus). *J Vet Diagn Invest* 25, 531–534, 2013.

Radomski N et al., Determination of genotypic diversity of Mycobacterium avium subspecies from human and animal origins by mycobacterial interspersed repetitive-unit-variable-number tandem-repeat and IS1311 restriction fragment length polymorphism typing methods. *J. Clin. Microbiol.* 48, 1026–1034, 2010.

2.14.3.3 Infection with M. avium subsp. paratuberculosis

M. avium subsp. *paratuberculosis* (MAP) has been known in veterinary medicine as an agent of chronic enteritis in cattle, sheep (Johne's disease), goats, and other wild or zoo ruminants. It has also been suspected to be the agent of Crohn's disease in humans where it has been found by cultural and molecular analysis in many but not all cases.

However, it has also been isolated, although rarely, from healthy people and from those with other diseases. It could be that MAP colonizes pre-damaged tissues and may not be a primary causative agent but rather an opportunist or just a commensal. How MAP is transmitted is not known. A direct infection from animals seems unlikely, as populations with and without animal contact are affected similarly by Crohn's disease. The only possible vehicle could be food from MAP-infected animals but there is no evidence that MAP occurs in meat products, while it has been found in raw milk and, in low counts, also in pasteurized and ultrahigh heated milk. A chain of transmission between animals/food and humans has not been elucidated.

REFERENCES

Collins MT et al., Results of multiple diagnostic tests for Mycobacterium avium subsp. paratuberculosis in patients with inflammatory bowel disease and in controls. *J. Clin. Microbiol.* 38, 4373–4381, 2000.

Eltholth M et al., Contamination of food products with Mycobacterium avium paratuberculosis: a systematic review. *J. Appl. Microbiol.* 107, 1061–1071, 2009.

Feller M et al., Mycobacterium avium subspecies paratuberculosis and Crohn's disease: a systematic review and meta-analysis. *Lancet Infect. Dis.* 7, 607–613, 2007.

Gao A et al., Effect of pasteurization on survival of Mycobacterium paratuberculosis in milk. *J. Dairy Sci.* 85, 3198–3205, 2002.

Grant IR, Zoonotic potential of Mycobacterium avium ssp. paratuberculosis: the current position. *J. Appl. Microbiol.* 98, 1282–1293, 2005.

Motiwala AS et al., Current understanding of the genetic diversity of Mycobacterium avium subsp. paratuberculosis. *Microbes Infect.* 8, 1406–1418, 2006.

Over K et al., Current perspectives on Mycobacterium avium subsp. paratuberculosis, Johne's disease, and Crohn's disease: a review. *Crit. Rev. Microbiol.* 37, 141–156, 2011.

Richter E et al., Mycobacterium avium subsp. paratuberculosis infection in a patient with HIV, Germany. *Emerg. Infect. Dis.* 8, 729–731, 2002.

Sechi LA et al., Identification of Mycobacterium avium subsp. paratuberculosis in biopsy specimens from patients with Crohn's disease identified by in situ hybridization. *J. Clin. Microbiol.* 39, 4514–4517, 2001.

Sidoti F et al., Validation and standardization of IS900 and F57 real-time quantitative PCR assays for the specific detection and quantification of Mycobacterium avium subsp. paratuberculosis. *Can. J. Microbiol.* 57, 347–354, 2011.

Waddell L et al., The zoonotic potential of Mycobacterium avium spp. paratuberculosis: a systematic review. *Can. J. Public Health.* 99, 145–155, 2008.

2.14.3.4 Infections with M. genavense

M. genavense also belongs to the NTM and it is regarded as an opportunistic agent in humans. Severe disseminated infections in immuno-suppressed patients with AIDS, sarcoidosis, transplantation, and thymectomy have been observed mostly in Europe, North America, Australia, and Taiwan. They became more frequent in HIV-infected patients until HAART was introduced. There is also a report of a lymphadenitis in an otherwise healthy 15-year-old boy.

This species may be more frequent as an agent of disease than is assumed. For culture, it needs mycobactin, a constant pH of ci. 6.0 and incubation for up to 8 weeks, conditions not generally met in the routine laboratory. It has been suspected that pet birds (who are frequently infected with M. genavense) and, on occasion, domestic and zoo animals (dogs, ferrets, rabbits, cats, monkeys) may be the source of human infections but this has not been proven beyond doubt.

REFERENCES

Arora M et al., GI involvement in disseminated: Mycobacterium genavense: endoscopy and histology. *Gastrointest. Endosc.* 74, 688–690, 2011.

Charles P et al., Mycobacterium genavense infections: a retrospective multicenter study in France, 1996–2007. *Medicine (Baltimore)* 90, 223–230, 2011.

Hillebrand-Haverkort ME et al., Generalized Mycobacterium genavense infection in HIV-infected patients: detection of the mycobacterium in hospital tap water. *Scand. J. Infect. Dis.* 31, 63–68, 1999.

Hughes M et al., Disseminated Mycobacterium genavense infection in a FIV-positive cat. *J. Feline Med. Surg.* 1, 23–29, 1999.

Kiehn TE et al., Mycobacterium genavense infections in pet animals. *J. Clin. Microbiol.* 34, 1840–1842, 1996.

Manarolla G et al., Avian mycobacteriosis in companion birds: 20-year survey. *Vet. Microbiol.* 133, 323–327, 2009.

Palmieri C et al., Avian mycobacteriosis in psittacines: a retrospective study of 123 cases. *J Comp Pathol* 148, 126–138, 2013.

Thomsen VO et al., Disseminated infection with Mycobacterium genavense: a challenge to physicians and mycobacteriologists. *J. Clin. Microbiol.* 37, 3901–3905, 1999.

2.15 Pasteurelloses

Pasteurelloses are diseases in animals caused by bacteria of the genus *Pasteurella*, which are transmitted to humans mostly by bite and scratch wounds. Diseases may be local or systemic.

Etiology. Pasteurellae are small, straight, non-motile, facultatively anaerobic Gram-negative rods. There are four species and four related species of uncertain taxonomic status. Disease in humans is primarily due to *P.multocida*, with the subspecies *multocida* and *septica*. There are 16 O-serotypes (Heddleston) and six capsular types (Carter) but many strains cannot be typed. Certain capsular and O types are highly virulent in some hosts causing primary infections, while others are less virulent and only cause opportunistic or secondary infections. Whether all strains can cause human disease is unknown.

Further zoonotic species are *P. dagmatis, P. canis,* and *P. stomatis*, and among the "related" species, *P. aerogenes, P. caballi,* and *P. pneumotropica*. The latter three may be more closely related to the genus *Actinobacillus*.

Occurrence. Pasteurellae are obligately parasitic, occur worldwide, and colonize the mucous membranes of the upper respiratory and gastrointestinal tracts and, more rarely, the urogenital tracts of many wild and domestic animals. In particular, *P. multocida* is a normal inhabitant of the nasopharynx in mammals and of nasopharynx and cloaca in birds. Approximately, 75 to 90% of cats and up to 55% of dogs carry *P. multocida* in the upper respiratory tract. The source for human infections is not only pets (cats, dogs, birds, rabbits, guinea pigs) but also farm animals (cattle, calves, pigs, sheep, poultry) and wild and zoo animals (buffalo, roebuck, panther, lion). *P. caballi* colonizes the respiratory tract of horses, and *P. pneumotropica* the respiratory, gastrointestinal and female genital tract of rodents. At particular risk for infection are people with intensive contact with animals, for example, animal care personnel, veterinarians, breeders, farmers, slaughterhouse workers, and butchers.

Transmission. Infection in humans occurs primarily in wounds caused by bites or scratches from the animals mentioned above. In cases of close contact with infected animals, a direct transmission into a wound is also possible. In very rare instances, aerogenic transmission seems possible; transmission through consumption of contaminated food (meat) is rare. In a few cases, transmission could not be explained.

In the US, ci. 1 million people per year are bitten by animals: 70 to 90% are dog bites and 3 to 15%, cat bites. The risk of acquiring an infection is 2 to 19% for dog bites and 20 to 50% for cat bites. The frequency of hospital visits for bites in England and Wales is ci. 200 000, in France, it is ci. 500 000 per year. In Germany, ci. 35 000 people are bitten every year and only 1 to 2% are treated on an outpatient basis.

Clinical Manifestations. The length of the incubation period depends on the portal of entry and generally extends from 2 to 14 days. Wound infections following superficial or deep bites or scratches show redness, swelling, and pain within hours. Frequently, there is a discrepancy between objective symptoms and subjective complaints. A phlegmonous or abscess-forming inflammation of the skin and subcutaneous tissues and a local lymphadenitis may develop. If the infection progresses tendon sheaths, tendons, periarticular tissues and bones may be affected resulting even in necrotizing fasciitis, periostitis, and osteomyelitis. Meningitis, encephalitis, sinusitis (e.g., following skull injuries) show no symptoms characteristic for *Pasteurella* infections. Acute and subacute infections of the lower respiratory tract may become manifest as chronic bronchitis, bronchiectasis, pneumonia, or asthma. Septic forms may occur in immunocompromised persons with AIDS, diabetic nephropathy, liver cirrhosis, or alcoholism. Individual cases of endophthalmitis, conjunctivitis, epiglottitis, peritonitis, intraabdominal abscesses, urogenital infections, myositis, and arthritis have been reported.

In animals, pasteurelloses are often clinically inapparent. Depending on the portal of entry, species and virulence of the isolate and the animal, and preexisting conditions (infectious or noninfectious primary diseases, stress) various clinical pictures may emerge. These are, for the most part, chronic diseases of the respiratory tract. Atrophic rhinitis and enzootic pneumonia of pigs, enzootic bronchopneumonia of cattle, and contagious catarrh of rabbits are frequent infectious diseases in which special capsular and somatic serotypes of *P. multocida* subsp. *multocida* may play an important role as secondary invaders. Conversely, fowl cholera and hemorrhagic septicemia of cattle are primary pasteurelloses caused by highly virulent subsp. *multocida* strains of capsular types A, B, and E. Fowl cholera is a peracute to chronic generalized disease with respiratory and gastrointestinal symptoms, inflammatory foci on the head, arthritis, conjunctivitis, meningitis, and sudden death. Hemorrhagic septicemia occurs in Africa, Asia, southeastern Europe, and the Middle East, affecting various ruminants and pigs and causing a severe illness.

Diagnosis. Depending on the location of the disease, the presence of pasteurellae can be proven in human and animal samples by microscopy and culture from wound swabs, bronchial secretions, sputum, nasal swabs, rinsings from sinuses, spinal fluid, blood, or autopsy material (lung). The presence of small Gram-negative rods, often with bipolar staining, is used as an initial screen. Most species diagnoses can be made from a culture with the help of biochemical tests. Pasteurellae grow on blood agar plates within 24 to maximally 72 h in a moist atmosphere. PCR techniques for direct diagnoses from clinical samples, and capsule typing as well as 16S rRNA gene sequencing for speciation have been developed. Determination of antibodies in serum samples is not possible in the routine laboratory as antigens are not available commercially. These tests also seem not to be of much value.

Differential Diagnosis. Depending on the clinical picture, staphylococcal and streptococcal infections may resemble *Pasteurella* infections, and, after animal bites, infections with *Capnocytophaga canimorsus, C. cynodegmi*, nonfermenters such as CDC group NO-1, *Neisseria canis, N. weaveri, Bergeyella zoohelcum,* and *Staphylococcus intermedius*, which may be commensals in the mouths of dogs and cats. Rat bite fever, cat scratch disease, pseudotuberculosis, tularemia, lymphocytic choriomeningitis, and salmonellosis should be considered in localized and generalized infections.

Therapy. If there is a monoinfection with *Pasteurella*, penicillin V $4 \times 500\,000$ IU/day p.o. or doxycycline 2×100 mg/day p.o. for 10 to 14 days are the antibiotics of choice. In case of mixed bite infections with anaerobes or other aerobes amoxicillin-clavulanic acid 2×1 g/day is recommended. Conservative and/or surgical therapy may be indicated as well. Tetanus and rabies vaccination should be kept in mind.

Prophylaxis. Intensive contact with animals requires following certain rules of hygiene. Bite wounds should be cleaned and disinfected.

REFERENCES

Albert TJ, Stevens DL, The first case of Pasteurella canis bacteremia: a cirrhotic patient with an open leg wound. *Infection* 38, 483–485, 2010.

Ashley BD et al., Fatal Pasteurella dagmatis peritonitis and septicaemia in a patient with cirrhosis: a case report and review of the literature. *J. Clin. Pathol.* 57, 210–212, 2004.

Bisgaard M, Heltberg O, Frederiksen W, Isolation of Pasteurella caballi from an infected wound on a veterinary surgeon. *APMIS* 99, 291–294, 1991.

Buma R et al., Pathogenic bacteria carried by companion animals and their susceptibility to antibacterial agents. *Biocontrol Sci* 11, 1–9, 2006.

Cohen-Adam D et al., Pasteurella multocida septicemia in a newborn without scratches, licks or bites. *Isr. Med. Assoc. J.* 8, 657–658, 2006.

Drabick JJ et al., Pasteurella multocida pneumonia in a man with AIDS and nontraumatic feline exposure. *Chest* 103, 7–11, 1993.

Ejlertsen T et al., Pasteurella aerogenes isolated from ulcers or wounds in humans with occupational exposure to pigs: a report of 7 Danish cases. *Scand J Infect Dis.* 28, 567–570, 1996.

Escande F, Vallee E, Aubart F, Pasteurella caballi infection following a horse bite. *Zentralbl. Bakteriol.* 285, 440–444, 1997.

Ewers C et al., Virulence genotype of Pasteurella multocida strains isolated from different hosts with various disease status. *Vet. Microbiol.* 114, 304–317, 2006.

Freeman AF et al., Pasteurella aerogenes hamster bite peritonitis. *Pediatr. Infect. Dis. J.* 23, 368–370, 2004.

Harper M, Boyce JD, Adler B, Pasteurella multocida pathogenesis: 125 years after Pasteur. *FEMS Microbiol. Lett.* 265, 1–10, 2006.

Henderson SR et al., Pig trotters lung-novel domestic transmission of Pasteurella multocida. *Clin. Med.* 10, 517–518, 2010.

Kobayaa H et al., Pasteurella multocida meningitis in newborns after incidental animal exposure. *Pediatr. Infect. Dis. J.* 28, 928–929, 2009.

Migliore E et al., Pasteurella multocida infection in a cirrhotic patient: case report, microbiological aspects and a review of literature. *Adv. Med. Sci.* 54, 109–112, 2009.

Pouëdras P et al., Pasteurella stomatis infection following a dog bite. *Eur. J. Clin. Microbiol. Infect. Dis.* 12, 65, 1993.

Sasaki H et al., Comparative analysis of Pasteurella pneumotropica isolates from laboratory mice and rats. *Antonie van Leeuwenhoek* 95, 311–317, 2009.

Satomura A et al., Peritonitis associated with Pasteurella multocida: molecular evidence of zoonotic etiology. *Ther. Apher. Dial.* 14, 373–376, 2010.

Wilson BA, Ho M, Pasteurella multocida: from zoonosis to cellular microbiology. *Clin Microbiol Rev.* 26, 631–655, 2013.

2.16 Plague

Plague is one of the oldest and most dangerous zoonoses. Three clinical forms can be distinguished: bubonic, pneumonic, and septicemic plague. Three pandemics, occurring in several waves, have probably claimed almost 100 million lives since the 6th century A.D.

Etiology. *Yersinia pestis* is a Gram-negative, straight, coccoid or pleomorphic rod that belongs to the genus *Yersinia* in the family *Enterobacteriaceae*. In contrast to other *Yersinia* species, which are motile below 30 °C, it is nonmotile, with a growth optimum at ci. 30 °C but is also able to grow at 4 °C and 41 °C. Phylogenetic data have suggested that *Y. pestis* represents a clone that emerged from *Y. pseudotuberculosis* 1 500 to 20 000 years ago.

The virulence of *Y. pestis* is determined mainly by the three plasmids, pFfra (ci. 100 kbp; syn. pMT1), pPst (ci. 9.5 kbp; syn. pPCP1), and PYV (ci. 70 kbp; syn. pCD1). pYV is also present in virulent strains of *Y. pseudotuberculosis* and *Y. enterocolitica*. Among the main virulence factors are Yops (Yersinia outer proteins), which are translocated into neutrophils, macrophages, and dendritic host cells through a pYV-coded type III secretion system. Furthermore, the antiphagocytic fraction 1 envelope antigen, Yersinia murine toxin (Ymt), plasminogen activator, pH 6 antigen, and LPS contribute to the parasitic existence of *Y.pestis* in vertebrates and arthropods.

Occurrence. *Y. pestis* may be found in >200 species or subspecies of free-living rodents and lagomorphs. The main reservoirs are rats, marmots, hares, ground and rock squirrels, hamsters, weasels, chipmunks, and prairie dogs, as well as their ectoparasites (fleas, ticks). Silvatic foci exist in Asia (Vietnam, China, Mongolia, Kasachstan, India, Myanmar) and in Africa (East and Central Africa, Uganda, Tanzania, Sambia, Democratic Repoublic of Kongo, Libya, Madagascar). In the past few decades, an increasing number of cases has been reported from the western and southwestern United States (New Mexico, Arizona, California, Colorado, Nevada, Wyoming, Oregon, Texas) and from South America (Brazil, Bolivia, Peru), which reflects the presence of natural foci in these areas. Europe and Australia are free of plague at present.

Today, plague is a sporadic disease. At particular risk are hunters, shepherds, farmers, cat owners, veterinarians, and tourists in areas of endemicity. Epidemics will arise if *Y.pestis* infects susceptible rodent populations living close to human habitats and is able to multiply there. The death of their main hosts forces the fleas to feed on other hosts, for example, humans. *Y. pestis* is a potential bioweapon. Biosafety level 3 laboratories are required for work with the agent.

Transmission. *Y. pestis* is primarily transmitted to humans by the bite of the rat flea (*Xenopsylla cheopis*) (Fig. 2.16). Other ectoparasites, for example, camel fleas, lice, blood-sucking bugs, mites, ticks, and the human flea (*Pulex irritans*) may also be transmitters. During one blood meal, a rat flea can take up as many as 300 bacteria from an infected host. These multiply within 3 to 9 days, mainly in the gut of the flea. Afterwards, up to 20 000 bacteria may be transmitted to a new host by a single flea bite.

Reports from the USA have emphasized the role of domestic cats in the transmission chain. They become infected by eating infected prey and transmit the organism to humans (e.g., veterinarians and cat owners) through aerosols or bite/scratch wounds. From 1977 to 1998, 297 people in the USA became infected with *Y. pestis*; in 23 cases (7.7%), cats were incriminated as the source.

The disease may also be transmitted when skin is removed from infected animals, either

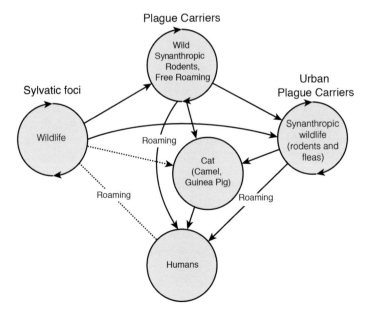

Figure 2.16 | Important transmission chains for *Yersinia pestis*.

Plague Carriers

Wild Synanthropic Rodents, Free Roaming

Sylvatic foci

Urban Plague Carriers

Wildlife

Roaming

Synanthropic wildlife (rodents and fleas)

Cat (Camel, Guinea Pig)

Roaming

Roaming

Humans

through blemishes or by inhaling infected dust. Rarely, consumption of meat from infected animals, for example, rabbits, may lead to human disease. Human-to-human transmission is possible for pneumonic plague but also after contact with pus containing yersiniae.

Clinical Manifestations. The clinical picture depends on the portal of entry. The incubation period of bubonic plague is 2 to 5 days, sometimes even 10 days. There is sudden fever up to 40° C, chills, headache, myalgias, and general malaise. At that time, or several hours later, a painful lymphadenopathy (bubo) develops proximal to the portal of entry, unilocular and mostly in the inguinal, axillar, or nuchal region. The surrounding tissue is edematous and inflamed and appears tight. The patient tries to minimize pain by flexion and external rotation of the thigh or by abduction of the arm. Intra-abdominal buboes mimic an acute abdomen with pain, nausea, vomiting, and diarrhea. Buboes may coalesce and perforate. The subsequent bacteremia leads to a septicemic picture with tachycardia, lethargy, somnolence, hypotension, hepatosplenomegaly, renal failure, disseminated intravascular coagulation, and gangrene of the extremities. The skin initially shows petechial hemorrhages (purpura), and later, necroses. Hematogenous spread leads to secondary pneumonic plague with chest pain, cough, and bloody or purulent, highly infectious sputum. Death is due to septic shock.

Fulminant septicemia without recognizable buboes is mostly diagnosed too late or not at all. The clinical picture is dominated by gastrointestinal symptoms (abdominal pain, nausea, vomiting, diarrhea), hypotension, ARDS, multiple organ failure, disseminated intravascular coagulation, and septic shock.

Symptoms of primary pneumonic plague appear after an incubation period of a few hours to 1 to 2 days with sudden fever, headache, myalgias, malaise, and pulmonary signs such as cough, chest pain, tachypnea, dyspnea, ARDS, hypotension and, eventually, shock. Initially, a single pulmonary lobe is involved, but rapid spread to other lobes may occur. Sputum

is initially mucoid, then thin and bloody, and contains large amounts of *Y. pestis* (danger!).

A rare form is primary cutaneous plague characterized by pustules, carbuncles, and necroses on skin and mucous membranes. Patients with a less threatening form of bubonic plague called pestis minor develop only lymphadenopathy or localized carbuncles without toxic symptoms.

The case-fatality rate of untreated bubonic plague is 40 to 60%, but only 5% if there has been early treatment. The case-fatality rate of untreated pneumonic plague and plague septicemia is close to 100%. Even if chemotherapy has been started early, up to 20% of patients will still die from cardiopulmonary failure. Plague leaves a long-lasting but incomplete immunity; therefore, reinfections are possible.

The course of plague in animals depends on species-susceptibility and individual immunity. The spectrum reaches from subclinical infections (in wild rodents constituting the reservoir) to fulminant hemorrhagic septicemia (in highly susceptible rodents, such as black rats). In domestic animals, such as camel, sheep, cattle, cats, and dogs, infection takes either the septicemic, bubonic, or pneumonic form. In cats, which are more susceptible than dogs, buboes develop preferentially on the head and neck.

Diagnosis. *Y. pestis* is highly infectious and must be handled at least under biosafety level 2 conditions (level 3 if aerosols may be formed). Because of the danger of spread, the diagnosis must be made as early as possible. The patient's history, particularly its epidemiological aspects, and suspicious symptoms, together with laboratory findings (leukocytosis with a left shift, dark urine with protein and red blood cells) should prompt the physician to collect specimens for microbiological analysis, that is, blood (three samples within 24 h), sputum, lymph node aspirates, tissues, or pus. Microscopy (Gram, Giemsa, methylene blue) shows small, bipolarly staining rods with a "safety pin" appearance. For culture, blood or brain heart infusion agar or, if a mixed flora is suspected, MacConkey agar or cefsulodin (4 mg/l)-irgasan-novobiocin (CIN) agar are used. Colonies show irregular edges after

48 h and a "fried egg" appearance after 72 h. *Y. pestis* is identified by biochemical and confirmed by other techniques (see Sentinel Level Clinical Lab Protocols for Suspected Biological Threat Agents and Emerging Infectious Diseases; www.asm/org/index.php/guidelines/sentinel-guidelines), such as slide agglutination, lysis by specific phages, or animal inoculation, but these tests should be performed in reference laboratories only. The envelope F1 antigen can be demonstrated in tissues by IF microscopy or ELISA; occasionally, however, it is not formed in sufficient amounts to be detected. Antibodies against F1 may be demonstrated in serum by agglutination, IHA (>1:10), CF, or ELISA from day 5 to day 10 on. Antibody tests, to be done every 1 to 2 weeks, are used for surveillance purposes only. A PCR has also been developed.

In animals, the diagnosis is made by culture of material from the carcass, such as heart blood, spleen, liver, lymph nodes, or bone marrow.

Differential Diagnosis. In the early stages, when lymph node swelling is not prominent, malaria, typhus, toxoplasmosis, brucellosis, cat scratch disease, typhoid, tularemia, lymphogranuloma inguinale, lymph node tuberculosis, and Morbus Hodgkin have to be considered. Pneumonic plague may resemble pulmonary anthrax, melioidosis, glanders, influenza, Hantavirus infection, and severe pneumonias of other origin.

Therapy. Antimicrobial treatment should start immediately when plague is suspected or after possible exposure. The antibiotics of choice are streptomycin (2×1 g/day i.m.) or gentamicin 5 mg/kg/day in 3 doses i.m. or i.v. and, as soon as clinically indicated, 3 mg/kg/day); or doxycycline 2×100 mg/day i.v. or p.o.; or chloramphenicol (check for availability!) 4×50 mg/kg/day i.v. or p.o. All of these are administered for 7 to 10 days.

Prophylaxis. Patients with plague or those suspected to be infected should be isolated and appropriate measures should be taken to protect the care personnel. The latter should receive doxycycline 2×100 mg/day p.o. or cotrimoxazole forte 2×1 tablet/day. Commercial vaccines are no longer available. Rat and insect control is important in urban areas. Free-living dogs and cats in endemic areas should be treated with insecticidal and akaricidal antiparasitic drugs. Official surveillance of natural foci has been effective in preventing an epizootic among wild animals and transmission to humans.

Reporting. Plague is a notifiable disease in the USA and in Canada.

REFERENCES

Achtman M et al., Yersinia pestis, the cause of plague, is a recently emerged clone of Yersinia pseudotuberculosis. *Mol. Microbiol.* 37, 316–330, 2000.

Ayyadurai S et al., Rapid identification and typing of Yersinia pestis and other Yersinia species by matrix-assisted laser desorption/ionization time-of-flight (MALDI-TOF) mass spectrometry. *BMC Microbiol.* 10, 285, 2010.

Bertherat E et al., Lessons learned about pneumonic plague diagnosis from 2 outbreaks, Democratic Republic of the Congo. *Emerg. Infect. Dis.* 17, 778–784, 2011.

Bin Saeed AA, Al-Hamdan NA, Fontaine RE, Plague from eating raw camel liver. *Emerg. Infect. Dis.* 11, 1456–1457, 2005.

Boisier P, Rahalison L, Rasolomaharo M et al., Epidemiologic features of four successive annual outbreaks of bubonic plague in Mahajanga, Madagascar. *Emerg. Infect. Dis.* 8, 311–316, 2002.

Butler T, Plague into the 21st century. *Clin. Infect. Dis.* 49, 736–742, 2009.

Cohn SKJr, Epidemiology of the Black Death and successive waves of plague. *Med. Hist.* Suppl. (27): 74–100, 2008.

Dennis DT et al., Plague manual–epidemiology, distribution, surveillance and control. *Wkly. Epidemiol. Rec.* 74, 447, 1999.

Fritz C et al., Surveillance for pneumonic plague in the United States during an international emergency: a model for control of imported emerging diseases. *Emerg. Infect. Dis.* 2, 30–36, 1996.

Gage KL et al., Cases of cat-associated human plague in the Western US, 1977–1998. *Clin. Infect. Dis.* 30, 893–900, 2000.

Gould L et al., Dog-associated risk factors for human plague. *Zoonoses Public Health.* 55, 448–454, 2008.

Kool JL, Risk of person-to-person transmission of pneumonic plague. *Clin. Infect. Dis.* 40, 1166–1172, 2005.

Monecke S, Monecke H, Monecke J, Modelling the black death. A historical case study and implications for the epidemiology of bubonic plague. *Int. J. Med. Microbiol.* 299, 582–593, 2009.

Orloski KA, Eidson M, Yersinia pestis infection in three dogs. *J. Am. Vet. Med. Assoc.* 207, 316–318, 1995.

Oyston PC, Williamson ED, Prophylaxis and therapy of plague. *Expert Rev Anti Infect Ther* 11, 817–829, 2013.

Perry RD, Fetherston JD, Yersinia pestis – etiologic agent of plague. *Clin. Microbiol. Rev.* 10, 35–66, 1997.

Riehm JM et al., Detection of Yersinia pestis using real-time PCR in patients with suspected bubonic plague. *Mol. Cell. Probes* 25, 8–12, 2011.

Rosenzweig JA et al., Progress on plague vaccine development. *Appl. Microbiol. Biotechnol.* 91, 265–286, 2011.

Rubin GJ, Dickmann P, How to reduce the impact of "low-risk patients" following a bioterrorist incident: lessons from SARS, anthrax, and pneumonic plague. *Biosecur. Bioterror.* 8, 37–43, 2010.

Ruiz A, Plague in the Americas. *Emerg. Infect. Dis.* 7, 539–540, 2001.

Splettstoesser WD et al., Evaluation of a standardized F1 capsular antigen capture ELISA test kit for the rapid diagnosis of plague. *FEMS Immunol. Med. Microbiol.* 41, 149–155, 2004.

Stenseth NC et al., Plague: past, present, and future. *PLoS Med.* 5, e3, 2008.

Tomaso H et al., Preliminary validation of real-time PCR assays for the identification of Yersinia pestis. *Clin. Chem. Lab. Med.* 46, 1239–1244, 2008.

Zhou D, Yang R, Molecular Darwinian evolution of virulence in Yersinia pestis. *Infect. Immun.* 77, 2242–2250, 2009.

2.17 Q Fever

Q fever (Q for query because of previously unclear etiology and pathogenesis) is a worldwide systemic zoonosis caused by the obligately intracellular bacterium, *Coxiella burnetii*.

Etiology. *C. burnetii* is a small, Gram-negative, nonmotile, oval to rod-like, pleomorphic bacterium that shows some similarity to the rickettsiae to whom it was thought to be related until recently. There are further similarities with Gram-negative rods as coxiellae also have an outer LPS membrane. Molecular taxonomy, however, has placed *Coxiella* in the Gamma subgroup of *Proteobacteria* while *Rickettsia* belongs to the Alpha-1-subgroup. *C. burnetii* is the only *Coxiella* species.

Coxiellae may go through a phase change comparable to the smooth-rough phase of *Enterobacteriaceae* caused by changes in the LPS membrane. Phase 1 (smooth) is characterized by a complete LPS membrane and is the natural, highly virulent form in humans, animals, and arthropods. Phase 2 (rough) forms after several passages in cell cultures or chicken eggs and has a LPS that is strain-specific and lacks certain protein and sugar determinants. Both phases are important for the serological diagnosis (see below). A further genus-specific characteristic is the development of two variants. The large cell variant (LCV) represents the intracellular vegetative (multiplying) stage with little resistance to environmental factors and disinfectants. When conditions are no longer conducive to growth the vegetative forms will split off at one end spore-like, electron-dense small cell variants (SCV) (Fig. 2.17a,b), which are resistant against drying, heat, and disinfectants. They are the extracellular forms that are transmitted through air, particularly in dust. They are highly infectious and the minimal dosis is probably close to 10 bacteria.

Occurrence. *C. burnetii* occurs worldwide (exception, New Zealand). Its host spectrum includes ticks, rodents, game, birds, most domestic animals, and humans. Natural reservoirs are >40 species of ticks that form, together with certain vertebrates such as rodents and game, the natural foci. Ticks remain infected throughout life but are also able to transmit the coxiellae transovarially. Coxiellae may multiply in the intestines of the ticks up to 10^{10} infectious units per g feces. In dry feces produced in large amounts by the tick *Dermacentor* coxiellae remain viable at average temperatures for at least 1 year and can be transmitted by air.

More recent investigations, however, have thrown some doubt on the central role of ticks and natural foci in the epidemiology of Q fever. An investigation of suspected natural foci in the Rhine and Kinzig valleys in Germany revealed that of 1060 *Dermacentor* ticks, not one carried coxiellae as determined by PCR, and none of the 119 rodents from these areas showed anti-Coxiella antibodies. It seems that in Central Europe, natural foci are sporadic, and that the role of *Dermacentor* is one of a multiplicator of coxiella.

The decisive factor in the epidemiology of Q fever is the susceptibility of domestic animals. In Central Europe, these are mainly sheep, goats, and cattle who become infected aerogenically. Their infection is generally inapparent but the bacteria are excreted, if only in small amounts, via feces and urine. If, however, the pregnant

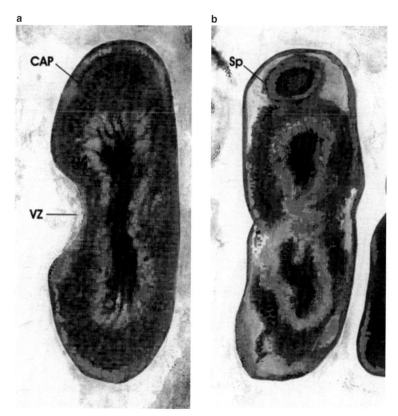

Figure 2.17 (a,b) | *Coxiella burnetii.* Spore-like bodies at the polar end of a vegetative cell (CAP, capping; VZ, vegetative cell, Sp, spore-like body). Modified from Bergey's *Manual of Systematic Bacteriology*, Vol 1, Krieg NR (ed.), p. 702. Williams & Wilkins, Baltimore/London, 1984, modified. Drawing by C. Lüttich, Gera, Germany.

uterus is infected where coxiellae multiply in the trophoblast, they may abort whereby large amounts of bacteria are excreted with the lochia (this could also occur during a seemingly normal delivery). In cattle, *C. burnetii* may be a causative agent of other disease such as metritis, retention of the placenta, and infertility. In the desiccated tissues, the SCV will form and contaminate the soil and environment. As they are resistant, and only minimally affected by weather changes, they form a highly infectious dust. Dry weather and strong winds favor the spread of *Coxiella* through dust.

Cattle may also develop nonpurulent mastitis that leads to contamination of milk; unpasteurized milk may contain more than 100 000 coxiellae per ml. In food prepared from unpasteurized milk, coxiellae can still multiply for 1 to 2 months. Tick-independent cycles have been

proven in cattle and it also seems likely in sheep. This is strongly suggested by Q fever epidemics in Soest and Jena, Germany where >300 cases were observed far outside the living area of *Dermacentor*. The significance of ticks for infection of these animals is regarded as minor.

Pigs, dogs, cats, and roaming animals are infected through the air and through consumption of *Coxiella*-containing placentas or prey. Wild animals and domestic birds (pigeons, sparrows) can be infected as well. Dogs and cats play a minor role in the epidemiology of human infections. *Coxiella burnetii* is a potential bioweapon, and work with it requires biosafety level 3 laboratories.

Transmission. Infection in humans is either airborne or results from direct or indirect contact with infected animals, their dried excreta

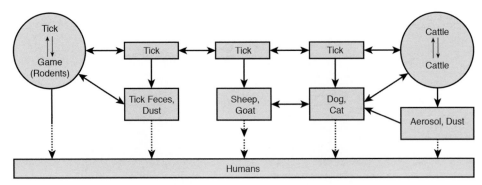

Figure 2.18 | Possible transmission chains, Q fever. The ticks are "multipliers" and are not mandatory for transmission.

(Fig. 2.18), or excreta of ticks. Consumption of unpasteurized milk or milk products leads to infection and seroconversion. A study of farmers in Southern Germany showed antibodies in 17% of those who drank raw milk vs. 7% who drank boiled milk only but there were no clinical symptoms in both groups. Alimentary Q fever should be more frequent in countries with primitive agricultural structures.

Clinical Manifestations. Following aerogenic or oral uptake coxiellae migrate via blood and lymph channels into the macrophages of the reticuloendothelial system, where they multiply in the phagolysosomes at pH 4.5 thanks to various mechanisms of evasion. The subsequent bacteremia may lead to organ manifestations with invasion of the alveolar macrophages and Kupffer cells, resulting in interstitial pneumonia and/or granulomatous hepatitis.

Human infections with *C. burnetii* are either subclinical, acute, or chronic. The discrepancy between the relatively large number of seropositive and the small number of overt clinical cases is probably due to inapparent or undiagnosed ("grippe") infections. A study of 2500 people in Southern Germany showed a mean seroprevalence of 7.5%; following epidemics, however, it was >30%. It is generally assumed that >60% of infections are subclinical, and that 10% of the acute infections involve organs.

Acute Q fever is a generalized infection resembling influenza. Depending on the infectious dose, the incubation period is 1 to 14 days. There is a sudden fever of 40 °C or higher, chills, severe malaise, arthralgias, myalgias, and photophobia. Headache, initially localized frontally and retroorbitally, become generalized later, persist during the course of the disease, and is not influenced by analgetics. Despite the high fever, the patient's face is pale grey, and the sclerae may be slightly yellow. The fever usually lasts for 1 to 2 weeks, sometimes longer in older patients. Loss of weight is another characteristic sign. The lungs are usually normal on percussion and auscultation but X-rays show an interstitial pneumonia in 30 to 50% of patients. Abnormal liver function tests such as bilirubin and alkaline phosphatase levels are frequent. Besides pneumonia and hepatitis, acute Q fever may manifest itself as meningoencephalitis, myocarditis, pericarditis, thromboses in several organs, granulomas and necrotic foci in the bone marrow, orchitis, and chorioamnionitis. Recovery may take several months.

C. burnetii infections in pregnancy may lead to prematurity, abortion, or stillbirth. While transplacental transmission is possible, malformations in newborns have not been reported. Due to the diminished T cell-mediated immune response, pregnancy causes enhanced susceptibility to *C. burnetii* infection as well as transition from acute to chronic disease.

Studies in animals have shown that *C. burnetii* is able to persist for long periods in the mammary glands, liver, spleen, lymph nodes, kidneys, bone marrow, and brain. The fact that the organism can be isolated from heart valves and livers of patients with chronic Q fever points to persistence in humans as well.

Chronic infections with *C. burnetii* appear mainly as endocarditis and/or chronic granulomatous hepatitis, more rarely as infections of vascular prostheses, osteomyelitis, or interstitial lung fibrosis. Q fever endocarditis may also follow an inapparent or subclinical infection and mainly affects the mitral and the aortic valve. The interval between the primary infection and the first symptoms of endocarditis may last between 6 months and 10 years. Usual symptoms are moderate fever, night sweats, anemia, arthralgias, and heart murmurs of variable character. Repeated blood cultures do not show growth; in fact, in cases of culture-negative endocarditis chronic Q fever must always be considered. Q fever hepatitis is histologically characterized by small granulomas with epithelioid cells in rosette formations (doughnut granulomas).

Diagnosis. In typical cases, the clinical diagnosis is usually made based on the patient's history and the triad of irregular fever, retrobulbar headache, and atypical pneumonia without catarrhal symptoms.

Microscopy is useful only in cases of high bacterial density and is only used in veterinary medicine, mostly on samples obtained at delivery. The test of choice in human infections is serology with phase I and phase II antigens that differentiate between acute, immediate past, and chronic disease. Among the techniques used, that is, ELISA, indirect immunofluorescence test (IIF), and CF, the latter has largely been abandoned because of low sensitivity and late positivity. Using appropriate conjugates, ELISA and IIF are able to differentiate between IgM, IgG, and IgA antibodies. The semiquantitative ELISA is the preferred test, while the more complicated quantitative IIF serves to follow the course of the disease and to rule out chronic infection. In acute Q fever, ELISA and IIF show phase II IgM antibodies 7 to 15 days after infection; a few days later phase II IgG antibodies become measurable. Both antibodies reach their highest titers during convalescence in the 6th to 8th week, and will slowly disappear (in

a new study, IgG phase II antibodies remained high even after 12 months). At this point, phase I and II IgM and IgG antibodies will be present in all patients, and in 20%, also phase I IgA antibodies, which should not be interpreted as persistent infection. Only if those antibodies fail to disappear, or increase in titer, chronic infection has to be considered. As this takes place only weeks to months after infection, a nested PCR that indicates the presence of circulating coxiellae has been developed; however, only positive results are meaningful. This PCR can also be tried for a diagnosis before antibodies are detectable.

Isolation of *C. burnetii* from blood (buffy coat) or biopsy material in cell cultures of embryonated chicken eggs should only be tried in biosafety level 3 laboratories.

Differential Diagnosis. Ornithosis, mycoplasmal, and other atypical pneumonias must be considered. In the initial stages, that is, before pulmonary symptoms arise, influenza and all systemic infections with a phase of generalization (bacteremia, viremia) should be included. In addition, malaria and dengue should be included in tropical areas.

Therapy. Acute Q fever: doxycycline 2×100 mg/day p.o. for 2 to 3 weeks, or moxifloxacin 1×400 mg/day or ciprofloxacin 2×500 to 750 mg/day p.o. for 2 to 3 weeks. In pregnancy, trimethoprim-sulfamethoxazole double strength 2×1 tablet/day, and after delivery, doxycycline as above. Children <8 years: trimethoprim-sulfamethoxazole 2×240 mg/day p.o. Chronic Q fever and endocarditis: doxycycline 2×100 mg/day p.o. plus hydroxychlorquine 600 mg/day p.o. for at least 1.5 to 2 years (hydroxychloroquine is a lysosomotropic and alkalizing agent).

Prophylaxis. Exposition can hardly be avoided. Even consequent avoidance of contact with sheep does not make sense because the SCV can persist in soil for months. Pasteurization or heating at 74 °C for 15 s is sufficient for killing coxiellae in milk. Proper hygiene in contact with infected cattle is indicated.

In Australia, an inactivated phase vaccine (Q-vax) has been developed and licensed for use in adults with a high risk of acquiring the infection (www.qfever.com.au). In the US, a noncommercial inactivated vaccine from embryonated eggs for laboratory personnel at risk is available and may be requested from the US Army Medical Research Institute at Fort Detrick, MD, USA (www.cdc.gov/qfever).

A vaccination with modern vaccines (Coxiella phase I) induces protective immunity in sheep, cattle, and goats, reduces the contamination of the environment and perhaps interrupts the infectious chains. Acaricidal treatment of domestic animals at the time of tick appearance should lead to the interruption of the chain that involves tick feces and should prevent further spread and multiplication of ticks.

Reporting. Q fever is a notifiable disease in the USA.

REFERENCES

Bernard H et al., High seroprevalence of Coxiella burnetii antibodies in veterinarians associated with cattle obstetrics, Bavaria, 2009. *Vector Borne Zoonotic Dis* 12, 552–557, 2012.

Boden K et al., Diagnosis of acute Q fever with emphasis on enzyme-linked immunosorbent assay and nested polymerase chain reaction regarding the time of serum collection. *Diagn Microbiol Infect Dis* 68, 110–116, 2010.

Domingo P et al., Acute Q fever in adult patients: report on 63 sporadic cases in an urban area. *Clin. Infect. Dis.* 29, 874–879, 1999.

European, Food Safety Authority, Scientific opinion on Q-fever. *EFSA Journal.* 8, 1595, 2010.

Fenollar F, Fournier PE, Raoult D, Molecular detection of Coxiella burnetii in the sera of patients with Q fever endocarditis or vascular infection. *J. Clin. Microbiol.* 42, 4919–4924, 2004.

Fournier PE, Marrie TJ, Raoult D, Diagnosis of Q fever. *J. Clin. Microbiol.* 36, 1823–1834, 1998.

Fournier PE, Raoult D, Comparison of PCR and serology assays for early diagnosis of acute Q-fever. *J. Clin. Microbiol.* 41, 5094–5098, 2003.

Hellenbrand W, Breuer T, Petersen L, Changing epidemiology of Q fever in Germany, 1947–1999. *Emerg. Infect. Dis.* 7, 789–7796, 2001.

Hoen B et al., Infective endocarditis in patients with negative blood cultures: analysis of 88 cases from a one-year nationwide survey in France. *Clin. Infect. Dis.* 20, 501–506, 1995.

Hogerwerf L et al., Reduction of Coxiella burnetii prevalence by vaccination of goats and sheep, The Netherlands. *Emerg. Infect. Dis.* 17, 379–386, 2011.

Levy PY, Carrieri P, Raoult D, Coxiella burnetii pericarditis: report of 15 cases and review. *Clin. Infect. Dis.* 29, 393–397, 1999.

Maurin M, Raoult D, Q-fever. *Clin. Microbiol. Rev.* 12, 518–553, 1999.

Pluta S et al., Prevalence of Coxiella burnetii and Rickettsia spp. in ticks and rodents in southern Germany. *Ticks Tick-borne Dis.* 1, 145–147, 2010.

Porten K et al., A super spreading ewe infects hundreds with Q fever at a farmers market in Germany. *BMC: Infect Dis* 6, 147, 2006.

Raoult D, Fenollar F, Stein A, Q-fever during pregnancy. *Arch Intern Med* 162, 701–704, 2002.

Rehacec J et al., Extensive examination of different tick species for infestation with Coxiella burnetii in Slovakia. *Eur. J. Epidemiol.* 7, 299–303, 1991.

Roest HI et al., Clinical microbiology of Coxiella burnetii and relevant aspects for the diagnosis and control of the zoonotic disease Q fever. *Vet Q* 33, 148–160, 2013.

Schack M et al., Coxiella burnetii (Q fever) as a cause of community-acquired pneumonia during the warm season in Germany. *Epidemiol Infect* 20, 1–6, 2013.

Stein A, Raoult D, Pigeon pneumonia in Provence: a bird-borne Q fever outbreak. *Clin. Infect. Dis.* 29, 617–620, 1999.

van der Hoek W et al., Follow-up of 686 patients with acute Q fever and detection of chronic infection. *Clin Infect Dis* 52, 1431–1436, 2011.

Wagner-Wiening C, Brockmann SO, Kimmig P, Serological diagnosis and follow-up of asymptomatic and acute Q-fever infections. *Int. J. Med. Microbiol.* 296(Suppl. 40), 294–296, 2006.

Wegdam-Blans MC et al., Chronic Q fever: review of the literature and proposal of new diagnostic criteria. *J Infect* 64, 247–259, 2012.

2.18 Rat Bite Fever

Rat bite fever, known in Japan as Sodoku, is a rare disease caused either by *Streptobacillus moniliformis* or by *Spirillum minus*. These bacteria are mostly transmitted by rat bites and induce a local or generalized infection. The form transmitted by the oral-alimentary way is called Haverhill fever.

Etiology. *Streptobacillus moniliformis* is a Gram-negative pleomorphic nonmotile rod that can be cultured on aerobic blood (optimal, 15%) agar with 5 to 10% CO_2 and may form filaments, particularly in older cultures. *Spirillum minus* is a motile, Gram-negative spiral-shaped bacterium that cannot be cultured on artificial media. Its taxonomic position is unclear, and its biochemical and molecular characteristics are incompletely known.

Occurrence. Rat bite fever occurs worldwide, particularly in Japan, the US, Eastern Africa, Australia, and India, and is underestimated and underdiagnosed. The reservoir are house (*R. rattus*) and migratory (*R. norvegicus*) rats. The agents have also been found in other rodents (mice, gerbils, squirrels, ferrets, weasels) and occasionally in dogs and cats. *S. moniliformis* occurs worldwide, *S. minus* mainly in North America, Southeast Asia, and Europe.

At risk are people having professional or other contact with rats, that is, canal or farm workers, animal dealers, those working with experimental animals, laboratory workers, pet owners, and veterinarians. In the US, the majority of cases occur in children <12 years.

Transmission. The agents are mostly transmitted through the bite of wild or experimental rats. *S. moniliformis* belongs to the normal pharyngeal flora of the rodents mentioned. *S. minus*, which does not occur in saliva but does in blood and eye secretions, is transported via lesions in the oral mucosa or via the lacrimal canal into the oral cavity. Human contact infection through feces or saliva is possible as well. When animals are fed or their cages are cleaned, the agents can enter the skin through small blemishes. Contaminated milk and other food, as well as drinking water, can also be sources.

Clinical Manifestations. *S. moniliformis* infections have an incubation period of 3 to 5 (1 to 10) days. There follows an abrupt onset of fever up to 40 °C, with chills, regional lymphadenopathy, vomiting, headache, lethargy, arthralgia, and myalgia. In >75% of cases, a dark red morbilliform exanthema arises on the dorsal surface of the extremities and joints that disappears within a few days. Painful mono- or polyarticular arthritides of several joints (e.g., knees, wrists, elbows) follows.

Haverhill, MA, gave its name to Haverhill fever, which is caused by oral uptake of *S.moniliformis*. It shows up as tonsillitis with dysphagia and diffuse redness without lymphadenitis,

as well as painful laryngitis with cough, hoarseness, and changes in the voice. These symptoms may last for 2 to 3 weeks; exanthema and polyarthritis may follow.

Possible complications of *S.moniliformis* disease are endocarditis, pancarditis, abscesses in internal organs, pneumonia, hepatitis, nephritis, pancreatitis, meningitis, prostatitis, and septicemia. The case-fatality rate without therapy is 7 to 13%.

Infections with *S. minus* have an incubation period of 2 to 3 weeks; however, sometimes be up to 4 months. Around the area of the bite, painful, edematous, purple-colored inflammatory foci with blebs and subsequent ulceration develop. Regional lymph nodes are enlarged. Fever for 3 to 5 days, chills, headaches, and general malaise are frequent. After a fever-free interval of 3 to 7 days, the fever returns. These intervals are repeated but decrease in intensity with the duration of the disease, which may last for weeks or months. In the area surrounding the bite there may be maculopapulous or urticarial exanthemas. Accompanying this, there may be headache, myalgias, diarrhea, vomiting, arthralgias, neuralgias, or CNS symptoms. Endocarditis, myocarditis, hepatitis, and meningitis are possible complications. With appropriate early therapy, prognosis is good and the case-fatality low.

In animals, *S. minus* infections are latent. In rodents, *S. moniliformis* is at best a secondary agent of conjunctivitis, otitis, and respiratory disease. Laboratory mice of certain lines, such as C57BL/6J Han, are particularly susceptible and may die with abortion, subcutaneous periarticular abscesses, lymphadenitis, septic arthritis/polyarthritis, nephritis, and septicemia. In turkeys, polyarthritis, bursitis, tenovaginitis, and lymphadenitis have been observed.

Diagnosis. After an animal bite, symptoms of the infection caused by the two organisms are similar. The diagnosis is confirmed by finding *S. moniliformis* during febrile episodes in blood wound secretions, pus, or joint fluid on blood agar (see above). Culture in liquid media shows the characteristic "puff balls." The organism is biochemically inert. A PCR has been developed.

Serological tests have only been used on SPF laboratory animals.

S. minus is detected in Giemsa-stained blood smears or in unstained smears by darkfield microscopy. It is corkscrew-like, motile, and has two or more spirals. Upon s.c. or i.p. injection of mice or guinea pigs with material containing the organisms, they may be found in blood or lymph node material 4 to 10 days later.

Differential Diagnosis. A broad spectrum has to be considered: staphylococcal and streptococcal infections, tularemia, tuberculosis, cat scratch disease, pasteurelloses, lues, rickettsioses, relapsing fever, brucellosis, ehrlichiosis, leptospirosis, and malaria.

Therapy. The drug of choice is penicillin G 3 × 1 mio. IU/day i.v. for 7 days, afterwards penicillin V 4 × 500 mg/day for another 7 days. Alternatives are tetracycline 4 × 500 mg/day or doxycycline 2 × 100 mg/day p.o. for 10 to 15 days.

Prophylaxis. The best prophylaxis is rat control and wearing gloves when handling rats in the laboratory. A bite wound from rodents should be cleaned and disinfected. Tetanus prophylaxis is indicated.

REFERENCES

Azimi P, Pets can be dangerous. *Pediatr. Infect. Dis. J.* 9, 670–684, 1990.

Banerjee P, Ali Z, Fowler DR, Rat bite fever, a fatal case of Streptobacillus moniliformis infection in a 14-month-old boy. *J. Forensic Sci.* 56, 531–533, 2011.

Boot R et al., An enzyme-linked immunosorbent assay (ELISA) for monitoring rodent colonies for Streptobacillus moniliformis antibodies. *Lab. Anim.* 27, 350–357, 1993.

Boot R, Oosterhuis A, Thuis HC, PCR for the detection of: Streptobacillus moniliformis. *Lab. Anim.* 36, 200–208, 2002.

Dendle C, Woolley IJ, Korman TM, Rat-bite fever septic arthritis: illustrative case and literature review. *Eur. J. Clin. Microbiol. Infect. Dis.* 25, 791–797, 2006.

Dubois D et al., Streptobacillus moniliformis as the causative agent in spondylodiscitis and psoas abscess after rooster scratches. *J. Clin. Microbiol.* 46, 2820–2821, 2008.

Elliott SP, Rat bite fever and Streptobacillus moniliformis. *Clin. Microbiol. Rev.* 20, 13–22, 2007.

Gaastra W et al., Rat bite fever. *Vet. Microbiol.* 133, 211–228, 2009.

Holroyd KJ, Reiner AP, Dick JD, Streptobacillus moniliformis polyarthritis mimicking rheumatoid arthritis: an urban case of rat bite fever. *Am. J. Med.* 85, 711–714, 1988.

Khatchadourian K et al., The rise of the rats: a growing paediatric issue. *Paediatr Child Health* 15, 131–134, 2010.

McEvoy MB, Noah ND, Pilsworth R, Outbreak of fever caused by Streptobacillus moniliformis. *Lancet* 2, 1361–1363, 1987.

McKee G, Pewarchuk J, Rat bite fever. *CMAJ* 185, 1346, 2013.

Ojukwu IC, Christy C, Rat-bite fever in children: case report and review. *Scand. J. Infect. Dis.* 34, 474–477, 2002.

Rordorf T et al., Streptobacillus moniliformis endocarditis in an HIV-positive patient. *Infection* 28, 393–394, 2000.

Sens MA et al., Fatal Streptobacillus moniliformis infection in a two-month-old infant. *Am. J. Clin. Pathol.* 91, 612–616, 1989.

Wang TK, Wong SS, Streptobacillus moniliformis septic arthritis: a clinical entity distinct from rat-bite fever? *BMC Infect. Dis.* 7, 56, 2007.

Wullenweber M, Streptobacillus moniliformis—a zoonotic pathogen. Taxonomic considerations, host species, diagnosis, therapy, geographical distribution. *Lab. Anim.* 29, 1–15, 1995.

2.19 Rickettsioses

2.19.1 GENERAL FEATURES

Rickettsioses are vector-associated bacterial infections for which mammals, primarily rodents, are the animal reservoir. Vectors are arthropods. Depending on the bacterial agent, these might be lice, fleas, mites, or ticks. All rickettsial infections are zoonoses, including epidemic typhus for which sporadic infections from natural foci are known. Epidemics of typhus (anthroponoses) have become rare today and occur only locally.

Rickettsia spp. are small, pleomorphic, round (diameter, 0.3 μm) or oval (0.3 × 0.5 μm), nonmotile, Gram-negative bacteria with an inner cytoplasmic membrane, a peptidoglycan layer, and an outer membrane with LPS and two immunodominant membrane proteins, rOmpA (190 kDa) and rOmpB (135 kDa). Frequently, rickettsiae are surrounded by a microcapsule and a mucin layer. They are obligately intracellular parasites of eukaryotes (vertebrates and arthropods), multiplying either in their cytoplasm or, more rarely, in their nuclei.

16S rDNA analysis has changed their taxonomy. *Rickettsia* spp. are now in the family *Rickettsiaceae* of the Alpha-1-subgroup of the *Proteobacteria*. The former *Rickettsia/Rochalimaea quintana* (agent of trench fever) is now in the family *Bartonellaceae* of the same subgroup, while the former *Coxiella burnetii* (agent of Q fever) is in the Gamma-Proteobacteria, order *Legionellales*. Within the family *Rickettsiaceae*, the agent of tsutsugamushi (scrub) fever is in a new genus, *Orientia*, which lacks LPS and contains unrelated proteins. The genus *Rickettsia* is divided into the typhus group, the spotted fever group, the phylogenetically oldest group, including *R. bellii* and *R. canadensis*, and a transitional group including *R. felis, R. australis,* and *R. akari*. Since 1985, more than 12 new potentially human pathogens have been delineated so that the genus now numbers >20 species, with >6 also being reported from Central Europe (Tab. 2.8). Independent of the new taxonomic positions, the above subdivision has maintained its value in clinical practice and serological diagnosis.

Rickettsiae infect the endothelial cells of small vessels causing vasculitides with hypoperfusion and anoxia, increased vascular permeability with edema, hypovolemia, hypotension, hypalbuminemia, hyponatremia and increased platelet adherence. Manifestations of rickettsioses vary depending on virulence and tropism of the species.

Target organs may be the skin (with development of exanthemas, petechiae, necroses due to microinfarcts), the lung (interstitial pneumonia and pulmonary edema), the heart (interstitial myocarditis), the brain (meningoencephalitis), the gastrointestinal tract (diarrhea), the pancreas (pancreatitis), the liver (hepatitis), and blood coagulation (thrombocytopenia, hemorrhages, and ecchymoses).

Laboratory Diagnosis. Rickettsial isolation must be performed in specialized biosafety level

Tab.2.8a | Human pathogenic *Rickettsia* spp.: spotted fever group, typhus group, and tsutsugamushi fever

SPECIES	DISEASE	SYMPTOMATOLOGY	VECTORS	OCCURRENCE
R. rickettsii	Rocky Mountain spotted fever	Frequently severe febrile disease, exanthema	*Dermacentor variabilis, D. andersoni* and others	North/South America
R. conorii	Mediterranean spotted fever	Moderately severe febrile disease, eschar, exanthema	*Rhipicephalus sanguineus* and others	Mediterranean area, Mideast, India
R. africae	African spotted fever	Moderately severe febrile disease, eschar, local exanthema	*Amblyomma hebraeum, A. variegatum* and others	Subsaharean Africa, Caribbean
R. acari	Rickettsialpox	Mild disease, eschar, varicella like exanthema	*Allodermanyssus sanguineus*	Probably worldwide, single foci
R. prowazekii	Epidemic typhus	High fever, exanthema, hemorrhagias, encephalitis, mortality 10 to 40%	*Pediculus humanus humanus*	Worldwide in moderate climates
R. typhi	Endemic typhus	Fever, exanthema Mortality 1 to 8%	*Xenopsylla cheopis* and other fleas	Worldwide single foci
Orientia tsutsugamushi	Tsutsugamushi fever	Frequently severe febrile disease, eschar, exanthema	*Leptotrombidium* spp. and other mites	East/South-east Asia

Modified from Dobler G and Wölfel R: Deutsches Aerzteblatt 106, 348–354, 2009; and from Knobloch R and Löscher T: Rickettsiosen, in: Löscher T and Burchard G-D (eds.): Tropenmedizin in Klinik und Praxis, Thieme, Stuttgart, Germany, 2010.

Table 2.8b | Human pathogenic *Rickettsia* spp. in Central Europe

SPECIES	DISEASE	SYMPTOMATOLOGY	VECTORS	OCCURRENCE
R. slovaca	Tick bite lymphadenitis		*Dermacentor marginatus*	Europe, Asia
R. raoultii	In single cases, tick bite lymphadenitis		*Dermacentor reticulatus*	France, Germany
R. helvetica	Noneruptive tick bite fever	In single cases, perimyocarditis, meningitis	*Ixodes ricinus*	Europe, Asia
R. monacensis	Tick bite fever	In single cases, fever, exanthema	*Ixodes ricinus*	Bavaria, Spain
R. massiliae	Tick bite fever	In single cases, fever, exanthema	*Rhipicephalus sanguineus, Ixodes ricinus*	Mediterranean area, Bavaria
R. felis	Cat-flea typhus	Fever, exanthema	*Ctenocephalides felis*	Probably worldwide

Modified from Dobler G and Wölfel R: Deutsches Aerzteblatt 106, 348–354, 2009; and from Knobloch R and Löscher T: Rickettsiosen, in: Löscher T and Burchard G-D (eds.): Tropenmedizin in Klinik und Praxis, Thieme, Stuttgart, Germany, 2010.

3 laboratories. Nowadays, culture is done in various (e.g., Vero) cell lines using shell vials that have supplanted embyonated eggs and animal inoculation (except for mice in suspected cases of *O. tsutsugamushi*).

The diagnosis is labor-intensive, expensive, and promising only if the material (biopsy, eschar material, blood) has been taken early. PCR serves to identify rickettsial isolates directly (e.g., from blood leukocytes) or in cell cultures. The sensitivity for the latter is as high as 70%. For some species specific primers are available; otherwise, genus-specific primers with subsequent DNA sequence analysis have to be employed. Work with rickettsiae must be performed in a biosafety 3 laboratory. They are also potential bioweapons.

Most frequently, however, the diagnosis is made by IFA with rickettsial antigens. The Weil-Felix reaction with cross-reacting *Proteus* antigens is obsolete. Western blot techniques with pre-absorption of antibodies are reserved for specialized laboratories. Within a group, rickettsiae show serological cross reactions; species differentiation can be attempted by comparison of titers with different antigens. Antibodies can be expected at the earliest 7 to 10 days after the onset of symptoms and they may not appear if antibiotic treatment has begun early.

Therapy. All rickettsioses react favorably to early antibiotic treatment, the drug of choice being doxycycline. Alternatives are ciprofloxacin or chloramphenicol (check for availability!), and in children <8 years and pregnant patients, macrolides (clarithromycin, azithromycin).

Prophylaxis. As vaccines have been discontinued and were never officially licensed, the only prophylactic measure to take is avoidance of tick exposure (see Borreliosis). In infested rooms, acaricides can be tried. Control of the brown dog tick with silicates requires specialists. If lice or fleas are vectors, systematic delousing or flea control are required. Rodenticides can be used if the reservoir involves rodents. Elimination of infected or stray dogs is a possibility but it would most likely meet resistance.

Reporting. The spotted fever rickettsioses are notifiable diseases in the USA and in Canada.

REFERENCES

Anonymous, Epidemic typhus in Rwandan refugee camps. *Wkly. Epid. Rec.* 69, 259, 1994.

Appel KE et al., Risk assesment of Bundeswehr (German Federal Armed Forces) permethrin −impregnated battle dress uniforms (BDU). *Int.J.Hyg. Environ. Health*, 211, 88–104, 2008.

Beati L, Raoult D, Rickettsia massiliae sp. nov., a new spotted fever group rickettsia. *Int. J. Syst. Bacteriol.* 43, 839–840, 1993.

Bise G, Coninx R, Epidemic typhus in a prison in Burundi. *Trans. R. Soc. Trop. Med. Hyg.* 91, 133–134, 1997.

Blanton LS, Rickettsial infections in the tropics and in the traveler. *Curr Opin Infect Dis* 26, 435–440, 2013.

Boostrom A et al., Geographic association of Rickettsia felis infected opossums with human murine typhus, Texas. *Emerg. Infect. Dis.* 8, 549–554, 2002.

Burgdorfer W et al., Ixodes ricinus: vector of a hitherto undescribed spotted fever group agent in Switzerland. *Acta Trop* 36, 357–67, 1979.

Cascio A et al., Clarithromycin versus azithromycin in the treatment of Mediterranean spotted fever in children: a randomized controlled trial. *Clin. Infect. Dis.* 34, 154–158, 2002.

Duma RJ et al., Epidemic typhus in the United States associated with flying squirrels. *J. Am. Med. Assoc.* 245, 2318–2323, 1981.

Dupon M et al., Scrub typhus: an imported rickettsial disease. *Infection.* 20, 153–154, 1992.

Fournier PE et al., Evidence of Rickettsia helvetica infection in humans, eastern France. *Emerg. Infect. Dis.* 6, 389–392, 2000.

Fournier PE et al., Outbreak of Rickettsia africae infections in participants of an adventure race in South Africa. *Clin. Infect. Dis.* 27, 316–323, 1998.

Gillespie JJ et al., Plasmids and rickettsial evolution: insights from Rickettsia felis. *PLoS One* 2(3), e266, 2007.

Hartelt K et al., Pathogens and symbionts in ticks: prevalence of Anaplasma phagocytophilum (Ehrlichia sp.), Wolbachia sp., Rickettsia sp., and Babesia sp. in Southern Germany. *Int. J. Med. Microbiol.* 293(Suppl. 37), 86–92, 2004.

Higgins JA et al., Rickettsia felis: a new species of pathogenic rickettsia isolated from cat fleas. *J. Clin. Microbiol.* 34, 671–674, 1996.

Jado I et al., Rickettsia monacensis and human disease, Spain. *Emerg. Infect. Dis.* 13, 1405–1407, 2007.

Jelinek T, Löscher T, Clinical features and epidemiology of tick-typhus in travellers. *J. Travel. Med.* 8, 57–59, 2001.

Kass EM et al., Rickettsialpox in a New York City hospital, 1980–1989. *New Engl. J. Med.* 331, 1612–1617, 1994.

Marquez FJ et al., Presence of Rickettsia felis in the cat flea from southwestern Europe. *Emerg. Infect. Dis.* 8, 89–91, 2002.

McDade JE et al., Evidence of Rickettsia prowazekii infections in the United States. *Am. J. Trop. Med. Hyg.* 29, 277–284, 1980.

Mediannikov O et al., Rickettsia raoultii sp. nov., a spotted fever group rickettsia associated with Dermacentor ticks in Europe and Russia. *Int. J. Syst. Evol. Microbiol.* 58, 1635–1639, 2008.

Nilsson K, Elfvig K, Pahlson C, Rickettsia helvetica in patient with meningitis, Sweden, 2006. *Emerg. Infect. Dis.* 16, 490–492, 2010.

Nilsson K, Lindquist O, Pahlson C, Association of Rickettsia helvetica with chronic perimyocarditis in sudden cardiac death. *Lancet* 354, 1169–1173, 1999.

Oteo JA, Portillo A, Tick-borne rickettsioses in Europe. *Ticks Tick Borne Dis* 3, 271–278, 2012.

Pai H et al., Central nervous system involvement in patients with scrub typhus. *Clin. Infect. Dis.* 24, 436–440, 1997.

Parola P, Davoust B, Raoult D, Tick-and flea-borne rickettsial emerging zoonoses. *Vet. Res.* 36, 469–492, 2005.

Parola P, Paddock CD, Raoult D, Tick-borne rickettsioses around the world: emerging diseases challenging old concepts. *Clin. Microbiol. Rev.* 18, 719–756, 2005.

Parola P, Raoult D, Tropical rickettsioses. *J. Clin. Dermatol.* 24, 191–200, 2006.

Parola P et al., Rickettsia slovaca and R. raoultii in tick-borne rickettsioses. *Emerg. Infect. Dis.* 15, 1105–1108, 2009.

Parola P et al., Update on tick-borne rickettsioses around the world: a geographic approach. *Clin Microbiol Rev* 26, 657–702, 2013.

Perine PL et al., A clinico-epidemiological study of epidemic typhus in: Africa. *Clin. Infect. Dis.* 14, 1149–1158, 1992.

Pluta S et al., Prevalence of Coxiella burnetii and Rickettsia spp. in ticks and rodents in southern Germany. *Ticks Tickborne Dis.* 1(3), 145–147, 2010.

Pluta S et al., Rickettsia slovaca in Dermacentor marginatus ticks, Germany. *Emerg. Infect. Dis.* 15, 2077–2078, 2009.

Raoult D et al., A new tick-transmitted disease due to: Rickettsia slovaca. *Lancet* 350, 112–113, 1997.

Raoult D, Roux V, Rickettsioses as paradigms of new or emerging infectious diseases. *Clin. Microbiol. Rev.* 10, 694–719, 1997.

Rehacek J, Rickettsiae of the spotted fever isolated from Dermacentor marginatus ticks in South Germany. *Zbl. Bakt. Hyg. I Abt. Orig. A* 239, 275–281, 1977.

Schex S et al., Rickettsia spp. in wild small mammals in lower Bavaria, South-Eastern Germany. *Vector Borne Zoonotic Dis.* 11, 493–502, 2011.

Seong SY, Choi MS, Kim IS, Orientia tsutsugamushi infection: overview and immune responses. *Microb Infect* 3, 11–21, 2001.

Simser JA et al., Rickettsia monacensis sp. nov., a spotted fever group Rickettsia, from ticks (Ixodes ricinus) collected in a European city park. *Appl. Environ. Microbiol.* 68, 4559–4566, 2002.

Thorner AR, Walker DH, Petri WA, Rocky Mountain spotted fever. *Clin. Infect. Dis.* 27, 1353–1359, 1998.

Vestris G et al., Seven years experience of isolation of Rickettsia spp. from clinical specimens using the shell vial cell culture assay. *Ann. N.Y. Acad. Sci.* 990, 371–374, 2003.

Walker DH, Rocky Mountain spotted fever: a seasonal alert. *Clin. Infect. Dis.* 20, 1111–1117, 1995.

Wölfel R et al., Rickettsia spp. in Ixodes ricinus ticks in Bavaria, Germany. *Ann. N. Y. Acad. Sci.* 1078, 509–511, 2006.

Yamashita T et al., Transmission of Rickettsia tsutsugamushi strains among humans, wild rodents, and trombiculid mites in an area of Japan in which tsutsugamushi disease is newly endemic. *J. Clin. Microbiol.* 32, 2780–2785, 1994.

2.19.2 ROCKY MOUNTAIN SPOTTED FEVER

RMSF is the most important rickettsiosis in the Western Hemisphere and the most severe one among those transmitted by ticks. It is a systemic febrile disease with a hemorrhagic exanthema. Due to the existence of natural foci, it has not lost in significance. The course is frequently severe and fatal without antibiotic treatment.

Etiology. The causative agent is *Rickettsia rickettsii.*

Occurrence. Natural foci are present in almost all states of the US, Canada, Central America (Mexico, Costa Rica, Panama), and in the northern countries of South America (Colombia, Brazil) but not in Europe, Africa, and Asia. Reservoirs are hard ticks (in the eastern US, *Dermacentor variabilis*; in the western states, *D. andersonii*; in Mexico, *Rhipicephalus sanguineus*, the brown dog tick; there and in Central and South America, *Amblyomma cayennense*) which, together with rabbits, field mice and other rodents form natural foci. Ticks

remain infectious throughout their lives and transmit the agent transovarially to their progeny. Among domestic animals, dogs may acquire the disease.

Transmission. Infection of humans and dogs occurs through the bite of infected ticks. At the earliest 6 h after being infected, the tick transmits the organism with its saliva. Infections occur mostly between April and October and in warm areas, also in winter. Dogs are frequently responsible for transmission (Fig. 2.19).

Clinical Manifestations. The incidence of RMSF is highest in individuals aged 5 to 9 years and in those >60 years. Risk factors are outdoor activities and contact with tick-infested dogs. In almost all patients, a history of tick exposure can be elicited; 60% even remember a tick bite. In contrast to other tick-borne fevers, primary lesions are rarely seen.

The incubation period is 3 to 12 (average, 7) days. Infection may be asymptomatic, light, or, fulminant. The latter generally starts acutely with high fever up to 40 °C, severe headache (90%), malaise and myalgias (80%), anorexia,

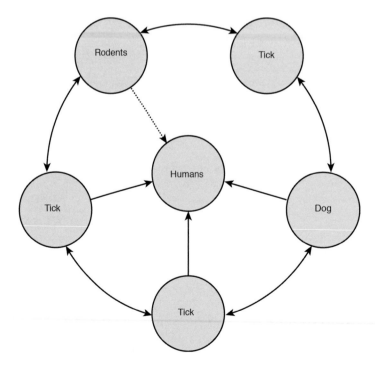

Figure 2.19 | Possible transmission chains, Rocky Mountain spotted fever.

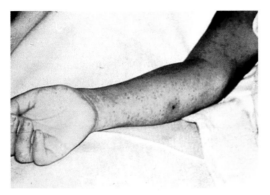

Figure 2.20 | Exanthema and primary lesion, Rocky Mountain spotted fever (Dr. H. Lieske, Hamburg, Germany).

nausea, vomiting (86%), and abdominal pain (50%). The rash (Fig. 2.20), initially pink, becoming maculo-papular and finally petechial with hemorrhages, is present on the first day only in every sixth patient but on the third day in every other patient. Occasionally, there are only a few spots, and 10 to 15% of the patients exhibit no rash at all, which does not point to a better prognosis, however. The rash generally starts over the joints of hands and feet, blanches on pressure, and intensifies with a rise in temperature. Within a few hours, it progresses centripetally and affects axilla, hip, the torso, and sometimes, the palms and soles. Complications are shock, skin gangrene, pulmonary edema, ARDS, acute renal failure, hepatosplenomegaly, focal hepatitis, pancreatitis, disseminated intravascular coagulation, hemorrhages in the gastrointestinal and urogenital tracts, and CNS symptoms, such as stupor, delirium, coma, and convulsions. The case-fatality rate is 10 to 60% in untreated cases, with early antibiotic treatment, it is 5 to 10%. Fulminant courses may lead to death within >5 days. Clinical symptoms in dogs are high fever, anorexia, general weakness, abdominal pain, and hemorrhages.

Diagnosis. The diagnosis may be difficult in the first few days. Even if a rash is absent, RSMF should be considered in patients who have been to areas of endemicity with tick exposure and who have a high fever, severe headache, myalgias, and malaise. The appearance of the rash during the following days would allow for a tentative diagnosis. The laboratory could confirm it by PCR of a skin biopsy or of peripheral leukocytes. Serology provides only for a group diagnosis (see 2.20.1).

Differential Diagnosis. During the initial, often oligosymptomatic phase influenza, enterovirus infections, typhoid fever, infectious mononucleosis, septicemia, and ehrlichiosis have to be taken into consideration. Depending on the localization of symptoms, acute bronchitis, bacterial or viral pneumonia, gastroenteritis, an acute abdomen, or meningoencephalitis may also be considered. The typical rash may resemble that of meningococcal septicemia, second-stage lues, toxic shock syndrome, and rubella.

Therapy. Early antimicrobial therapy is mandatory, even if the diagnosis has not been confirmed in the laboratory, because it will help to prevent dangerous complications. Optimal is doxycycline 2×100 mg/day i.v. or p.o. for 7 days. Pregnant patients receive chloramphenicol (check for availability!) 4×15 mg/kg/day i.v. or p.o. for 7 days. If therapy starts later, rickettsiae may still be eliminated but organ damage may nevertheless lead to a fatal outcome. In severe cases, admission to an intensive care unit is necessary.

Prophylaxis. See 2.19.1.

2.19.3 MEDITERRANEAN SPOTTED FEVER

Mediterranean spotted fever (Fièvre boutonneuse) belongs to the most frequent rickettsioses in Southern Europe and may affect tourists from Central Europe as well. The generally benign disease is characterized by a primary lesion, fever for up to 10 days, and a maculopapular rash.

Etiology. The causative agent is *R. conorii*, which is now considered a complex with a variety of subspecies.

Occurrence. *R. conorii* is endemic in the entire Mediterranean area. The yearly incidence in Portugal could extend to 10 per 100 000 inhabitants. Sporadic cases from Africa below the Sahara and from the Black Sea have been known but may have to be reassessed in view of the new taxonomy. The reservoir is primarily ticks (*Rhipicephalus sanguineus*) that are able to transmit the agent transovarially. The animal reservoir is in small rodents (rats) and, particularly in Mediterranean countries, in dogs who have shown seroprevalence rates of up to 70%. Mass imports of dogs from this area involve the danger of importing *R. conorii*, and *Rhipicephalus* would be brought along which, as a thermophilic species, could survive indoors for long periods. This way, endemic foci of *R. conorii* would be created.

Transmission. Infected ticks cause human infection through their saliva that is transmitted by the bite. Most infections take place during summer, the time of the highest activity of ticks. Although 5 to 12% of *R. sanguineus* are infested with *R. conorii*, humans are relatively rarely affected because of the high host specificity of the brown dog tick. The most likely mode of infection is through living with dogs or through collection of their ticks. Other ways, for example,

direct contact with infected dogs, are being discussed (Fig. 2.21).

Clinical Manifestations. The incubation period is between 2 and 7 days. In >50% of the cases, there is a pea-size primary lesion with a central necrosis (eschar), which may ulcerate and is covered with a black scab ("tache noire"; Fig. 2.22). However, a tick bite cannot be seen in every case of Mediterranean fever. Most cases show a regional lymphadenitis and fever of >39 °C lasting for 1 to 2 weeks associated with head, joint and muscle aches, and a generalized papulous rash ("boutonneuse") that develops on the third to fifth day but may not show at all. This rash will disappear without desquamation at the end of the febrile period.

Changes in cytokines, hypercoagulability, and deep venous thromboses may occur. In severe cases, particularly in older patients or those with alcoholism, diabetes or heart failure, meningoencephalitis with coma and convulsions or disseminated vasculitis in heart, lungs, kidneys, liver, and pancreas may occur. The case-fatality rate is 1 to 5% and higher in severe cases.

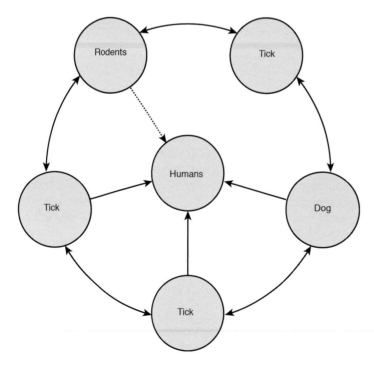

Figure 2.21 | Possible transmission chains, Mediterranean spotted fever.

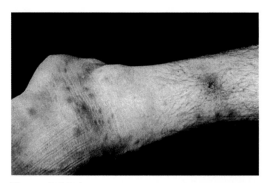

Figure 2.22 | Tache noire and exanthema, Mediterranean spotted fever (Dr. B. Stenglein, Institut für Infektions und Tropenmedizin, Ludwig Maximilians Universität, Munich, Germany).

Diagnosis. The diagnosis should be based on a history of tick exposure and the clinical symptoms (tache noire, rash). The laboratory diagnosis uses PCR from biopsies of a tache noire or the area of the rash. Serological tests are group-, not species-specific (see 2.20.1)

Differential Diagnosis. If there is no primary lesion, murine and classical typhus and other diseases that go along with a rash have to be considered. In areas where malaria occurs, it has to be ruled out.

Therapy. Doxycyline 2×100 mg/day p.o. for 7 days. Children <8 years and pregnant women may be treated with azithromycin 1×10 mg/kg/day p.o. for 3 days, unless there is a severe course.

Prophylaxis. See 2.19.1.

2.19.4 AFRICAN TICK BITE FEVER AND OTHER SPOTTED FEVER DISEASES

African tick bite fever is being increasingly diagnosed in tourists visiting South African national parks. The characteristics of African tick bite fever are multiple primary lesions due to multiple tick bites, as well as a local rash; the disease, however, is benign. Several similar diseases of the spotted fever group have been observed in various continents but have only local significance.

Etiology. The agent of African tick fever is *R. africae*. Initially, it was thought to be *R. conorii* but separation of the two species was accomplished in 1990. Other agents of the spotted fever group have been observed in various regions: *R. australis*, *R. marmionii* (Australia), *R. honei* (Flinders Island), *R. sibirica*, *R. mongolotimonae* (North and Central Asia), *R. japonica* (Japan), *R. aeschlimannii* (Africa), and *R. parkeri* (North and South America). Their pathogenicity has only been proven in the past few years. Description of new species on the basis of molecular differentiation is likely.

Occurrence. *R. africae* occurs primarily in South Africa and Zimbabwe. Endemic areas are the national parks. It has, however, also been found in many other countries south of the Sahara, with a seroprevalence in the population as high as 30 to 80%. It is assumed that *Amblyomma* ticks and *R. africae* were introduced to Guadeloupe through the export of cattle, and from there spread to other West Indian islands.

Transmission. The most important vector in South Africa is the cattle tick, *Amblyomma hebraeum*. In northern areas, there is *A. variegatum* and *A.lepidum*. *Amblyomma* ticks are aggressive in searching out hosts, therefore, multiple infections are not rare. In South Africa, the attack rate can be close to 100%, which explains the high seroprevalence rates.

Clinical Manifestations. African tick fever is rare in the indigenous population and it is almost only travelers from North America or Europe who are affected. The seroprevalence rate is ci. 10% in tourists from Africa. Approximately 50 cases per year are reported in Germany. After an incubation period of 5 to 7 days, fever, multiple eschars, lymphadenitis and, in 50% of cases, a rash will develop (Fig. 2.23) Fatal cases have never been reported. The disease is generally mild but frequent in travelers.

Diagnosis, Differential Diagnosis, Therapy, Prophylaxis. Similar to that of Mediterranean spotted fever.

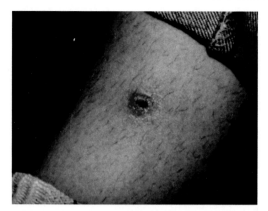

Figure 2.23 | African tick bite fever. Tache noire (eschar) on the left ankle (Dr. D. Hassler, Kraichtal, Germany).

2.19.5 RICKETTSIOSES IN CENTRAL EUROPE

Rickettsioses in Central Europe had not been known since the end of the typhus epidemics. Only in the 1970s, rickettsial species were detected in *Dermacentor* and *Ixodes* spp. and in some rodents. Initially, they were thought to be apathogenic for humans but this proved to be an error.

Etiology. These rickettsiae have been mostly reported from Southern Germany but sporadically also from Central Germany. This may have been due to the fact that investigations centered on those areas.

Transmission. Rickettsiae were found in only three tick species: *D. marginatus, D. reticulatus,* and *I. ricinus. D. marginatus* is host-specific, *D. reticulatus* occurs mostly in dogs, and only *I. ricinus* has a wide host spectrum that includes humans. The patients' histories mention tick bites.

Clinical Manifestations. These infections have been sporadic. In Rhineland-Palatinate, a bite of *D. marginatus* has caused lymphadenitis and local erythema (Tick-borne lymphadenopathy, TIBOLA) due to *R. slovaca*. Disease due to *R. raoultii, R. helvetica, R. monacensis, R. massiliae,* and *R. felis* have not been seen in Germany. Diseases in other areas, however, have shown their

human pathogenicity: *R. raoultii* has also caused lymphadenitis, *R. helvetica* was found associated with perimyocarditis, meningitis, and a febrile generalized infection; *R. monacensis, R. massiliae,* and *R. felis* caused a febrile disease with a maculopapular rash (Tab. 2.8b).

Diagnosis. Tick bite, fever, lymphadenopathy. For the laboratory diagnosis, see 2.19.1.

Differential Diagnosis, Therapy, Prophylaxis. As for 2.19.3.

2.19.6 RICKETTSIALPOX

Rickettsialpox is a rare, sporadic, benign febrile infection characterized by a primary lesion and a varicella-like rash.

Etiology. The causative agent is *R. akari* that belongs to the transitional group of rickettsiae (see 2.19.1). As it shares antigens with organisms of the spotted fever group, which leads to cross reactions, it is, for practical reasons, often listed as a member of that group.

Occurrence. Rickettsialpox has thus far only been found in the USA (primarily in New York State) and in Russia, while the causative agent has also been isolated in Croatia, Southern Europe, South Africa, and Korea. The disease remains local and occurs mainly in spring and summer.

The reservoir are small, colorless, bloodsucking mites (*Liponyssoides (formerly Allodermanyssus) sanguineus*), which transmit the rickettsiae transovarially. Infected mites and their natural hosts, mice and rats, are natural foci. In mice, *R. akari* remains alive for about 1 month.

Transmission. *R. akari* is transmitted to humans by the bite of infected mites or direct skin contact with them (Fig. 2.24). The presence of natural hosts is a requirement, for example, mice who are attracted by the garbage shoots and ovens of modern cooperative dwellings. Aerogenic transmission has taken place in laboratories.

Clinical Manifestations. The incubation period is 7 to 14 days. At the site of the bite, a painful papule will develop that ulcerates and leaves a

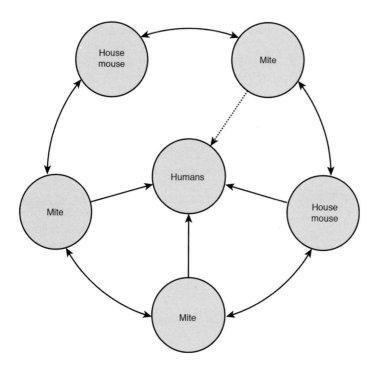

Figure 2.24 | Possible transmission chains, rickettsialpox.

black eschar. Regional lymph nodes are swollen but are painless. Some days later, fever, chills, headache, myalgia, and photophobia appear. After several hours or days, a varicella-like rash develops with initial erythematous papules and later blisters that form crusts and heal. The course is benign but without treatment, the disease may last for several weeks.

Diagnosis. The clinical symptoms alone may lead to a diagnosis, which is to be confirmed by a laboratory (see 2.19.1).

Differential Diagnosis. Tick bite fever, varicella, eczema herpeticum, and eczema vaccinatum have to be considered.

Therapy and Prophylaxis. See 2.19.3.

2.19.7 EPIDEMIC TYPHUS

Epidemic (louse-borne) typhus is one of the oldest and most dangerous plagues of humankind. Its occurrence, often in the form of pandemics, has always been associated with hunger, war, and human misery. At the time of the Napoleonic wars in the 19th century, it was of considerable significance. DNA analyses have shown that ci. one-third of all sodiers were infected with *R. prowazekii*. From 1918 to 1922, 30 million people acquired the disease in Russia and 3 million died. From 1981 to 1990 over 20 000 cases were reported worldwide. In 1997 and 2000, there were outbreaks in Russia and Kazakhstan, respectively.

Etiology. The agent is *R. prowazekii*, the prototype of the typhus group. It is closely related to *R. mooseri*, the agent of endemic typhus that belongs to the same group.

Occurrence. The classical epidemic form (case-fatality rate without treatment, 10 to 40%) is encountered today in Northern and Central Africa (Ethiopia, Sudan, Somalia, Kenya, Uganda, Ruanda, Burundi), Central and South America (Mexico, Colombia, Peru, and Bolivia), the countries of the former USSR, and in the Himalaya region including Pakistan and Afghanistan.

Massive and constantly worn clothing, and particularly congested living conditions due to war, dislocation, and refugee existence, favor outbreaks. Sporadic cases have occurred in some states of the USA (Maine to Florida, Minnesota to eastern Texas), as there have been natural foci whose existence is independent of human settlements, and where *R. prowazekii* occurs widely in flying squirrels (*Glaucomys volans volans*) and their ectoparasites (lice and fleas). Following an infection, flying squirrels develop rickettsemia for 2 to 3 weeks. These strains, however, differ from classical ones insofar as they do not, as a rule, cause epidemics in humans but rather sporadic disease only, particularly in winter. In Ethiopia, a further animal reservoir was found in *Hyalomma* ticks infesting domestic animals, but their epidemiological significance is unclear.

Transmission. The classical epidemic form is transmitted by the human body louse (*Pediculus humanus corporis*), which only parasitizes humans, infects itself on bacteremic patients, and dies from the infection. It defecates when taking a blood meal. The bite causes itching and the subsequent scratching leads to inoculation of the rickettsiae into the skin. Dead lice and their excreta, for example, dried louse feces, may cause airborne infection if inhaled. This classical mode of transmission does not operate in sporadic cases that occur on contact with natural foci. As the lice parasitizing flying squirrels are host specific, it can be assumed that the flying squirrel flea, *Orchopeas howardii*, which may also infect humans, transmits the rickettsiae.

Clinical Manifestations. The incubation period is 10 to 14 days. After nonspecific prodromes, a febrile illness develops within 3 days, characterized by a continuous fever of 40 °C, conjunctivitis, severe headache, tachypnea, myalgias, arthralgias, dry cough, anorexia, nausea, vomiting, and diarrhea. From the 5th day on, the rash develops, which is first pink and spotted and later deep red and maculopapular, occasionally even confluent. It starts in the axillar region and spreads centrifugally.

The face, palms, and soles are not affected. Encephalitis with confusion, restlessness, excitation, changes in speech and motion, myocarditis with tachycardia of 120 to 140/min and hypotension are well-known complications. Kidney and liver function may be impaired. If the patient survives without treatment, a slow decrease in fever, bradycardia, and remission of the CNS symptoms occur after ci. 2 weeks of illness. Full recovery may take years. *R. prowazekii* may also persist in humans and later cause a mild recurrence called Brill-Zinsser disease. The symptoms of sporadic typhus resemble those of the classical form but the course is mostly benign; fatalities are not known.

Diagnosis. The diagnosis is suspected by the patient's history (lice) and the clinical symptoms (high fever, rash). The laboratory diagnosis involves PCR from skin biopsy specimens. The serological mainstays are IFA and EIA (see 2.19.1).

Differential Diagnosis. RMSF, relapsing fever, measles in adults (Africa!).

Therapy. Therapy must be started early in order to avoid irreversible organ damage. The drug of choice is doxycycline 2×100 mg/day for 7 to 10 days i.v. or p.o. Children and pregnant women receive chloramphenicol (check for availability!) 4×15 mg/kg/day i.v. or p.o. for 7 days. In late pregnancy, doxycycline may be used.

Prophylaxis. Production of a vaccine has been discontinued. For louse control permethrin, a contact poison with excellent stability is best suited. In some countries, permethrin impregnation of uniforms has been successful. In areas with high risk, 1×100 mg doxycycline /week until 1 week after leaving the area is recommended.

2.19.8 MURINE TYPHUS

Murine typhus (endemic typhus, Toulon typhus, tabardillo) is a rickettsial infection of rodents that can be transmitted to humans by fleas. Symptoms resemble that of classical typhus except that the course is milder.

Etiology. The agent is *R. typhi* (formerly, *R. mooseri*). Identical symptoms may be caused by *R. felis*, which is transmitted by cat fleas.

Occurrence. Murine typhus occurs primarily in the tropics and subtropics, either sporadically or in miniepidemics. In Europe, cases have been observed in the former Yugoslavia, Greece, Malta, and Sicily. Recently, a few cases were reported from Japan. In the US, simultaneous infections with *R. typhi* and *R. felis* have occurred in California and in Texas. Men are more frequently affected than women. Peak seasons are summer and fall. Human infections depend on the presence of a substantial rat population, for example, in port cities or in rural areas. In Los Angeles, urban opossums have been implicated as hosts.

Transmission. Reservoirs and vectors are rat fleas (*Xenopsylla cheopis* and *Leptopsylla segnis*) in which a transovarial cycle (of lesser significance) may also occur (Fig. 2.25). Cat fleas (*Ctenocephalides felis*) are rare vectors. Fleas remain infected for their entire lives and they are only slightly affected by the presence of the rickettsiae, which is in contrast to lice. Humans become infected from flea feces by killing an infected flea or through inhalation of contaminated dust in which rickettsiae can remain alive for years.

Clinical Manifestations. After an incubation period of 7 to 14 days, fever, headache, anorexia, myalgias, epistaxis, and in 60 to 80% of patients, a rash is observed. This is initially spotted, later becoming maculopapular in 50% of the patients and mostly present on the torso. Murine typhus is benign (see above) and has a case-fatality rate of <1% even without treatment.

Diagnosis. As for the other rickettsioses. Antibodies are rarely detected during the acute phase; therefore, the laboratory diagnosis is mostly a retrospective one.

Therapy. As for 2.19.7.

Prophylaxis. In endemic areas, use of insecticides and rodenticides.

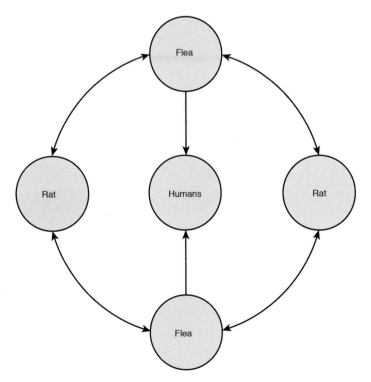

Figure 2.25 | Transmission chains, endemic typhus.

2.19.9 TSUTSUGAMUSHI FEVER (SCRUB TYPHUS)

Tsutsugamushi fever (kedani disease, chigger-borne rickettsiosis, scrub typhus) is a frequently severe rickettsial disease. It is characterized by a primary lesion, fever lasting for 1 to 2 weeks, and a rash that starts toward the end of the first week.

Etiology. The agent, *Orientia tsutsugamushi*, is a small (0.3 to 0.5 × 0.8 to 1.5 µm) Gram-negative bacterium of the family *Rickettsiaceae*. It differs from the other members of the genus *Rickettsia* in its genetic makeup and its wall structure as LPS, peptidoglycan, and the outer mucus layer are missing. Instead it has a large (56 kDa) and several smaller (110, 80, 46, 43, 39, 35, 28, 25 kDa) surface proteins. There is considerable variation between strains as regards their virulence and antigenic composition. Immunity is type-specific and allows repeated infections.

Occurrence. Scrub typhus is endemic in Southern and Eastern Asia, in the Pacific Islands, and in Northern Australia, with ci. 1 million cases per year. The most important reservoir are rats, mice, rabbits, and marsupials. Mites (*Trombicula* spp.) also act as reservoirs as they transmit the agent transovarially (nymphs and adults live on the ground and are predators). Areas with a moist climate and bush vegetation are natural habitats for the vectors. Humans acquire the disease by walking through those natural habitats. At special risk are participants in adventure travels in the Far East, the Pacific area, and in Australia, if they rest or sleep in the open.

Transmission. Transmission occurs through the bite of *Trombicula* mites whose larvae digest the upper layers of human skin with the help of infected saliva (Fig. 2.26).

Clinical Manifestations. The incubation period lasts from 8 to 10 (6 to 21) days. At the site of inoculation, mostly on moist parts of the skin, a papule develops that ulcerates and heals with the formation of a scab (eschar). The

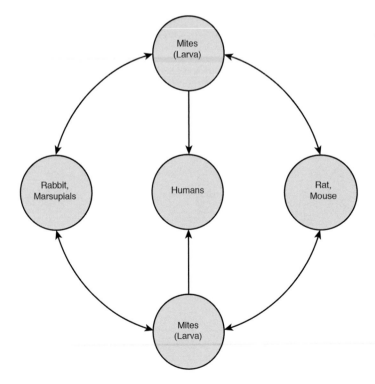

Figure 2.26 | Transmission chains, Tsutsugamushi fever.

regional lymph nodes are swollen. A generalized stage follows with acute fever >40 °C with relative bradycardia, severe headache, apathy, myalgias, generalized lymphadenopathy, photophobia, and a dry cough. Approximately 1 week later, initially a spotted, then a maculopapular rash will develop which starts on the torso and spreads to the extremities but blanches after a few days. Complications are interstitial pneumonia (30 to 65% of patients), meningoencephalitis, and myocarditis. Even without treatment, the symptoms will start to disappear after 2 weeks. The case-fatality rate can be up to 30% if complications arise.

Diagnosis. If history and symptoms are typical (presence in an endemic area, primary lesion, and local lymphadenitis), the diagnosis may already be suspected. Later, the high fever and the rash at the end of the first week provide further evidence. The organism can be diagnosed by PCR from eschar or from the patient's blood. Most cases are diagnosed by serology with IFA or EIA.

Differential Diagnosis. Other diseases with lymphadenopathy, for example, infectious mononucleosis, dengue fever, typhoid fever, and malaria tropica. In India and Southeast Asia, there are also various tick fevers and murine typhus.

Therapy. Doxycycline or chloramphenicol (check for availability!) as in 2.19.7. If resistance has developed, for example, in Northern Thailand, doxycycline should be combined with rifampicin 1×600 to 900 mg/day p.o. for 7 days. Uncomplicated illness in children and in pregnancy can be treated with azithromycin: children 1×10 mg/kg/day p.o. for 3 days, pregnant women 1×500 mg as a single dose p.o. Treatment for up to 2 weeks minimizes the risk of a relapse.

Prophylaxis. Rodenticides, insecticides, protective clothing with a mite repellent. Chemoprophylaxis with 200 mg doxycycline per week for up to 6 weeks can be tried.

2.20 Salmonelloses

For epidemiological and nosological reasons, salmonellosis may be subdivided into the systemic typhoid and paratyphoid diseases (occur in humans only) and the acute enteritides. The latter are important as zoonoses and are increasing in frequency.

Etiology. *Salmonella* is a genus of facultatively anaerobic Gram-negative rods that comprises two species: *S. enterica* (with five subspecies: *enterica* (I), *salamae* (II), *arizonae* (IIIa), *diarizonae* (IIIb), *houtenae* (IV), *indica* (VI); and *S. bongori* (subspecies V). The heterogeneity of salmonellae with their cell wall polysaccharides and flagellar proteins (O and H antigens) is the basis for the Kauffmann-LeMinor (formerly Kauffmann-White) scheme, which at present comprises >2610 serovars.

Most, and possibly all, serovars are human pathogens and may cause acute gastroenteritis in humans. There are, however, differences in virulence between serovars and strains. In most countries, almost all human salmonelloses can be traced to 20 to 30 nonhost-adapted serovars. Until the mid-1980s, serovar *S.* Typhimurium was the predominating one; since then it has been overtaken by *S.* Enteritidis. These serovars are responsible for >80% of all reported *Salmonella* infections in the countries of the European Union.

Salmonellae are invasive and lead a facultatively intracellular existence. Their ability to invade and penetrate intestinal epithelial cells by way of a trigger mechanism and to survive and multiply in macrophages are important factors in establishing their cycle in vertebrates. They have at their disposal a substantial array of virulence factors many of which are encoded by genes that are chromosomally located in groups called "pathogenicity islands." Important virulence factors of salmonellae are adhesive fimbriae (SEF, LPF, Tafi), nonfimbrial adhesins (SdhA, SiiE, BapA), LPS, and various effector proteins that are translocated by the SPI-1 and SPI-2 encoded type III secretion systems into the cytosol of the host cell (SopB, SopD, SopE, SopE2, SipA, SipC, SptP, SpiC, SseF, SpvB, SpvC).

Occurrence. The host spectrum of most salmonellae is wide but individual serovars are adapted by various degrees to certain hosts. This adaptation is reflected in the frequency in which certain serovars occur in certain hosts. Serovars of *S. enterica* subsp. *enterica* prefer warm-blooded vertebrates, other serovars are preferentially found in reptiles. Some *S. enterica* subsp. *enterica* serovars are adapted to a smaller number of hosts or even to one host species only, and found preferentially or exclusively in those hosts. Examples are *S.* Typhi and *S.* Paratyphi A, B, C (human, chimpanzee), *S.* Gallinarum (chicken), *S.* Choleraesuis and *S.* Typhisuis (pig), *S.* Abortusequi (horse), and *S.* Abortusovis (sheep). Among *S.* Typhimurium, which generally has a wide host spectrum, there are variants that are highly adapted to pigeons (phage types DT2 and DT99).

Nontyphoidal salmonellae occur worldwide with various frequencies in all species of vertebrates (mammals, birds, reptiles, amphibias, fish) and arthropods. Sources of infection for humans are domestic animals (calves, pigs), poultry (chicken, turkeys, geese, ducks), free-living birds (seagulls, pigeons), pets (dogs, cats, turtles, iguanas, snakes), rodents (mice, rats), and also humans. The natural habitat of salmonellae is the intestinal tract. They enter the environment via sewage and sludge and are able to remain infective there for months and even years under optimal conditions, for example, in contaminated lakes, brooks, rivers, soil, and on plants. Pandemic spread is possible through international traffic of merchandise, animals, and plants. An example is the multiresistant *S.* Typhimurium DT 104 clone that has been found worldwide since the 1990s.

Salmonelloses occur sporadically, as small-group epidemics (e.g., in families) or epidemically. Epidemics may affect several hundred people in different countries and, under those circumstances, could be difficult to trace. In 2009, the incidence of registered new cases of salmonellosis in the European Union was 23.7 per 100 000 inhabitants (2 to 100, depending on the country register), with a falling tendency.

There is probably a considerable number of unreported cases. Salmonelloses occur during the entire year but are more frequent during the summer months, particularly those due to *S.* Enteritidis, whose frequency in August is 3 to 6 times that of February or March.

Transmission. Animals infected with *Salmonella* excrete the organism mainly through their feces; urine, milk, oro- and nasopharyngeal secretions, as well as material from abortion or amniotic fluid, which on occasion may contain salmonellae as well. Some serovars (e.g., *S.* Enteritidis) can be transmitted transovarially in chicken, infecting eggs and progeny.

In humans, salmonelloses are mostly due to consumption of contaminated foodstuffs. Insufficiently heated chicken eggs and meals prepared with raw egg or egg powder (mayonnaise, icecream, crèmes, sabaione) are the most frequent sources of infection. However, meat and meat products, such as mincemeat, meat salad, and poultry, as well as raw milk and raw milk products, are significant sources. Vegetables and their products, such as tomatoes, rucola, sprouts, paprika, basil, herb teas, chocolate, paprika-spiced potato chips, melons, and unpasteurized fruit juices, are also significant sources. While animal products can occasionally be infected with salmonellae at the time of slaughter, in most instances, contamination of food occurs through fecal or cross contamination during cultivation, harvesting, processing, or cooking. The number of salmonellae transmitted is mostly low and below the minimum infective dose (MID) of 10 000 to 100 000 bacteria. As salmonellae are able to multiply outside hosts in moist environments rich in nutritive material and at temperatures starting at 7 °C (optimally between 35° and 40 °C), certain breaks in food hygiene (interruption of the cold chain, insufficient heating, warming) can lead to higher numbers of bacteria within a few hours. If salmonellae are taken up with chocolate, cheddar cheese, or other food rich in fats, or if infants, small children, older or immunocompromised persons consume salmonellae with their food, even <10 bacteria of some serovars may suffice to cause enteritis.

Humans may also become infected by contact with excreta of infected animals or contaminated items. Human-to-human transmission has taken place in hospitals, old age homes, kindergartens, and schools. A source of growing importance for small children and immunocompromised persons in Europe and North America are hedgehogs and pet reptiles (snakes, iguanas, turtles) that are frequently (sometimes to 100%) and latently infected with salmonellae. In Canada, 3 to 5% of human salmonelloses have arisen from these animals. Dogs, cats, guinea pigs, hamsters, rabbits, and pet birds are further possible sources.

The epidemiological connection between animal hosts and survival of salmonellae in the environment (see above) is responsible for the buildup of complex and difficult-to-trace infectious chains in which humans can, but do not have to, be the terminal link (Fig. 2.27).

Clinical Manifestations. The incubation period of nontyphoidal *Salmonella* enteritis depends on the number of bacteria ingested and their virulence (see above) and varies from 5 to 72 h. There is sudden nausea, vomiting, and watery, foul-smelling diarrhea, which, in most cases, last only for a few hours. If the colon is affected,

the stool may contain blood and/or mucus. The patients feel weak, frequently there is fever, sometimes >39 °C. Convalescence starts within 1 to 2 days but, depending on disposition and constitution of the patient, the illness may last for 5 to 7 days. If the infecting serovar is particularly invasive or if the patient is immunocompromised, the infection may spread and lead to septicemia, abscess formation, meningitis, osteomyelitis, arthritis, pyelonephritis, urinary tract infection, cholecystitis, pneumonia, and endo/peri/myocarditis. Once cured, patients will excrete salmonellae for 1 to 2 months. Permanent excretors (>10 months) are rare in nontyphoidal disease. The case-fatality in Germany is below 0.1%.

In animals, particularly in reptiles, salmonelloses with nonadapted strains remain mostly latent but may persist for weeks to months and are accompanied by (intermittent) excretion of salmonellae. Acute enteritis and, occasionally, fatal septicemia have been observed in calves, piglets, and young animals of other species. Arthritis, abortion, and, more rarely, omphalitis and pneumonia have also been reported. In chickens, symptoms are mostly limited to the

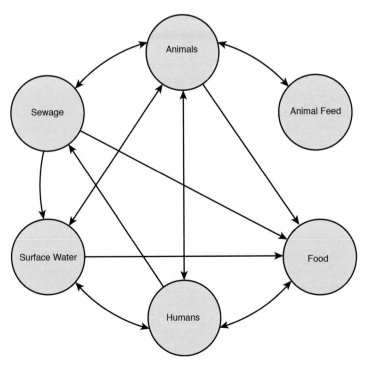

Figure 2.27 | Important transmission chains and avenues of contamination for nontyphoidal salmonellae.

first weeks of life and are nonspecific (delayed growth, weakness, diarrhea, dehydration).

Diagnosis. An unequivocal diagnosis of *Salmonella* infection can be provided by isolation of the organism from stool or vomit, and in cases of septicemia also from blood. Stool samples have to be taken early after the first symptoms have appeared. For culture, selective media are obligatory [Rambach, xylose-lysine-deoxycholate, Salmonella-Shigella (SS) or Hektoen enteric agars; tetrathionate, selenite, or Vassiliades-Rappaport broths]. Suspicious isolates are tested for certain biochemical characteristics; some laboratories also use the bacteriophage 0-1 that lyses 95% of clinical strains. Serotyping uses commercial omni/poly/monovalent antisera. A detailed determination of serovars is often done by national reference laboratories only. A rapid diagnostic means is provided by PCR (marker genes *invA, stn*). In recent years, MALDI-TOF mass spectrometry and DNA microarrays have been used in diagnostic laboratories. The Widal agglutination test, formerly mostly used for serology of typhoid fever, lacks sensitivity and specificity.

In animals, the diagnosis rests on isolating salmonellae from stool or intestines, meconium, organs (liver, spleen), eggs, and possibly from urine and milk, and from dust and dirt for control purposes. The techniques follow those described above. Serological ELISA tests have been used for herd diagnostic in pigs, chickens (also egg yolk), and cattle but cannot provide information on the infectious status of single animals or a group. Epidemiological investigations nowadays require typing techniques beyond those of serotyping, such as phage typing, PFGE, and others.

Differential Diagnosis. Acute enteritides can also be caused by other bacterial agents, for example, *Campylobacter jejuni*, enteropathogenic *Escherichia coli*, *Shigella* spp., *Yersinia enterocolitica*, *Y. pseudotuberculosis*, *Aeromonas* spp., as well as rotavirus, norovirus, and various parasites. In addition, poisoning by mushrooms or heavy metals (arsenic, mercury) has to be ruled out. The definite diagnosis is based on the isolation of a diarrhogenic agent or the demonstration of a poison.

Therapy. Mild infections in patients not belonging to a risk group do not require antimicrobials but there should be fluid and electrolyte substitution (oral polyelectrolyte rehydration solution as recommended by WHO).

Antibiotics are indicated only for infants, small children, immunocompromised individuals, severe cases and those with extraintestinal (incl. systemic) complications. Recommended are ciprofloxacin 2 × 500 mg/day, or trimethoprim-sulfamethoxazole double strength 2 × 1 tablet/day, or amoxicillin 4 × 0.5 to 1 g/day p. o. for 3 to 7 days. Permanent excretors receive ciprofloxacin 2 × 500 mg/day for 10 days. However, it should be kept in mind that an increasing percentage of salmonellae, particularly of *S.* Typhimurium, has acquired multiple antibiotic resistance and that antibiotics should only be used according to the results of an antibiogram.

In animals, uncomplicated salmonellosis and clinically inapparent *Salmonella* excretion are no indication for antibiotic treatment. In severe cases or those with extraintestinal complications, antibiotic treatment can be undertaken following testing for antibiotic resistance.

If salmonelloses occur in cattle herds or chicken coops, measures in accordance with legal requirements have to be instituted. If permitted, Salmonella live vaccines are used. In Europe, the use of antibiotics in Salmonella-infested chicken is restricted by law and has to be approved by a veterinary authority.

Prophylaxis. In view of the wide dissemination of salmonellae, it is impossible to eliminate reservoirs and infection. Preventive measures, at best, can minimize the possibility of transmission.

The countries of the European Union have instituted surveillance and control programs in order to lower *Salmonella* prevalence in domestic animals, and thus, the possible entry of the bacterium into the food chain. In this program, salmonellae are also being controlled in cattle, fattening pigs, chicken, laying hens, and broiler chicken with the help of live and inactivated vaccines. A prophylactic vaccination of juvenile laying hens is mandatory.

In the food industry, that is, in dairies, butcheries, restaurants, and large kitchens, legally required hygienic measures have to be applied in order to avoid cross-contamination and unintended multiplication of salmonellae. Eggs, egg products, and foodstuffs prepared with raw eggs are not to be traded or sold unless certain legal requirements have been fulfilled.

As other foodborne infections, *Salmonella* infections can be kept in check by thorough handwashing with warm water and soap after contact with animals (reptiles!) and items in contact with them. The same holds true after the use of toilets and the preparation and consumption of meals (children!). Sufficient heating of food (for at least 10 min at 70 °C) prior to consumption, boiling of raw milk and cooking of duck eggs for at least 10 min are mandatory. Meat, particularly mincemeat and poultry, as well as vegetable sprouts, should be well cooked. Raw foodstuffs should be kept separately from food that will not be heated again before consumption. Items in use, work surfaces and hands should be washed with hot water between different cooking procedures. Food should be kept in a refrigerator (<7 °C) or should be cooked at least at 70 °C. Raw vegetables and fruit should be washed thoroughly. Pregnant women and small children should not have contact with reptiles.

In Germany, children below 6 years of age who have salmonellosis must stay away from kindergartens, schools, and other teaching institutions, and people with *Salmonella* infections are not allowed to work in the food processing industry or in kitchens serving communal food if they are in contact with food of any kind.

Reporting. Salmonelloses are notifiable diseases in the USA and in Canada.

REFERENCES

Aiken AM, Lane C, Adak GK, Risk of Salmonella infection with exposure to reptiles in England, 2004–2007. *Euro Surveill.* 15, 19581, 2010.

Berger CN et al., Fresh fruit and vegetables as vehicles for the transmission of human pathogens. *Environ. Microbiol.* 12, 2385–2397, 2010.

Blaser MJ, Newman LS, A review of human salmonellosis: I.: infective dose. *Rev. Infect. Dis.* 4, 1096–1106, 1982.

Centers for: Disease Control and Prevention(CDC). Multistate outbreak of human Salmonella typhimurium infections associated with aquatic frogs – United States, 2009. MMWR Morb. Mortal. Wkly. Rep. 58, 1433–1436, 2009.

Dontsenko I et al., Outbreak of salmonellosis in a kindergarten in Estonia, May 2008. *Euro Surveill.* 13, pii18900, 2010.

EFSA, The European Union Summary Report on Trends and Sources of Zoonoses, Zoonotic Agents and Foodborne Outbreaks in 2009. *The EFSA Journal* 9, 2090, 2011.

Evans HS, Maguire H, Outbreaks of infectious intestinal disease in schools and nurseries in England and Wales 1992 to 1994. *Commun. Dis. Rep. CDR Rev.* 6, R103–108, 1996.

Fernandez Guerrero ML et al., The spectrum of cardiovascular infections due to Salmonella enterica: a review of clinical features and factors determining outcome. *Medicine (Baltimore).* 83, 123–138, 2004.

Gerlach RG, Hensel M, Salmonella pathogenicity islands in host specificity, host pathogen-interactions and antibiotics resistance of Salmonella enterica. *Berl. Munch. Tierarztl. Wochenschr.* 120, 317–327, 2007.

Guibourdenche M et al., Supplement 2003–2007 (No. 47) to the: White-Kauffmann-Le Minor scheme. *Res. Microbiol.* 161, 26–29, 2010.

Hohmann EL, Nontyphoidal salmonellosis. *Clin. Infect. Dis.* 32, 263–269, 2001.

Hopkins KL et al., Multiresistant Salmonella enterica serovar 4,[5],12:i:- in Europe: a new pandemic strain? *Euro Surveill.* 15, 19580, 2010.

Jackson Br et al., Outbreak-associated Salmonella enterica serotypes and food commodities, United States, 1998–2008. *Emerg Infect Dis* 19, 1239–1244, 2013.

Kagambega A et al., Prevalence and characterization of Salmonella enterica from the feces of cattle, poultry, swine, and hedgehogs in Burkina Faso and their comparison to human Salmonella isolates. *BMC Microbiol* 13, 253, 2013.

Lee K et al., A novel multiplex PCR assay for: Salmonella subspecies identification. *J. Appl. Microbiol.* 107, 805–811, 2009.

Lehmacher A, Bockemühl J, Aleksic S, Nationwide outbreak of human salmonellosis in Germany due to contaminated paprika and paprika-powdered potato chips. *Epidemiol. Infect.* 115, 501–511, 1995.

Nowak B et al., Salmonella contamination in pigs at slaughter and on the farm: a field study using an antibody ELISA test and a PCR technique. *Int J FoodMicrobiol* 115, 259–267, 2007.

Olsen SJ et al., The changing epidemiology of Salmonella: trends in serotypes isolated from humans in the United States, 1987–1997. *J. Infect. Dis.* 183, 753–761, 2001.

Olsen SJ et al., A nosocomial outbreak of fluoroquinolone-resistant: Salmonella infection. *N. Engl. J. Med.* 344, 1572–1579, 2001.

Rabsch W et al., Salmonella enterica serotype Typhimurium and its host-adapted variants. *Infect. Immun.* 70, 2249–2255, 2002.

Ribot EM et al., Salmonella enterica serotype Typhimurium DT104 isolated from humans, United States, 1985, 1990, and 1995. *Emerg. Infect. Dis.* 8, 387–391, 2002.

Singh A et al., Dynamic predictive model for the growth of Salmonella spp. in liquid whole egg. *J. Food Sci.* 76, M225–232, 2011.

Standaert SM, Hutcheson RH, Schaffner W, Nosocomial transmission of Salmonella gastroenteritis to laundry workers in a nursing home. *Infect. Control Hosp. Epidemiol.* 15, 22–26, 1994.

Tindall BJ et al., Nomenclature and taxonomy of the genus Salmonella. *Int. J. Syst. Evol. Microbiol.* 55, 521–524, 2005.

Valdez Y, Ferreira RB, Finlay BB, Molecular mechanisms of Salmonella virulence and host resistance. *Curr. Top. Microbiol. Immunol.* 337, 93–127, 2009.

Wagner C, Hensel M, Adhesive mechanisms of Salmonella enterica. *Adv. Exp. Med. Biol.* 715, 17–34, 2011.

Wales AD et al., Review of the carriage of zoonotic bacteria by arthropods, with special reference to Salmonella in mites, flies and litter beetles. *Zoonoses Public Health* 57, 299–314, 2010.

2.21 Staphylococcal Infections

There has been a growing number of reports of zoonotic human infections with staphylococci.

Etiology. *Staphylococcus* is a genus of nonmotile, facultatively anaerobic, catalase-positive Gram-positive cocci.

The most important zoonotic staphylococci are the coagulase-positive *S. aureus* and *S. pseudintermedius*. The zoonotic significance of *S. intermedius* and *S. delphini* has not been clear at this time as earlier research did not separate the species *S. intermedius, S. pseudintermedius,* and *S. delphini*, which can only be separated with confidence by molecular techniques.

Only a few years ago it was assumed that humans and animals are colonized or infected by specific eco/biovars of *S. aureus*. Molecular genetic analyses undertaken to solve problems with methicillin-resistant *S. aureus* (MRSA) strains confirmed that there are such adapted types that rarely pass the species barrier. However, other types occur in humans and animals (horses, dogs, cats, turtles, bats, pigs, parrots) and they can easily be transmitted to each other.

Prominent among them is the clonal cluster CC/ST 398, which occurs in many countries and is, above all, associated with pigs, calves and poultry but has also been isolated with increased frequency from humans. Conversely, certain human *S. aureus* types, such as MRSA-ST1 and ST22, can be transmitted to animals, which are likely to be a source for human infections. The molecular mechanisms of different adaptations of *S. aureus* "ecovars" are being investigated in several laboratories. The variable presence of certain virulence factors of *S. aureus*, which may be affecting hosts to different degrees, seems to play an important role. Among these factors are the Panton-Valentine leukocidin, protein A and variants of the hemoglobin receptor (iron surface determinant, IsdB) that the staphylococci need for iron uptake. According to recent research, the coagulase-negative opportunistic species *S. haemolyticus* and *S. sciuri* may also be zoonotic agents.

Occurrence. *S. aureus* has a wide distribution and colonizes transiently or permanently skin and mucous membranes of numerous mammals, birds, and reptiles. The most important site in humans are the nares. *S. pseudintermedius* (formerly identified as *S. intermedius*) occurs primarily in dogs and cats. Staphylococci of the *S. intermedius* group are also found in foxes, ferrets, horses, donkeys, dolphins, and pigeons.

Transmission. Zoonotic staphylococcal infections occur when the bacteria enter skin wounds, for example, during work with animal tissues or bones, or through bites or scratch wounds brought about by contact with colonized or infected animals. Smear infections following contact with purulent infections in animals are also possible. At special risk are people who keep or take care of animals, veterinarians, butchers, and others who are in frequent contact with raw meat. Through dirt or smear infections, the organisms can be transmitted to others.

Clinical Manifestations. Unless the staphylococci are inoculated through a traumatic wound, colonization is the first step. Infections occur only when there is trauma to the skin or to mucous membranes, for example, through accidents, surgical operations, or catheterizations.

The spectrum of presumably zoonotic staphylococcal infections is wide. Immunocompetent hosts react with local inflammation, such as impetigo, folliculitis, cellulitis, abscesses, furuncles/carbuncles, or a generalized pyoderma. If the infection spreads, it may lead to bacteremia, pneumonia, osteomyelitis, sinusitis, mastoiditis, otitis, endocarditis, and brain abscess.

In animals, *S. aureus* causes infections similar to those of humans, that is, purulent or occasionally granulomatous inflammation of skin and mucous membranes. Frequent manifestations are mastitis (in cattle, sheep, and goats), external otitis, sinusitis, arthritis, anal gland inflammation (dogs), osteomyelitis, pneumonias, and septicemia.

S. pseudintermedius is an opportunist and one of the most frequent agent of purulent skin infections, external otitis, wound infections, abscesses, pyometra, and mastitis in dogs and cats. It is also the most frequent agent of pyoderma in dogs.

Diagnosis. The etiological diagnosis is done by microscopy and culture of pus, exudates, secretions, blood, or material from organs. The species diagnosis involves colonial morphology and pigmentation, NaCl tolerance, certain virulence-associated factors (hemolysin, coagulase, clumping factor, thermonuclease), biochemical reactions, and susceptibility to novobiocin. For epidemiological investigations, typing techniques such as pulsed field gel electrophoresis (PFGE) of *Sma*I macrorestriction fragments, multilocus sequence typing (MLTS), multilocus enzyme electrophoresis (MLEE), *SCCec* and *spa* typing have been used.

Differential Diagnosis. Other agents causing similar infections (streptococci, pasteurellae, pseudomonads) have to be considered.

Therapy. As multiple resistance is frequent in staphylococci, an antibiogram prior to the start of therapy is mandatory. The rare beta-lactamase negative strains are best treated with benzyl penicillin, those producing a beta-lactamase with isoxazolyl penicillin. If there is a penicillin allergy or if a MRSA is the infecting agent, vancomycin, linezolid or daptomycin are indicated (attention: rare resistant strains!).

Prophylaxis. Contact with, or care of, animals includes the usual precautions, in some cases even the use of gloves. Bite and scratch wounds should be cleansed and disinfected.

REFERENCES

Atalay B et al., Brain abscess caused by Staphylococcus intermedius. *Acta Neurochir. (Wien)* 147, 347–348;discussion 348, 2005.

Cuny C et al., Emergence of methicillin-resistant Staphylococcus aureus (MRSA) in different animal species. *Int. J. Med. Microbiol.* 300, 109–117, 2010.

Cuny C et al., Nasal colonization of humans with methicillin-resistant Staphylococcus aureus (MRSA) CC398 with and without exposure to pigs. *PLoS One* 4, e6800, 2009.

Fluit AC., Livestock-associated Staphylococcus aureus. *Clin Microbiol Infect* 18, 735–744, 2012.

Gomez-Sanz E et al., Clonal dynamics of nasal Staphylococcus aureus and Staphylococcus pseudintermedius in dog-owning household members. Detection of MSSA ST (398). *PloS One.* 8, e69337, 2013.

Guardabassi L, Loeber ME, Jacobson A, Transmission of multiple antimicrobial-resistant Staphylococcus intermedius between dogs affected by deep pyoderma and their owners. *Vet. Microbiol.* 98, 23–27, 2004.

Hanselman BA et al., Coagulase positive staphylococcal colonization of humans and their household pets. *Can. Vet. J.* 50, 954–958, 2009.

Kehrenberg C et al., Methicillin-resistant and -susceptible Staphylococcus aureus strains of clonal lineages ST398 and ST9 from swine carry the multidrug resistance gene cfr. *Antimicrob. Agents Chemother.* 53, 779–781, 2009.

Kikuchi K et al., Molecular confirmation of transmission route of Staphylococcus intermedius in mastoid cavity infection from dog saliva. *J Infect Chemother* 10, 46–48, 2004.

Lee J, Staphylococcus intermedius isolated from dog-bite wounds. *J. Infect.* 29, 105, 1994.

Loeffler A et al., Prevalence of methicillin-resistant Staphylococcus aureus among staff and pets in a small animal referral hospital in the UK. *J. Antimicrob. Chemother.* 56, 692–697, 2005.

Lowy FD, How Staphylococcus aureus adapts to its host. *N. Engl. J. Med.* 364, 1987–1990, 2011.

Moodley A, Guardabassi L, Clonal spread of methicillin-resistant coagulase-negative staphylococci among horses, personnel and environmental sites at equine facilities. *Vet. Microbiol.* 137, 397–401, 2009.

Nannini E, Murray BE, Arias CA, Resistance or decreased susceptibility to glycopeptides, daptomycin, and linezolid in methicillin-resistant Staphylococcus aureus. *Curr. Opin. Pharmacol.* 10, 516–521, 2010.

Paul NC et al., Carriage of methicillin-resistant Staphylococcus pseudintermedius in small animal veterinarians: indirect evidence of zoonotic transmission. *Zoonoses Public Health* 58, 533–539, 2011.

Pilla R et al., Methicillin-resistant Staphylococcus pseudintermedius as causative agent of dairy cow mastitis. *Vet Rec* 173, 19, 2013.

Riegel P et al., Coagulase-positive Staphylococcus pseudintermedius from animals causing human endocarditis. *Int. J. Med. Microbiol.* 301, 237–239, 2011.

Rutland BE et al., Human-to-dog transmission of methicillin-resistant Staphylococcus aureus. *Emerg. Infect. Dis.* 15, 1328–1330, 2009.

Sasaki T et al., Reclassification of phenotypically identified Staphylococcus intermedius strains. *J. Clin. Microbiol.* 45, 2770–2778, 2007.

Strommenger B et al., Molecular characterization of methicillin-resistant Staphylococcus aureus strains from pet animals and their relationship to human isolates. *J. Antimicrob. Chemother.* 57, 461–465, 2006.

Talan DA et al., Bacteriologic analysis of infected dog and cat bites. Emergency Medicine Animal Bite Infection Study Group. *N. Engl. J. Med.* 340, 85–92, 1999.

Tanner MA, Everett CL, Youvan DC, Molecular phylogenetic evidence for noninvasive zoonotic transmission of Staphylococcus intermedius from a canine pet to a human. *J. Clin. Microbiol.* 38, 1628–1631, 2000.

van Belkum A et al., Methicillin-resistant and -susceptible Staphylococcus aureus sequence type 398 in pigs and humans. *Emerg. Infect. Dis.* 14, 479–483, 2008.

Van Hoovels A et al., First case of Staphylococcus pseudintermedius infection in a human. *J. Clin. Microbiol.* 44, 4609–4612, 2006.

Walther B et al., Staphylococcus aureus and MRSA colonization rates among personnel and dogs in a small animal hospital: association with nosocomial infections. *Berl. Munch. Tierarztl. Wochenschr.* 122, 178–185, 2009.

Weese JS, van Duijkeren E, Methicillin-resistant Staphylococcus aureus and Staphylococcus pseudintermedius in veterinary medicine. *Vet. Microbiol.* 140, 418–429, 2010.

2.22 Streptococcal Infections

Pathogenic streptococci are obligately parasitic and are, as a rule, adapted to certain animal species. Some species, however, can be zoonotic and, on contact with infected animals, could be transmitted to humans.

2.22.1 GENERAL FEATURES

The genus *Streptococcus* consists of nonmotile, facultatively anaerobic, catalase-negative Gram-positive ovoid or, rarely, round bacteria with a tendency to produce chains. Species differentiation in the medical/veterinary laboratory is based on biochemical and hemolytic properties, as well as antigenic cell wall polysaccharides, which serve as the basis for the Lancefield serogroups.

Taxonomy and nomenclature of streptococci have changed in the past years due to chemotaxonomic analyses, DNA-DNA hybridizations, and 16 S rRNA gene sequencing. Accordingly, the genus *Streptococcus* can be divided into several species groups: the pyogenic (including those of Lancefield groups A, C, and G), the *mutans* (with, among others, *S. hyovaginalis*), the *mitis* (with *S. sanguinis* and *S. pneumoniae*), the *salivarius, anginosus,* and *bovis* groups with individual species.

The natural habitat of most streptococcal species are skin and mucous membranes of vertebrates. Outside of their hosts, they do not multiply under natural conditions and their tenacity is low. Host spectra vary widely in range from species to species; only a few species are zoonotic.

2.22.2 STREPTOCOCCUS EQUI INFECTIONS (GROUP C)

In humans, infections with these zoonotic agents occur only sporadically and with variable clinical symptoms.

Etiology. *S. equi* subsp. *zooepidemicus* is more frequent as a zoonotic agent than *S. equi* subsp. *equi*; *S. equi* subsp. *ruminatorum* may also be zoonotic.

Occurrence. Within the genus *Streptococcus*, *S. equi* subsp. *zooepidemicus* is the infectious agent with the widest host spectrum. Animals are frequent carriers of this bacterium, above all, horses in which it colonizes the respiratory and genital tracts. Diseases in animals (also cattle) include wound infections, endometritis, arthritis, mastitis, and septicemias. In horses, it is a frequent agent of respiratory (pharyngitis, bronchopneumonia), genital tract infections (endometritis, abortion), and septic arthritis of foals. In dog kennels and dog breeding establishments *S.equi* subsp. *zooepidemicus* is the cause of severe hemorrhagic pneumonias.

S. equi subsp. *equi* is almost exclusively found in equines and is the agent of strangles, an acute and febrile disease of the upper respiratory tract with regional abscess-forming lymphadenitis. The bacterium, however, can also be isolated from the nasopharynx, the guttural pouch, from pulmonary mucus, and from the genital tract of healthy horses.

S. equi subsp. *ruminatorum* was first described in 2004 as the third subspecies of *S. equi* that was found in Spain in milk of sheep and goats with mastitis. Additional detection in free-living but diseased hyenas and zebras in Tanzania point to a wider host spectrum. Reports of a fatal generalized infection and a case of bacteremia with endocarditis in France show the pathogenicity of this subspecies for humans. Infection from animals was suspected but not proven.

In humans, 0.25 to 7% of all streptococcal infections can be traced to group C streptococci. A British study showed 9 to 17% of all beta-hemolytic streptococci isolated from humans belong to serogroup C, and 3% of these were *S. equi* subsp. *zooepidemicus*. At special risk are animal care personnel, farmers, animal dealers, and other people who are in frequent contact with horses and domestic animals.

Transmission. Primarily through intensive contact with infected animals who excrete the organisms in large amounts via nasal secretions, pus from wounds, or through consumption of raw milk or its products. Dog and cat bites involve mostly *S. dysgalactiae* subsp. *equisimilis*.

Clinical Manifestations. Wound infections (impetigo), upper respiratory infections, lymphadenopathy, pneumonia, pleuritis, endocarditis, septicemia, meningitis, arthritis, and streptococcal toxic shock syndrome. Immunocompromised patients seem to be affected more often. A late complication may be glomerulonephritis. The case-fatality rate can be as high as 29%.

Diagnosis. Culture of clinical specimens is the method of choice.

Differential Diagnosis. Depending on the localization of the disease, many bacterial and viral agents have to be ruled out.

Therapy. Penicillin G 4×2 to 5 mio. IU/day i.v.; aminoglycosides have a synergistic effect. Third generation cephalosporins have also been recommended.

Prophylaxis. Close contact with infected animals should be avoided, also consumption of nonpasteurized milk.

REFERENCES

Abbott Y et al., Zoonotic transmission of Streptococcus equi subsp. zooepidemicus from a dog to a handler. *J. Med. Microbiol.* 59, 120–123, 2010.

Bordes-Benitez A et al., Outbreak of Streptococcus equi subsp. zooepidemicus infections on the island of Gran Canaria associated with the consumption of inadequately pasteurized cheese. *Eur. J. Clin. Microbiol. Infect. Dis.* 25, 242–246, 2006.

Bradley SF et al., Group C streptococcal bacteremia: analysis of 88 cases. *Rev. Infect. Dis.* 13, 270–280, 1991.

Collazos J et al., Streptococcus zooepidemicus septic arthritis: case report and review of group C streptococcal arthritis. *Clin. Infect. Dis.* 15, 744–746, 1992.

Dolinski SY et al., Group C streptococcal pleurisy and pneumonia: a fulminant case and review of the literature. *Infection* 18, 239–241, 1990.

Downar J et al., Streptococcal meningitis resulting from contact with an infected horse. *J. Clin. Microbiol.* 39, 2358–2359, 2001.

Edwards AT, Roulson M, Ironside MJ, A milk-borne outbreak of serious infection due to: Streptococcus zooepidemicus (Lancefield Group C). *Epidemiol. Infect.* 101, 43–51, 1988.

Elsayed S et al., Streptococcus equi subspecies equi (Lancefield group C) meningitis in a child. *Clin. Microbiol. Infect.* 9, 869–872, 2003.

Eyre DW et al., Streptococcus equi subspecies zooepidemicus meningitis–a case report and review of the literature. *Eur. J. Clin. Microbiol. Infect. Dis.* 29, 1459–1463, 2010.

Friederichs J et al., Human bacterial arthritis caused by Streptococcus zooepidemicus: report of a case. *Int. J. Infect. Dis.* 14 (Suppl 3), e233–235, 2010.

Kuusi M et al., An outbreak of Streptococcus equi subspecies zooepidemicus associated with consumption of fresh goat cheese. *BMC Infect. Dis.* 6, 36, 2006.

Meyer A et al., Second reported case of human infection with Streptococcus equi subsp. ruminatorum. *Joint Bone Spine* 78, 303–305, 2011.

Priestnall S, Erles K, Streptococcus zooepidemicus: an emerging canine pathogen. *Vet. J.* 188, 142–148, 2011.

2.22.3 *STREPTOCOCCUS SUIS* INFECTIONS (GROUPS R, S, AND T)

S. suis infections have been reported in humans with increasing frequency. They often involve the meninges and the eighth cranial nerve.

Etiology. The infectious agent is *S. suis*, with 35 serovars recognized by now. The main zoonotic serovar is serovar 2. Strains of serovars 1, 4, 14, and 16 are rarely isolated from patients. Most sporadic cases are sequence type ST-1.

Occurrence. As far as is known, pigs are the main reservoir for *S. suis* serovar 2, with frequencies varying from herd to herd. Infected pigs harbor the organism mainly in the tonsils but may also have their oronasal and genital mucous membranes and intestinal tracts colonized with the organism. On occasion, serovar 2 has been found in wild boars, ruminants, horses, dogs, cats, and birds.

Individual cases have also been reported from Germany, Danmark, France, the UK, the Netherlands, Sweden, North America, Australia, and New Zealand. Most cases have thus far been reported from Southeast Asia. There have been two epidemics in China: in 1998 with 25 patients and 14 fatalities and in 2005 with 215 patients and 38 fatalities. At special risk are butchers, meat vendors, farmers, veterinarians, and people who process pork.

Transmission. Human infections are primarily smear infections that arise from contact with live or slaughtered pigs or with pork. Conjunctivitis and small blemishes serve as portals of entry but contaminated instruments (e.g., knives) can also transmit the organism in cut, sting, or tear wounds. At this point, it cannot be excluded that infection takes place through consumption of raw or insufficiently cooked pork.

Clinical Manifestations. Following an incubation period of several hours to 14 days, patients show signs of meningitis; in >50%, the eighth cranial nerve is involved with loss of hearing and balance. Deafness may ensue. Fatalities have been recorded (see above). Septicemic infections without meningitis have also been reported. The spectrum of potential complications includes uveitis, endophthalmitis, pneumonia, endocarditis, myocarditis, arthritis (knee joints), spondylodiscitis, ophthalmoplegia (3rd cranial nerve), epidural abscess, and streptococcal toxic shock syndrome.

In pigs, the infection is mostly inapparent, with persistence of the organism for weeks and months. Weaning piglets and young fattening pigs are primarily affected. High density, low ceilings, and poor aeration in stables favor infections that include arthritis, meningitis, serositis, endocarditis, and otitis.

Diagnosis. History (contact with pigs or pork) and the clinical picture of meningitis accompanied by hearing loss and disturbed balance are suspicious. The diagnosis is confirmed by culture of spinal fluid, blood, and perhaps, synovial fluid. *S. suis* shows alpha hemolysis on sheep blood agar. Species identification requires biochemical testing. *S. suis* belongs to serogroups R, S, or T. Serotyping is done by reference laboratories. A rapid diagnosis may be accomplished by a *S. suis* type 2 specific PCR.

Differential Diagnosis. Agents of meningitis (*Neisseria meningitidis, Streptococcus pneumoniae, Haemophilus influenzae, Listeria monocytogenes, Mycobacterium tuberculosis, Cryptococcus neoformans,* and viruses, such as enteroviruses, herpes simplex, and mumps virus).

Therapy. Penicillin G 4×2 to 5 mio. IU/day is the drug of choice. As there have been penicillin-resistant strains, an antibiogram would be required prior to the start of chemotherapy. Ampicillin in combination with aminoglycosides is also effective. The outlook is favorable if the diagnosis is made early and therapy started immediately.

Prophylaxis. Gloves should be worn on contact with infected pigs and pork. Hands and wounds should be cleaned and disinfected. Pork must be heated before consumption to at least 70 °C for 10 min.

REFERENCES

Allgaier A et al., Relatedness of Streptococcus suis isolates of various serotypes and clinical backgrounds as evaluated by macrorestriction analysis and expression of potential virulence traits. *J. Clin. Microbiol.* 39, 445–453, 2001.

Baums CG, Valentin-Weigand P, Surface-associated and secreted factors of Streptococcus suis in epidemiology, pathogenesis and vaccine development. *Anim. Health Res. Rev.* 10, 65–83, 2009.

Feng Y et al., Uncovering newly emerging variants of Streptococcus suis, an important zoonotic agent. *Trends Microbiol.* 18, 124–131, 2010.

Ho DT et al., Risk factors of Streptococcus suis infection in Vietnam. A case-control study. *PLoS ONE* 6, e17604, 2011.

Navacharoen N et al., Hearing and vestibular loss in Streptococcus suis infection from swine and traditional raw pork exposure in northern Thailand. *J. Laryngol. Otol.* 123, 857–862, 2009.

Nga T et al., Real-time PCR for detection of: Streptococcus suis serotype 2 in cerebrospinal fluid of human patients with meningitis. *Diagn. Microbiol. Infect. Dis.* 70, 461–467, 2011.

Nghia H et al., Human case of Streptococcus suis serotype 16 infection. *Emerg. Infect. Dis.* 14, 155–157, 2008.

Staats JJ et al., Streptococcus suis: past and present. *Vet. Res. Commun.* 21, 381–407, 1997.

Tambyah PA et al., Streptococcus suis infection complicated by purpura fulminans and rhabdomyolysis: case report and review. *Clin. Infect. Dis.* 24, 710–712, 1997.

Tang J et al., Streptococcal toxic shock syndrome caused by Streptococcus suis serotype 2. *PLoS Med.* 3, e151, 2006.

Teekakirikul P, Wiwanitkit V, Streptococcus suis infection: overview of case reports in Thailand. *Southeast Asian J. Trop. Med. Public Health* 34(Suppl 2), 178–183, 2003.

Varela NP et al., Antimicrobial resistance and prudent drug use for Streptococcus suis. *Anim. Health Res. Rev.* 14, 68–77, 2013.

Wangsomboonsiri W et al., Streptococcus suis infection and risk factors for mortality. *J. Infect.* 57, 392–396, 2008.

Wertheim HF et al., Streptococcus suis: an emerging human pathogen. *Clin. Infect. Dis.* 48, 617–625, 2009.

Yu H et al., Human Streptococcus suis outbreak, Sichuan, China. *Emerg. Infect. Dis.* 12, 914–920, 2006.

2.22.4 *STREPTOCOCCUS PYOGENES* (SEROGROUP A) INFECTIONS

S. pyogenes causes severe and life-threatening infections in humans, for example, scarlet fever, erysipelas, pharyngitis, cellulitis, necrotizing fasciitis, streptococcal toxic shock, the sequelae of rheumatic fever glomerulonephritis, and chorea minor. In animals, A streptococci have occasionally been isolated from cattle, dogs, and apes. It is assumed that these animals could also serve as sources but probably via the chain human-animal-human.

REFERENCES

Copperman SM, Cherchez le chien: household pets as reservoirs of persistent or recurrent streptococcal sore throats in children. *N. Y. State J. Med.* 82, 1685–1687, 1982.

Falck G, Group A streptococci in household pets' eyes—a source of infection in humans? *Scand. J., Infect. Dis.* 29, 469–471, 1997.

Johansson L et al., A. Norrby-Teglund: Getting under the skin: the immunopathogenesis of Streptococcus pyogenes deep tissue infections. *Clin. Infect. Dis.* 51, 58–65, 2010.

Mayer G, Van Ore S, Recurrent pharyngitis in family of four. Household pet as reservoir of group A streptococci. *Postgrad. Med.* 74, 277–279, 1983.

2.22.5 *STREPTOCOCCUS AGALACTIAE* (SEROGROUP B) INFECTIONS

S. agalactiae has been regarded for quite some time as zoonotic because of its occurrence in animals, particularly in cattle (mastitis) and humans (septicemia and meningitis in newborns, pneumonia, urinary tract infection). Comparative analyses of pheno- and genotypes and complete sequencing of clinical isolates, however, has shown that most *S. agalactiae* strains from cattle and humans differ considerably and that the species consist of two "ecovars." Only in a very few instances, identity between human and animal strains was found, so that *S. agalactiae* infections in cattle seem to play a minor, if any, role as causes of human infections.

REFERENCES

Manning SD et al., Association of Group B Streptococcus colonization and bovine exposure: a prospective cross-sectional cohort study. *PLoS One* 5, e8795, 2010.

Richards VP et al., Comparative genomics and the role of lateral gene transfer in the evolution of bovine adapted Streptococcus agalactiae. *Infect. Genet. Evol.* 11, 1263–1275, 2011.

2.22.6 INFECTIONS WITH OTHER *STREPTOCOCCUS* SPP.

The literature contains a good number of articles on human infections with streptococci other than those mentioned previously, which are caused by strains from animals.

Etiology. Individual cases of zoonotic streptococci of groups G, L, E, P, U, and V and of *S. iniae* have been reported.

Occurrence. Group G streptococci (part of *S. dysgalactiae subsp. equisimilis, S. canis*) cause infections in many animal species, for example, in dogs and cats (respiratory and urogenital infections, otitis externa, wound infections, mastitis, pyoderma, endocarditis, septicemia) and in cattle (mastitis).

In Europe, streptococci of the serogroup L (part of *S. dysgalactiae subsp. dysgalactiae*) have been isolated from pigs (associated with septicemia, arthritis, endocarditis, lymphadenitis, meningitis), dogs (urinary tract and skin infections), and poultry (nasopharyngeal infections). Streptococci of the serogroups E, P, U, and V (*S. porcinus*) have been isolated from pig tonsils in Scandinavia and they have caused sporadic septicemias in humans.

S. iniae (no Lancefield antigens) was first described in 1976 as the cause of subcutaneous abscesses in freshwater dolphins in the Amazonas region. It may also affect other fresh and salt water fish (tilapia, yellowtail, rainbow trout, and coho salmon) as well as frogs and it has a worldwide distribution. As a causative agent of meningoencephalitis, necrotizing myositis, and septicemia, it has been of increasing economic significance for fisheries in North America, Japan, and Europe.

At special risk for infections with the above streptococci are people who have intensive contact with pigs (butchers, abattoir workers), dogs, cats, poultry, and fish (fishers, fishmongers).

Transmission. Streptococci of the serogroups E, G, L, P, U, and V can be transmitted by direct contact with infected animals and their secretions and through bites and scratches. *S. iniae* infections are brought about by wounds arising from handling fish or contaminated items.

Clinical Manifestations. In humans, subspecies of *S. dysgalactiae* (serogroups G and L) have caused pharyngitis, pleuritis, arthritis, endocarditis, and septicemia, and, in particular *S. dysgalactiae subsp. dysgalactiae*, skin infections in slaughterhouse workers transmitted from pigs.

S. porcinus has been found sporadically in women with urogenital infections and in patients with bacteremia and wound infections. Infections with *S. iniae* comprised bacteremia, cellulitis, endocarditis, meningitis, osteomyelitis, and septic arthritis.

Diagnosis. Culture and subsequent biochemical tests for species/subspecies. Serogroup determination with appropriate antibodies (no result for *S. iniae*!).

Differential Diagnosis. Depending on the symptomatology, bacterial, and viral infections.

Therapy. Penicillin G 4 ×2 to 5 mio. IU/day i.v.; depending on the illness, other antibiotics, possibly combined with aminoglycosides, have to be used.

Prophylaxis. As for 2.22.3.

REFERENCES

Agnew W, Barnes AC, Streptococcus iniae: an aquatic pathogen of global veterinary significance and a challenging candidate for reliable vaccination. *Vet. Microbiol.* 122, 1–15, 2007.

Baiano JC, Barnes AC, Towards control of Streptococcus iniae. *Emerg. Infect. Dis.* 15, 1891–1896, 2009.

Chen C et al., A glimpse of streptococcal toxic shock syndrome from comparative genomics of S. suis 2 Chinese isolates. *PLoS ONE* 2, e315, 2007.

Duarte RS et al., Phenotypic and genotypic characteristics of Streptococcus porcinus isolated from human sources. *J. Clin. Microbiol.* 43, 4592–4601, 2005.

Galpérine T et al., Streptococcus canis infections in humans: retrospective study of 54 patients. *J. Infect.* 55, 23–26, 2007.

Koh TH et al., Streptococcal cellulitis following preparation of fresh raw seafood. *Zoonoses Public Health* 56, 206–208, 2009.

Lam MM et al., The other group G Streptococcus: increased detection of Streptococcus canis ulcer infections in dog owners. *J. Clin. Microbiol.* 45, 2327–2329, 2007.

Lamm CG et al., Streptococcal infection in dogs: a retrospective study of 393 cases. *Vet. Pathol.* 47, 387–395, 2010.

Lau SK et al., Invasive Streptococcus iniae infections outside North America. *J. Clin. Microbiol.* 41, 1004–1009, 2003.

Martin C et al., Streptococcus porcinus as a cause of spontaneous preterm human stillbirth. *J. Clin. Microbiol.* 42, 4396–4398, 2004.

Reitmeyer JC, Guthrie RK, Steele JH, Biochemical properties of group G streptococci isolated from cats and man. *J. Med. Microbiol.* 35, 148–151, 1991.

Takahashi T, Ubukata K, Watanabe H, Invasive infection caused by Streptococcus dysgalactiae subsp. equisimilis: characteristics of strains and clinical features. *J. Infect Chemother* 17, 1–10, 2010.

Takeda N et al., Recurrent septicemia caused by Streptococcus canis after a dog bite. *Scand. J. Infect. Dis.* 33, 927–928, 2001.

Tessier J et al., Zoonotic infection with group G streptococcus. *Clin. Infect. Dis.* 28, 1322–1323, 1999.

Timoney JF, The pathogenic equine streptococci. *Vet. Res.* 35, 397–409, 2004.

Vieira VV et al., Genetic relationships among the different phenotypes of Streptococcus dysgalactiae strains. *Int. J. Syst. Bacteriol.* 48(Pt 4), 1231–1243, 1998.

Weinstein MR et al., Invasive infections due to a fish pathogen, Streptococcus iniae. S. iniae Study Group. *N. Engl. J. Med.* 337, 589–594, 1997.

2.23 Tularemia

Tularemia is a plague-like contagious disease involving lymph nodes that affects many animal species. In some populations of wild-living rodents and lagomorphs, it can cause septicemias and epidemics.

The infection is transmissible from animals to humans. In humans, it may remain asymptomatic or symptomatic, from skin ulcers with regional lymphadenopathy to severe pleuropulmonary and typhoid-like generalized illness. In many parts of the world, tularemia is known by special names: Francis' disease, market men's disease, rabbit fever; Pahvant Valley plague or deerfly fever (USA), Yato-byo or Ohara's disease (Japan), lemming fever (Norway).

Etiology. *Francisella tularensis* is a Gram-negative, aerobic, nonmotile coccoid to pleomorphic rod, which requires special media containing cystine or cysteine for culture. There are five species: *F. tularensis, F. philomiragia, F. noatunensis, F. hispaniensis,* and *F. asiatica. F. tularensis* comprises four subspecies:

- The subspecies *tularensis* (*nearctica*; biovar type A) occurs only in North America and is highly virulent for most mammals. On occasion, it has been isolated in Austria and Slovakia, possibly imported from North America;

- The subspecies *holarctica* (*palaearctica*; biovar type B) occurs in North America, Europe, Siberia, Israel, Iran, and Japan. In both subspecies, several subpopulations with different geographical distributions and different host preferences can be distinguished;

- The subspecies *mediasiatica* has thus far only been observed in the Central Asian republics of the former Soviet Union.

- The subspecies *novicida* was found in the US, Canada, and Spain, as well as in Australia as the only country in the Southern hemisphere. The two latter subspecies are pathogenic for humans and animals with a moderate to low virulence.

F. philomiragia is relatively rare, less virulent and causes granulomatous inflammations in animals and humans; in the latter, immunocompromised patients who had contact to brackish or salt water have been at particular risk. There is only one report extant about the isolation of *F. hispaniensis* from blood of a patient. *F. noatunensis* and *F. asiatica* are fish pathogens.

Occurrence. More than 125 animal species may be natural hosts for *F. tularensis.* Wild-living hare and rodents, such as wild rabbits, hamster, rats, mice, lemmings, and squirrels are natural reservoirs. Infections have also been observed in weasels, foxes, bears, coyotes, opossums, various wild birds (pheasant, quail, partridge), farm animals (cattle, sheep), and pets (dogs, cats). The agent is an obligate parasite but in endemic areas, it may also be found in surface waters and water sediments. At least the subspecies *holarctica* is able to multiply in aquatic protozoa. In vertebrates, *F. tularensis* leads a facultatively intracellular life.

Tularemia occurs in countries of the Northern Hemisphere; human cases correspond to the geographical distribution in animals. The epidemiologically important foci are in the USA and in Russia. In, Europe, tularemia occurs in all countries except the UK, Iceland, and Portugal. Endemic foci are in Scandinavia, the Czech Republic, Slovakia, Austria, Switzerland, and Germany (North Sea coast, Mecklenburg,

Franconia). Cases in humans are either rare individual ones or affect small groups; however, epidemics with >100 cases have been documented. At special risk are hunters, taxidermists, cooks, and people working with game, on farms, and in laboratories. *F. tularensis* is a potential bioweapon. Cultures should be handled in a biosafety 3 laboratory.

Transmission. The organism is highly virulent for humans. Under natural conditions, the disease, originating in vertebrates, is transmitted through direct contact with excreta, blood, or organs of infected game or wild animals (Fig. 2.28). The bacterium is able to enter the human body, not only through minimal blemishes (MID 10 organisms), but also through mucous membranes (mostly conjunctivae). Most infections come about through carving or processing meat of infected hares, as well as through bites or stings of blood-sucking arthropods (ticks, fleas, lice, horseflies) or bites of cats or squirrels. Inhalation of dust contaminated with excreta of infected rodents (MID 10 to 50 organisms), as may occur during harvest time, may also lead to infection. Oral infection through ingestion of contaminated food (MID 10^8 organisms) or drinking water is also possible. Human-to-human transmission has thus far not been observed.

Clinical Manifestations. Following an incubation period of 1 to 21 (3 to 10) days, the disease starts with sudden head- and muscle ache, fever, chills, and weakness. Further symptoms depend on virulence and portal of entry of the organism.

In the external form of tularemia, there is a red papule at the portal of entry that becomes enlarged and necrotic (Fig. 2.29). Within 2 to 4 days, a primary complex will form with enlarged local lymph nodes, which necrotize and ulcerate (ulcero-glandular tularemia). The primary complex may not form so that there is only lymph node enlargement, mostly in the axillar or inguinal region (glandular form). If the portal of entry is in the conjunctiva, the oculo-glandular form (Parinaud conjunctivitis) will develop.

The internal forms may manifest themselves as stomatitis, pharyngitis/tonsillitis, otitis, cervical lymphadenopathy (oropharyngeal form) and/or as pneumonia and pleuritis with retrosternal pain (pleuropulmonary form) and/or with abdominal pain, nausea, vomiting, gastrointestinal bleeding, and diarrhea (gastrointestinal form).

The typhoidal form without skin lesion or lymphadenopathy may be manifested by a systemic inflammatory response syndrome with a persistent high or intermittent fever, chills,

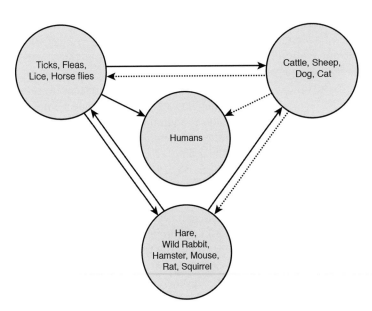

Figure 2.28 | The most important transmission chains for *Francisella tularensis*.

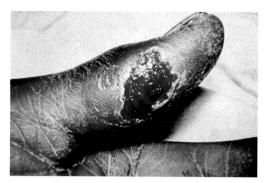

Figure 2.29 | Primary lesion following infection with *Francisella tularensis* (Prof. W. Knapp, Erlangen, Germany).

headache, meningitis, myalgia, lassitude, abdominal pain, diarrhea, hepatosplenomegaly, renal failure, and multiorgan failure.

Unless treated, tularemia lasts for 2 to 3 weeks followed by a long convalescence. In spite of appropriate therapy, the case-fatality rate is 4 to 6% and even 30% in the typhoidal form. The subspecies *holarctica* rarely causes severe cases or fatalities. There is a life-long immunity.

In animals, the spectrum of infection spans from a mild regional lymphadenopathy to a fulminant hemorrhagic septicemia that is fatal within a few days. In susceptible and nonimmune populations of hares and rodents, morbidity and mortality (hare plague) can be high. Diseased wild animals lose their natural shyness, look shaggy, and have an unsteady gait. Chronically ill animals lose weight and present on autopsy with a tuberculous/pseudotuberculous disease with enlarged lymphnodes, splenomegaly, and miliary white to yellowish, sometimes caseating foci in lymph nodes, liver, spleen, and bone marrow. Pregnant sheep may suffer from late abortions and delivery of extremely weak lambs.

Diagnosis. The diagnosis can be suspected from the history (contact with wild animals) and clinical symptoms. For culture, swabs from ulcers, pus, lymph node biopsy material, conjunctival secretions, sputum, and blood may be submitted. The special media (see above), possibly with antibiotics, have to be incubated for 2 days or longer but success may not ensue. PCR may be more successful.

Serology is helpful as well, using agglutination and ELISA testing for IgM, IgA, and IgG. Antibodies may be detected as early as 1 week after the onset of symptoms; by two weeks, they are detected in the large majority of cases. Antibiotics may inhibit the antibody response. Titers of 1:40 in the agglutination test are suspicious but should be checked every 8 to 10 days so that significant elevations (1:160 to 1:5120) are not missed. Care should be taken with interpretation, as *F. tularensis* possesses cross-reactive antigens with *Brucella* and *Yersinia enterocolitica*. The infecting subspecies (*tularensis* and *holarctica*) cannot be distinguished by serology. Western blots and lymphocyte stimulation tests can be helpful.

In animals, the diagnosis is made by culture or PCR from blood or biopsy specimens or in materials from autopsy (lung, liver, spleen, kidney, lymph nodes). Microagglutination or intradermal tests with tularin/tularemin (suspension of killed *F. tularensis*, positive from 5th day of disease) are further diagnostic steps.

Differential Diagnosis. Glandular and ulceroglandular form: infections with staphylococci, streptococci and pasteurellae, infectious mononucleosis, toxoplasmosis, lymphogranuloma venereum, cat scratch disease, plague, and sporotrichosis. Typhoidal form: typhoid fever, salmonellosis, brucellosis, malaria, Q fever, psittacosis/ornithosis, Legionnaire's disease, and hantavirus infection. Oropharyngeal form: streptococcal infections and diphtheria. If the history provides evidence for tick or insect bites and fever Lyme borreliosis, tick encephalitis, and, in particular geographical locations, RMSF and Colorado tick fever have to be considered.

Therapy. Recommended are gentamicin 5 mg/kg/day in three doses i.v. or i.m., or streptomycin 2 × 10 mg/kg/day i.m. for 10 days, or ciprofloxacin 2 × 400 mg/day i.v. or 2 × 750 mg/day p.o., or doxycycline 2 × 100 mg/day i.v. or p.o. for 14 to 21 days. In animals, oxytetracycline 10 mg/kg/d has been used in some cases.

Prophylaxis. Vaccines are not approved in Europe and in the US, but in some countries of the former USSR, live vaccines are admitted for prophylactic purposes. Vaccination with an attenuated *F. tularensis* strain can lead to a cell-mediated and humoral immunity that will last for several years. In the US, it has only been used in research because of possible complications and limited effectiveness.

People at special risk (see above) must follow appropriate rules when handling game and when in contact with rodents or other wild animals. Game imported from endemic areas must be thoroughly cooked before consumption. Laboratories working with *F. tularensis* must have biosafety level 3 facilities.

Reporting. Tularemia is a notifiable disease in the USA and in Canada.

REFERENCES

Abd H et al., Survival and growth of Francisella tularensis in Acanthamoeba castellanii. *Appl. Environ. Microbiol.* 69, 600–606, 2003.

Anda P et al., Waterborne outbreak of tularemia associated with crayfish fishing. *Emerg. Infect. Dis.* 7, 575–582, 2001.

Anonymous, *Tularemia*. The Center for Food Security and Public Health, Iowa State University. http://www.cfsph.iastate.edu/Factsheets/pdfs/tularemia.pdf. 2009.

Busse H et al., Objections to the transfer of Francisella novicida to the subspecies rank of Francisella tularensis - response to Johansson et al. *Int. J. Syst. Evol. Microbiol.* 60, 1718–1720, 2010.

Capellan JI, Fong W, Tularemia from a cat bite: case report and review of feline-associated tularemia. *Clin. Infect. Dis.* 16, 472–475, 1993.

Centers for: Disease Control and Prevention (CDC). Tularemia – United States, 2001–2010. Morb Mortal Wkly Rep MMWR. 62, 963–966, 2013.

Dennis DT et al., Tularemia as a biological weapon: medical and public health management. *JAMA* 285, 2763–2773, 2001.

Eliasson H et al., The 2000 tularemia outbreak: a case-control study of risk factors in disease-endemic and emergent areas, Sweden. *Emerg. Infect. Dis.* 8, 956–960, 2002.

Ellis J et al., Tularemia. *Clin. Microbiol. Rev.* 15, 631–646, 2002.

Eneslatt K et al., Persistence of cell-mediated immunity three decades after vaccination with the live vaccine strain of Francisella tularensis. *Eur. J. Immunol.* 41, 974–980, 2011.

Farlow J et al., Francisella tularensis strain typing using multiple-locus, variable-number tandem repeat analysis. *J. Clin. Microbiol.* 39, 3186–3192, 2001.

Feldman KA et al., An outbreak of primary pneumonic tularemia on Martha's Vineyard. *N. Engl. J. Med.* 345, 1601–1606, 2001.

Fredricks DN, Remington JS, Tularemia presenting as community-acquired pneumonia. Implications in the era of managed care. *Arch. Intern. Med.* 156, 2137–2140, 1996.

Gyuranecz M et al., Phylogeography of Francisella tularensis subsp. holarctica, Europe. *Emerg Infect Dis* 18, 290–293, 2012.

Hauri AM et al., Investigating an airborne tularemia outbreak, Germany. *Emerg. Infect. Dis.* 16, 238–243, 2010.

Kaysser PE et al., Re-emergence of tularemia in Germany: presence of Francisella tularensis in different rodent species in endemic areas. *BMC Infect. Dis.* 8, 157, 2008.

Kugeler KJ et al., Molecular epidemiology of Francisella tularensis in the United States. *Clin. Infect. Dis.* 48, 863–870, 2009.

O'Toole D et al., Tularemia in range sheep: an overlooked syndrome? *J. Vet. Diagn. Invest.* 20, 508–513, 2008.

Oyston PC, Francisella tularensis: unravelling the secrets of an intracellular pathogen. *J. Med. Microbiol.* 57, 921–930, 2008.

Perez-Castrillon JL et al., Tularemia epidemic in northwestern Spain: clinical description and therapeutic response. *Clin. Infect. Dis.* 33, 573–576, 2001.

Petersen JM, Molins CR, Subpopulations of Francisella tularensis ssp. tularensis and holarctica: identification and associated epidemiology. *Future Microbiol.* 5, 649–661, 2010.

Reintjes R et al., Tularemia outbreak investigation in Kosovo: case control and environmental studies. *Emerg. Infect. Dis.* 8, 69–73, 2002.

Sjostedt A et al., Detection of Francisella tularensis in ulcers of patients with tularemia by PCR. *J. Clin. Microbiol.* 35, 1045–1048, 1997.

Tärnvik A, WHO, Guidelines on Tularaemia. Vol. WHO/CDS/EPR/2007.7. World Health Organization, Geneva, 2007.

Urich SK, Petersen JM, In vitro susceptibility of isolates of Francisella tularensis types A and B from North America. *Antimicrob. Agents Chemother.* 52, 2276–2278, 2008.

Vogler AJ et al., Phylogeography of Francisella tularensis: global expansion of a highly fit clone. *J. Bacteriol.* 191, 2474–2484, 2009.

Weber IB et al., Clinical recognition and management of tularemia in Missouri: a retrospective record review of 121 cases. *Clin Infect Dis* 55, 1283–1290, 2012.

Wik O, Large tularaemia outbreak in Varmland, central Sweden, 2006. *Euro Surveill.* 11, E060921 060921, 2006.

2.24 Vibrioses

Vibrio spp. cause various diseases such as cholera, gastroenteritis, wound infection, and septicemia.

2.24.1 CHOLERA

Cholera, an infectious intestinal disease, is an anthroponosis whose transmission from fish to human justifies its classification as a zoonosis. Whether *V. cholerae* only uses fish as a vehicle or whether it actually infects fish is not clear at the present time. The chain from vertebrate to human, however, plays a minor role in the epidemiology of cholera.

Etiology. *V. cholerae* is a curved, motile, facultatively anaerobic Gram-negative rod of the size 0.5 to 0.8 × 1.3 µm. It possesses one polar flagellum and somatic polysaccharide antigens that allow the differentiation into >200 serogroups. Until now, only the toxin-encoding strains of serogroup O1 and, since 1992, O139 have been associated with epidemics.

Based on further antigenic determinants, there are three serovars/subtypes in *V. cholerae* O1 and, based on biochemical parameters, two biovars. Serovar Inaba carries O antigens A and C, serovar Ogawa O-antigens A and B, and serovar Hikojima O antigens A, B, and C. The biovars "classic" and "El Tor" differ, among others, in phage susceptibility, polymyxin B susceptibility, and hemolysis.

The most important virulence factors are the cholera toxin (CTX) and the toxin-coregulated pilus (TCP). CTX is a hetero-hexameric protein with AB5 structure and ADP ribosyltransferase activity, TCP is a type IV fimbria which serves to attach the organisms to the intestinal mucosa. Moreover, *V. cholerae* produces the zona occludens toxin, the accessory cholera enterotoxin, and a cytotoxin, which forms anion-permeable channels in the membrane of its target cells.

Occurrence. *V. cholerae* O1/O139 and non-O1/non-O139 live mostly together in their natural reservoir, that is, fresh or brack water habitats in areas of river estuaries. The nontoxigenic non-O1/non-O139 are numerically superior to the toxigenic O1/139 strains. In endemic areas, epidemiologically relevant reservoirs for *V. cholerae* are asymptomatic patients.

V. cholerae lives in its natural aquatic environment in close association with algae, shellfish, and copepods (zooplankton). Under favorable temperature and concentration of salt and nutrients, *V. cholerae* will multiply and survive for years. However, it can also make a transition from a metabolically active to a resting state in which it is able to survive under unfavorable circumstances but cannot be cultured even in enriched media ("viable but nonculturable" state). *V. cholerae* has not only been isolated from water sources but also from birds and plant-eating mammals who live in considerable distance from water.

Non-O1/non-O139 *V. cholerae* occur worldwide in water sources. O1 cholera is found in Africa, Asia, and South and Central America, while O-139 has been limited to Southeast Asia, India, and Pakistan. Cholera presents a considerable health problem in developing countries, above all, in poor and crisis areas in which large epidemics can begin suddenly. The WHO estimates that every year ci. 3 to 5 million people become infected with cholera and that more than 100 000 will die.

Transmission. For humans, the oral uptake of contaminated water is the primary way of infection but fecally or otherwise contaminated food is a frequent source as well. Epidemics can be caused by consumption of raw fish, insufficiently heated shellfish, and raw fresh or salt water mussels or oysters. Human-to-human transmission is possible. Epidemics are more frequent during the warm months.

Clinical Manifestations. The incubation period depends on the number of bacteria ingested and ranges from several hours to 5 days. The MID in persons with normal stomach acidity is ci. 10^{11} bacteria but in people with hypochlorhydria or stomach acid buffered by food, *Helicobacter pylori*, or antacid it may be considerably lower, for example, 10^6 at neutral stomach pH.

Severe cases of cholera begin with sudden profuse painless watery diarrhea and vomiting, whereby the fluid loss may amount to up to 25 l per day. The stool is typically a grey, slightly flocculated fluid with some mucus but without blood (rice water stool). Very quickly symptoms of dehydration will develop: extreme thirst, dry mucous membranes, decreasing turgor of the skin, deep-seated eyeballs, hypotension, weak pulses, tachycardia, tachypnea, a raw or soundless voice, oliguria, renal failure, convulsions, drowsiness, coma, and, finally, death. Without treatment, the case-fatality rate may reach 50%. WHO estimates that 90% of all cases show a mild or moderate course and are frequently caused by biovar El Tor.

Non-O1/non-O139 strains cause a foodborne gastroenteritis but also otitis media, wound infections, and bacteremia. The incubation period is >2 days. Stools are watery, occasionally bloody or mucoid. This illness lasts for 2 to 7 days. Patients with extraintestinal infections often give a history of contact with surface waters, mostly seawater.

In herbivores (horse, cattle, sheep, bison), non-O1/non-O139 *V. cholerae* infection is associated with sudden death, watery or bloody diarrhea, and abortion. In Japan and Australia, septicemia was observed in some species of fish, with loss of eel and ayu populations.

Diagnosis. In endemic as well as in epidemic areas, full-blown cases are being diagnosed clinically. Direct detection in stools by use of darkfield microscopy or immobilization with antibody requires considerable experience. On selective media, such as thiosulfate-citrate-bile salts-sucrose, *V. cholerae* forms yellow colonies but there should be confirmation by biochemical tests. PCR methods are also available.

Differential Diagnosis. Cholera-like diarrhea can also be caused by *Cryptosporidium* spp. and enterotoxigenic *Escherichia coli*.

Therapy. Electrolyte and fluid loss must be substituted immediately. Intravenous Ringer lactate plus potassium is indicated in dehydrated patients with >10% loss of body weight. The fluid deficit can be compensated within the first 4 h and half of it within the first hour. Afterwards, peroral treatment should be continued with the WHO cholera drink (WHO Oral Dehydration Solution, ORS) which contains Na+ 75 mMol/l, K+ 20 mMol/l, Cl- 65 mMol/l, citrate 10 mMol/l, and glucose 75 mMol/l. This peroral rehydration is more secure than intravenous one as it uses the patient's thirst and urine production as guidelines, and thus, avoids hyperhydration with pulmonary edema.

Antibiotics shorten the duration of illness, bacterial excretion, and fluid loss. The drug of choice is doxycycline 1 × 300 mg/day p.o. or azithromycin 1 × 1 g/day p.o., each as a single dose; in pregnancy, azithromycin 1 × 1 g/day p.o. as a single dose or erythromycin 500 mg/day for 3 days; for children, azithromycin 20 mg/kg/day p.o. as a single dose.

Prophylaxis. The most important steps are providing the population with safe drinking water and good sewage disposal. Furthermore, personal and food hygiene are mandatory. In some countries, peroral whole cell inactivated vaccines are available. Safety and efficacy of the most recent vaccines are 66 to 85% after two doses. The use of chemoprophylaxis (ciprofloxacin) is controversial.

Reporting. Cholera is a notifiable disease in both the USA and Canada.

REFERENCES

Alam M et al., Diagnostic limitations to accurate diagnosis of cholera. *J Clin Microbiol* 48, 3918–3922, 2010.

Alam M et al., Viable but nonculturable Vibrio cholerae O1 in biofilms in the aquatic environment and their role in cholera transmission. *Proc. Natl. Acad. Sci. U. S. A.* 104, 17801–17806, 2007.

Albert MJ, Neira M, Motarjemi Y, The role of food in the epidemiology of cholera. *World Health Stat. Q.* 50, 111–118, 1997.

Austin B, Vibrios as causal agents of zoonoses. *Vet. Microbiol.* 140, 310–317, 2010.

Bharati K, Ganguly NK, Cholera toxin: a paradigm of a multifunctional protein. *Indian J. Med. Res.* 133, 179–187, 2011.

Bhattacharya SK, An evaluation of current cholera treatment. *Expert Opin. Pharmacother.* 4, 141–146, 2003.

Cho YJ et al., Genomic evolution of Vibrio cholerae. *Curr. Opin. Microbiol.* 13, 646–651, 2010.

Echevarria J et al., Efficacy and tolerability of ciprofloxacin prophylaxis in adult household contacts of patients with cholera. *Clin. Infect. Dis.* 20, 1480–1484, 1995.

Kaper JB, Morris JGJr, Levine MM, Cholera. *Clin. Microbiol. Rev.* 8, 48–86, 1995.

Lizárraga-Partida ML et al., Association of Vibrio cholerae with plankton in coastal areas of Mexico. *Environ. Microbiol.* 11, 201–208, 2009.

Luquero FJ et al., Use of Vibrio cholera vaccine in an outbreak in Guinea. *N Engl J Med* 370, 2111–2120, 2014.

Nelson EJ et al., Cholera transmission: the host, pathogen and bacteriophage dynamic. *Nat. Rev. Microbiol.* 7, 693–702, 2009.

Ogg JE, Ryder RA, Smith HLJr, Isolation of Vibrio cholerae from aquatic birds in Colorado and Utah. *Appl. Environ. Microbiol.* 55, 95–99, 1989.

Pape JW, Rouzier V, Embracing oral cholera vaccine – the shifting response to cholera. *N Engl J Med* 370, 2067–2069, 2014.

Raufman JP, Cholera. *Am. J. Med.* 104, 386–394, 1998.

Rhodes JB, Schweitzer D, Ogg JE, Isolation of non-O1 Vibrio cholerae associated with enteric disease of herbivores in western Colorado. *J. Clin. Microbiol.* 22, 572–575, 1985.

Safa A, Nair GB, Kong RY, Evolution of new variants of Vibrio cholerae O1. *Trends Microbiol.* 18, 46–54, 2010.

Schild S, Bishop A, Camilli A., Ins and outs of V. cholerae. *Microbe* 3, 131–136, 2008.

Seas C et al., Practical guidelines for the treatment of cholera. *Drugs* 51, 966–973, 1996.

Shahinian ML et al., Helicobacter pylori and epidemic Vibrio cholerae O1 infection in Peru. *Lancet* 355, 377–378, 2000.

Visser IJ et al., Isolation of Vibrio cholerae from diseased farm animals and surface water in The Netherlands. *Vet. Rec.* 144, 451–452, 1999.

WHO, Cholera, 2010. *WHO: Weekly Epidemiological Record* 31, 325–340, 2011.

WHO/UNICEF, *Oral Rehydratation Salts. Production of the New ORS.* WHO/FCH/CAH/06, Geneva, 2006.

Zuckerman JN, Rombo L, Fisch A, The true burden and risk of cholera: implications for prevention and control. *Lancet Infect. Dis.* 7, 521–530, 2007.

2.24.2 DISEASE DUE TO OTHER *VIBRIO* SPP. AND CLOSELY RELATED SPECIES

In seawater close to coasts and in brackish waters of estuaries other, often halophilic, vibrios and related bacteria are able to multiply above temperatures of 10 to 20 °C. Crustaceans and copepods, such as oysters, crabs, and crayfish, are "filters" who take up vibrios and enrich them in their organs, particularly during warm seasons. Some of these bacteria are human pathogens and may even be transmitted from fish to human.

Most reports on infections come from East Asia and from US coasts, particularly from the coast at the Gulf of Mexico. V. *parahaemolyticus, V. mimicus, V. fluvialis, V. furnissii*, and

Grimontia hollisae (formerly *V. hollisae*) can cause gastroenteritis following consumption of insufficiently heated or recontaminated shellfish. Wound and ear infections, cellulitis, and septicemia may be caused by these species but are mostly due to *V. vulnificus, V. alginolyticus, V. metschnikovii, V. harveyi* (Syn. *V. carchariae*), and *Photobacterium damselae*. Infection results from contamination of open wounds with seawater, in the case of *P. damselae*, also after contact with damselfish and in *V. harveyi*, after shark bites. These wound infections can lead to fulminant, deep soft tissue infections to necrotizing fasciitis, and osteomyelitis. Septicemia occurs primarily in immunocompromised individuals with liver and kidney disease, tumors, diabetes, thalassemia, iron overload, coronary insufficiency, and leg ulcers. Particularly virulent is *V. vulnificus*, which causes life-threatening septicemia within hours after percutaneous or oral uptake.

Enteritis due to these organisms is mostly self-limited and does not require antibiotic treatment. For wound infections and in suspected cases of septicemia, however, early antibiotic treatment is important. Ceftazidime 3×2 gm/day i.v. plus doxycycline 2×100 mg/day i.v.or p.o., provided the bacteria have proven to be susceptible.

Seafood and food washed with seawater should not be consumed raw or insufficiently heated. People at special risk should not expose their wounds to seawater.

REFERENCES

Aigbivbalu L, Maraqa N, Photobacterium damsela wound infection in a 14-year-old surfer. *South. Med. J.* 102, 425–426, 2009.

Austin B, Vibrios as causal agents of zoonoses. *Vet. Microbiol.* 140, 310–317, 2010.

Bisharat N et al., Clinical, epidemiological, and microbiological features of Vibrio vulnificus biogroup 3 causing outbreaks of wound infection and bacteraemia in Israel. Israel Vibrio Study Group. *Lancet* 354, 1421–1424, 1999.

Broberg CA, Calder TJ, Orth K, Vibrio parahaemolyticus cell biology and pathogenicity determinants. *Microbes Infect.* 13, 992–1001, 2011.

Derber C et al., Vibrio furnissii: an unusual cause of bacteremia and skin lesions after ingestion of seafood. *J. Clin. Microbiol.* 49, 2348–2349, 2011.

Gomez JM et al., Necrotizing fasciitis due to Vibrio alginolyticus in an immunocompetent patient. *J. Clin. Microbiol.* 41, 3427–3429, 2003.

Gras-Rouzet S et al., First European case of gastroenteritis and bacteremia due to Vibrio hollisae. *Eur. J. Clin. Microbiol. Infect. Dis.* 15, 864–866, 1996.

Igbinosa EO, Okoh AI, Vibrio fluvialis: an unusual enteric pathogen of increasing public health concern. *Int. J. Environ. Res. Public. Health* 7, 3628–3643, 2010.

Kim HR et al., Septicemia progressing to fatal hepatic dysfunction in a cirrhotic patient after oral ingestion of Photobacterium damsela: a case report. *Infection* 37, 555–556, 2009.

Kuo CH et al., Septic arthritis as the initial manifestation of fatal Vibrio vulnificus septicemia in a patient with thalassemia and iron overload. *Pediatr. Blood Cancer* 53, 1156–1158, 2009.

Miron D et al., Vibrio vulnificus necrotizing fasciitis of the calf presenting with compartment syndrome. *Pediatr. Infect. Dis. J.* 22, 666–668, 2003.

Nair GB et al., Global dissemination of Vibrio parahaemolyticus serotype O3: K6 and its serovariants. *Clin Microbiol Rev* 20,39–48, 2007.

Nakamura Y et al., Necrotizing fasciitis of the leg due to Photobacterium damsela. *J. Dermatol.* 35, 44–45, 2008.

Schets FM et al., Potentially human pathogenic vibrios in marine and fresh bathing waters related to environmental conditions and disease outcome. *Int. J. Hyg. Environ. Health* 214, 399–406, 2011.

Shimohata T, Takahashi A, Diarrhea induced by infection of Vibrio parahaemolyticus. *J. Med. Invest.* 57, 179–182, 2010.

Tebbs R et al., Design and validation of a novel multiplex real-time PCR assay for Vibrio pathogen detection. *J. Food Prot.* 74, 939–948, 2011.

Tena D et al., Fulminant necrotizing fasciitis due to Vibrio parahaemolyticus. *J. Med. Microbiol.* 59, 235–238, 2010.

2.25 Yersinioses (Enteric Infections due to *Yersinia enterocolitica* and *Y. pseudotuberculosis*)

The agents of enteric yersinioses are widespread in animals but transmission from animals to humans has not been proven beyond doubt because of the similarity of regionally circulating strains. Transmission, however, offers the most plausible explanation for the existence of human infections. Enteric yersinioses are almost always foodborne infections.

Etiology. *Yersinia* is a genus of Gram-negative rods in the family *Enterobacteriaceae*. With the exception of *Y. pestis* they are motile below 30 °C and can be speciated according to biochemical traits and antigenic characteristics. Their growth optimum is at 28 °C but they are able to multiply at 4 °C as psychotrophs and at 41 °C. Besides *Y. enterocolitica*, *Y. pseudotuberculosis*, and *Y. pestis* (see 2.16), *Y. frederiksenii*, *Y. kristensenii*, *Y. intermedia*, *Y. mollaretii*, *Y. bercovieri*, *Y. aldovae*, and *Y. rhodei* have been isolated from human specimens but they can so far be called neither human pathogens nor zoonotic species. *Y. ruckeri* causes enteric red mouth disease of rainbow trout and other salmonides and is not a zoonotic agent either.

The virulence of *Y. enterocolitica* and *Y. pseudotuberculosis* is, among other factors, caused by a 70 kbp plasmid bYV that encodes components of a type III protein secretion system and effector proteins (*Yersinia* outher proteins YopE, YopH, YopO, YopP/YopJ, YopM, YopT) translocated by this system into host cells. Strains without this plasmid are avirulent.

Occurrence. Human infections with *Y. enterocolitica* and *Y. pseudotuberculosis* are found worldwide but are more frequent in areas with moderate or cool climates than in warm ones. In the European Union, the yearly incidence of registered cases between 2005 and 2009 was between 1.6 and 3.0 per 100 000 inhabitants. Among the >50 known serogroups and the six biochemically defined biovars of *Y. enterocolitica*, only biovars/serogroups 4/O:3, 2/O:9 and 2/O:5,27 are of significance as human pathogens. In the US, there were mainly 4/O:3 and 1B/O:8; in Japan and Canada, mainly 2/O:5,27.

Y. pseudotuberculosis has 21 O groups and subgroups that occur with variable frequency in the various continents: in Europe, O:1a and O:1b cause ci. 60%, O:2a, O:2b, and O:3 ci. 30%, and O:4a, O:5a, and others ci. 10% of the enteric yersinioses; the latter groups are more frequent in Japan where the other groups occur as well. *Y. pseudotuberculosis* can be subdivided into four biotypes based on utilization of melibiose, raffinose, and citrate.

Enteric infections with *Y.enterocolitica* are observed during the entire year but are more frequent during (late) summer and in January/

February. *Y. pseudotuberculosis* infections show peaks in late fall, winter, and spring. Enteric yersinioses are mostly observed as singular cases or small (family) epidemics; larger epidemics are rare.

Virulent and avirulent strains of *Y. enterocolitica* have been isolated from many domestic and wild animals' intestines and feces. Pigs in whom var 4/O:3 has been isolated from 30 to 60% of the tonsils are regarded as the main reservoir of *Y. enterocolitica*. *Y. pseudotuberculosis* infections occur in a wide spectrum of vertebrates. An epidemiologically important reservoir seems to be wild living rodents and birds but domestic animals, particularly ruminants and pigs are also sources.

Following excretion, yersiniae can survive for up to several weeks in the environment, for example, in soil even for several months. Whether they can multiply there is unclear. Virulent yersiniae are found in food of animal origin (milk, meat) and in surface waters with surprising regularity.

At special risk are immunocompromised people. Whether people with frequent contact to pigs, such as butchers, are also at risk has not been determined with certainty.

Transmission. Enteric yersinioses are mainly transmitted by the fecal-oral route. Uptake occurs through fecally contaminated food and water. Epidemics in children have been caused by secondarily contaminated pasteurized milk or chocolate milk, tofu, beans, carrots, iceberg salad, raw or insufficiently heated pork or chitterlings, and surface waters, although a source could often not be determined. Oral smear infections may also play a role (Fig. 2.30); human-to-human transmission may occur that way. Iatrogenic *Y. enterocolitica* septicemias due to transfusion of contaminated blood stored under refrigeration are well known.

Clinical Manifestations. *Y. enterocolitica* infection has an incubation period of between 1 and 11 days; that of *Y. pseudotuberculosis* is probably between 7 and 21 days. Clinical symptoms are similar for both diseases while there are differences in frequency, age, and gender distributions (Table 2.9).

The most frequent manifestation is enteritis or enterocolitis. Initial symptoms are vomiting and very soft or watery stools that may contain blood or mucus in 30 to 50% of cases. There may be fever up to 39 °C. Colicky pain may

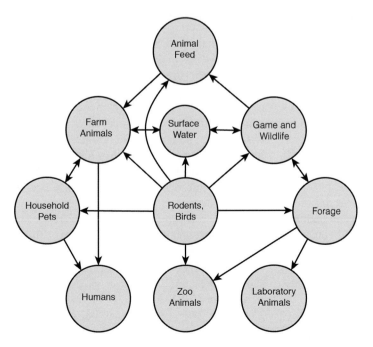

Figure 2.30 | Possible transmission chains for *Yersinia enterocolitica* and *Y. pseudotuberculosis*.

Table 2.9 | Frequent Manifestations of Enteral Yersinioses with Regard to Species and also to Age and Sex of Patients.

CLINICAL MANIFESTATION	Y. ENTEROCOLITICA PREFERENCE FOR		Y. PSEUDOTUBERCULOSIS PREFERENCE FOR	
	AGE	SEX	AGE	SEX
Enteritis, enterocolitis, febrile diarrhea	1 to 10 y, >30 y	NS	>18 y	NS
Mesenterial lymphadenitis, terminal ileitis, pseudoappendicitis	10 to 30 y	NS	6 to 18 y	M > F
Arthritis, arthralgias	25 to 35 y	NS	>10 y	NS
Erythema nodosum	>40 y	F>M	<20 y	NS

F, female; M, male; NS, no significant differences; y, years. From Knapp, W: Deutsches Aerzteblatt 77:1671–1676, 1980.

occur in the right lower or the entire abdominal area. "Pseudoappendicitis" due to mesenterical lymphadenitis (more frequent in *Y. pseudotuberculosis*) or due to terminal ileitis (more frequent in *Y. enterocolitica*) may give rise to laparotomies, which do not show an inflamed appendix but rather enlarged and inflamed lymphnodes or clusters of them causing invagination.

Following the enteritic or pseudoappendicitic course (with a good prognosis), symptoms of a reactive arthritis may arise within 1 to 3 weeks. There may be mono- or asymmetrical polyarthritis (with 40 to 80% of the patients being HLA-B27positive), arthralgias, or erythema nodosum preferentially located on the lower extremities. These illnesses are due to immunopathological processes and do not occur in the enteric phase. In individual cases, colicky abdominal pain without diarrhea, symptoms of pharyngotonsillitis, a complete or incomplete Reiter syndrome with conjunctivitis or uveitis, urethritis, and/or carditis, are the sole prodromi of arthritis. In general, they will last for 3 to 6 months, in 20% of the patients >12 months, and in individual cases up to 5 years.

Septicemic infections with both *Yersinia* species occur with particular frequency in patients with thalassemia, sickle cell anemia, hemochromatosis, those on hemodialysis, with liver disease, iron overload, and diabetes. Unless early antibiotic treatment is initiated, the case fatality rate of these patients can go up to 50%.

In individual cases, *Y. enterocolitica* was found as the agent of meningitis, endophthalmitis, conjunctivitis, myocarditis, pneumonia, abscesses in lung, liver and kidney, hepatitis, cholangitis, peritonitis, glomerulonephritis, urethritis, cellulitis, osteomyelitis, septic arthritis, hemolytic anemia, and arterial aneurysms. Rare diseases due to *Y. pseudotuberculosis* are Parinaud's conjunctivitis and interstitial nephritis.

In the Far East, a scarlet fever-like syndrome due to *Y. pseudotuberculosis* has been observed. Those strains possess a superantigen YPM (*Y. pseudotuberculosis* derived mitogen) encoded by a gene present in 95% of the Far Eastern strains.

In animals, *Y. enterocolitica* infections are mostly latent and only in single cases manifested as febrile enteritis, organ involvement, or septicemia. Infections with *Y. pseudotuberculosis* are acute, subacute, or chronic generalized diseases. In rodents, the disease will lead to granulomas in internal organs (called pseudotuberculosis) and to death within 10 to 14 days. Acute septicemic courses with high case-fatality rates have been observed in rabbits, hares, guinea pigs, and birds. In wild populations of rodents and lagomorphs, epidemics have occurred ("rodentiosis"). In domestic animals, the disease occurs sporadically.

Diagnosis. A definite diagnosis requires culture and perhaps proof of the presence of antibodies. The bacteria are best cultured from diarrhoic stool on cefsulodin (4 g/l)-irgasan-novobiocin (CIN) agar at 30 °C for 48 h or at 37 °C for 24 h followed by 48 to 72 h at room temperature. Cold enrichment at 4 °C for 3 weeks in phosphate-buffered saline (with weekly subcultures on CIN agar) is used only for carriers or people with reactive arthritis. While CIN agar yields better results than Mac-Conkey, SS agar, or SS agar with desoxycholate plus 0.1% $CaCl_2$ for *Y. enterocolitica*, MacConkey agar is the preferred medium for isolation of *Y. pseudotuberculosis*. Other specimens used for culture are lymphnodes, material from resections, pus, or blood, the latter in cases of septicemia. Speciation is done with biochemical tests. Commercial galleries may not always yield correct diagnoses. Virulence genes can be detected by PCR.

Antibodies are detectable within the first week of illness by agglutination (titer 1:160 or higher) but specificity is hampered by cross-reactivity to *Brucella*, *Francisella*, *Vibrio*, certain *Salmonella* groups, *Borrelia burgdorferi*, *Chlamydia pneumoniae*, some *E. coli* groups, as well as to nonpathogenic *Yersinia* species. ELISA is able to separate IgM, IgA, and IgG antibodies. An immunoblot using antigens encoded by pYV avoids cross reactions. In animals, yersiniae are cultured from feces or organ material.

Differential Diagnosis. Infections with salmonellae, shigellae, *Campylobacter* spp., and clostridia have to be considered. Pseudoappendicitis must be separated from Crohn's disease by pathologic anatomy, if necessary. Arthritis has a host of differential diagnoses, mainly from the rheumatic syndromes. If generalized yersinioses, particularly those with abscess formation in abdominal organs, are suspected amebiasis, typhoid fever, and malaria should be considered.

Therapy. Antibiotic treatment is indicated only in septicemia or in chronic or recurring disease. The drug of choice is doxycycline 2×100 mg/ day i.v. plus gentamicin or tobramycin 5 mg/ kg/day i.v. Alternatives are trimethoprim-sulfamethoxazole double strength 2×1 tablet/d or ciprofloxacin 2×500 mg/day for 3 to 7 days. Uncomplicated courses and arthritis require symptomatic treatment only. In animals, oxytetracycline may lead to a cure.

Prophylaxis. A specific prophylaxis cannot be recommended at this time because of lack of epidemiological data. Avoidance of smear infection and general hygienic measures to be taken when treating diarrhoic patients are to be followed.

REFERENCES

Ackers ML et al., An outbreak of Yersinia enterocolitica O:8 infections associated with pasteurized milk. *J. Infect. Dis.* 181, 1834–1837, 2000.

Aleksić S, Bockemühl J, Wuthe HH, Epidemiology of Y. pseudotuberculosis in Germany, 1983–1993. *Contrib. Microbiol. Immunol.* 13, 55–58, 1995.

Batzilla J et al., Yersinia enterocolitica palearctica serobiotype O:3/4 - a successful group of emerging zoonotic pathogens. *BMC Genomics* 12, 348, 2011.

Carniel E et al., Yersinia enterocolitica and Yersinia pseudotuberculosis. In: The Prokaryotes, Vol. 6: Proteobacteria: Gamma Subclass. Dworkin M, and Falkow S (eds.), pp. 270–398. Springer, Heidelberg, Germany, 2006.

Dube P, Interaction of Yersinia with the gut: mechanisms of pathogenesis and immune evasion. *Curr. Top. Microbiol. Immunol.* 337, 61–91, 2009.

Fenwick SG, Madie P, Wilks CR, Duration of carriage and transmission of Yersinia enterocolitica biotype 4, serotype 0:3 in dogs. *Epidemiol. Infect.* 113, 471–477, 1994.

Fredriksson-Ahomaa M, Epidemiology of human Yersinia pseudotuberculosis infection. *Arch. Lebensmittelhyg.* 60, 82–87, 2009.

Fredriksson-Ahomaa M, Stolle A, Korkeala H, Molecular epidemiology of Yersinia enterocolitica infections. *FEMS Immunol. Med. Microbiol.* 47, 315–329, 2006.

Fredriksson-Ahomaa M et al., Sporadic human Yersinia enterocolitica infections caused by bioserotype 4/O: 3 originate mainly from pigs. *J. Med. Microbiol.* 55, 747–749, 2006.

Heesemann J, Sing A, Trülzsch K, Yersinia's stratagem: targeting innate and adaptive immune defense. *Curr. Opin. Microbiol.* 9, 55–61, 2006.

Laukkanen R et al., Contamination of carcasses with human pathogenic Yersinia enterocolitica 4/O:3 originates from pigs infected on farms. *Foodborne Pathog. Dis.* 6, 681–688, 2009.

Kaasch AJ et al., Yersinia pseudotuberculosis bloodstream infection and septic arthritis: case report and review of the literature. *Infection* 40, 185–190, 2012.

Long C et al., Yersinia pseudotuberculosis and Y. enterocolitica infections, FoodNet, 1996–2007. *Emerg. Infect. Dis.* 16, 566–567, 2010.

Neubauer HK, Sprague LD, Epidemiology and diagnostics of Yersinia infections. *Adv. Exp. Med. Biol.* 529, 431–438, 2003.

Nowgesic E et al., Outbreak of Yersinia pseudotuberculosis in British Columbia–November 1998. *Can. Commun. Dis. Rep.* 25, 97–100, 1999.

Ong KL et al., Changing epidemiology of Yersinia enterocolitica infections: markedly decreased rates in young black children, Foodborne Diseases Active Surveillance Netwoek (FoodNet), 1996–2009. *Clin Infect Dis 54/S* 385–390, 2012.

Rimhanen-Finne R et al., Yersinia pseudotuberculosis causing a large outbreak associated with carrots in Finland, 2006. *Epidemiol. Infect.* 137, 342–347, 2009.

Rosner BM, Stark K, Werber D, Epidemiology of reported Yersinia enterocolitica infections in Germany, 2001–2008. *BMC Public Health* 10, 337, 2010.

Thompson JS, Gravel MJ, Family outbreak of gastroenteritis due to Yersinia enterocolitica serotype 0:3 from well water. *Can. J. Microbiol.* 32, 700–701, 1986.

Tipple MA et al., Sepsis associated with transfusion of red cells contaminated with Yersinia enterocolitica. *Transfusion (Paris)* 30, 207–213, 1990.

Viboud GI, Bliska JB, Yersinia outer proteins: role in modulation of host cell signaling responses and pathogenesis. *Annu. Rev. Microbiol.* 59, 69–89, 2005.

Virdi JS, Sachdeva P, Molecular heterogeneity in Yersinia enterocolitica and "Y. enterocolitica-like" species – implications for epidemiology, typing and taxonomy. *FEMS Immunol. Med. Microbiol.* 45, 1–10, 2005.

2.26 Rare and Potential Agents of Bacterial Zoonoses

2.26.1 *ACTINOBACILLUS* INFECTIONS

Zoonotic infections with *Actinobacillus spp.* occur only sporadically in humans, mostly through bite wounds.

Etiology. The Gram-negative rods, *Actinobacillus lignieresii, A. equuli,* and *A. suis.*

Occurrence. These bacteria are part of the normal oropharyngeal flora of horses, cattle, sheep, and pigs.

Transmission. Mostly through animal bites. It seems possible that touching the animals and close contact with meat products causes infections via conjunctivae or skin lesions. At special risk are people with intensive contact to those animals.

Clinical Manifestations. Most frequent are wound infections, particularly on hands and lower arms with abscess formation, and in individual cases, there can also be septicemia.

Diagnosis. Culture and speciation with biochemical tests.

Differential Diagnosis. Bite wounds caused by other bacterial agents, such as staphylococci, streptococci, pasteurellae, *S. moniliformis*, and *Capnocytophaga* spp.

Therapy. Treatment with beta lactam antibiotics or fluoroquinolones is recommended.

Prophylaxis. Hygienic measures, avoidance of bites, and cleaning and disinfection of bite wounds.

REFERENCES

Ashhurst-Smith C et al., Actinobacillus equuli septicemia: an unusual zoonotic infection. *J. Clin. Microbiol.* 36, 2789–2790, 1998.

Benaoudia F, Escande F, Simonet M, Infection due to Actinobacillus lignieresii after a horse bite. *Eur. J. Clin. Microbiol. Infect. Dis.* 13, 439–440, 1994.

Brook I, Management of human and animal bite wound infection: an overview. *Curr. Infect. Dis. Rep.* 11, 389–395, 2009.

Dibb WL, Digranes A, Tonjum S, Actinobacillus lignieresii infection after a horse bite. *Br. Med. J. (Clin. Res. Ed.)* 283, 583–584, 1981.

Escande F et al., Actinobacillus suis infection after a pig bite. *Lancet.* 348, 888, 1996.

Peel MM et al., Actinobacillus spp. and related bacteria in infected wounds of humans bitten by horses and sheep. *J. Clin. Microbiol.* 29, 2535–2538, 1991.

Rycroft AN, Garside LH, Actinobacillus species and their role in animal disease. *Vet J* 159, 18–36, 2000.

2.26.2 *AEROMONAS* INFECTIONS

Etiology. The genus *Aeromonas* comprises by now more than 20 species of which *A. hydrophila*, *A. caviae*, and *A. veronii* (with two biovars) are most frequently found in humans and warm-blooded animals; however, in cold-blooded animals, *A. salmonicida* is frequent.

Occurrence. Aeromonads are widespread in humans and in animals (fish, reptiles, amphibians, pigs, cattle, dogs, cats, horses, foxes, mice, monkeys, rabbits, birds, etc.), mostly in the intestinal flora. They are normally found in many water sources but also in food items, probably through contact with water.

Transmission. Aeromonads are primarily transmitted from water or from moist soil to human tissues. Transmission from animals or through foods has been postulated but has not been documented beyond doubt except in infections caused by the clinical use of leeches (*Hirudo medicinalis*). They carry aeromonads in their gut and they have given rise to infections ranging from cellulitis to myonecrosis and septicemia.

Clinical Manifestations. *Aeromonas* spp. may cause infections in animals and in humans; in the latter particularly septicemia in immuno-compromised individuals and wound infections from contact with contaminated water sources. Whether aeromonads are causative agents of diarrhea is still under discussion; it seems that the presence of certain enterotoxins (Act, Alt, Ast) is necessary to elicit diarrhea.

Diagnosis. Culture (selective media) and biochemical tests for speciation; however, for accurate identification of some species molecular methods have to be employed.

Differential Diagnosis. This depends on the site from which the organism has been isolated.

Therapy. Although aminoglycosides, ciprofloxacin, carbapenems, and trimethoprim-sulfamethoxazole have been active against most strains, susceptibility testing is mandatory in view of recent reports of resistance to these compounds.

Prophylaxis. None.

REFERENCES

Giltner CL et al., Ciprofloxacin-resistant Aeromonas hydrophila cellulitis following leech therapy. *J Clin Microbiol.* 51, 1324–1326, 2013.

Janda JM, **Abbott SL**, The genus Aeromonas: taxonomy, pathogenicity, and infection. *Clin Microbiol Rev* 23, 35–73, 2010.

Lineweaver WC, Aeromonas hydrophila infections following clinical use of medicinal leeches: a review of published cases. *Blood Coagul Fibrinolysis* 2, 201–203, 1991.

Pablos M et al., Identification and epidemiological relationships of Aeromonas isolates from patients with diarrhea, drinking water, and foods. *Int J Food Microbiol* 147, 2013–210, 2011.

von Graevenitz A, The role of Aeromonas in diarrhea – a review. *Infection* 35, 59–64, 2007.

2.26.3 *ARCOBACTER* INFECTIONS

Etiology. These are slender, motile Gram-negative curved or helical rods closely related to *Campylobacter*. They are able to multiply under microaerobic conditions at 15 to 30 °C, may grow aerobically at 30 °C, and do not require an increased hydrogen concentration for growth.

Of the 12 *Arcobacter spp.* known by now, *A. butzleri* and *A. cryaerophilus* have been found in association with human infections. The role of *A. skirrowii* in human disease remains unclear. All three species have also been incriminated in infections in animals but animal-human transmission has not been proven beyond doubt.

Occurrence. The three species mentioned occur worldwide and have been isolated from feces or intestinal contents of pets and domestic animals. Some have been isolated from preputial and vaginal samples of healthy cattle and pigs, as well as from the oral cavities of dogs and cats. They occur with high frequency in the gastrointestinal tract of birds which is a potentially important reservoir. Whether open water sources from which *Arcobacter spp.* have been isolated frequently are natural habitats for potentially pathogenic *Arcobacter spp.* or whether these species originate from excreta of infected animals or humans is uncertain. Ground water may be contaminated with *Arcobacter spp.* as well.

Transmission. Human infection is probably preceded by oral uptake of contaminated foodstuffs (meat, milk, oysters, shrimp) or drinking water. One case of intrauterine infection of a fetus has been reported but the exact route of infection could not be determined.

Clinical Manifestations. *A. butzleri* and *A. cryaerophilus* are causative agents of bacteremia, endocarditis, peritonitis, and gastrointestinal infections in humans. The latter are manifested by nausea, vomiting, and watery diarrhea, but occasionally by abdominal cramps without diarrhea. Predisposing ailments have not been conspicuous. There is only one report of a chronic diarrhea from which *A. skirrowii* was isolated.

In animals, abortion and diarrhea seem to be associated with *Arcobacter spp. A. cryophilus* is found much more frequently in material from abortions in cattle, sheep, and pigs than *A. butzleri* and *A.skirrowii*. The latter is presumed to be the causative agent of diarrhea and hemorrhagic colitis in cattle, sheep, and goats. *A. butzleri* is found more often than the other species in the feces of diarrhoic pigs, cattle, horses, monkeys, ostriches, and turtles. Experimentally, *A. cryaerophilus* was able to produce mastitis in cattle and a fatal generalized disease in rainbow trout.

Diagnosis. Proof is provided by culture from feces, blood or organs. Addition of antibiotics to the media, sometimes combined with filtration, increases the chances of isolation. Speciation follows biochemical tests. PCR (amplification of 16S or 23S rDNA) techniques have been developed as well.

Differential Diagnosis. Infectious gastroenteritis due to *Campylobacter, Salmonella, Shigella, Yersinia,* and *C. difficile.*

Therapy. Antibiotic treatment with fluoroquinolones or tetracyclines is recommended only for severe, long-lasting or bacteremic infections. Antibiotic resistance may develop.

REFERENCES

Anderson KF et al., Arcobacter (Campylobacter) butzleri-associated diarrheal illness in a nonhuman primate population. *Infect. Immun.* 61, 2220–2223, 1993.

Collado L, Figueras MJ, Taxonomy, epidemiology, and clinical relevance of the genus Arcobacter. *Clin. Microbiol. Rev.* 24, 174–192, 2011.

Higgins R et al., Arcobacter butzleri isolated from a diarrhoeic non-human primate. *Lab. Anim.* 33, 87–90, 1999.

Ho HT, Lipman LJ, Gaastra W, Arcobacter, what is known and unknown about a potential foodborne zoonotic agent. *Vet. Microbiol.* 115, 1–13, 2006.

Houf K et al., Dogs as carriers of the emerging pathogen Arcobacter. *Vet. Microbiol.* 130, 208–213, 2008.

Houf K et al., Antimicrobial susceptibility patterns of Arcobacter butzleri and Arcobacter cryaerophilus strains isolated from humans and broilers. *Microb. Drug Resist.* 10, 243–247, 2004.

Hsueh PR et al., Bacteremia caused by Arcobacter cryaerophilus 1B. *J. Clin. Microbiol.* 35, 489–491, 1997.

Levican A, Figueras MJ, Performance of five molecular methods for monitoring arcobacter spp. *BMC Microbiol* 13, 220, 2013.

On SL, Stacey A, Smyth J, Isolation of Arcobacter butzleri from a neonate with bacteraemia. *J. Infect.* 31, 225–227, 1995.

Patyal A et al., Prevalence of Arcobacter spp. in humans, animals and foods of animal origin including sea food from India. *Transbound Emerg Dis* 58, 402–410, 2011.

Vandenberg O et al., Antimicrobial susceptibility of clinical isolates of non-jejuni/coli campylobacters and arcobacters from Belgium. *J. Antimicrob. Chemother.* 57, 908–913, 2006.

van Driessche E et al., Isolation of Arcobacter species from animal feces. *FEMS Microbiol. Lett.* 229, 243–248, 2003.

Wybo I et al., Isolation of Arcobacter skirrowii from a patient with chronic diarrhea. *J. Clin. Microbiol.* 42, 1851–1852, 2004.

2.26.4 *BORDETELLA* INFECTIONS

Infections with *Bordetella bronchiseptica* that originate in animals occur only sporadically in humans and show variable symptoms.

Etiology. *B. bronchiseptica*, a coccoid, strictly aerobic Gram-negative rod, is an agent of respiratory infections in domestic animals, and *B. avium* an agent of similar infections in turkeys. *B.hinzii*, which has been found in the respiratory tract of birds but also, albeit rarely, in humans is regarded as an opportunist with a hitherto unknown potential for zoonotic infections.

Occurrence. *B. bronchiseptica* has been proven as an agent of respiratory infections in horses, pigs (atrophic rhinitis), dogs (kennel cough), cats, rabbits, and guinea pigs. Under normal circumstances it is a commensal on the mucous membranes of the upper respiratory tract and causes inflammatory processes only if there is a concomitant infection with another bacterial or a viral agent, or if the environment in the stable is inadequate (poor climatization, overcrowding).

In humans, *B. bronchiseptica* has caused infections in patients with AIDS and other immune defects associated with hemodialysis,

Crohn's disease, endotracheal intubation, and following heart transplantation.

Transmission. Transmission is accomplished most likely via air or through direct contact.

Clinical Manifestations. In humans, a pertussis-like disease has been observed, mostly in immunocompromised individuals.

Diagnosis. Culture and, if a zoonotic origin is suspected, typing techniques.

Differential Diagnosis. Bacterial agents of respiratory disease: *B. pertussis, B. parapertussis, Streptococcus pneumoniae, Haemophilus influenzae, Mycoplasma pneumoniae,* and *Chlamydia pneumoniae.*

Therapy. As *B. bronchiseptica* is erythromycin-resistant, treatment with aminoglycosides, penicillins or cephalosporins is recommended.

Prophylaxis. Immunocompromised patients should avoid contact with the animal species mentioned above.

REFERENCES

Choy KW et al., Bordetella bronchiseptica respiratory infection in a child after bone marrow transplantation. *Pediatr. Infect. Dis. J.* 18, 481–483, 1999.

Gisel JJ, Brumble LM, Johnson MM, Bordetella bronchiseptica pneumonia in a kidney-pancreas transplant patient after exposure to recently vaccinated dogs. *Transpl. Infect. Dis.* 12, 73–76, 2010.

Goldberg JD et al., "Kennel cough" in a patient following allogeneic hematopoietic stem cell transplant. *Bone Marrow Transplant.* 44, 381–382, 2009.

Gore TM et al., Intranasal kennel cough vaccine protecting dogs from experimental Bordetella bronchiseptica challenge within 72 hours. *Vet. Rec.* 156, 482–483, 2005.

Gueirard PC et al., Human Bordetella bronchiseptica infection related to contact with infected animals: persistence of bacteria in host. *J. Clin. Microbiol.* 33, 2002–2006, 1995.

Harrington AT et al., Isolation of Bordetella avium and novel Bordetella strain from patients with respiratory disease. *Emerg Infect Dis* 15, 72–74, 2009.

Hemsworth S, Pizer B, Pet ownership in immunocompromised children–a review of the literature and survey of existing guidelines. *Eur. J. Oncol. Nurs.* 10, 117–127, 2006.

Huebner ES et al., Hospital-acquired Bordetella bronchiseptica infection following hematopoietic stem cell transplantation. *J. Clin. Microbiol.* 44, 2581–2583, 2006.

Libanore M et al., Bordetella bronchiseptica pneumonia in an AIDS patient: a new opportunistic infection. *Infection* 23, 312–313, 1995.

Ner Z et al., Bordetella bronchiseptica infection in pediatric lung transplant recipients. *Pediatr. Transplant.* 7, 413–417, 2003.

Redelman-Sidi G, Grommes C, Papanicolaou G, Kitten-transmitted Bordetella bronchiseptica infection in a patient receiving temozolomide for glioblastoma. *J. Neurooncol.* 102, 335–339, 2011.

Register KB et al., Bordetella bronchiseptica in a paediatric cystic fibrosis patient: possible transmission from a household cat. *Zoonoses Public Health* 59, 246–250, 2012.

Stefanelli PP et al., Molecular characterization of two Bordetella bronchiseptica strains isolated from children with coughs. *J. Clin. Microbiol.* 35, 1550–1555, 1997.

Wernli D et al., Evaluation of eight cases of confirmed Bordetella bronchiseptica infection and colonization over a 15-year period. *Clin. Microbiol. Infect.* 17, 201–203, 2011.

Woolfrey BF, Moody JA, Human infections associated with Bordetella bronchiseptica. *Clin. Microbiol. Rev.* 4, 243–255, 1991.

2.26.5 *CAPNOCYTOPHAGA* INFECTIONS

Capnocytophaga canimorsus and *C. cynodegmi* are able to cause a wide spectrum of diseases from local bite wounds to fulminant, frequently lethal illnesses with septicemia, meningitis, and disseminated intravascular coagulation.

Etiology. The genus *Capnocytophaga* (formerly DF-1 and DF-2), family *Flavobacteriaceae*, contains nine species of facultatively anaerobic, fastidious, Gram-negative, mostly fusiform rods. They are members of the normal oral flora, have been isolated from dental plaque, and are associated with periodontitis. Zoonotic are *C. canimorsus* and *C. cynodegmi.*

Occurrence. *C. canimorsus* and *C. cynodegmi* belong to the normal oral flora of dogs and, more rarely, to that of cats and rabbits. In immunosuppressed, but also in immunocompetent patients, *C. canimorsus* is able to cause septicemia and other severe diseases, such as endocarditis, osteomyelitis, and peritonitis. People in close contact with dogs and cats are at particular risk.

Transmission. Transmission occurs mainly by bites (which can also transmit other aerobic and anaerobic bacteria), rarely by licking of wounds.

Clinical Manifestations. The average incubation time from bite to clinical symptoms is 5 days (1 to 8, rarely up to 30 days). Patients who see their physicians within 8 to 12 h after the bite show only circumscribed lesions without signs of local inflammation. Later, localized cellulitis, pain, purulent secretion, and lymphangitis with regional lymph node swelling are seen in those who have been splenectomized, are alcoholics, or under steroid therapy. The disease can take a severe and fulminant course with septicemia, meningitis, endocarditis, pneumonia, arthritis, purpura fulminans, disseminated intravascular coagulation, peripheral gangrene, and shock. Signs of septicemia are fever, chills, headache, myalgia, vomiting, diarrhea, abdominal pain, severe malaise, dyspnea, and confusion. The case-fatality rate may be as high as 30%.

Diagnosis. Culture on rich media with 5 to 10% CO_2 and biochemical differentiation. PCR techniques have been developed.

Differential Diagnosis. Infections with streptococci (e.g., *S. milleri* group), staphylococci, and nonfermenters, for example, group NO-1 and other bacteria associated with dog and cat bites.

Therapy. *Capnocytophaga* spp. are susceptible to beta lactam antibiotics (although a few strains have been beta-lactamase-positive), macrolides, clindamycin, tetracycline, fluoroquinolones but are resistant to aminoglycosides. Therapy with amoxicillin-clavulanic acid 2 to 3×1 g/day p.o. or 2 to 3×1.2 g/day i.v. has to be started immediately if an infection with *C. canimorsus* is suspected, particularly in immunocompromised or splenectomized patients.

REFERENCES

Chary S et al., Septicemia due to Capnocytophaga canimorsus following dog bite in an elderly male. *Indian J. Pathol. Microbiol.* 54, 368–370, 2001.

Christiansen CB et al., Two cases of infectious purpura fulminans and septic shock caused by Capnocytophaga canimorsus transmitted from dogs. *Scand J Infect Dis* 44, 635–639, 2012.

Ciantar M et al., Assessment of five culture media for the growth and isolation of Capnocytophaga spp. *Clin. Microbiol. Infect.* 17, 158–160, 2011.

Dilegge SK, Edgcomb VP, Leadbetter ER, Presence of the oral bacterium Capnocytophaga canimorsus in the tooth plaque of canines. *Vet. Microbiol.* 149, 437–445, 2011.

Gaastra W, Lipman LJ, Capnocytophaga canimorsus. *Vet. Microbiol.* 140, 339–346, 2010.

Gerster JC, Dudler J, Cellulitis caused by Capnocytophaga cynodegmi associated with etanercept treatment in a patient with rheumatoid arthritis. *Clin. Rheumatol.* 23, 570–571, 2004.

Janda JM et al., Diagnosing Capnocytophaga canimorsus infections. *Emerg Infect Dis* 12, 340–442, 2006.

Le Meur A et al., Acute tenosynovitis of the ankle due to Capnocytophaga cynodegmi/canimorsus as identified by 16S rRNA gene sequencing. *Joint Bone Spine* 75, 749–751, 2008.

Le Moal G et al., Meningitis due to Capnocytophaga canimorsus after receipt of a dog bite: case report and review of the literature. *Clin. Infect. Dis.* 36, e42–46, 2003.

O'Rourke GA, Rothwell R, Capnocytophaga canimorsus a cause of septicaemia following a dog bite: a case review. *Aust. Crit. Care* 24, 93–99, 2011.

Oehler RL et al., Bite-related and septic syndromes caused by cats and dogs. *Lancet Infect. Dis.* 9, 439–447, 2009.

Pers C, Gahrn-Hansen B, Frederiksen W, Capnocytophaga canimorsus septicemia in Denmark, 1982–1995: review of 39 cases. *Clin. Infect. Dis.* 23, 71–75, 1996.

Pers C et al., Capnocytophaga cynodegmi peritonitis in a peritoneal dialysis patient. *J. Clin. Microbiol.* 45, 3844–3846, 2007.

Sandoe JA, Capnocytophaga canimorsus endocarditis. *J. Med. Microbiol.* 53, 245–248, 2004.

Suzuki M et al., Prevalence of Capnocytophaga canimorsus and Capnocytophaga cynodegmi in dogs and cats determined by using a newly established species-specific PCR. *Vet. Microbiol.* 144, 172–176, 2010.

Sarma PS, Mohanty S, Capnocytophaga cynodegmi cellulitis, bacteremia, and pneumonitis in a diabetic man. *J. Clin. Microbiol.* 39, 2028–2029, 2001.

2.26.6 *CORYNEBACTERIUM PSEUDOTUBERCULOSIS* INFECTIONS

Natural hosts of this Gram-positive rod are sheep, horse, and cattle. In sheep, *C. pseudotuberculosis* (syn. *C.ovis*) is the agent of pseudotuberculosis (caseous lymphadenitis) which, at this time, is most prominent in Australia. Rare infections in cattle have been described in Denmark, Israel, and California, as well as in buffalo in Egypt. There have also been reports from Germany of infections in zoo animals, particularly in pet zoos.

Single cases of human infection (granulomatous necrotizing lymphadenitis in neck, axillar and groin) have been reported from Australia and New Zealand. Some cases were probably associated with professional exposure in shepherds, shearers, slaughterhouse personnel, and butchers, therefore, contact transmission was most likely; however, there have also been cases associated with the consumption of raw milk. Surgical excision and treatment with erythromycin or tetracycline are recommended.

REFERENCES

Baird GJ, **Fontaine MC**. Corynebacterium pseudotuberculosis and its role in ovine caseous lymphadenitis. *J Comp Pathol* 137, 179–210, 2007.

Dorella FA et al., Corynebacterium pseudotuberculosis: microbiology, biochemical properties, pathogenesis and molecular studies of virulence. *Vet. Res.* 37, 201–218, 2006.

Hémond V et al., Axillary lymphadenitis due to Corynebacterium pseudotuberculosis in a 63-year-old patient. *Med. Mal. Infect.* 39, 136–139, 2009.

Join-Lambert OF et al., Corynebacterium pseudotuberculosis necrotizing lymphadenitis in a twelve-year-old patient. *Pediatr. Infect. Dis. J.* 25, 848–851, 2006.

Liu DT et al., An infected hydrogel buckle with Corynebacterium pseudotuberculosis. *Br. J. Ophthalmol.* 89, 245–246, 2005.

Mills AE, **Mitchell RD**, **Lim EK**, Corynebacterium pseudotuberculosis is a cause of human necrotising granulomatous lymphadenitis. *Pathology (Phila.)* 29, 231–233, 1997.

Peel MM et al., Human lymphadenitis due to Corynebacterium pseudotuberculosis: report of ten cases from Australia and review. *Clin. Infect. Dis.* 24, 185–191, 1997.

2.26.7 *CORYNEBACTERIUM ULCERANS* INFECTIONS

This Gram-positive rod is primarily known as an animal pathogen causing sporadic cases of mastitis in cattle but the bacterium has also been found in domestic and wild pigs, dogs, and cats. In humans, strains able to produce diphtheria toxin and, rarely, atoxinogenic strains have been described as infectious agents. These

infections were rare until the 1990s. However, between 1975 and 1993, 81 cases were registered in the UK, mostly in children between 5 and 14 years of age. Since then, there have been more reports, particularly from countries of the Northern Hemisphere (USA, Netherlands, Switzerland, Italy, Germany, and Japan). Those due to toxigenic strains cause respiratory diseases resembling diphtheria, rarely pneumonia, sinusitis, or ulcerating lesions on the hands and arms. Severe cases were usually observed in patients who had not been vaccinated, or who had been incompletely vaccinated against diphtheria. The bacterium has also been reported as an agent of peritonitis. Transmission is most likely via raw milk or close contact with animals. Treatment with erythromycin has been recommended; in severe respiratory infections, diphtheria antitoxin has been used.

REFERENCES

Contzen M et al., Corynebacterium ulcerans from diseased wild boars. *Zoonoses Public Health* 58, 479–488, 2011.

de Carpentier JP et al., Nasopharyngeal Corynebacterium ulcerans: a different diphtheria. *J. Laryngol. Otol.* 106, 824–826, 1992.

Dewinter LM, **Bernard KA**, **Romney MG**, Human clinical isolates of Corynebacterium diphtheriae and Corynebacterium ulcerans collected in Canada from 1999 to 2003 but not fitting reporting criteria for cases of diphtheria. *J. Clin. Microbiol.* 43, 3447–3449, 2005.

De Zoysa A et al., Characterization of toxigenic Corynebacterium ulcerans strains isolated from humans and domestic cats in the United Kingdom. *J. Clin. Microbiol.* 43, 4377–4381, 2005.

Dias AA et al., Strain-dependent arthritogenic potential of the zoonotic pathogen Corynebacterium ulcerans. *Vet. Microbiol.* 153, 323–331, 2011.

Hatanaka AA et al., Corynebacterium ulcerans diphtheria in Japan. *Emerg. Infect. Dis.* 9, 752–753, 2003.

Hogg RA et al., Possible zoonotic transmission of toxigenic Corynebacterium ulcerans from companion animals in a human case of fatal diphtheria. *Vet. Rec.* 165, 691–692, 2009.

Kimura Y et al., Acute peritonitis due to Corynebacterium ulcerans in a patient receiving continuous ambulatory peritoneal dialysis: a case report and literature review. *Clin. Exp. Nephrol.* 15, 171–174, 2011.

Lartigue MF et al., Corynebacterium ulcerans in an immunocompromised patient with diphtheria and her dog. *J. Clin. Microbiol.* 43, 999–1001, 2005.

Mattos-Guaraldi AL et al., First detection of Corynebacterium ulcerans producing a diphtheria-like toxin in a case of human with pulmonary infection in the Rio de Janeiro metropolitan area, Brazil. *Mem. Inst. Oswaldo Cruz* 103, 396–400, 2008.

Schuhegger R et al., Pigs as source for toxigenic Corynebacterium ulcerans. *Emerg. Infect. Dis.* 15, 1314–1315, 2009.

Tiwari TS et al., Investigations of 2 cases of diphtheria-like illness due to toxigenic Corynebacterium ulcerans. *Clin. Infect. Dis.* 46, 395–401, 2008.

von Hunolstein C et al., Molecular epidemiology and characteristics of Corynebacterium diphtheriae and Corynebacterium ulcerans strains isolated in Italy during the 1990s. *J. Med. Microbiol.* 52, 181–188, 2003.

Wagner J et al., Infection of the skin caused by Corynebacterium ulcerans and mimicking classical cutaneous diphtheria. *Clin. Infect. Dis.* 33, 1598–1600, 2001.

Wagner KS et al., Diphtheria in the United Kingdom, 1986–2008: the increasing role of Corynebacterium ulcerans. *Epidemiol. Infect.* 138, 1519–1530, 2010.

Wellinghausen N et al., A fatal case of necrotizing sinusitis due to toxigenic: Corynebacterium ulcerans. *Int. J. Med. Microbiol.* 292, 59–63, 2002.

2.26.8 *DERMATOPHILUS CONGOLENSIS* INFECTIONS

Etiology. *Dermatophilus congolensis* belongs to the order *Actinomycetales*. It is a facultatively anaerobic Gram-positive rod that forms 1 to 5 μm thick, branching mycelia-like filaments, which divide longitudinally and transversely so that parallel rows of coccoid cells result. These develop into motile zoospores that grow out to filaments and repeat the cycle.

Occurrence. *D. congolensis* is an obligately pathogenic skin bacterium that causes an acute to chronic, purulent-exudative skin disease (dermatophilosis) in many wild and domestic animals, particularly cattle, sheep, horses, camels, and salt water crocodiles (Fig. 2.31). This disease is widespread in tropical and subtropical areas of Africa, Australia, New Zealand, and India and it has impacted on the economics of these countries. In countries with moderate climates (USA, Argentina, UK, France, Germany) the disease occurs sporadically. Human infections are rare.

Transmission. The bacterium is transmitted through contact with infected animals or their products. It seems possible that flies and ectoparasites act as vectors. People at risk are those in close contact with infected animals.

Clinical Manifestations. Human dermatophilosis is preferentially localized on the hand and forearm. There are either eczematous lesions, or multiple pea-size pustules or furuncles, or pin-needle sized crater-like areas of keratolysis (pitted keratolysis) and leukoplakia (in immunosuppressed patients). The lesions generally heal within 2 to 3 weeks.

Diagnosis. Microscopy (Giemsa) of exudate, scabs, crusts, skin scrapings, or excised pustules (Fig. 2.32). Most strains grow well under microaerophilic conditions. Colonies form short aerial hyphae and are surrounded by a zone of beta hemolysis.

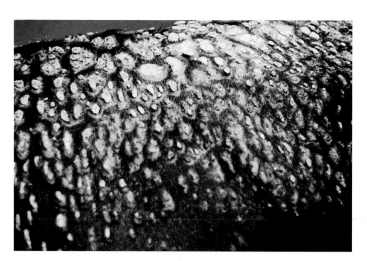

Figure 2.31 | Dermatophilosis. Massive crust formation (up to 2 cm) in cattle.

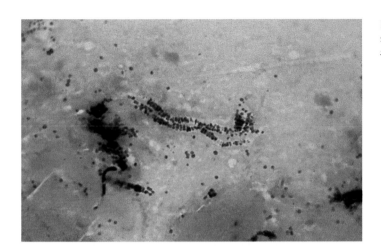

Figure 2.32 | Typical microscopy of *Dermatophilus congolensis* (Gram stain of skin lesion).

Therapy. Skin lesions are treated with disinfecting soaps or antibacterial creams. Parenteral antimicrobials (penicillin V, tetracyclines, streptomycin, erythromycin) are rarely indicated.

REFERENCES

Amor A et al., Is infection by Dermatophilus congolensis underdiagnosed? *J. Clin. Microbiol.* 49, 449–451, 2011.

Buenviaje GN et al., Isolation of Dermatophilus sp. from skin lesions in farmed saltwater crocodiles (Crocodylus porosus). *Aust. Vet. J.* 75, 365–367, 1997.

Burd EM et al., Pustular dermatitis caused by Dermatophilus congolensis. *J. Clin. Microbiol.* 45, 1655–1658, 2007.

Gitao CG, Agab H, Khalifalla AJ, Outbreaks of Dermatophilus congolensis infection in camels (Camelus dromedaries). from the Butana region in eatern Sudan. *Rev Sci Tech.* 17, 743–748, 1998.

Harman M, Sekin S, Akdeniz S, Human dermatophilosis mimicking ringworm. *Br. J. Dermatol.* 145, 170–171, 2001.

Norris BJ, Colditz IG, Dixon TJ, Fleece rot and dermatophilosis in sheep. *Vet. Microbiol.* 128, 217–230, 2008.

Towersey L et al., Dermatophilus congolensis human infection. *J. Am. Acad. Dermatol.* 29, 351–354, 1993.

Zaria, LT., Dermatophilus congolensis infection (Dermatophilosis) in animals and man. An update. *Comp. Immunol. Microbiol. Infect. Dis.* 16, 179–222, 1993.

2.26.9 *HELICOBACTER* INFECTIONS

Helicobacter pylori, a Gram-negative species in the order *Campylobacteriales*, is an organism adapted to the human stomach, which is able to cause chronic gastritis of types B or A/B, as well as stomach and duodenal ulcers that may, in turn, foster the development of gastric cancer and lymphomas of the mucosa-associated lymph tissue (MALT). Humans take up the organism by the oral route. *H. pylori* is one of the most frequent bacterial agents in humans with a worldwide prevalence of ci. 50%.

Sporadic findings of *H. pylori* in cats and dogs with gastritis seem to indicate that the agent may "transgress" the barrier to some animal species and cause disease in them. Conversely, certain farm animals (pigs, cattle) and pets (dogs, cats) have been suspected to act as sources for *H. pylori*-related species that have been found with variable frequencies in the gastric mucosa of animals. These species are *H. canis, H. felis, H. fennelliae, H. bizzozeronii, H. salomonis, Candidatus H. heilmannii, H.cinaedi,* and *H. suis.* In a few cases, these bacteria have been associated in humans with bacteremia, cellulitis, gastroenteritis, stomach ulcers, and septic shock.

For treatment of *H. pylori* infections, combinations of two or three antimicrobials (amoxicillin with or without clavulanic acid, clarithromycin, metronidazole) and a proton pump inhibitor (PPI) have been used. Failure with this therapy and recurrences call for higher dosages, extension of treatment, addition of bismuth subcitrate potassium plus metronidazole plus tetracycline plus a PPI (pantoprazole or rabeprazole), or adjustment of therapy after a check of antimicrobial resistance.

REFERENCES

De Bock MK et al., Peptic ulcer disease associated with Helicobacter felis in a dog owner. *Eur. J. Gastroenterol. Hepatol.* 19, 79–82, 2007.

De Groote D, Ducatelle R, Haesebrouck F, Helicobacters of possible zoonotic origin: a review. *Acta Gastroenterol. Belg.* 63, 380–387, 2000.

El-Zaatari FA et al., Failure to isolate Helicobacter pylori from stray cats indicates that H. pylori in cats may be an anthroponosis–an animal infection with a human pathogen. *J. Med. Microbiol.* 46, 372–376, 1997.

Fox JG et al., Helicobacter pylori-induced gastritis in the domestic cat. *Infect. Immun.* 63, 2674–2681, 1995.

Goldman CG, Mitchell HM, Helicobacter spp. other than Helicobacter pylori. *Helicobacter* 15 (Suppl 1), 69–75, 2010.

Haesebrouck F et al., Gastric helicobacters in domestic animals and nonhuman primates and their significance for human health. *Clin. Microbiol. Rev.* 22, 202–223, 2009.

Handt, LK et al., Helicobacter pylori isolated from the domestic cat: public health implications. *Infect. Immun.* 62, 2367–2374, 1994.

Hsueh P et al., Septic shock due to Helicobacter fennelliae in a non-human immunodeficiency virus-infected heterosexual patient. *J. Clin. Microbiol.* 37, 2084–2086, 1999.

Jalava K et al., A cultured strain of "Helicobacter heilmannii", a human gastric pathogen, identified as H. bizzozeronii: evidence for zoonotic potential of: Helicobacter. *Emerg. Infect. Dis.* 7, 1036–1038, 2001.

Joosten M et al., Case report: Helicobacter suis infection in a pig veterinarian. *Helicobacter* 18, 392–396, 2013.

Leemann C et al., First case of bacteremia and multifocal cellulitis due to Helicobacter canis in an immunocompetent patient. *J. Clin. Microbiol.* 44, 4598–4600, 2006.

Marshall BJ, Windsor HM, The relation of Helicobacter pylori to gastric adenocarcinoma and lymphoma: pathophysiology, epidemiology, screening, clinical presentation, treatment, and prevention. *Med. Clin. North Am.* 89, 313–344, 2005.

Solnick JV, Schauer DB, Emergence of diverse Helicobacter species in the pathogenesis of gastric and enterohepatic diseases. *Clin. Microbiol. Rev.* 14, 59–97, 2001.

Warren J, Helicobacter: the ease and difficulty of a new discovery (Nobel lecture). *Chemmedchem* 1, 672–685, 2006.

2.26.10 MELIOIDOSIS (*BURKHOLDERIA PSEUDOMALLEI* INFECTIONS)

Melioidosis is an infectious disease of animals and humans in tropical and subtropical areas and is most prevalent in Southeast Asia (Vietnam, Cambodia, Laos, Thailand, Malaysia) and northern Australia. It seems to be a sapronosis (possibly saprozoonosis) rather than a pure zoonosis and comprises a broad spectrum of acute and chronic local and systemic manifestations, for example, abscesses in various organs, pneumonia, necrotic lesions in the gastrointestinal tract, meningoencephalitis, and septicemia.

Etiology. *Burkholderia pseudomallei* is a motile, nonfermentative, facultatively intracellular Gram-negative rod that is able to penetrate and multiply in epithelial and phagocytic cells. Among the most important virulence factors are type III (gene cluster Bsa, *Burkholderia* secretion apparatus) and type VI protein secretion systems, as well as a polysaccharide capsule.

Occurrence. *B. pseudomallei* belongs to the flora of soil and surface water between 20° south and 20° north (Southeast Asia, Brazil, Central and South America, West and East Africa), is able to survive for months in these areas and can be isolated from ponds, swamps, rivers, rice paddies, and produce. Optimal are low-lying plains in a high moisture climate. Infections have been observed in pigs (Vietnam), horses, sheep (Australia), goats, cattle, rodents, cats and ci. 200 other animals, occasionally also in birds and reptiles. In the recent past, infections in horses, monkeys and other animals imported under poor surveillance have been reported from France and Spain. Melioidosis is mostly encountered as a sporadic and only rarely as a group disease. There is a numerical increase in cases after heavy rainfalls. People at risk are travelers in endemic areas and those exposed to tsunamis. Several hundred cases of overt melioidosis have been recorded in French and US soldiers during the wars in Vietnam. Moreover, it seems that several US war veterans with latent infections came down with overt melioidosis as an opportunistic infection years after their return. *B. pseudomallei* is a potential bioweapon.

Transmission. Humans contract the disease by contamination of skin abrasions with soil, contaminated drinking or surface water, and by aerosolization of these fomites. Portals of entry are skin lesions, mouth, and the respiratory tract. Possible infections from animal contacts, consumption of meat or milk and from laboratory work have been recorded. In cats and goats, diaplacentar transmission has been described.

Clinical Manifestations. Many infections take a clinically inapparent course and they are only detected by seropositivity or abnormal routine chest roentgenograms. The main risk factors are diabetes, renal failure, and alcoholism.

Overt infection may take several forms. The incubation period of the acute form is probably 2 to 14 days but may extend to several months and even years. Acute cutaneous melioidosis manifests itself in single or multiple tender nodules or abscesses with lymphangitis and lymphadenopathy, high fever, and malaise that may rapidly progress to septicemia. The acute pulmonary form varies in severity from mild bronchitis to fulminating necrotizing lobar or bronchopneumonia with an abrupt onset of fever, headache, anorexia, and myalgia, dyspnea, tachypnea, productive cough, and pleural effusions. Cavitation resembling tuberculosis is possible. Mechanical ventilation may be required. Acute septicemia due to hematogenous spread may rapidly follow the cutaneous or pulmonary form. In addition to the symptoms mentioned, there may be hepatosplenomegaly, diarrhea, or meningoencephalitis. The skin may appear cyanotic with pustular lesions on hand, trunk, and extremities. Shock and death will follow within a few days.

Subacute and chronic forms manifest themselves in febrile alternating with afebrile periods and abscess formation in various organs, that is, brain, lungs, pleura, peritoneum, liver, spleen, kidneys, prostate, bones, muscles, and skin. The overall case-fatality rate is between 15% and 20% (localized infection, 9 to 17%; multifocal infection with septicemia, 87%).

In animals, melioidosis resembles human disease with abscess formation in many organs, especially in lung, spleen, liver, and local lymph nodes. In some animals, aortic aneurysms (in goats) and CNS lesions have been observed. The main animals affected are sheep, goats, and pigs. There is trembling gait, torticollis, nystagmus, salivation, nasal discharge, cough, polyarthritis, paresis of the hind legs, and mastitis.

While sheep and goats have mostly severe disease with a fatal outcome, abscesses in internal organs of pigs are often discovered at the time of slaughter only. In horses, acute melioidosis manifests itself with fever, sweats, anorexia, edematous mucous membranes, and pulmonary edema, with death occurring within hours or days. Symptoms of chronic melioidosis are nasal discharge, pulmonary abscesses, and necroses in the gastrointestinal tract.

Diagnosis. Melioidosis should be considered in patients originating from regions of endemicity presenting with fever, fulminant respiratory infection with tachypnea, pulmonary infiltrates resembling tuberculosis, and cutaneous or subcutaneous pustules or necrotic lesions. Microbiological samples show small Gram-negative rods with irregular bipolar staining that will grow on routine enteric media (e.g., MacConkey agar) within 24 to 48 h with a variable colonial morphology. Materials likely to be mixed (sputum, stool, bronchial secretions, pus, ulcers) are best cultured on selective media such as Ashdown's medium, which contains crystal violet and gentamicin and is superior to MacConkey agar with colistin. By using an enrichment broth with the ingredients of Ashdown's medium plus colistin, the recovery rate can still be increased. Biochemical tests are used for the species diagnosis. A PCR has been developed.

Of the serological tests, the IHA is the most widely used test although not available commercially. It becomes positive in the second to third week of the disease and allows a diagnosis of melioidosis if there is a 4-fold or higher increase in titer. Serological tests on individuals from endemic areas are of limited value because healthy persons may be seropositive.

Differential Diagnosis. In acute and subacute cases, cholera, shigellosis, amebiasis, typhoid fever, plague, tularemia, military tuberculosis, malaria, syphilis, glanders, and systemic mycoses have to be considered. The skin lesions may resemble those of actinomycosis.

Therapy. Either ceftazidime 3×30 to 50 mg/kg/day (maximally 6 g/day) i.v., or imipenem 3×20 mg/kg/day i.v. for at least 2 to 4 weeks or until clinical improvement has set in. Afterwards, trimethoprim-sulfamethoxazole 2×5 mg (TMP component)/day combined with doxycycline 2×100 mg/day for 3 to 5 months. The recurrence rate with this treatment is ci. 10%.

Prophylaxis. No vaccine is available. In endemic areas, repeated contact with soil or surface water, particularly following rainy periods, should be avoided by people with breaks in the skin, as should be drinking of raw sheep or goat milk. Water from suspicious sources should be disinfected with chlorine. For postexposition prophylaxis, trimethoprim-sulfamethoxazole 2×960 mg/day for 3 weeks is recommended.

REFERENCES

Cheng AC, Melioidosis: advances in diagnosis and treatment. *Curr. Opin. Infect. Dis.* 23, 554–559, 2010.

Choy JL et al., Animal melioidosis in Australia. *Acta Trop.* 74, 153–158, 2000.

Currie BJ et al., Endemic melioidosis in tropical northern Australia: a 10-year prospective study and review of the literature. *Clin. Infect. Dis.* 31, 981–986, 2000.

Currie BJ, **Ward L**, **Cheng AC**, The epidemiology and clinical spectrum of melioidosis: 540 cases from the 20 year Darwin prospective study. *PLoS Negl. Trop. Dis.* 4, e900, 2010.

Dance DA, Melioidosis: the tip of the iceberg? *Clin. Microbiol. Rev.* 4, 52–60, 1991.

Draper AD et al., Association of the melioidosis agent Burkholderia pseudomallei with water parameters in rural water supplies in Northern Australia. *Appl. Environ. Microbiol.* 76, 5305–5307, 2010.

Galyov EE, **Brett PJ**, **DeShazer D**, Molecular insights into Burkholderia pseudomallei and Burkholderia mallei pathogenesis. *Annu. Rev. Microbiol.* 64, 495–517, 2010.

Hodgson K et al., A comparison of routine bench and molecular diagnostic methods in the identification of: Burkholderia pseudomallei. *J Clin Microbiol* 47, 1578–1580, 2009.

Ip ML et al., Pulmonary melioidosis. *Chest* 108, 1420–1424, 1995.

Millan JM et al., Clinical variation in melioidosis in pigs with clonal infection following possible environmental contamination from bore water. *Vet. J.* 174, 200–202, 2007.

Norazah A et al., Indirect hemagglutination antibodies against Burkholderia pseudomallei in normal blood donors and suspected cases of melioidosis in Malaysia. *Southeast Asian J. Trop. Med. Public Health* 27, 263–266, 1996.

Walsh AL et al., Selective broths for the isolation of Pseudomonas pseudomallei from clinical samples. *Trans. R. Soc. Trop. Med. Hyg.* 89, 124, 1995.

Wiesinga WJ, **Currie BJ**, **Peacock SJ**. Melioidosis. *N Engl J Med.* 387, 1035–1044, 2012.

Wuthiekanun V et al., Rapid immunofluorescence microscopy for diagnosis of melioidosis. *Clin. Diagn. Lab. Immunol.* 12, 555–556, 2005.

2.26.11 *RHODOCOCCUS EQUI* INFECTIONS

Rhodococcus equi, a Gram-positive, facultatively intracellular rod, causes pneumonia in foals and it has been isolated from other animal species, such as cattle, sheep, and pigs.

Human infections with *R. equi* are mainly granulomatous, often caseating pneumonias in immunocompromised patients. Extrapulmonary infections (e.g., abscesses) are rare. Most patients had contact to animals but transmission has never been proven beyond doubt. The natural habitat for *R. equi* is soil; therefore, infections may be sapronoses. For therapy, erythromycin and rifampicin have been recommended.

REFERENCES

Akilesh S et al., Pseudotumor of the tracheal-laryngeal junction with unusual morphologic features caused by Rhodococcus equi infection. *Head Neck Pathol* 5, 395–400, 2011.

Guerrero R, **Bhargava A**, **Nahleh Z**, Rhodococcus equi venous catheter infection: a case report and review of the literature. *J. Med. Case Reports* 5, 358, 2011.

Letek M et al., The genome of a pathogenic Rhodococcus: cooptive virulence underpinned by key gene acquisitions. *PLoS Genetics* 6, e1001145, 2010.

Makrai L et al., Characterisation of Rhodococcus equi strains isolated from foals and from immunocompromised human patients. *Acta Vet. Hung.* 48, 253–259, 2000.

Meijer WG, **Prescott JF**, Rhodococcus equi. *Vet. Res.* 35, 383–396, 2004.

Ocampo-Sosa AA et al., Molecular epidemiology of Rhodococcus equi based on traA, vapA, and vapB virulence plasmid markers. *J. Infect. Dis.* 196, 763–769, 2007.

Perez MG, **Vassilev T**, **Kemmerly SA**, Rhodococcus equi infection in transplant recipients: a case of mistaken identity and review of the literature. *Transpl. Infect. Dis.* 4, 52–56, 2002.

Pusterla N et al., Diagnostic evaluation of real-time PCR in the detection of Rhodococcus equi in faeces and nasopharyngeal swabs from foals with pneumonia. *Vet. Rec.* 161, 272–275, 2007.

Roda RH et al., Rhodococcus equi pulmonary-central nervous system syndrome: brain abscess in a patient on high-dose steroids – a case report and review of the literature. *Diagn. Microbiol. Infect. Dis.* 63, 96–99, 2009.

Rodríguez-Lázaro D et al., Internally controlled real-time PCR method for quantitative species-specific detection and vapA genotyping of Rhodococcus equi. *Appl. Environ. Microbiol.* 72, 4256–4263, 2006.

Scott M et al., Rhodococcus equi – an increasingly recognized opportunistic pathogen. Report of 12 cases and review of 65 cases in the literature. *Am. J. Clin. Pathol.* 103, 649–655, 1995.

Topino S et al., Rhodococcus equi infection in HIV-infected individuals: case reports and review of the literature. *AIDS Patient Care STDS* 24, 211–222, 2010.

Vazquez-Boland JA et al., Rhodococcus equi: the many facets of a pathogenic actinomycete. *Vet. Microbiol.* 167, 9–33, 2013.

2.26.12 *TRUEPERELLA PYOGENES* INFECTIONS

The Gram-positive rod, *Trueperella pyogenes* (formerly *Arcanobacterium pyogenes*), is a commensal of mucous membranes of cattle, sheep, and pigs and may cause abortion, mastitis, and abscesses of skin and various organs in those animals. *T. pyogenes* has been found as an agent of septicemia, endocarditis, meningitis, empyema, arthritis, pneumonia, and abscess formation on the hands, lower arms, and legs. Patients often suffer from underlying diseases, such as cancer or diverticulitis. An animal-human chain has not been proven but it seems likely. Flies can transmit the bacterium. Treatment is with penicillin G, V, or ampicillin/amoxicillin.

REFERENCES

Brook I, Dohar JE, Management of group A beta-hemolytic streptococcal pharyngotonsillitis in children. *J. Fam. Pract.* 55, S1–11; quiz S12, 2006.

Dias CAG, Cauduro PF, Mezzari A, Actinomyces pyogenes isolated from a subcutaneous abscess in a dairy farmer. *Clin Microbiol Newsl* 18, 38–40, 1996.

Gahrn-Hansen B, Frederiksen W, Human infections with Actinomyces pyogenes (Corynebacterium pyogenes). *Diagn. Microbiol. Infect. Dis.* 15, 349–354, 1992.

Hijazin M et al., Molecular identification and further characterization of Arcanobacterium pyogenes isolated from bovine mastitis and from various other origins. *J. Dairy Sci.* 94, 1813–1819, 2011.

Jost BH, Billington SJ, Arcanobacterium pyogenes: molecular pathogenesis of an animal opportunist. *Antonie van Leeuwenhoek* 88, 87–102, 2005.

Kavitha K et al., Three cases of Arcanobacterium pyogenes-associated soft tissue infection. *J. Med. Microbiol.* 59, 736–739, 2010.

Lynch M et al., Actinomyces pyogenes septic arthritis in a diabetic farmer. *J. Infect.* 37, 71–73, 1998.

Plamondon M et al., A fatal case of: Arcanobacterium pyogenes endocarditis in a man with no identified animal contact: case report and review of the literature. *Eur. J. Clin. Microbiol. Infect. Dis.* 26, 663–666, 2007.

Fungal Zoonoses | 3

3.1 Introduction

Dermatophytoses are chronic fungal infections caused by dermatophytes, that is, keratinophilic fungi that are able to utilize keratin-containing structures (hair, nails, scales, etc.) from humans and animals. They belong to the genera *Epidermophyton*, *Microsporum*, and *Trichophyton* of the family *Arthrodermataceae*. Individual species may be anthropophilic, zoophilic, or geophilic. Zoophilic species from warm-blooded animals with overt or latent infections may, if transmitted to humans, give rise to severe cases of dermatitis. Transmission from human to human is possible, although infectivity decreases with each passage and dies out after three to four passages. Anthropophilic dermatophytes, such as *Trichophyton rubrum*, *T. tonsurans*, and *Epidermophyton floccosum*, can also (although rarely) be transmitted from humans to animals, in whom they may cause skin diseases. In turn, these animals could be a source for human infections. The same chain may operate in primarily geophilic species, such as *Microsporum racemosum* and *M. gypseum*.

Mycoses due to *Cryptococcus neoformans*, *Blastomyces dermatitidis*, *Histoplasma capsulatum*, *Coccidioides immitis*, *Paracoccidioides brasiliensis*, and *Rhinosporidium seeberi* will not be discussed here. Although they may cause latent infections in animals, direct transmission from animals to human has not been proven. Infections with these agents should be called geonoses/sapronoses because the natural habitat of the fungi is in the soil.

REFERENCES

Bergmans AM et al., Evaluation of a single-tube real-time PCR for detection and identification of 11 dermatophyte species in clinical material. *Clin. Microbiol. Infect.* 16, 704–710, 2010.

Seebacher C, Bouchara JP, Mignon B, Updates on the epidemiology of dermatophyte infections. *Mycopathologia* 166, 335–352, 2008.

Weitzman I, Summerbell RC, The dermatophytes. *Clin. Microbiol. Rev.* 8, 240–259, 1995.

3.2 Dermatophytoses Caused by *Microsporum* spp

Microsporum spp. cause infectious dermatophytoses in animals and humans. Two clinical forms, tinea capitis and tinea corporis, are known.

Etiology. At this time, 16 species of *Microsporum* have become known. The most important

293

Table 3.1 | Zoophilic Zoonotic Species of Dermatophytes

SPECIES	OCCURRENCE IN ANIMALS
Microsporum canis	Cat, dog, horse, pig, cattle, sheep, goat, rabbit, hamster, rat, zoo animals (mostly monkeys, tiger, jaguar, lynx)
M. nanum	Pig, rabbit
M. gallinae	Chicken, duck, other birds
M. distortum	Monkeys, dog, rabbit, guinea pig, rat
M. persicolor	Vole
M. racemosum	Rat
M. equinum	Horse
M. amazonicum	Rat
Trichophyton mentagrophytes (formerly *T. mentagrophytes* var. *quinckeanum*)	Mouse (mouse favus), guinea pig, rat, rabbit, occasionally dog, cat, horse, cattle, sheep, pig, zoo animals (mostly monkeys)
T. interdigitale (formerly *T. mentagrophytes*: occasionally var. *granulosum*)	Mouse, gold hamster, guinea pig, chinchilla, rat, rabbit, dog, cat, occasionally horse, cattle, sheep, pig, zoo animals (mostly monkeys)
T. erinacei	Hedgehog
T. equinum	Horse
T. gallinae	Chicken
T. simii	Primates, carnivores, birds
T. verrucosum	Cattle, occasionally other ruminants, solipeds,
Arthroderma benhamiae (teleomorph of *Trichophyton sp.*)	Guinea pig, cat
A. vanbreuseghemii (teleomorph of *T. interdigitale*, zoophilic)	Dog, cat

zoophilic species and their occurrence in animals are listed in Table 3.1.

Occurrence. *Microsporum* infections occur world-wide. Cats and dogs are the most important source for human infections as >90% of feline and >50% of canine dermatophytoses are caused by *M. canis*. In addition, transmission of *M. nanum* from pigs, of *M. persicolor* from voles, and *M. amazonicum* from rats to humans has been proven.

At special risk are people in close contact with animals, particularly children.

Transmission. Human infection occurs through direct contact with manifestly ill or latently infected animals. *Microsporum* spp. can also be spread via lice, flies, fleas, and mites, and indirectly via fomites.

Clinical Manifestations. The slow development of *Microsporum* lesions makes an exact determination of the incubation period difficult as it probably extends between several days and a few weeks. Depending on the localization, two different forms can be distinguished.

Tinea capitis occurs on the head as single or multiple round or ovoid lesions of different size (Fig. 3.1) in areas covered by hair. Hairs break off at a distance of 2 to 4 mm from the skin. The stumps lose their shiny appearance and they become covered with a gray film. Signs of inflammation are mostly absent; occasionally, however, erythema and swelling may occur at the margins of the lesions.

Tinea corporis occurs on areas covered with lanugo (very fine hair) and on areas not covered by clothing, such as hands, forearms, neck, and face (Fig. 3.2). Lesions are flat and often wet

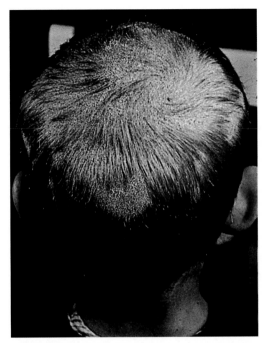

Figure 3.1 | Tinea capitis (Alopecia areata) caused by *Microsporum canis*. (Archives of the Dermatology Department, Justus Liebig University, Giessen, Germany.)

and are covered with crusts and scales. The latter are fatty and grey to yellowish. The margins of the lesions are often red and coalescing.

In both forms, lesions start healing from the center and the outlook is favorable. Endemic or even epidemic situations, for example, in kindergartens, are not rare.

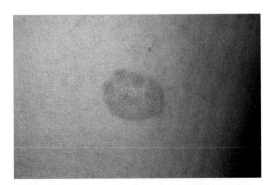

Figure 3.2 | Tinea corporis. Patch of a *Microsporum canis* infection following contact with an infected cat. (Courtesy of Prof. W. Meinhof, Dermatology Department, Rheinisch-Westfälische Technische Hochschule, Aachen, Germany.)

In animals, lesions resemble those of tinea capitis in humans, with thick, crusty, sticky scales that are yellowish-grey to asbestos-like and fatty. They are mostly, but not exclusively, found on the head and they may cause itching; in severe cases, they can be large and deep with eumycetoma-like nodules. Latent infections occur, particularly in cats.

Diagnosis. The clinical picture, particularly in tinea corporis, allows only for a suspicion. Microscopic examination of hair, crusts, or scales in an unstained preparation (following KOH treatment) provides for a diagnosis of fungal elements only, whereby brighteners, such as Blankophor-P liquid, cellufluor, Uvitex 2B, or glucan-binding dyes, for example congo red, can be of help. A reliable diagnosis, however, can only be provided by culture of hair stumps taken from the transitional zone between infected and healthy areas, or of scales or crusts.

Culture is done on Sabouraud dextrose agar with added chloramphenicol, cycloheximide, and gentamicin. Less suitable are dermatophyte test medium (DTM) and dermatophyte indicator medium (DIM), which can lead to false-positive results. A species diagnosis using morphological criteria such as macro- and microconidia takes between 1 and 4 weeks. Sensitive and specific molecular biological methods (RFLP, PCR, ELISA) kits have been developed in the past few years.

Cats, dogs, and rabbits infected with *M. canis* can be diagnosed with the help of Wood's lamp. Hair infected by this species show a greenish fluorescence in UV light. However, only positive results are proof of the presence of *M. canis*. Otherwise, the diagnosis is made by culture. In other animal species, and in humans, the diagnostic use of Wood's lamp is unreliable.

Differential Diagnosis. Depending on the localization of the infection, trichophytosis, alopecia areata, syphilitic alopecia, erythema chronicum, psoriasis, granuloma anulare, pityriasis versicolor, seborrhoic eczema, and candidiasis have to be taken into consideration.

Therapy. The recommended therapy uses terbinafine 1 × 250 mg/day orally (p.o.) for 2 to 4 weeks; in children, 5 mg/kg/day for 4 weeks; or itraconazole 1 × 200 mg/day p.o. for 4 weeks; or griseofulvin 1 × 500 mg/day p.o., in children 10 mg/kg/day for 4 to 6 weeks (the only therapeutic modality allowed for children in Germany). Adjuvant topical application of keto-conazole or of selenium-containing shampoos will decrease the risk of transmission of tinea capitis. The course of treatment should be monitored by the mycological laboratory.

Infected animals should be treated with anti-mycotics by a veterinarian.

Prophylaxis. Proper hygiene should be used when in contact with animals, particularly with those that show suspicious skin changes. They should be examined promptly and treated if infected.

REFERENCES

Chermette R, Ferreiro L, Guillot J, Dermatophytoses in animals. *Mycopathologia* 166, 385–405, 2008.

Gräser Y, Scott J, Summerbell R, The new species concept in dermatophytes – a polyphasic approach. *Mycopathologia* 166, 239–256, 2010.

Kefalidou S et al., Wood's light in Microsporum canis positive patients. *Mycoses* 40, 461–463, 1997.

Pönnighaus JM, Warndorff D, Port G, Microsporum nanum – a report from Malawi (Africa). *Mycoses* 38, 149–150, 1995.

Skerley M, Miklic P, The changing face of Microsporum spp infections. *Clin Dermatol* 28, 146–150, 2010.

3.3 Dermatophytoses Caused by *Trichophyton* spp.

Trichophytosis is an infectious skin condition in humans and animals caused by dermatophytes of the genus *Trichophyton* and manifests itself in cutaneous or subcutaneous foci.

Etiology. At this time, 26 different *Trichophyton* spp. are known. Zoonotic agents are the species listed in Table 3.1, with their names as used at present based on molecular biology and some on earlier names. The teleomorphs, *Arthroderma benhamiae* and *A. vanbreuseghemii*, have become more conspicuous in the last decade.

Occurrence. Trichophytoses occur worldwide and the zoophilic species have been observed in many animal species (Table 3.1).

At particular risk are children who are in close contact with pet animals (guinea pigs, rabbits, etc.), animal care personnel, farmers, veterinarians, animal owners, fur traders, butchers, and hunters.

Transmission. Human infections are mostly caused by direct contact with animals that are either latently or overtly infected with *Trichophyton* spp. In cattle, trichophytosis is highly contagious. Indirect transmission through fomites, such as bridles, saddles, stable posts, brushes, wood splinters, and straw, is possible. Flies, mites, lice, fleas, and spiders may play a role in spread and transmission.

Clinical Manifestations. The incubation period is between 2 and 4 weeks. Uncovered parts of the body (face, neck, beard, extremities, etc.) are most frequently affected.

Tinea barbae (deep trichophytosis) is a deep, abscess-forming folliculitis of the beard hair, caused by *T. verrucosum* and the zoophilic *T. interdigitale*. It starts with a few single purulent foci from that the infection spreads through shaving. Initially superficial with redness, scaling and pustules, the infection penetrates rapidly into the hair follicles whereby soft, infiltrated, furuncle-like nodules arise with follicular pustules on their surfaces (Fig. 3.3). The most severe form with fever and generalized symptoms arises through colliquation of cutaneous/subcutaneous confluent, abscess-forming, secreting, and painful tumor-like infiltrates, combined with regional lymphadenitis. Epilation of beard hair for diagnostic and therapeutic purposes is painless.

Superficial trichophytosis starts with a circumscribed folliculitis in several patches (Fig. 3.4). If there is exudation and formation of crusts and scales, the picture may resemble impetigo.

If the mouse favus agent *T. mentagrophytes* infects human skin, the typical trichophytotic foci with a characteristic mouse urine-like smell will be formed. They do not show the "scutulae" typical of favus but multiple pustules or smaller follicular abscesses with yellowish scales and

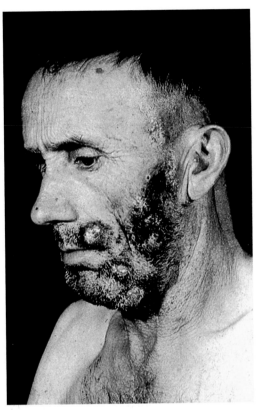

Figure 3.3 | Deep trichophytosis in a farmer, caused by *Trichophyton verrucosum* following contact with infected cattle. (Archives of the Dermatology Department, Justus Liebig University, Giessen, Germany.)

crusts. The infected patches show a sharper demarcation than in infections with other zoonotic *Trichophyton* spp. (Fig. 3.5).

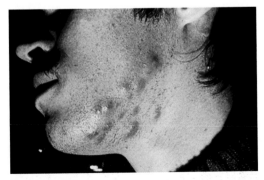

Figure 3.4 | Superficial trichophytosis in an animal caretaker caused by *Trichophyton mentagrophytes* following contact with infected rabbits. (Courtesy of Dr H Mayer, Heidelberg, Germany.)

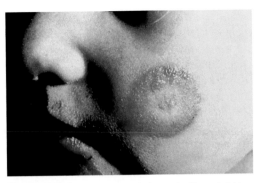

Figure 3.5 | Trichophytosis (scutula-like patch) in a child caused by *Trichophyton quinckeanum* following contact with infected guinea pigs. (Archive of the Institute of Parasitology, Justus Liebig University, Giessen, Germany.)

In animals, trichophytotic symptoms extend from superficial, slightly scaling, hairless patches to deep granulomatous, sometimes purulent inflammatory foci. Besides skin, hair and even claws, clutches, or hooves may be affected. In hunting dogs, the head (nose, ears, and eyes) is frequently the site of infection. In cattle, there is a characteristic trichophytosis (ringworm-like, in German: Teigmaul, Glatzflechte) with round (diameter 2 to 10 cm) hairless patches with scabs, also mostly on the head. Mouse favus with heavy scutula formation caused by *T. mentagrophytes* and chicken favus with scutulae on the comb caused by *T. gallinarum* are characteristic diseases as well. Trichophytosis in animals is frequently a latent infection; overt diseases are more frequent in the young. Immunosuppressive treatment (e.g., glucocorticoids) and underlying endocrine disorders (e.g., Morbus Cushing) may contribute to overt disease or lead to exacerbations.

Diagnosis. Clinical symptoms allow only for a tentative diagnosis. Microscopic examination of hair, crust, or scales after treatment with 10 to 20% KOH will show fungal elements but their presence does not allow a genus diagnosis for which culture on Sabouraud dextrose agar with antibiotics (see above) is necessary. A species diagnosis by way of the morphology of macroconidia will take several weeks; molecular methods will shorten this interval.

In animals, culture is necessary as well, except if the typical symptoms of cattle trichophytosis or mouse/chicken favus are present.

Differential Diagnosis. Depending on the symptoms, one has to consider infections with *Microsporum* spp. or *Epidermophyton*, erythema migrans, psoriasis, pityriasis versicolor, seborrhoic eczema, allergic contact eczema, and candidiasis.

In cases of suspected tinea barbae, bacterial follicultits, *Candida* folliculitis, actinomycosis, and skin tuberculosis have to be considered.

Therapy. A successful therapy has to be based on the exact diagnosis. The drug of choice is terbinafine; alternatively, itraconazole. For topical monotherapy in uncomplicated infections or as an adjuvant to systemic therapy, terbinafine crème is applied 2 ×/day for 2 to 3 weeks. If the infection is extensive or if topical treatment has been unsuccessful: terbinafine 1 × 250 mg/day p.o.; for children, 5 mg/kg/day for 4 weeks; or itraconazole 1 × 100 mg/day p.o. for 2 to 4 weeks; or fluconazole 1 × 50 mg/day p.o. for 2 to 7 weeks. If pruritus becomes irritating, antihistaminics or glucocorticoids should be considered.

Infected domestic animals should be treated with antimycotics by a veterinarian.

Prophylaxis. As for diseases due to *Microsporum* spp, in cattle, trichophyton vaccines have been used with good success for treatment and prophylaxis.

REFERENCES

Brilhante RS et al., Canine dermatophytosis caused by anthropophilic species: molecular and phenotypical characterization of Trichophyton tonsurans. *J Med Microbiol* 55, 1583–1586, 2006.

Chermette R, Ferreiro L, Guillot J, Dermatophytoses in animals. *Mycopathologia* 166, 385–405, 2008.

Drouot S et al., Pets as the main source of two zoonotic species of the Trichophyton mentagrophytes complex in Switzerland, Arthroderma vanbreuseghemii and Arthroderma benhamiae. *Veterinary Dermatology* 20, 13–18, 2009.

Fumeaux J et al., First report of Arthoderma benhamiae in Switzerland. *Dermatology* 208, 244–250, 2004.

Gräser Y, Scott J, Summerbell R, The new species concept in dermatophytes – a polyphasic approach. *Mycopathologia* 166, 239–256, 2010.

Gründer S et al., Mycological examinations on the fungal flora of the chicken comb. *Mycoses* 48, 114–119, 2005.

Kick G, Korting HC, Tinea barbae due to Trichophyton mentagrophytes related to persistent child infection. *Mycoses* 41, 439–441, 1998.

Liu D et al., Use of arbitrarily primed polymerase chain reaction to differentiate Trichophyton dermatophytes. *FEMS Microbiol. Lett.* 136, 147–150, 1996.

Romano C et al., Case reports. Six cases of infection due to Trichophyton verrucosum. *Mycoses* 44, 334–337, 2001.

Salkin IF, Padhye AA, Kemna ME, A new medium for the presumptive identification of dermatophytes. *J. Clin. Microbiol.* 35, 2660–2662, 1997.

3.4 Sporotrichosis

Sporotrichosis is a subacute to chronic granulomatous systemic mycosis in animals and humans. The cutaneous form manifests itself by papulous, occasionally ulcerating lesions at the site of inoculation and along the local lymph channels. In aerogenic infections, such foci are present in the upper airways. Hematogenous spread will lead to local or multifocal sporotrichosis in a variety of organs.

Etiology. *Sporothrix schenckii*, a dimorphic fungus.

Occurrence. Sporotrichosis occurs worldwide. It is dependent on relative humidity (92 to 100%) and temperature (26 to 29 °C) and is mostly seen in moist tropical and subtropical zones, that is, Brazil, Colombia, Venezuela, Costa Rica, Guatemala, Mexico, the Mississippi delta, in Southeast Asia (particularly Indonesia), South Africa, and Australia. There have even been epidemics with several hundred cases. Since 1998, there has been a large outbreak in Rio de Janeiro in which cats played an important role as reservoirs and transmitters. In Europe, sporotrichosis has been observed in increased numbers in Italy for the past 30 years (more than 70 cases in Apulia), whereas in other countries there have only been sporadic cases.

The geophilic fungus is ubiquitous in nature, that is, in soil, on rotten wood, on dead plants, in surface waters, and occasionally even in swimming pools. Besides humans, animals may catch the disease, particularly cats, horses, mules, and dogs. At particular risk are workers in farms and forests and persons in contact with contaminated plants (sphagnum moss, roses), wood, and infected animals (e.g., cats).

Transmission. As a zoonotic disease, sporotrichosis has been observed after a person has been scratched or bitten by a cat or, occasionally, by a dog, rat, armadillo, or squirrel. Small wounds created by splinters, thorns, or insect bites may serve as portals of entry. Aerogenic infection and transmission from human to human are rare.

Clinical Manifestations. The incubation period is 3 to 21 days, sometimes up to 3 months. There are a number of different forms.

Most frequent is lymphocutaneous sporotrichosis, above all, on uncovered parts of the body. At the site of infection, a painless, initially well movable papule develops that later becomes firmly attached to the surrounding pale gray tissue, necrotizes, ulcerates, and secretes a serous or purulent fluid. Further nodes will develop within a few days to weeks alongside the lymph channels and may ulcerate as well. The general health of the patient is little affected. The primary foci usually heal spontaneously but may leave disfiguring scars. Secondary foci may persist for years.

The mucosal form is characterized by nodules in the mouth, nose, oropharynx, larynx, and trachea, and thus, it may resemble tonsillitis, stomatitis, glossitis, laryngitis, or rhinitis of other origin. If the disease is allowed to progress, ulcers with irregular contours and elevated margins as well as granulomas accompanied by local lymphadenopathy develop and they heal with the formation of soft scars.

In rare cases, sporotrichosis in humans will affect one or, particularly in immunocompromised patients, multiple internal organs: lung, bones (osteitis, osteo/periosteal gummas), joints (synovitis), muscles, eyes (chorioretinitis),

testicles, and epididymis. This form will be fatal unless treated.

In animals, particularly in cats and dogs, sporotrichosis may take one of three forms. The cutaneous, localized form is characterized by single or multiple nodules in the skin or in the nasal mucosa that tend to ulceration and formation of fistulae. In the lymphocutaneous form, the nodular or ulcerating granulomatous and purulent foci affect skin, subcutaneous tissues, and draining lymph channels. The systemic or disseminated form is often a consequence of the localized or lymphocutaneous disease in which the infection extends to internal organs, mostly the lower respiratory tract and the liver. In endemic areas one can isolate *S. schenckii* from the skin and the mucous membranes of mouth and nose of healthy cats.

Diagnosis. The diagnosis of sporotrichosis is made by histology and/or culture of biopsy samples. Histology (periodic acid-Schiff or Grocott stain) reveals a purulent to granulomatous inflammation and the causative agent in the yeast form as round to oval and typical cigar-shaped cells. The fungus grows on Sabouraud dextrose agar as a yeast at 37 °C and as the mycelial form at 22 °C but without the typical mold appearance. The dimorphism becomes manifest by incubation at 25° and 37 °C on brain heart infusion agar, chocolate agar, or potato dextrose agar in a 5% CO_2 atmosphere.

A latex agglutination test (Immuno Mycologics, Norman, OK, USA) can be used to detect antibodies. Titer of >1:4 are suspicious, and even at >1:8 false positive titers cannot be ruled out. Therapy has little influence on antibody titers. Other serological tests, for example, agglutination and precipitation reactions and the intracutaneous sporotrichin skin test may be positive in patients from areas of endemicity without overt signs of sporotrichosis.

Differential Diagnosis. Tuberculosis, swimming pool granuloma (*Mycobacterium marinum*), leprosy, tularemia, lues, coccidiomycosis, blastomycosis, and leishmaniasis.

Therapy. Lymphocutaneous sporotrichosis: itraconazole 1 to 2 × 200 mg/day p.o., or terbinafine

2×500 mg/day p.o. for 3 to 6 months, or at least for 2 to 4 weeks after all lesions have healed. Alternative (mostly for cost considerations): saturated potassium iodide solution, initially 3×5 to 10 drops/day in milk or juice, then increasing dosages from 3 to 5 drops/day up to 3×40 to 50 drops/day; total duration of treatment 4 to 8 weeks. If side effects, such as increased production of tears or saliva or iodine acne occur, therapy should be discontinued for a few days and then continued at a lower dosage.

Joint, bone or lung sporotrichosis: Itraconazole 2×200 mg/day p.o. for 12 months.

Disseminated, severe pulmonary, and central nervous system (CNS) sporotrichosis: liposomal amphotericin B 5 mg/kg/day intravenously (i.v.) for 4 to 6 weeks until improvement occurs, then itraconazole 2×200 mg/day p.o. Total time, 12 months.

Localized sporotrichosis (e.g., lung caverns): surgery (lobectomy).

Prophylaxis. Care in handling rotted wood, plant material (gloves!), and infected animals.

REFERENCES

Alves SH et al., Sporothrix schenckii associated with armadillo hunting in Southern Brazil: epidemiological and antifungal susceptibility profiles. *Rev. Soc. Bras. Med. Trop.* 43, 523–525, 2010.

Aung AK et al., Pulmonary sporotrichosis: case series and systematic analysis of literature on clinical-radiological patterns and management outcomes. *Med Mycol* 51, 534–544, 2013.

Barros MB, de Almeida Paes R, Schubach AO. Sporothrix schenckii and sporotrichosis. *Clin Microbiol Rev* 24, 633–654, 2011.

Bonifaz A, Vázquez-González D, Perusquia-Ortiz AM, Subcutaneous mycoses: chromoblastomycosis, sporotrichosis and mycetoma. *J. Dtsch. Dermatol. Ges.* 8, 619–627, 2010.

Carlos IZ et al., Current research on the immune response to experimental sporotrichosis. *Mycopathologia* 168, 1–10, 2009.

Crothers SL et al., Sporotrichosis: a retrospective evaluation of 23 cases seen in northern California (1987–2007). *Vet. Dermatol.* 20, 249–259, 2009.

Fleury RN et al., Zoonotic sporotrichosis. Transmission to humans by infected domestic cat scratching: report of four cases in Sao Paulo, Brazil. *Int. J. Dermatol.* 40, 318–322, 2001.

Kaddad V et al., Localized lymphatic sporotrichosis after fish-induced injury (Tilapia sp.). *Med. Mycol.* 40, 425–427, 2002.

Kauffman CA, Bustamante B, Chapman SW, Clinical practice guidelines for the management of sporotrichosis. 2007 update of the Infectious Diseases Society of America. *Clin. Infect. Dis.* 45, 1255–1265, 2007.

Noguchi H, Hiruma M, Kawada A, Sporotrichosis successfully treated with itraconazole in Japan. *Mycoses* 42, 571–576, 1999.

Ramos-e-Silva M et al., Sporotrichosis. *Clin. Dermatol.* 25, 181–187, 2007.

Reed KD et al., Zoonotic transmission of sporotrichosis: case report and review. *Clin. Infect. Dis.* 16, 384–387, 1993.

Reis RS et al., Molecular characterisation of Sporothrix schenckii isolates from humans and cats involved in the sporotrichosis epidemic in Rio de Janeiro, Brazil. *Mem. Inst. Oswaldo Cruz.* 104, 769–774, 2009.

Saravanakumar PS, Eslami P, Zar FA, Lymphocutaneous sporotrichosis associated with a squirrel bite: case report and review. *Clin. Infect. Dis.* 23, 647–648, 1996.

Schubach A, Barros MB, Wanke B, Epidemic sporotrichosis. *Curr. Opin. Infect. Dis.* 21, 129–133, 2008.

3.5 Pneumocystosis (*Pneumocystis* Pneumonia) as a Potential Zoonotic Mycosis

Pneumocystosis caused by *Pneumocystis carinii* occurs primarily in malnourished children and immunosuppressed persons (e.g., AIDS patients) as an interstitial plasmacellular pneumonia [*Pneumocystis* pneumonia (PCP)], and more rarely as extrapulmonary disease with abscesses in lymph nodes, liver, spleen, and bone marrow.

Etiology. *P. carinii* was, for a long time, regarded as a protozoon on account of morphological criteria and susceptibility to antimicrobials until molecular biological and structural investigations suggested its taxonomic position among the fungi. However, it lacks ergosterol, the characteristic component of the cell membrane in fungi, this being the reason why inhibitors of ergosterol synthesis are ineffective against it. Conversely, its cell wall contains beta-1,3 glucan and fungicidal antibiotics active against its synthesis are highly effective *in vivo*.

P. carinii is involved in a developmental cycle, the details of which are not fully known at present but can be described in parasitological as well as in mycological terms. From mature cysts with eight round, oval or spindle-shaped intracystic bodies (young trophozoites/spores) small (1 to 2 μm) or larger (3 to 5 μm) haploid trophozoites/trophic forms are released through a burst. A Giemsa stain shows their red nucleus and blue cytoplasm. In the asexual phase, two of these haploid trophozoites fuse and form a diploid zygote that is surrounded by a thin cyst wall and is called pre-cyst/sporocyst (4 to 5 μm). Two meiotic divisions and mitosis yield eight haploid nuclei. Division of the cytoplasm again yields intracystic bodies (young trophozoites/spores), with the pre-cyst/sporocyst becoming a thick-walled mature cyst (5 to 8 μm), which can be stained by methenamin-silver nitrate. Either this stage is eliminated or the cyst wall bursts in the lung of the host and leads to autoinfection, which can lead to fungemia with high counts, for example, in AIDS patients.

Occurrence. *P. carinii* is widespread in nature but seems to be an obligate parasite that can multiply only in a host. Domestic and zoo animals as well as free-living rodents have been regarded as possible sources for human infection: pigs, rabbits, sheep, goats, dogs, mice, and rats. Different protein patterns and detailed DNA and RNA sequence analyses have, in the meantime, shown a distinct host specificity of the variants so that a host-dependent classification has been proposed, for example, *P. carinii* formae specialis (f.c.) *ratti* (rat as host), *P. carinii* f.c. *muris* (mouse as host), *P. carinii* f. c. *suis* (pig as host). The agent of human infection, initially named *P. carinii* f.c. *hominis*, has now been named *P. jirovecii*.

An animal reservoir for this species has not been found thus far, therefore, one can assume that human pneumocystosis is not a zoonosis. The reservoirs are presumably patients with clinically inapparent infection and those with overt disease.

Pneumocystosis is usually a disease of immunocompromised patients (AIDS) or of malnourished children up to the 4th month of life or of patients under immunosuppressive treatment, for example, following transplantation.

Transmission. Seroepidemiological investigations have shown that most (70 to 100%) children up to their 4th year of life have been infected with *Pneumocystis* without presenting overt disease. Transmission from human to human has been proven; however, the agent seems to occur in the environment as well, albeit in small numbers. Human infection is aerogenic through inhalation of contaminated dust particles or aerosols. Diaplacentar transmission into the fetal lung has been recorded and interpreted as an expression of organotropism of the agent.

It is still unclear whether the early contact with *Pneumocystis* is only a transient colonization or whether it leads to a lifelong latent infection, which later, for example, under immunosuppressive conditions, leads to a clinically manifest pneumocytosis. The ability of the agent to change its superficial glycoproteins may contribute to its evasion of the body's immune mechanisms. As an alternative, reinfection ould occur later in life and lead to overt pneumocytosis under the conditions mentioned above.

Clinical Manifestations. Most infections are asymptomatic and become manifest only in immunocompromised patients. Clinical studies have suggested an incubation period of 4 to 8 weeks.

The main symptoms are fever, dyspnea, a nonproductive cough, occasional retrosternal pain, tachypnea, tachycardia, and cyanosis.

Auscultation generally yields nothing or, occasionally, rales. The X-ray picture, however, often shows bilateral diffuse, particularly perihilar infiltrates which correspond to the autoptic findings of alveoli and bronchioles filled with viscous, foamy exudate and large numbers of *Pneumocystis*. Seventy to eighty percent of all HIV-infected patients have at least one episode of PCP during the progress of their infection that will be the immediate cause of death in every 5th patient.

Extrapulmonary manifestations, for example, necrotic or hemorrhagic foci in lymph nodes, liver, spleen and bone marrow, as well as retinitis and vasculitis, have been rare in the past but have recently occurred more frequently in HIV patients.

Diagnosis. For a demonstration of the agent in sputum (following inhalation of 3% NaCl solution), tracheal secretions, bronchial lavage, or lung biopsy microscopy (Giemsa, Gram-Weigert, Grocott or fluorescein marked antibodies), as well as PCR, can be used. PCR is more sensitive but less specific than microscopy.

Differential Diagnosis. Pneumonias of other etiologies.

Therapy. The drug of choice is trimethoprim-sulfamethoxazole double strength 3×2 tablets/day p.o. for 21 days. Alternatives are dapsone 1×100 mg/day p.o. plus trimethoprim 3×5 mg/kg/day p.o.; or clindamycin 4×300 to 450 mg/day plus primaquin 1×15 mg base/day p.o.; or atovaquon 2×750 mg/day (with food intake), each for 21 days. In severe and acutely ill patients, trimethoprim-sulfamethoxazole is applied i.v.: trimethoprim 15 to 20 mg/kg/day plus sulfamethoxazole 75 to 100 mg/kg/day in 3 to 4 single doses. To prevent clinical deterioration, particularly during the first days of treatment, additional prednisone treatment is indicated: 15 to 30 min before trimethoprim-sulfamethoxazole, 2×40 mg/day p.o. for 5 days; afterwards, 1×40 mg/day for a further 5 days, and then 1×20 mg/day for another 11 days.

In HIV patients with PCP, the frequently severe infection often improves under antiretroviral treatment (HAART) and the case-fatality rate will decrease markedly.

Prophylaxis. Primary prophylaxis is indicated in all HIV patients with CD4 counts of >200/microliter; secondary prophylaxis is indicated in all HIV patients and patients with persistent depression of cell-mediated immunity. The drug of choice is trimethoprim-sulfamethoxazole double strength 1 tablet/day or 3 times a week p.o. permanently. Alternatives are dapsone 100 mg/day p.o., or a pentamidine aerosol.

REFERENCES

Agostoni F et al., Pneumocystis carinii diagnosis: an update. *Int. J. Antimicrob. Agents* 16, 549–557, 2000.

Beard CB et al., Strain typing methods and molecular epidemiology of Pneumocystis pneumonia. *Emerg. Infect. Dis.* 10, 1729–1735, 2004.

Cavallini Sanches EM et al., Pneumocystis sp. in bats evaluated by PCR. *J Mycol Med* 23, 47–52, 2013.

Chabé M et al., Pneumocystis: from a doubtful unique entity to a group of highly diversified fungal species. *FEMS Yeast Research* 11, 2–17, 2011.

Durand-Joly I et al., Pneumocystis carinii f. sp. hominis is not infectious for SCID mice. *J. Clin. Microbiol.* 40, 1862–1865, 2002.

Edman JC et al., Ribosomal RNA sequence shows Pneumocystis carinii to be a member of the fungi. *Nature* 334, 519–522, 1988.

Evans R, Ho-Yen DO, Nested PCR is useful to the clinician in the diagnosis of Pneumocystis carinii pneumonia. *J. Infect.* 40, 207–208, 2000.

Kling HM et al., Pneumocystis colonization in immunocompetent and simian immunodeficiency virus-infected cynomolgus macaques. *J Infect Dis* 199, 89–96, 2009.

Morris A, Beard CB, Huang L, Update on the epidemiology and transmission of Pneumocystis carinii. *Microb Infect* 4, 95–103, 2002.

Morris A et al., Improved survival with highly active antiretroviral therapy in HIV-infected patients with severe Pneumocystis carinii pneumonia. *AIDS* 17, 73–80, 2003.

Schliep TC, Yarrish RL, Pneumocystis carinii pneumonia. *Semin. Respir. Infect* 14, 333–343, 1999.

Stringer JR, Pneumocystis. *Int. J. Med. Microbiol.* 292, 391–404, 2002.

Stringer JR et al., A new name (Pneumocystis jiroveci) for Pneumocystis from humans. *Emerg. Infect. Dis.* 8, 891–896, 2002.

Parasitic Zoonoses | 4

4.1 Introduction

Parasitic zoonoses belong to the most important human diseases worldwide. They are caused by protozoa, helminths [trematodes (flukes), cestodes (tapeworms), and nematodes (round worms)], Acanthocephala (thorny-headed worms), pentastomids (tongue worms), and arthropods. The last of these plays an additional role as a transmitter of viruses, rickettsiae, bacteria, protozoa, and helminths.

A number of parasitic protozoa have gained importance in recent years as agents of opportunistic infections. This is true of some parasites, almost neglected in the past, now known as occasionally life-threatening opportunistic agents (e.g., cryptosporidia). In addition, the clinical picture of some established diseases has dramatically changed expression in immunocompromised patients when compared with immunologically competent individuals (e.g., toxoplasmosis in patients with HIV).

Parasites are eukaryotes and differ from prokaryotes, such as bacteria, by complex developmental cycles, which include morphologically, biologically, and biochemically different stages. Many zoonotic parasites involve one or more intermediate hosts in which further development and often multiplication take place. This is known for protozoa but also for the other groups of agents. Intermediate hosts may be invertebrates (molluscs or arthropods) or vertebrates, transmitting the parasites either in an active or in a passive fashion. In other cases, the infectious stages leave the intermediate host and invade the final host directly or are ingested. Humans may be involved in these cycles as final hosts, intermediate hosts (e.g., in echinococcosis) or paratenic (transport) hosts (e.g., *Toxocara* infections). In the last case, the parasites persist in the tissue in a usually arrested, mostly larval stage but capable of causing symptoms.

Parasites may damage their hosts by mechanical injury, metabolic products, or nutritional competition. They induce specific and nonspecific defense reactions in their hosts. However, many parasites developed effective evasion strategies (e.g., antigenic variation and immunological mimicry), which enable them to persist in a host in spite of humoral and cellular immune reactions. In addition, many parasites modulate immune responses of the host to their advantage. However, host hypersensitivity and autoimmunity may complicate the clinical picture of parasitic infections significantly.

When compared with previous editions of this book, a more itemized spectrum of agents is shown based on recent genetic studies (e.g., concerning zoonotic *Babesia* species or *Giardia* assemblages). These data give a more deversified picture and allow detailed insights into epidemiological relationships. The following sections, however, do not include diseases in which animal hosts may be involved but do not have a significant role in the epidemiology of the disease (e.g., infections with *Onchocerca volvulus* or *Mansonella perstans*). Diseases for which the zoonotic characteristic of an infection has not yet been proven are also omitted. For instance, it remains unsolved whether occasional reports of human infections with *Trichuris vulpis* and *T. suis*, globally common whipworms of dogs and pigs, respectively, are relevant. We have also not included infections with *Dientamoeba fragilis*, which causes diarrhea in humans. Indeed, there are reports on animal reservoirs; however, the eventual mode of transmission is unclear. *D. fragilis* does not develop cysts that are resistant to environmental influences like other ameba. Likewise, *Neospora caninum* remains unconsidered. This parasite is closely related to the zoonotic agent, *Toxoplasma gondii*; it shows a broad spectrum of intermediate hosts, such as *T. gondii*, and is a major cause of abortion in cattle. Indeed, specific antibodies to *N. caninum* have been repeatedly observed in humans but there is no evidence so far on pathogenicity in humans. Furthermore, we have disregarded infections that are extremely rare in humans. For example, there are reports that humans may be infected with *Metastrongylus apri*, a lungworm of pigs, at most a very sporadic, implausible event.

Otherwise, this does not mean that the list of relevant zoonotic agents can be closed. It can rapidly amplify under new ecological conditions. For instance, changes in animal production in terms of a more ecological livestock breeding may favor the development and propagation of at least particular, also zoonotic parasites and enhance the pressure of infection onto the animals. In addition, an uncontrolled utilization of aquaculture may be hazardous concerning several zoonoses.

The diagnostic methods in parasitology often differ considerably, for example, from those used in bacteriology. They are often specifically adapted to the various parasites. Thus, we have desisted from describing specific diagnostic techniques in parasitology and morphological aspects in detail because this would be beyond the scope of this book. We therefore refer to special publications on the diagnosis of parasitic infections below. Tab. 4.1 defines some parasitological terms used in this chapter.

REFERENCES

Anderson RC, *Nematode parasites of vertebrates. Their development and transmission*. CAB International, Wallingford, Oxon, 2000.

Anderson RC, Chabaud AG Willmot S, *Key to the nematodes of vertebrates*. CABI Publishing, Wallinford, UK, 2009.

Ash LR, Orihel TC, *Atlas of human parasitology*, 3rd edition. ASCP Press, Chicago, 1990.

Ash LR, Orihel TC *Parasites. A guide to laboratory procedures and identification*. ASCP Press, Chicago, 1987.

Barrat JL et al., The ambiguous life of Dientamoeba fragilis: the need to investigate current hypotheses on transmission. *Parasitology*. 135, 557–572, 2011.

Brown D et al., (eds.), *Zoonoses*. 2nd ed. Oxford University Press, Oxford, 2011.

Burgess NRH, Cowan GO, *A colour atlas of medical entomology*. Chapman & Hall, London, 1993.

Dorny P et al., Emerging food-born parasites. *Vet. Parasitol*. 163, 196–206, 2009.

Deplaces P et al., *Lehrbuch der Parasitologie für die Tiermedizin*. 3. Aufl. Enke-Verlag Stuttgart, 2012.

Garcia LN, Bruckner DA, *Diagnostic medical parasitology*, 4th edition. ASM Press, Washington, DC, 2001.

Hiepe T, Lucius R Gottstein B, *Allgemeine Parasitologie*. Parey, Stuttgart, 2006.

Isenberg HD (ed.), *Essential procedures for clinical microbiology*. ASM Press, Washington, DC, 1998.

Kenney M, Yermakov V, Infection of man with Trichuris vulpis, the whipworm of dogs. *Am. J. Trop. Med. Hyg*. 29, 1205–1208, 1980.

Kettle PS, *Medical and veterinary entomology*. CAB International, Wallingford, 1990.

Lane RP, Crossey RW (eds.), *Medical insects and arachnids*. Chapman & Hall, London 1995.

Lobato J et al., Detection of immunoglobulin G antibodies to *Neospora caninum* in humans: high seropositivy rates in patients who are infected by human immunodeficiency virus or have neurological disorders. *Clin. Vaccine Immunol*. 13, 84–89, 2006.

Macpherson CN, Human behaviour and the epidemiology of parasitic zoonoses. *Int. J. Parasitol*. 35, 1319–1331, 2005.

McCann CM et al., Lack of serologic evidence of *Neospora caninum* in humans, England. *Emerg. Infect. Dis*. 14, 978–980, 2008.

Mehlhorn H (ed.), *Encyclopedia of parasitology*. 3rd edition. Springer-Verlag Heidelberg, 2008.

Table 4.1 | Definitions of parasitological terms

TERM	DEFINITION
Amastigotes	Intracellular developmental stages of leishmaniae and *T. cruzi* in the vertebrate host; regression of the flagellum
Bradyzoite	Slowly multiplying stage in tissue cysts of cyst-forming Coccidia
Cercaria	Motile larval stage of digenean trematodes, infective for second intermediate or final hosts (the latter in case of schistosomes)
Coracidium	Ciliated first-stage larva developing in the eggs of cestodes of the order Pseudophyllidea
Cuticle	Acellular covering of nematodes, pentastomids, and arthropods (in case of arthropods reinforced with chitin)
Cyst	1. Stage of Giardia and amebae in the environment, enclosed by a resistant cyst wall 2. Tissue stage of cyst-forming Coccidia (e.g., *Toxoplasma gondii*, *Sarcocystis* spp.) in intermediate hosts
Cysticercoid	Second larva of some cyclophyllid cestodes which use invertebrates as intermediate hosts
Cysticercus	Second larva (bladder worm) of taeniid cestodes in mammals that do not multiply in the intermediate host
Cystozoite	See "bradyzoite"
Definitive host	Final (specific) host
Embryophore	Shell of tapeworm eggs enclosing the oncosphere
Endodyogeny	Type of asexual multiplication of cyst-forming Coccidia
Epimastigotes	Stage of trypanosomes and leishmaniae occurring in the arthropod vector
Final host	Host in the course of heterogenous development where sexual multiplication takes place
Gametes	Sexually determined stages of Apicomplexa (microgametes are "male," macrogametes are "female" gametes)
Gamogony	Sexual reproduction phase of Coccidia
Incubation period	Period of time between infection and occurrence of clinical symptoms
Intermediate host	Host in the course of heterogenous development in which asexual development (sometimes multiplication) takes place
Kinetoplast	DNA-containing portion of the mitochondrium of trypanosomes and leishmaniae (order Kinetoplastida) that is located close to the basal body of the flagellum
Merozoite	Motile stage of Coccidia developed in a schizont
Metacercaria	Persistent developmental stage of digenean trematodes formed by encapsulation of cercariae in the environment or in second intermediate hosts
Metacestode	Larval stage of cyclophyllidean cestodes in intermediate hosts
Microfilaria	First stage larva of filariae in the blood or skin of the final host; infectious stage for the intermediate host (arthropods)
Miracidium	First stage larva of (digenean) trematodes, developing in the egg
Oncosphere	First stage larva of cyclophyllidean cestodes (in the egg)
Oocyst	Stage in the life cycle of Coccidia, developing after fusion of gametes
Paratenic host	Host in which infective stages may accumulate but not develop further
Parthenogenesis	Egg production without fertilization
Patency	Period during which parasites or their sexual products can be detected

continued

Table 4.1 *continued*

TERM	DEFINITION
Plerocercoid	Third stage larva of pseudophyllidean cestodes
Prepatency	Period of time between infection and first appearance of parasites or sexual parasite products (eggs, larvae)
Procercoid	Second stage larva of pseudophyllidean cestodes
Proglottid	Segment of cestodes with own set of genitals
Promastigotes	Flagellated developmental stages of leishmaniae and *T. cruzi* in the intestine of vectors
Protoscolex	Larval stage of cestodes in an echinococcus or coenurus
Pseudopodia	Cytoplasm protrusions within the cell membrane used by amebae for a forward flow
Rostellum	Mostly armed (with hooks) protrudable extension of the scolex of cestodes
Schizont	Intracellular stage in the life cycle of Coccidia in which merozoites develop by asexual multiplication (schizogony)
Scolex	"Head" of cestodes
Sporogony	Development of spores (Microsporidia) or sporozoites (Coccidia)
Sporozoite	Motile infectious stage of sporozoa developing asexually from zygotes (sporogony)
Tachyzoite	Rapidly dividing stages of cyst-forming Coccidia
Trophozoite	Feeding stage of protozoa
Trypomastigotes	Free, flagellated stages of trypanosomes mostly in vertebrates
Zygote	Fusion product of gametes

Meyers WM (ed.), *Pathology of infectious diseases, Vol. I Helminthiases*. Armed Forces Institute of Pathology, Washington, DC, 2000.

Ministry of Agriculture, Fisheries and Food, *Manual of veterinary parasitological laboratory techniques*. Reference Book 418. London, Her Majesty's Stationary Office, 1986.

Orihel TC, Ash LA, *Parasites in human tissues*. ASCP Press, Chicago, 1995.

Petersen E et al. 1999. *Neospora caninum* infection and repeated abortions in humans. *Emerg. Infect. Dis.* 5, 278–280.

Pfaller MA, Garcia L (eds.), Parasitology. Section IX. In: Murray PR, Baron EJ, Pfaller MA et al. (eds.), *Manual of clinical microbiology*, 7th edition. ASM Press, Washington, 2006.

Price DL, *Intestinal protozoa in MIF. A reference set of photomicrographs of protozoa stained by the modified MIF method*. Marion. Scientific. Corp., Kansas City, 1978.

Schmidt GD, *Handbook of tapeworm identification*. CRC Press Inc., Boca Raton, 1986.

Schnieder T (Hrsg.), Veterinärmedizinische Parasitologie. *+6. Aufl.*, MVS Medizinverlage StuttgartGmbH&Co.KG., Stuttgart, 2006.

Singh S et al., *Trichuris vulpis* in an Indian tribal population. *J. Parasitol.* 79, 457–458, 1993.

Warren KS, Mahmoud AAF (eds.), *Tropical and geographical medicine*. 2nd edition. McGraw-Hill, New York, 1990.

Winzeler EA, Advances in parasite genomics: from sequences to regulatory networks. *PloS Pathog* 5, e1000649. doi: 10.1371/journal ppat.1000649, 2009.

WHO *Basic laboratory methods in medical parasitology*. WHO, 1991.

Yamaguti S, *Systema Helminthum*. Interscience Publ., New York, 1961.

Yorke W, Maplestone PA, *The nematode parasites of vertebrates*. Hafner Publishing Company, New York, 1962.

4.2 Zoonoses Caused by Protozoa

Protozoa are unicellular, eukaryotic (nucleus enclosed in a membrane), either free-living or parasitic organisms. Their sizes (approximately 1 to 300 μm) and shapes vary according to the various phyla and classes. The genomes of Protozoa are larger than those of viruses or bacteria and comprise about 10 to 80 Mb (for comparison: *Escherichia coli*: 4.2 Mb; mouse: 2700 Mb). Approximately 17 000 parasitic protozoan species are known. The parasites live either extracellularly in tissues or in hollow organs, or invade host cells and develop intracellularly. Some groups of Protozoa proliferate asexually by binary or multiple fissions, in most cases; however, the life cycle includes an alternation of asexual and sexual generations.

Life cycles are either direct, often including infective stages that are resistant to environmental influences (e.g., oocysts), or are indirect, including specific intermediate hosts, which may transmit the agent actively or passively after being, for example, ingested by the final host.

The following chapters are arranged alphabetically and and insofar the sequence disregards the taxonomic system.

4.2.1 AMEBIASIS

Amebiasis (amebic dysentery or invasive amebiasis) is an infectious disease caused by the intestinal protozoan parasite, *Entamoeba histolytica*. Most infections run a clinically asymptomatic course, and only about 10% cause a spectrum of diseases ranging from amebic dysentery to amebic abscesses of the liver and other organs.

In recent decades, severe disease due to free-living, water-born amebae of the genera *Naegleria* and *Acanthamoeba* (facultative parasitism) has been observed in humans and animals with increasing frequency. An often lethal amebic meningoencephalitis caused by *Balamuthia mandrillaris* occurs in animals and humans, predominantly in immunosuppressed patients.

Etiology. Entamebae are protozoan parasites of the class Entamoebidea. Formerly, it was assumed that the major parasite *E. histolytica* is the cause of both symptomatic and inapparent infections. Meanwhile, it is accepted that several, morphologically indistinguishable species of the genus *Entamoeba* are responsible for different manifestations. *E. histolytica* is the pathogenic species, whereas *E. dispar* and *E. moshkovskii are* not pathogenic. Molecular studies have shown that the former species is split into a variety of genotypes, although these could not be attributed to particular clinical pictures. Three stages of *E. histolytica* are found in humans:

1. Tissue or motile vegetative form (trophozoite: magna form), approximately 20 to 30 μm in size. Trophozoites move actively by means of pseudopodia (Fig. 4.1); invades the intestinal wall; phagocytise erythrocytes, leucocytes, and tissue debris; and cause the acute amebic dysentery with its sequelae.

2. Vegetative "intestinal lumen form" (minuta form), ca. 10 to 20 μm in size. These innocent commensales live freely in the intestinal lumen and are found predominantly in chronic infections.

3. Permanent form (cyst), ca. 10 to 15 μm in size, rounded, immotile. Due to a tough cyst wall, this form is highly resistant. Cysts are the sole infectious stages.

The developmental cycle of *E. histolytica* is demonstrated in Fig. 4.2. In individual cases, infection with *E. polecki* was supposed to be the reason of dysentery. In general, however, this worldwide distributed species with mononuclear cysts, which is mainly found in pigs, is not regarded pathogenic.

Free-living, optionally parasitic amebae are found occasionally in the human central nervous system (CNS) and in the brain of animals: *Naegleria fowleri*, *Acanthamoeba* spp., *Balamuthia mandrillaris* and *Sappinia diploidea*, and, probably, *S. pedata*. Several *Acanthameba* spp. and *Dictyostelium polycephalum* may induce keratitis in humans.

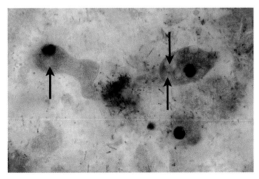

Figure 4.1 | *Entamoeba histolytica* trophozoites with phagocytized erythrocytes (arrows) in feces of a patient with invasive amebiasis (picture: N. Fiege, Giessen, Germany).

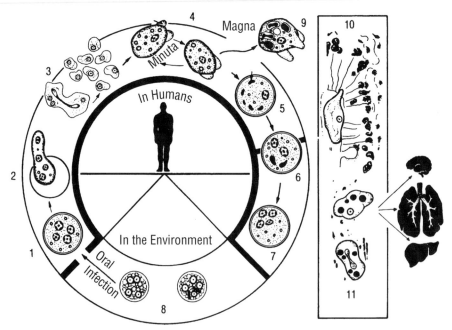

Figure 4.2 | Developmental cycle of *E. histolytica*. (1) Cyst with four nuclei is ingested orally; (2) trophozoite with four nuclei leaves cyst within small intestine; (3) both cytoplasm and nuclei divide to form eight small amebae; (4) mature trophozoites (i.e., minuta forms) reproduce by constant binary fission in intestinal lumen; (5) uninucleate cyst (precyst) with marginal chromatoid bodies; (6) cyst with two nuclei and chromatoid bodies; (7) mature cyst with four nuclei (metacyst); (8) infectious cysts are set free with feces; (9) during acute amebic dysentery, minuta forms enlarge to large vegetative forms, i.e., magna or tissue forms; (10) magna forms enter submucosa of intestinal wall; (11) hematogenous spread to brain, lung, liver, skin, and other organs, with invasive, extraintestinal amebiasis with abscess formation.

Occurrence. The prevalence of amebic infections depends on socioeconomic status, sanitation, and crowding. According to the World Health Organization (WHO), approximately 10% of the world population is infected with *Entamoeba* spp.; about 50 million cases of invasive disease occur each year, causing up to 100 000 deaths. The parasite occurs in all climatic zones. In some endemic areas of Africa and Asia >80% of the population shed cysts of *Entamoeba* spp.; 5 to 15% of them carry *E. histolytica*.

Dogs, monkeys and rodents are supposed to be the major animal reservoirs; however, most of these studies have been performed at times when the *Entamoeba* spp. had not yet been discriminated, that is, the situation is not clear. Most of the free-living amebic species that invade the human CNS or cause damage of the eyes are ubiquitous cosmopolits. *B. mandrillaris* is found in warm climates.

Transmission. Transmission of *Entamoeba* spp. occurs by oral ingestion of water and food, mainly of plant origin, contaminated with cysts. Flies and cockroaches play a role of mechanical vectors for infectious cysts. Infection of young children by their mothers excreting cysts and/or by manual feeding with contaminated fingers is frequent. Infections transmitted by anilingus are common in homosexuals.

Naegleria spp. invade the organism via the olfactory mucosa by small (20 by 7 µm) flagellated stages with large pseudopods, for example, during swimming in stagnating freshwater. Points of entry of *Acanthamoeba* organisms and *D. polycephalum* are respiratory tract, urogenital tract, and the skin. Amebic keratitis is mostly found in carriers of soft contact lenses and transmission occurs predominantly due to insufficient cleaning of the lenses. Free cysts containing ameboid stages are the infectious forms. *B. mandrillaris* has not yet been found in the environment. The transmission route is unknown.

Clinical Manifestations. *E. histolytica* infections remain asymptomatic in 15 to 25% of cases. The incubation period of amebic dysenteria varies, it is usually 2 to 6 weeks after ingestion of cysts before acute invasive dysentery starts gradually, with mild gastrointestinal symptoms, such as diarrhea, sometimes alternating with constipation. Severe mucoid blood-tinged diarrhea with spasms, colics, and tenesmus may develop. Patients pass 10 to 12 stools per day. Rarely, in malignant or complicated cases, high fever (toxemia), ileus, electrolyte imbalances, and cachexia occur.

The course of amebic dysentery varies between spontaneous recovery within a few days or weeks to chronicity and recrudescence, that is, relapsing colitis lasting months or years. A typical complication is an ameboma, a localized, tumor-like inflammatory, colonic granuloma, which resembles a carzinoma.

Intestinal amebic infection may be complicated by metastasis in the liver. The so-called "tropical liver abscess" may develop just a few weeks after a previously acquired intestinal infection but usually occurs after a period of 2 to 5 months and manifests itself as either solitary or multiple hepatic lesions. In 80 to 90% of cases, it is found in the right liver lobe, and it is 10 times more common in men than in women. A single liver abscess may reach the size of a fist or even a child's head, while multiple foci are smaller, but rarely observed. Most patients present with an acute or subacute onset of fever and abdominal pain localized in the right upper quadrant, sometimes radiating to the right shoulder. Tenderness over the liver, hepatomegaly, and right-sided rales are common. However, clinical diagnosis may be difficult: 10 to 15% of patients present with fever only.

Pleuropulmonary amebiasis may complicate amebic liver abscess, mostly due to abscess rupture through the diaphragm. Pleural empyema and intrapulmonary abscesses may ensue; patients have fever, dyspnea, pleuritic pain, and cough. Mortality may reach >30%. Amebic liver abszesses may also rupture into the peritoneal cavity and pericardium, thus inducing peritonitis and pericarditis, both associated with high mortality. Hematogenous spread may result in cerebral, splenic, and genitourinary amebiasis.

Cutaneous amebiasis is frequently the result of intestinal amebiasis and manifests itself in painful ulcerations and condyloma-like lesions in the anal and perianal skin regions. Free-living amebae of the genera *Naegleria*, *Acanthamoeba*, and *Balamuthia* have been identified as agents causing infections of the CNS of humans and other vertebrates. They may be responsible for mild or severe disease.

Naegleria spp. enter the olfactory mucosa and through the cribiform plate gain access to the CNS, causing primary meningoencephalitis (PAM). The incubation time is 1 to 9 days. Symptoms are severe and include headache, high fever, nausea, vomiting, photophobia, stiff neck, and coma, leading to death (95%) within 3 to 10 days after onset. Acanthamoebae and *Sappinia* spp. invade people with chronic disease or immunodeficiency via the respiratory or urogenital tract or skin, followed by hematogenous spread to the CNS. They cause acute or chronic granulomatous encephalitis (GAE), inflammation of inner organs, and diarrhea. Several *Acanthamoeba* spp. and *D. polycephalum* cause a painful keratitis, especially in wearers of certain types of contact lenses, which can result in permanent visual impairment and even blindness. GAE patients show usually progredient courses of disease. Prognoses are generally poor. *B. mandrillaris* causes a subacute or chronic granulomatous encephalitis in both immunocompetent and immunosuppressed patients. The prognosis is poor.

Diagnosis. Intestinal amebiasis: History and clinical signs allow a presumptive diagnosis. Endoscopic examination (sigmoidoscopy and colonoscopy) may reveal petechiae and small, solitary, rarely confluent ulcers with exudative centers and edematous, hyperemic rims. The colonic mucosa is hyperemic and edematous, occasionally covered with pseudomembranes.

Microscopic detection of trophozoites and cysts establishes the diagnosis. Liquid feces and samples taken by endoscopy (biopsy, ulcer secretion, and swab specimens) are suitable materials. Samples must be fresh and should be examined within 30 min after suspension in physiological saline by phase contrast microscopy showing trophozoites with linear movement. Samples may also be examined after fixation in polyvinyl alcohol and staining with Heidenhain's iron-hematoxylin or Wheatley trichrome stain, the latter being the more commonly used approach. Microscopic detection of hematophagous trophozoits (Fig. 4.1) is pathognomonic for *E. histolytica* infection. Using fluorescein labeled monoclonal antibodies, *E. histolytica*, *E. dispar*, and *E. moshkovskii* may be differentiated. Fecal samples may also be examined after flotation and concentration by sodium acetate-acetic acid formaldehyde (SAF) or merthiolate-iodine formaldehyde techniques. For subjects with clinical signs but negative results of microscopic examination of fecal samples, the examination should be repeated at least three times to avoid false-negative results.

In vitro cultivation of amebae is costly and available only in specialized laboratories, but may be useful in chronic ambeiais with few cysts. It is required for zymodeme determination (isoenzyme pattern). Defined parasitic antigens can be detected in feces and serum by enzyme linked immunosorbent assay (ELISA). PCR is also suitable for detection and differentiation of *Entamoeba* spp.

Specific antibodies, which can be demonstrated by ELISA and indirect hemagglutination assay (IHA), may persist for many years after recovery and are of limited diagnostic value. Asymptomatic cyst carriers are usually serologically negative.

Extraintestinal amebiais: Humoral antibodies against defined *Entamoeba* surface antigens are found in almost all patients with extraintestinal amebiasis. Abscesses in liver, lung or other organs may be localized by sonography, computed tomography (CT) scan, magnetic resonance imaging (MRI), and scintigraphy (technetium and gallium isotopes).

For diagnostic purposes, or in case of imminent rupture of an abscess, fine-needle biopsy aspiration under sonographic guidance may be helpful. A bacteriologically sterile, odorless, yellow-brown liquid that yields trophozoites rarely on microscopy but occasionally by *in vitro* cultivation may be obtained by this approach. Amebic antigens can be detected by ELISA, amebic DNA by PCR.

PAM: Microscopic detection of amebic organisms in the CSF leads to diagnosis. A wet mount of CSF is examined for the presence of motile *N. fowleri* amebae. Monoclonal antibodies and PCR can be used for doubtless identification.

Primers for PCR-diagnosis of free-living ameba are available. Iron-hematoxilin staining is recommended for direct demonstration. In GAE, *Acanthamoeba* trophozoites are rarely, if ever, seen in CSF. Culture techniques with biopsy specimens and corneal scrapings use agar plates with *E. coli* lawn (incubation at 35 to 42 °C for 3 weeks). *B. mandrillaris* grows *in vitro* on mammalian cells (not on agar) and it can be transmitted to mice.

Differential Diagnosis. Intestinal amebiasis has to be distinguished from colitis of other etiology, schistosomiasis, ulcerative colitis, Crohn's disease, colonic carcinoma, and balantidiasis. In case of extraintestinal manifestations, abscesses of other etiology and malignant tumors must be excluded; in case of liver and lung lesions, especially cystic echinococcosis, tuberculosis, brucellosis, and Hodgkin's disease must be excluded.

Therapy.

- Asymptomatic intestinal carriers: Paronomycin, 25 to 35 mg/kg three times a day orally for 7 days, or iodoquinol, 650 mg three times a day orally for 20 days, or diloxanidfuroate, 500 mg three times a day orally for 10 days;

- Amebic dysentery and amebic abscess: metronidazole, 750 mg three times a day orally for 7 to 10 days, or tinidazole, 2 g per day orally for 3 days; subsequently, for elimination of intestinal cysts: paronomycin, 25 to 35 mg/kg three times a day orally for 7 days, or iodoquinol, 650 mg three times a day orally for 20 days;

- Heavy extraintestinal infection: Metronidazole, 750 mg three times a day intravenously for 10 days, or tinidazole, 2 g per day intravenously for 5 days; subsequently, for elimination of intestinal cysts: paronomycin, 25 to 35 mg/kg three times a day orally for 7 days, or iodoquinol, 650 mg three times a day orally for 20 days;
- PAM due to *N. fowleri*. Amphotericin B, 1.5 mg/kg per day in two doses intravenously for 3 days; subsequently 1 mg/kg per day intravenously for 6 days; in addition 1.5 mg per day intrathecally for 2 days, subsequentially 1 mg per day intrathecally for 8 days.
- GAE by*Acanthamoeba* spp.: Pentamidine plus sulfadiazine plus flucytosine plus (fluconazole or itraconazole) intravenously;
- Amebic keratitis: Miltefosine or voriconazole.
- *B. mandrillaris* infection: Patients may be treated with pentamidine plus clarithromycine plus azithromycin plus fluconazole plus sulfadiazine plus flucytosine.

Prophylaxis. General hygienic measures include prevention of contamination of water and food by amebic cysts, use of insecticides (flies and cockroaches play a role as mechanical vectors), improvement of sanitary hygiene (toilets), and change of living conditions in areas of endemicity.

Travelers in the tropics should avoid raw food and fruits that cannot be peeled and they should never drink uncooked or unfiltered water. Amebic cysts are not destroyed by low concentrations of chlorine or iodine in drinking water. Heating to 50 °C kills amebic cysts in water within 5 min. Chemoprophylaxis or vaccination against amebic infection is not available.

Known carriers should not be employed in eating establishments or water sanitation until after appropriate therapy and laboratory confirmation of cure. Proper cleaning of contact lenses minimizes the risk of amebic keratitis. Hydrogen-peroxide based cleaning solutions are effective in disinfection.

REFERENCES

Ali IK, Clark CG, Petri WA Jr, Molecular epidemiology of amebiasis. *Infect. Genet. Evol.* 8, 698–707, 2008.

Bakardjiev A et al., Amebic encephalitis caused by *Balamuthia mandrillaris*: report of four cases. *Pediatr. Infect. Dis. J.* 22, 447–453, 2003.

Blessmann J, Le Van A, Tannich E, Hepatic ultrasound in a population with high incidence of invasive amoebiasis: evidence for subclinical, self-limited amoebic liver abscesses. *Trop. Med. Int. Health* 8, 231–233, 2003.

Cordel H et al., Imported amoebic liver abscess in France. *PLoS Negl. Trop. Dis.* 7, e2333, 2013.

Dart JK, Saw VP, Kilvington S, *Acanthamoeba* keratitis: diagnosis and treatment update 2009. *Am. J. Ophthalmol.* 148, 487–499, 2009.

Das K et al., Multilocus sequence typing system (MLST) reveals a significant association of *Entamoeba histolytica* genetic patterns with disease outcome. *Parasitol. Int.* 63, 308–314, 2014.

Fotedar R et al., PCR detection of *Entamoeba histolytica, Entamoeba dispar*, and *Entamoeba moshkovskii* in stool samples from Sidney, Australia. *J. Clin. Microbiol.* 45, 1035–1037, 2007.

Heggie TW, Swimming with death: *Naegleria fowleri* infections in recreational waters. *Travel Med. Infect. Dis.* 8, 201–206, 2010.

Lamb CA et al., Sexually transmitted infections manifesting as proctitis. *Frontline Gastrooenterol.* 4, 32–40, 2013.

Leippe M et al., Ancient weapons: the three-dimensional structure of amoebapore A. *Trends Parasit.* 21, 5–7, 2005.

Mortimer L, Chadee K, The immunopathogenesis of *Entamoeba histolytica*. *Exp. Parasitol.* 126, 366–380, 2010.

Murakawa GJ et al., Disseminated acanthamebiasis in patients with AIDS. A report of five cases and a review of the literature. *Arch. Dermatol.* 131, 1291–1296, 1995.

Nishise S et al., Mass infection with *Entamoeba histolytica* in a Japanese institution for individuals with mental retardation: epidemiology and control measures. *Ann. Trop. Med. Parasitol.* 104, 383–390, 2010.

Reddy AK et al., *Dictyostelium polycephalum* infection of human cornea. *Emerg. Infect. Dis.* 18, 1644–1645, 2010.

Sateriale A, Roy NH, Huston CD, SNAP-tag technology optimized for use in *Entamoeba histolytica*. *PLoS One* 8, e83997, 2013.

Visvesvara GS, Amebic meningoencephalitis and keratitis: challenges in diagnosis and treatment. *Curr. Opin. Infect. Dis.* 23, 590–594, 2010.

Visvesvara GS, Moura H, Schuster FL, Pathogenic and opportunistic free-living amoeba: *Acanthamoeba* spp., *Balamuthia mandrillis, Naegleria fowleri*, and *Sappinia diploidea*. *FEMS Immunol. Med. Microbiol.* 50, 1–26, 2007.

Walochnick J, Wylezich C, Michel R, The genus *Sappinia*: history, phylogeny and medical relevance. *Exp. Parasitol.* 126, 4–13, 2011.

Zhou F et al., Seroprevalence of *Entamoeba histolytica* infection among chinese men who have sex with men. *PLoS Negl. Trop. Dis.* 7, 32232, 2013.

4.2.2 BABESIOSIS

Babesiosis in humans has gained increasing attention as an emerging zoonosis caused by animal-specific protozoan parasites of the family Babesiidae (order Piroplasmida). *Babesia* spp. are transmitted by "hard ticks" (Ixodidae; see chapter 4.7.1.1), invade erythrocytes and may induce a febrile disease with hemolytic anemia, hemoglobinuria, and in severe cases, acute respiratory distress syndrome (ARDS), shock and death.

Etiology. The taxonomy of Babesiidae is in discussion. According to 18S rDNA sequences, the agents are divided into *Babesia* species sensu stricto (s.s.), mostly so-called large babesia (>2.5 μm) including the cattle babesia *B. divergens* and into members of the *B. microti* group, so-called small babesia (<2.5 μm). A previously suggested unique species *B. microti* in microtine rodents does not exist. The *B. microti* group is currently divided into strains that contain (i) genotypes in rodents, which include the majority of the zoonotic genotypes; (ii) genotypes in carnivorous animals; and (iii) rodent parasites without zoonotic potential. *Babesia*

s.s. may invade the oocytes of female ticks so that all subsequent tick stages may be infected (transovarial transmission). In contrast, parasites of the *B. microti* group are only passed in a transstadial manner, that is, the tick larvae hatching the eggs do not become infected. Both groups of *Babesia* spp. contain parasites of different pathogenicity and geographical distribution that have been found in humans (Tab. 4.2). The developmental cycle of Babesia spp. s.s. is shown in Fig. 4.3.

Occurrence. Human babesiosis is a comparatively rare, but probably underreported disease. Cases were mainly observed in the United States and in Europe.

Human infections in the US are predominantly caused by members of the *B. microti* group. Distinctly >300 clinical cases are documented, especially from the East Coast. Both immunocompetent and immunosuppressed persons were affected. Furthermore, sporadic infections are reported especially in splenectomized patiens with *B. duncani* and *Babesia* sp. MO1, which is related to *B. divergens* (*B. divergens* s.s. is obviously not existing in North America).

Table 4.2 | *Babesia* spp. found in humans

SPECIES/TYPE	OCCURRENCE	VERTEBRATE HOSTS(S)	VECTOR(S)
Babesia spp. sensu stricto			
B. divergens	Europe	Cattle (other ruminants)	*Ixodes ricinus*
B. venatorum[1]	Europe	Roe deer	*I. ricinus*
Babesia sp. (M01)[2]	North America Europe	Unknown	Unknown
Babesia sp. (K01)[3]	Korea, Asia (?)	Unknown	Unknown
B. microti Group			
B. microti	North America Asia	Rodents	*I. scapularis*[4], *I. trianguliceps*[5],
B. microti-like	Europe		*I. ricinus*[6], *I. persulcatus*[7]
B. duncani[8]	North America	Unknown	Unknown

[1] Synonym with *Babesia* sp. EU1-3, genetically closely related with *B. divergens*.
[2] Close relationship with *B. divergens*.
[3] Genetically closely related with *Babesia*.sp. from sheep (*Babesia* sp. BQ1) in China.
[4] In North America.
[5,6] In Eurasia.
[7] In East Asia.
[8] Synonym with various isolates (WA1, CA1, CA5 and others) in the United States.

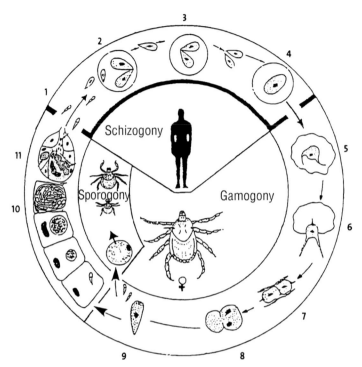

Figure 4.3 | Developmental cycle of *Babesia* spp. (1) Sporozoites in saliva of feeding tick and invasion of erythrocytes of the vertebrate host; (2 and 3) asexual reproduction in erythrocytes by binary fission (formation of merozoites); (4) intraerythrocytic ovoid gamont develops (sexually differentiated stage); (5) after ingestion by ticks, gamonts form radiate protrusions in intestinal cells; (6) gamete ("ray body" as fertile stage); (7) fusion of two gametes; (8) formation of zygotes; (9) formation of sporokinetes (motile invasive forms); (10) sporokinetes leave intestinal cells and enter cells of various organs, e.g., epidermis, muscle, hemolymph, and ovaries and eggs; (11) invasion of salivary glands and formation of sporozoites; (12) transovarial transmission (transmission of sporozoites to next tick generation by infested eggs, heavy multiplication in gut epithelia of tick larvae and nymphs, and settlement in tick salivary glands).

Human *Babesia* infections in Europe were caused in approximately 40 people by *B. divergens* s.s. from cattle. Most cases were reported in France and the UK; however, the parasite is widely spread in other areas of Central Europe and Scandinavia. Infections concerned predominantly splenectomized patients (>80% of the cases). Sporadically, *B. venatorum* and parasites of the *B. microti* group were found in humans in Europe. Reports on human infections with *B. canis* from dogs and *B. bovis* from cattle have not been confirmed.

The reservoir of *B. microti* are microtine rodents (=rodents of the genus *Microtus*), which generally show high *Babesia* prevalences throughout the world. On average 1 to 1.5% of the ticks of involved species (see Tab. 4.2) are infected but there are high variations depending on the geographic area.

The relatively small numbers of documented cases of human babesiosis may mislead over the real occurrence. In Switzerland, for example, 1.5% of the human population show antibodies to *B. microti*, and the prevalence of specific antibodies in humans in New England (USA) has reached a level approaching that of borreliosis.

Transmission. Vectors are hard ticks (Ixodidae) specific for *Babesia* species (Tab. 4.2). Infection occurs by inoculation of sporozoites with tick saliva, when infected ticks feed on their animal hosts or on humans (Fig. 4.3). It remains unclear why, in contrast to North America, *B. microti* is only rarely found in humans in Europe, although there are no significant differences between the infection rates in respective rodent populations. Apart from dark figures in Europe, one reason might be that *I. trianguliceps*, the main vector in Europe, inhabits the burrows of rodents. However, *B. microti* is increasingly found in *I. ricinus* (see chapter 4.7.1.1). Accordingly, with the life cycles of ticks, the major risk for infection must be expected in Europe and North America between May and October.

Apart from tick bites, babesia are also transmitted by blood transfusion and congenitally. Babesiosis is considered the most frequent transfusion transmitted human infection with >160 cases since 1980. *B. microti* survives in erythrocytes for 35 days under blood storing conditions (4 °C) and indefinitely in cryopreserved red blood cells. According to estimates, up to 3.7% of blood products in *B. microti* endemic areas of the United States may contain babesia. Babesiosis after organ transplantation seems to be also mainly associated with blood transfusions.

Clinical Manifestations. *B. microti* infections in immunocompetent patients are often asymptomatic (one-third of the cases). Clinical manifestations were observed mainly in patients with immunosuppression, such as that following splenectomy. After an incubation period of 1 to 9 weeks, patients have fever (~39 °C), severe malaise, dyspnea, arthralgias, myalgias, hemolytic anemia, hemoglobinuria, thrombocytopenia, and elevated levels of serum liver transaminases. The percentage of erythrocytes parasitized is between 1 and 10% (rarely as high as 85%), with especially high numbers in splenectomised, older, immunosuppressed patients and in those infected with HIV. Mortality rates of approximately 20% are observed in this population. Surviving patients often develop a long-lasting disease with relapses.

B. divergens infections occur predominantly in asplenic persons and after incubation periods of 1 to 3 weeks give rise to often fulminant courses of disease with high fever (40 to 41 °C), headache, chills, sweating, myalgias, arthralgias, and hemolytic anemia; within 1 week pulmonary edema, ARDS, and kidney failure may occur, with a mortality rate of 40%.

Concerning infections with other *Babesia* spp., the numbers of cases are too small to show general tendencies; however, severe courses and deaths have to be expected in every case.

Diagnosis. Babesiosis in humans is based on the history and it should be suspected in cases of febrile disease after a tick bite. For laboratory diagnosis, Giemsa-stained thin blood smears are examined for intraerythrocytic merozoites (Fig. 4.4). PCR techniques are sensitive and helpful in subclinical infections (they have low parasitemia) and are essential for species determination.

Serological methods, that is, IHA, immunofluorescence assay (IFA), and ELISA, are useful but specific antibodies are not detected until 7 to 10 days after a tick bite.

Differential diagnosis. All diseases with fever, anemia, and hemoglobinuria, for example, malaria, have to be considered in differential diagnosis. Intraerythrocytic trophozoites multiply by binary fission, forming two or four merozoites, at times in a configuration resembling a

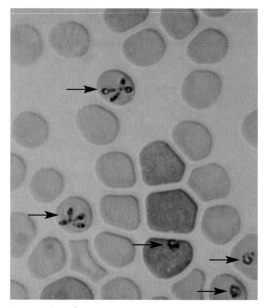

Figure 4.4 | *Babesia divergens.* Thin blood smear from an experimentally infected bird; aberrant forms, partly Maltese cross forms as occurring in human blood (picture: Ute Mackenstedt, Hohenheim, Germany).

Maltese cross (Fig. 4.4). They do not form multi-nuclear schizonts and pigment in erythrocytes as *Plasmodium* spp. do. A history of tick contact, splenectomy, or the diagnosis of Lyme disease is important.

Therapy. A combination of clindamycin (in adults, 600 mg three or four times a day, intravenously (i.v.); in children, 20 mg/kg/d, i.v.) plus quinine sulphate (in adults, 650 mg/kg three or four times a day, orally; in children, 25 mg/kg/d orally for 7 to 10 days) is effective. As an alternative, atovaquone, 750 mg twice a day orally, plus azithromycin, 500 mg on the first day and 250 to 1000 mg a day thereafter orally for 7 to 10 days is recommended. In severe cases with high parasitemia and hemolysis, in addition to chemotherapy, blood exchange transfusion (2 to 3 times the blood volume) can be life-saving.

Prophylaxis. Chemoprophylaxis and vaccination used in veterinary medicine are not available for humans. In areas of endemicity, tick bites can be prevented by proper clothing and use of repellents. In such areas, at times of heavy tick activity, individuals with a history of tick bites should be excluded from blood donation (a donor questionnaire is currently the only measure to avoid *Babesia*-contaminated blood donations in the US).

REFERENCES

Asad S, Sweeney J, Mermel LA, Transfusion-transmitted babesiosis in Rhode Islands. *Transfusion* 49, 2564–2573, 2009.

Bonnet S et al., Experimental in vitro transmisson of *Babesia* sp. EU1 by *Ixodes ricinus*. *Vet. Res.* 40, 21, 2009.

Centers for Disease Control and Prevention (CDC), Babesiosis surveillance - 18 states, 2011. *MMWR Morb. Mortal. Wkly. Rep.* 61, 505–509, 2012.

Cieniuch S, Stanczak J, Ruczaj A, The first detection of *Babesia* EU1 and *Babesia canis canis* in *Ixodes ricinus* ticks (Acari, Ixodidae) collected in urban and rural areas in northern Poland. *Pol. J. Microbiol.* 58, 231–236, 2009.

Conrad PA et al., Description of *Babesia duncani* n. sp. (Apicomplexa: Babesiidae) from humans and its differentiation from other piroplasms. *Int. J. Parasitol.* 36, 779–789, 2006.

Foppa IM et al., Entomologic and serologic evidence of zoonotic transmission of *Babesia microti*; Eastern Switzerland. *Emerg. Inf. Dis.* 8, 722–726, 2002.

Fox LM et al., Neonatal babesiosis: case report and review of the literature. *Pediatr. Infect. Dis.* 25, 169–173, 2006.

Gubernot DM et al., *Babesia* infection through blood transfusions: reports received by the US Food and Drug Administration, 1997–2007. *Clin. Infect. Dis.* 48, 25–30, 2009.

Hersh MH et al., Reservoir competence of wildlife host species for *Babesia microti*. *Emerg. Infect. Dis.* 18, 1951–1957, 2012.

Herwaldt BL et al., Molecular characterization of a Non-*Babesia divergens* organism causing zoonotic babesiosis in Europe. *Emerg. Inf. Dis.* 9, 942–948, 2003.

Herwaldt BL et al., A fatal case of babesiosis in Missouri: identification of another piroplasm that infects humans. *Ann. Inter. Med.* 124, 643–650, 1996.

Joseph JT et al., Vertical transmission of *Babesia microti*, United States. *Emerg. Infect. Dis.* 18, 1318–1321, 2012.

Kirby CS 3rd. et al., Expansion of human babesiosis and reported cases, Connecticut, 2001–2010. *J.Med. Entomol.* 51, 245–252, 2014.

Kjemtrup AM, Conrad PA, Human babesiosis: an emerging tick-borne disease. *Int. J. Parasitol.* 30, 1323–1337, 2000.

Krause PJl et al., 2008. Persistent and relapsing babesiosis in immunocompromised patients. *Clin. Infect. Dis.* 46, 370–376, 2008.

Walsh GM, The relevance of forest fragmentation on the incidence of human babesiosis: investigating the landscape epidemiology of an emerging tick-borne disease. *Vector Borne Zoonotic Dis.* 13, 250–255, 2013.

Wei Q et al., Human babesiosis in Japan: isolation of *Babesia microti*-like parasites from a asymptomatic transfusion donor and from a rodent from an area where babesiosis is endemic. *J. Clin. Microbiol.* 39, 2178–2183, 2001.

Yabsley MJ, Shock BC, Natural history of zoonotic babesia: role of wildlife reservoirs. *Int. J. Parasitol. Parasites Wildl.* 2, 18–31, 2012.

4.2.3 BALANTIDIASIS

Balantidiasis, caused by the ciliate *Balantidium coli*, occurs sporadically in humans. Most infections are asymptomatic. Signs of disease are abdominal pain, weight loss, intermittent diarrhea, and occasionally, severe colitis, with stools containing mucus and blood.

Etiology. *B. coli* (class Ciliophora) is the only known ciliate pathogenic for humans. In its developmental cycle, two forms are recognized, trophozoites (25 to 120 μm in size) and cysts (40 to 60 μm in diameter), the latter being the infectious stage. The trophozoit has a characteristic oval shape and it is covered with cilia. The cytoplasm contains two distinct nuclei, a bean-shaped macronucleus and a smaller, globular micronucleus, located along the concave side of the former. A contractile vacuole is seen in unstained preparations.

Occurrence. *B. coli* occurs worldwide, especially in countries with a temperate or warm climate, in people living under poor hygienic conditions with animal contact, especially pigs. Areas where it is endemic are the People's Republic of China, the Philippines, Indonesia, Japan, the South Pacific islands, Brazil, Peru, Panama, and Cuba. The main animal host for *B. coli* is the domestic pig, in which the infection is asymptomatic. Usually, the parasite lives as a cecal commensal. The rate of infection may reach 40 to 80%. Other common animal hosts are wild boars, rabbits, rats, monkeys (rhesus and New World monkeys), and primates (chimpanzees and orangutans). Cattle, sheep, and horses are rarely infected and of no epidemiological significance. For the developmental cycle, see Fig. 4.5.

Transmission. Transmission occurs by oral ingestions of cysts, for example, through food contaminated with pig feces. Flies may transmit the agent mechanically. Transmission from human to human is rare but has been described.

After digestion of cysts, the developing trophozoites excrete hyaluronidase, which enables the parasite to invade tissues.

Clinical Manifestations. The incubation time depends on the infective dose and patient's health. Cyst ingestion often induces an intraluminal, clinically asymptomatic intestinal infection. Depending upon promoting factors, for example, food rich in carbohydrates, hypoacidity, dyspepsia, and the patient's general condition, mild or severe disease may develop.

Acute disease presents with violent bouts of colitis with abdominal pain, tenesmus, nausea, vomiting, headache, anorexia, and diarrhea that may be bloody, with copious mucus, and malodorous. Fluid loss may be considerable. Later on fever occurs. Fatal infections may occur in untreated children. Mortality rates of 30% have been reported.

In chronic infections, intermittent diarrhea, alternating with consistent constipation, is observed. Stools are loose, without blood and mucus. After invasion of the submucosa, perforations may lead to diffuse peritonitis. Hematogenous dissemination of the parasite into other organs is rare.

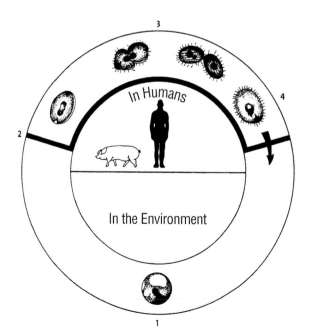

Figure 4.5 | Developmental cycle of *B. coli*. (1) Cysts (40 to 60 μm) are excreted with feces; (2) cysts are ingested with food; (3) vegetative forms reproduce by repeated transverse binary fission and genetic information is exchanged by conjugation; (4) cyst formation is initiated by dehydration within feces in the rectum.

Diagnosis. Occupational contact with pigs may be an important hint in the diagnosis. By microscopy (60- to 100-fold magnification) of fresh fecal samples, trophozoits with typical ciliary movement are detected. Cysts are rarely found in human feces.

B. coli may be concentrated from more solid feces by submersion of fecal samples, enclosed in gauze, into saline. Due to the positive geotactic reaction of the parasites, they may be detected at the bottom of the test tube. Endoscopy of the colon reveals ulcerations with crater-like margins. Serological methods for detection of humoral antibodies are of no significance for routine diagnosis.

Differential Diagnosis. Acute balantidiasis must be differentiated from dysentery caused by *Shigella* spp., *E. histolytica*, and *Salmonella* spp.

Therapy. Infection with *B. coli*, including asymptomatic forms, should be treated. Patients are treated with tetracycline, 500 mg four times a day orally, or metronidazole, 750 mg three times a day orally over 7 to 10 days, or with iodoquinol, 650 mg three times a day, over 20 days.

Prophylaxis. As infection of pigs with *B. coli* is common, hygienic measures must be taken to avoid transmission from pigs. Manure from pigs should not be used as fertilizer. Under moist conditions, cysts of *B. coli* remain infectious for several weeks in the environment. In regions of endemicity, food and drinking water must be adequately protected.

REFERENCES

Anargyrou K et al., Pulmonary *Balantidium coli* infection in a leukemic patient. *Am J. Hematol.* 73, 180–183, 2003.

Bellanger AP et al., Dysenteric syndrome due to *Balantidium coli*: a case report. *New Microbiol.* 36, 203–205, 2013.

Damriyasa IM, Bauer C, Prevalence and age-dependent occurrence of intestinal protozoan infections in suckling piglets. *Berl. Münch. Tierärztl. Wochenschr.* 119, 287–290, 2006.

Kaur R et al., Intestinal parasites in children withe diarrhea in Delhi, India. *Southeast Asian J. Trop. Med. Public Health* 33, 725–729, 2002.

Nakauchi K et al., The prevalence of *Balantidium coli* infection in fifty-six mammalian species. *J. Vet. Med. Sci.* 61, 63–65, 1999.

Schuster FL, Ramirez-Avila L, Current world status of *Balantidium coli. Clin. Microbiol. Rev.* 212, 626–638, 2008.

Solaymani-Mohammadi S, Rezaian M, Ali Anwar M, Human balantidiasis in Iran: an unsolved enigma. *Trends Parasitol.* 21, 160–161, 2005.

4.2.4 CHAGAS' DISEASE (AMERICAN TRYPANOSOMIASIS)

Chagas' disease is named after the Brazilian physician, Carlos Chagas, who, in 1909, was the first person to describe the flagellated parasite *Trypanosoma cruzi* as a pathogen for humans and animals. The American form of trypanosomiasis is a serious public health problem in Central and South American countries and considered the third largest parasitic disease after malaria and schistosomiasis.

Etiology. *Typanosoma cruzi* is found early after infection of vertebrates in the blood in a nonpropagating trypomastigote stage as a large flagellate (17 to 20 μm by 2 μm) with an undulating membrane and a flagellum. After penetration into cells of the reticuloendothelial system (RES) and other tissues of the host, the parasite differentiates into its productive amastigote form, a small oval protozoon (5 by 1.5 μm) with a round nucleus and a distinct stick-shaped kinetoplast (part of the mitochondrium); the flagellum is almost completely reduced. In this stage of development, the flagellate propagates by binary fission as long as the host cell survives. The parasite lives directly in the host cell cytoplasma, that is, unlike other important intracellular parasites as *Babesia* spp., *Toxoplasma gondii*, or *Plasmodium* spp. is not included in a parasitophorous vacuole. After rupture of the host cell, the freed parasites transform back into trypomastigotes and invade other local cells or spread via circulation to distant tissue cells, for example, muscle cells, where they initiate further cycles of reproduction. Trypomastigotes are the infective stages for the intermediate hosts.

T. cruzi is a multiclonal parasite with marked genetic diversity. A complex of six evolutionary lineages or "discrete typing units" (DTUs), *Tc*I to *Tc*VI, are currently assumed on the basis of isoenzyme and RAPD analyses. A seventh lineage deriving from bats (*Tc*bat) is discusseed. *Tc*I to *Tc*IV (and *Tc*bat) are distinctly homozygot, *Tc*V and *Tc*VI show heterozygocity, are hybrids, and derive from *Tc*II and *Tc*III. The basic nuclear fusion mechanisms in the mammalian stage are not yet understood. *Tc*I contains >25 genotypes, that is, more than any other of the other five DTUs

A second species of trypanosomes, *T. rangeli*, occurs in humans in Central and South America. It shares the invertebrate hosts with *T. cruzi*. The life cycle of *T. rangeli* in the vertebrate host is still unclear, but it is nonpathogenic in vertebrates. In certain areas, the number of asymptomatic infections with this parasite is five to six times higher than infections with *T. cruzi*. *T. rangeli* may be found for more than 1 year within the blood of infected persons.

Occurrence. Chagas' disease is endemic throughout the whole of the Latin American continent, except Cuba; autochthonous cases are also found in the southern United States, for example, Texas, Virginia, and California. According to Pan American Health Organization/WHO estimates (2006), 75 million people from Mexico to Argentina are at risk of infection. Currently, 300 000 new infections are assumed per year; 8 to 12 million people suffer from chronic infections; about 11 000 people died from Chagas' disease in 2008. The geographic distribution of the disease is determined by the occurrence of hematophagous triatomine (reduviid) bugs. High infection rates are found among poor people living in rural areas and in slums under poor sanitary conditions. Highest seroprevalences within 22 American countries, where Chagas' disease is endemic, were observed in Bolivia (6.75%), Argentina (4.13%), El Salvador (3.37%), Honduras (3.05%), and Paraguay (2.54%); in the other countries prevalence rates of 0.7 to 2.0% are reported. Seroprevalences of up to >70% were observed in hyperendemic areas of, for example, Columbia.

The various DTUs, which are of basic importance in the epidemiology and outcome of *T. cruzi* infections, show relatively specific geographical distributions. In general, *Tc*I predominates and is abundant north of the Amazon basin

(United States, Mexico, Central America, northern South American countries). Human infections in Central and the north of South America are associated with cardiomyopathy. *Tc*II predominates in the southern and central region of South America. It is associated with cardiac alterations and concomitant intestinal megasyndroms. *Tc*III occurs mostly in Brazil and adjacent countries. Relatively few human infections due to this DTU have been documented. *Tc*IV shows a similar distribution as *Tc*III but is rare in the Chaco area. It is relatively frequently found in humans. *Tc*V and *Tc*VI are associated with human Chagas' disease in Southern and Central South America.

T. cruzi has been detected in more than 150 domestic and wild animal species that act as natural hosts and reservoirs, for example, bats, armadillos, opossums, and rodents in sylvatic cycles; dogs, cats, and pigs are epidemiologically important, particularly in domestic cycles. Birds are resistant, but they may be hosts of reduviid bugs.

Natural vectors and intermediate hosts of *T. cruzi* are >35 species of blood sucking, winged reduviid bugs (vinchugas, kissing bugs) of the subfamily Triatominae (family Reduviidae). They suck blood at all stages (five larval stages and adults) and reach sizes up to 28 mm. They live in burrows, birds' nests, and hideouts of wild animals. Some species, such as *Triatoma infestans, Rhodnius prolixus, Panstrongylus megistus*, populate houses and stables in rural areas, but have also found habitats in towns. The prevalence of infection within a population of bugs varies but may approximate 100%. Various haplotypes of *T. cruzi* are associated with specific vector species.

In the United States, infections with *T. cruzi* have been detected in 24 species of wildlife mammals; woodrats (*Neotoma* spp.) are the most common reservoir in the southwestern states; in eastern countries mostly raccoons, opossums, armadillos, and skunks are infected. Eleven species of triatome bugs were found. Presumably, due to low reduviid vector density and good housing, human infections are rare in the United States. By testing blood donors, 23 chronic autochthonous cases were reported from 1987 to 2008. The general prevalence was 1 in 354 000 blood donors. However, imported cases (in immigrants from Latin American countries) are numerous: more than 300 000 immigrants are assumed to be chronically infected with *T. cruzi*.

Transmission. Transmission of *T. cruzi* to humans takes place by several routes: (i) by infected reduviid bugs, (ii) by transfusion of blood products or (iii) organ transplants, (iv) congenitally, and (v) orally.

i. In spite of successful control measures against the vectors in several South American countries, transmission by reduviid bugs is still the most important mode of infection (80 to 90% of all cases). Specific characteristics are allocated in natural cycles to the various DTUs. *Tc*I is commonly associated with sylvatic cycles of transmission and arboreal animals as reservoirs whereas the lineages, which predominate more south, have more terrestrial reservoirs and are often transmitted in domestic cycles. Cumulative analyses suggest arborean hosts as original hosts for *Tc*I, for example, opossums (*Didelphis* spp.) and burrowing animals, for example, armadillos, as natural terrestrial hosts of the other DTUs.

Triatomine bugs are infected by feeding on mammals, including humans, which harbor the trypomastigote stage in the blood (see life cycle: Fig. 4.6). In the anterior midgut (stomach) of the vector, parasites differentiate into another characteristic morphological stage, the so-called epimastigote stage (kinetoplasts are in close proximity to the nucleus). Extensive binary fissions of the trypanosomes ensue in the intestine of the bug, predominantly at the posterior end. [According to the mode of transmission by their vector, *T. cruzi* has been classified into the major group Stercoraria (transmitted via feces), in contrast to the African *Trypanosoma* spp., which belong to the Salivaria (transmitted with saliva)]. Finally, the epimastigotes in the rectal contents differentiate into a trypomastigote (metacyclic) form, which is infectious for the vertebrate host.

Transmission of infective, metacyclic trypanosomes to humans (or animals) takes place after a blood meal of the infected bugs, which then defecate before leaving the (sleeping) prey. Trypanosomes are shed in large numbers with the liquid fecal material. The painful stab wound causes rubbing/scratching, bringing the parasites into the wound or onto mucous membranes of the eye, mouth, or nose (smear

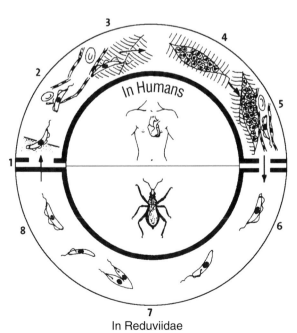

In Reduviidae

Figure 4.6 | Developmental cycle of *T. cruzi*. (1) Metacyclic (infectious) trypanosomes are transmitted by contaminated feces of triatomine bugs to humans. They enter the body through feeding lesions or via intact mucosa. (2) They spend a short time in the peripheral blood (no reproduction). (3) Parasites enter myocardial and endothelial cells of internal organs, e.g., spleen, RES, and liver. (4) Parasites reproduce in the amastigote (unflagellated) stage and form cysts. (5) Parasitized cells burst; organisms are transformed into trypomastigote (flagellated) forms, with a temporary appearance in the peripheral blood. Host cells are infected further. (6) Triatomine bugs ingest parasitized blood. (7) Parasites transform into epimastigote forms and rapidly reproduce in intestine of bugs. (8) Organisms are transformed into metacyclic trypanosomes and colonize the rectal ampoule.

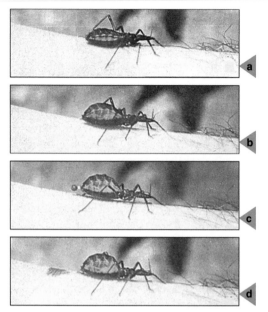

Figure 4.7 | Infection of humans with *T. cruzi*. An infected triatomine bug pierces the skin (**a**) and sucks blood and increases in size while feeding (**b**). After feeding, the bug sheds a fecal droplet containing infectious trypanosomes (**c**), which spreads on the skin (**d**). Through feeding lesions, abrasions, or mucous membranes (conjunctiva, etc.), trypanosomes reach blood vessels. (From product information for Lampit [nifurtimox; Bayer].)

infection); from where they start to invade the host (see Fig. 4.7). The parasites invade macrophages, muscle cells, neuroglia and other cell types, transform to amastigots, and multiply by binary fission within a doubling time of approximately 12 h. After 4 to 5 days the parasites transform to trypomastigotes again; the host cell ruptures and releases the parasites into the blood, from where they may be ingested again by blood sucking bugs or infect new cells.

ii. Transmission via transfusion of blood products was a frequent mode of transmission, causing 5 to 20% of human infections. The importance, however, decreased, as almost all Latin American countries have introduced a compulsory screening of donated blood and blood products for *T. cruzi*. The current risk in Latin America in countries where screening is implemented is estimated to be 1 in 200 000.

iii. Naturally, *T. cruzi* infections by organ transplants are rare events. Nevertheless, a considerable number of parasite transmissions to uninfected recipients by transplants is documented. Otherwise, it is not an inevitable consequence; in several cases, individual recipients of organs from a common, infected donor remained either free of *T. cruzi* or became infected. Also, the kind of organs plays a role in this respect. Due to these observations, and in consideration of the general shortage of suitable donor organs, guidelines of the "Chagas Disease Argentine Collaborative Transplant Consortium" (2010) recommend relaxing the selection criteria for deceased donors in a way that organs from infected donors can be used under certain circumstances.

iv. One to 10% of infants from *T. cruzi* infected mothers are born with congenital Chagas' disease, but high regional differences are reported. HIV infection of the mother increases the risk of the fetus. Congenital infections amount to >15 000 cases per year in the Americas, representing 5 to 10% of total new infections. They are responsible for spreading the disease also to areas of nonendemicity, for example, to Europe. Cases of galactogenous transmission of *T. cruzi* to children are documented too.

v. Oral transmission of *T. cruzi* has been increasingly reported in recent years. Fruit juices, fruits, or sweets contaminated with feces of infected reduviid bugs seem to be the major sources. Metacyclic stages of *T. cruzi* survive, for example, on pieces of sugar cane for at least 24 h. The largest outbreak known after oral infection happened in a school in Caracas (Venezuela) and concerned >100 scholars and staff persons.

Clinical Manifestations. Chagas' disease is complex. In principle, four different phases must be differentiated in its course, that is, an early locally expressed chancre stage, a succeeding acute phase, a usually long lasting intermediate phase, and a chronic phase with destructive pathology. The severity of symptoms and the individual outcome underlie various factors with parasite and host genetics playing central roles. As a general tendency, chronic megasyndroms are relatively rare in the northern Amazon area but common in the southern part of South America, possibly associated with the geographical predominance of TcI and TcII-VI, respectively (TcIII is rarely found in humans). Otherwise, acute disease types seem to be often associated with TcI. Particular interest is attracted by the observation that in mixed *T. cruzi* infections, parasites of different genotypes accumulate in different host tissues. The role of host factors [e.g., of major histocompatibility complex (MHC)] in the course of Chagas' disease is only partly evaluated and complicated by often contradictory results. In fact, some data suggest that cardiotropism of the parasites is influenced by host genetics at the MHC locus; however, due to the genetic complexicity of both parasite and host the underlying causal mechanisms are still not understood.

Clinical disease starts about 7 days post infection (p.i.), when a chancre (chagoma), an erythematous, indurated, slightly painful swelling, and a regional lymphadenopathy develop at the cutaneous site of parasite entry. If the parasite enters via the conjunctiva, the so-called Romana sign is observed, a unilateral, painless edematous swelling of eyelids and periocular tissue (Fig. 4.8).

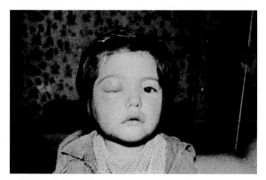

Figure 4.8 | Edema of the eyelids in a child with acute Chagas' disease as an early symptom of infection with *T. cruzi* (Romaña sign), a reaction to local multiplication of parasites.

Within 10 to 30 days p.i., about 30% of the patients develop an acute, generalized disease. Patients suffer from fever (at first intermittent), general malaise, anorexia, edema of face and lower extremities, occasionaly generalized lymphadenopathy, hepatosplenomegaly, and a measles-like exanthema. In some cases, especially in young children, severe myocarditis with congestive heart failure (mortality, 2 to 3%) or meningoencephalitis (mortality in children, 50%) may occur.

With development of cellular and humoral immune responses, symptoms resolve slowly, within 2 to 3 months, even without treatment, and acute disease enters the indeterminate (latent) phase, with asymptomatic low-grade parasitemia, and positive antibody responses to *T. cruzi* antigens. This stage may persist lifelong.

Ten to 20 years after infection, however, in 10 to 30% of the patients (mostly middle-aged people), chronic Chagas' disease develops as a result of progressive cell destruction, especially of mycardial and autonomous ganglion cells, due to the parasites and, presumably, also by autoimmune processes. Clinical symptoms are cardiomyopathy (in 30% of patients); ventricular arrhythmia, especially right bundle-branch block; biventricular heart failure; thromboembolism; gastrointestinal megasyndrome (in 6% of patients), that is, megaesophagus, megagaster (symptoms: dysphagia, regurgitation, achalasia, cachexia, aspiration, and aspiration pneumonia), and megacolon (symptoms: severe constipation, obstruction, intestinal volvulus, and septicemia); meningoencephalitis (in 3% of patients) (symptoms: dementia and psychotic changes of personality); and endocrinopathies (symptoms: adrenal insufficiency and myxedema due to parasitic thyroiditis).

HIV infection or immunosuppression after organ transplantation may lead to early recrudescence, rapid progression, and adverse course of chronic Chagas' disease. In patients with HIV, brain abscesses due to *T. cruzi* are frequently observed.

Congenital infections in 1 to 10% of pregnancies of chronically infected mothers cause abortion and intrauterine fetal death or neonatal *T. cruzi* infection with fever, icterus, anemia, thrombocytopenia, splenomegaly, skin lesions containing parasites, myocarditis, pneumonia, and meningoencephalitis. Exceptionally severe courses are observed in HIV-coinfected neonates.

Diagnosis. Clinical symptoms and epidemiological history, especially of areas of endemicity with poor living conditions, allow a presumptive diagnosis. Diagnostic proof of Chagas' disease is the microscopic detection of *T. cruzi*. Parasites can be demonstrated at the earliest 1 to 2 weeks p.i.; highest levels of parasitemia are found between 30 and 90 days after infection. Especially in the acute stage with high parasitemia, the parasites can be detected in anticoagulated peripheral blood or in buffy coat or in thick blood films. Unstained preparations (motile trypanosomes) of fresh, anticoagulated blood or Giemsa-stained blood smears may be used. In patients with low parasitemia (latent or chronic phase), biopsies of lymph nodes or bone marrow aspirates may yield more positive results. Alternatively, *in vitro* culture techniques [e.g., Novy-McNeal-Nicolle (NNN) medium, 25 °C, 30 days of incubation], animal inoculation [intraperitoneal (i.p.) injection of blood into mice], or xenodiagnosis may be used. For xenodiagnosis, laboratory-reared bugs are fed on a patient suspected of being infected with *T. cruzi*. It takes at least a month to complete (specifity, 100%; sensitivity, 50 to 70%). Highest specifity and sensitivity is reached by PCR techniques, which are currently standardized by international cooperations. DTU determination uses PCR based techniques.

T. cruzi must be differentiated from the apathogenic species *T. rangeli*. The latter is larger (26 to 36 μm) than *T. cruzi* (17 to 20 μm) and shows a distinctly smaller subterminal kinetoplast. Molecular biological techniques are more satisfying than morphological differentiation.

Serologic techniques are important during latent and chronic phases. Particularly ELISAs and IFAs are largely standardized, sold as kits, and give reliable results in individual cases, including in monitoring of pregnant women and in the control of blood donors. In most endemic countries, two independent assays are applicable as a standard procedure in screening. To determine connatal infections as early as possible, umbilical cord blood and tissue are investigated by PCR. In case of negative results in suspected cases, repeated subsequent examinations are recommended as parasitemia increases within 4 to 10 weeks in neonates. In addition, it should be attempted to detect specific IgM antibodies in the neonate (no intrauterine transfer of IgM to fetuses).

Differential Diagnosis. Typhus, influenzal syndrome, visceral leishmaniasis, malaria, schistosomiasis, brucellosis, and infectious mononucleosis have to be considered in the acute and early chronic stage. In the chronic stage, cardiomyopathy and congestive heart failure of other etiologies, achalasia and pseudo-obstruction due to various neoplasms, cytomegalovirus (CMV) infection, myotonic dystrophy, and von Recklinghausen neurofibromatosis must be excluded.

Therapy. The drugs of choice are nifurtimox and benznidazole, which are especially effective during the acute phase of Chagas' disease. They eliminate the parasites in 70 to 80% of the patients and reduce the severity and duration of the disease and the mortality. Whether these drugs are also effective during the intermediate and chronic phases is still not clear. However, as *T. cruzi* is present in the myocardium of chronically sick patients and long-term treatment reduces duration of symptoms and parasitemia and decreases mortality, treatment of all stages of Chagas' disease is strongly recommended.

Nifurtimox should be administered orally in four divided doses for 90 to 120 days as follows: for adults, 8 to 10 mg/kg/day; for adolescents (>11 to 16 years), 12.5 to 15 mg/kg/day; for children (<11 years old), 15 to 20 mg/kg/day. Similar efficacy is obtained with benznidazole, 5 to 7 mg/kg/day in two divided doses, orally over a period of 30 to 90 days. Neonates and children <1 year are treated with 10 mg/kg/day and 10 to 15 mg/kg/day, respectively, for 60 days. Take drugs with meals!

Side effects of treatment are gastrointestinal disturbances, including abdominal pain, vomiting, nausea, anorexia, and weight loss. Neurological side effects include insomnia, restlessness, twitching, paresthesias, and seizures. These symptoms are reversible by reduction of dose or suspension of therapy.

Additional application of recombinant gamma interferon showed favorable effects in some patients with acute Chagas' disease and is presumably indicated for immunosuppressed patients.

Surgical intervention is indicated for patients with megaesophagus and megacolon. Cardiomyopathy and cardiac arrhythmias are treated by cardiologists (with medication or peacemaker or, if needed, by cardiac transplantation). Due to indispensable postoperative immunosuppression, Chagas' disease may be reactivated, but is preventable by nifurtimox therapy.

Prophylaxis. Chemoprophylaxis is not possible and an effective vaccine is not available. The main control measures are efficient vector control and improvement of housing and living conditions for people in rural areas to avoid infestation with triatomine bugs. For example, *T. cruzi* transmission by *T. infestans* has been at least partly interrupted in Argentina, Paraguay, and Chile. Travelers in countries where Chagas' disease is endemic should avoid potentially bug-infested areas and should use insect repellents. However, resistances must be expected.

REFERENCES

Almeida AE et al., Chagas' disease and HIV co-infection in patients without effective antiretroviral therapy: prevalence, clinical presentation and natural history. *Trans. R. Soc. Trop. Med. Hyg.* 104, 447–452, 2010.

Andrade M et al., Clinical and serological evaluation in chronic Chagas disease patients in a 4 year pharmacotherapy follow up: a preliminary study. *Rev. Soc. Bras. Med. Trop.* 46, 706–708, 2013.

Bern C et al., Congenital *Trypanosoma cruzi* transmission in Santa Cruz, Bolivia. *Clin. Infect. Dis.* 49, 1667–1674, 2009.

Blanco SB et al., Congenital transmission of *Trypanosoma cruzi*: an operational outline for detecting and treating infected infants in north-western Argentina. *Trop. Med. Int. Health* 5, 293–301, 2000.

Britto CC, Usefulness of PCR-based assays to assess drug efficacy in Chagas disease chemotherapy: value and limitations. *Mem. Inst. Oswaldo Cruz* 104, Suppl. 1, 122–135, 2009.

Bruckner FS, Navabi N, Advances of Chagas disease drug development: 2009-2010. *Curr. Opin. Infect. Dis.* 23, 609–616, 2010.

Carod-Artal FJ, Stroke: a neglected complication of American trypanosomiasis (Chagas' disease). *Trans. R. Soc. Trop.Med. Hyg.* 10, 1075–1080, 2007.

Chippaux JP et al., Antibody drop in newborns congenitally infected by *Trypanosoma cruzi* treated with benznidazole. *Trop. Med. Int. Health* 15, 87–93, 2010.

Córdova E et al., Neurological manifestations of Chagas' disease. *Neurol. Res.* 32, 238–244,2010.

Diazgranados CA et al., Chagasic encephalitis in HIV patients: common presentation of an evolving epidemiological and clinical association. *Lancet Infect Dis.* 9, 324–330, 2009.

Dutra WO, Rocha MOC, Teixeira MM, The clinical immunology of human Chagas disease. *Trends Parasitol.* 21, 581–587, 2005.

Espinoza N et al., Chagas disaese vector control in a hyperendemic setting: the first 11 years after intervention in Cochabamba, Bolivia. *PLoS Negl. Trop. Dis.* 8, e2782, 2014.

Frade AF et al., Genetic susceptibility to Chagas disease cardiomyopathy: involvement of several genes of the innate immunity and chemokine dependent migration pathways. *BMC Infect. Dis.* 13, 587, 2013.

Garcia Borrás S et al., Distribution of HLA-DRB1 alleles in Argentinean patients with Chagas' disease cardiomypathy. *Immunol. Invest.* 38, 268–275, 2009.

Gomes YM, Lorena VMB, Luquetti AO, Diagnosis of Chagas disease: what has been achieved? What remains to be done with regard to diagnosis and follow up studies. *Mem. Inst. Oswaldo Cruz* 104, Suppl 1, 115–121, 2009.

Gutierrez FRS et al., The role of parasite persistence in pathogenesis of Chagas heart disease. *Parasite Immunol.* 31, 673–685, 2009.

Kirchhoff LV, Epidemiology of American trypanosomiasis (Chagas disease). *Adv. Parasitol.* 75, 1–18, 2011.

Kjos SA et al., Distribution and characterization of canine Chagas disease in Texas. *Vet. Parasitol.* 152, 249–256, 2008.

Kransdorf P et al., Heart transplantation for Chagas cardiomyopathy in the United States. *Am. J. Transplant.* 13, 3262–3268, 2013.

Marin-Neto JA et al., Pathogenesis of chronic Chagas heart disease. *Circulation* 115, 1109–1123, 2007.

Meneghelli UG, Chagasic enteropathy. *Rev. Soc. Bras. Med. Trop.* 37, 252–260, 2004.

Mejia-Jaramillio A et al., Genotyping of *Trypanosoma cruzi* in a hyperendemic area of Columbia reveals an overlap among domestic and sylvatic cycles of Chagas disease. *Parasites & Vectors* 7, 108, 2014.

Nieto A et al., HLA haplotypes are associated with differential susceptibility to *Trypanosoma cruzi* infection. *Tissue Antigens* 55, 195–198, 2000.

Punukollu G et al., Clinical aspects of the Chagas' heart disease. *Int. J. Cardiol.* 115, 279–283, 2007.

Rosecrans K et al., Opportunities for improved Chagas disease vector control based on knowledge, attitudes and practices of communities in the Yucatan Peninsula, Mexico. *PLoS Negl. Trop. Dis.* 8, e2763, 2014.

Schmunis GA, Epidemiology of Chagas disease in non-endemic countries: the role of international migration. *Mem. Inst. Oswaldo Cruz* 102, Suppl.1, 75–85, 2007.

Schmunis GA, Cruz JR, Safety of the blood supply in Latin America. *Clin. Microbiol. Rev.* 18, 12–29, 2005.

Solari A et al., Treatment of *Trypanosoma cruzi*-infected children with nifurtimox: a 3 year follow-up by PCR. *J. Antimicrob. Chemother.* 48, 515–519, 2001.

Sosa-Estani S, Viotti R, Segura EL, Therapy, diagnosis and prognosis of chronic Chagas disease: insight gained in Argentina. *Mem. Inst. Oswaldo Cruz* 104, Suppl. 1, 167–1180, 2009.

Urbina JA, Specific chemotherapy of Chagas disease: relevance, current limitations and new approaches. *Acta Trop.* 115, 55-68, 2009.

4.2.5 CRYPTOSPORIDIOSIS

The genus *Cryptosporidium*, first described as *Cryptosporidium muris* in the beginning of the last century, was neglected for a long time, until it turned out that cryptosporidia are the agents of an economically important diarrheic disease of very young calves and, in particular, causes life-threatening diseases in immunocompromised humans.

Etiology. The protozoa of the genus *Cryptosporidium* are classified as eukaryotes in the phylum Apicomplexa as a special form of the "single host" coccidian parasites. On the basis of DNA sequence analyses, and considering host preferences, morphological criteria (oocyst size), and other characteristics, currently 30 species are distinguished, in mammals, birds, fishes, reptiles, and amphibians. In addition, >60 genotypes are known with uncertain status. More than 150 animal species were described shedding *Cryptosporidium* oocysts.

Fourteen *Cryptosporidium* species have been found in humans (see Tab. 4.3). By far the most common agents in humans are *C. hominis* (previously genotype Human I or anthroponotic type of *C. parvum*), and *C. pestis* (previously Bovine II genotype of *C. parvum*). These species are responsible for >90% and 80% of infections in immunocompetent and immunocompromised patients, respectively. *C. hominis* is a pathogenic species in humans and occurs rarely in calves and lambs. *C. pestis* is found predominantly in young calves, but also in lambs and other ungulates. Furthermore, *C. meleagridis* (a species infecting birds and mammals), *C. felis* (from cats), *C. viatorum*, an obviously worldwide distributed species, which was recently detected in humans (animal reservoir hosts are unknown), and *C. cuniculus* from rabbits are species that infect immunocompetent and immunocompromised humans and may be of some public health significance. In contrast, *C. ubiquitum* (various mammals), *C. canis* (from

Table 4.3 | *Cryptosporidium* spp. found in humans

SPECIES	NATURAL HOSTS	IMPORTANCE IN HUMANS
C. hominis	Humans, rarely ruminants	+++
C. pestis	Calves (<2 weeks of age), other mammals, humans	+++
C. meleagridis	Various birds and mammals	++
C. felis	Cats	++
C. viatorum	?	++
C. cuniculus	Rabbits, other mammals	++
C. canis	Dogs, other canids	+
C. ubiquitum	Mammals	+
C. muris	Mice, various mammals, birds	+
C. andersoni	Cattle (heifers and older animals)	(+)
C. parvum	Mice, various mammals	(+)
C. fayeri	Marsupials	(+)
C. scrofarum	Domestic and wild pigs	(+)
C. suis	Pigs (<5 weeks of age)	(+)

dogs and other canids), *C. muris* (from rodents), *C. andersoni* (from cattle), *C. parvum* (previously the Mouse I genotype of *C. parvum*), *C. fayeri* (from marsupials) and the pig infesting species, *C. scrofarum* and *C. suis*, are of minor importance, with rare or very rare human infections. Moreover, several other genotypes were found in human feces, for example, the Chipmunk genotype I in Sweden, and a horse genotype in the United States.

Occurrence. Human infections with cryptosporidia occur worldwide, either sporadical or endemic. The estimated incidence of confirmed or probable cases of cryptosporidiosis in the United States is 4 per 100 000 population. The prevalence in Central Europe (determined by oocyst excretion) is about 2%, and in developing countries, it is approximately 10%. Children are involved more often than adults are and a higher prevalence is found in AIDS patients. Diarrheic immunocompetent and HIV infected patients shed *Cryptosporidium* oocysts by 5% and >25%, respectively. Cryptosporidiosis was observed after transmission in swimming pools and by contaminated drinking water. In 1993, an outbreak in Milwaukee, WI, caused by contaminated drinking water resulted in diarrhea in more than 400 000 people. In general, *Cyptosporidium* infections in humans may be underdiagnosed, because usual methods used for routine coproscopical surveys are not suited for the detection of the oocysts.

Cryptosporidia have been found in >150 mammalian species. Predominantly young animals are infected. For example, in Central Europe >50% of healthy calves shed *Cryptosporidium* oocysts with the feces during their first weeks of life. Predominantly calves and lambs are clinically threatened up to the 4th week of life. The animals usually recover after a period of diarrhea of 4 to 6 days, although in some stocks, persistent problems with severe diseases are reported.

Transmission. Infection occurs by ingestion of thick-walled oocysts that are shed with the feces by infected hosts (Fig. 4.9). *Cryptosporidium* oocysts are already sporulated, that is,

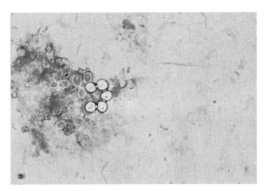

Figure 4.9 | Cryptosporidia (unstained oocysts) and yeasts in calf feces and "negative staining" with carbolfuchsin (picture: Institute for Parasitology, Giessen, Germany).

infectious, when they are excreted, and may survive in the environment for months. The human disease is frequently associated with traveling, contact with livestock, or person-to-person transmission, for example, in day care centers and medical institutions. The 50% infective dose for humans is between 50 and 100 oocysts or even lower in particular parasite strains. Routes of transmission are person-to-person, by direct or indirect contact, including homosexual activities (anilingus); animal to human; contaminated water (drinking water, water in swimming pools, or sewage); and food-borne by surface contamination of vegetables, fruits, meat, and seafood. There are also numerous reports of airborne transmission of the disease by aerosols, predominantly in children and immunocompromised persons (lethal respiratory cryptosporidiosis).

In addition to thick-walled oocysts, a second type of oocysts develops (Fig. 4.10), which is thin-walled and hardly resists environmental effects. However, these oocysts may lead to endogenous autoinfections and are probably the cause of persistent infection and disease in immunocompromised patients.

Clinical Manifestations. Cryptosporidia primarily infect the intestinal epithelium but may be disseminated to epithelial cells of other organs, for example, the bile duct or the respiratory tract. In immunocompetent people, infection is frequently asymptomatic; however, the

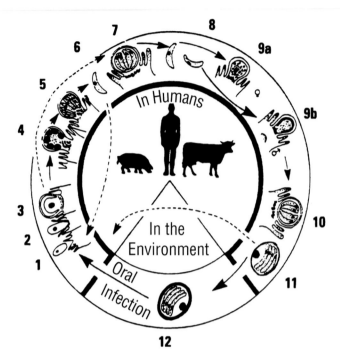

7
8
6
9a
5
9b
In Humans
4
3
10
2
In the
Environment
1
Oral
Infection
11
12

Figure 4.10 | Developmental cycle of *Cryptosporidium* spp. (modified from Eckert, 1984). (1) Sporozoite set free in stomach and duodenum approaching intestinal epithelium; (2) sporozoite with basal adhesive zone between microvilli of an intestinal cell; (3) young schizont within vacuole; (4) dividing schizont; (5) mature schizont with eight merozoites (type I meront); (6) free merozoite becomes attached to epithelial cell; (7) mature schizont with four merozoites (type II meront) (repeat of schizogonic process); (8) free merozoites; (9a) macrogamete; (9b) microgamont with nonflagellated microgametes; (10) thick-walled oocyst (permanent stage in environment); (11) thin-walled oocyst leading to endogenous autoinfection (ca. 20% of formed cysts); (12) sporulated oocyst containing four sporozoites, shed with feces (thick walled; oral infection).

clinical course partially depends on the parasite species. *C. pestis* infections, for example, in general tend to more inapparent courses than *C. hominis* infections. Clinically, overt disease develops after an incubation period of 5 to 28 days. Symptoms are profuse watery diarrhea without blood, epigastric pain, nausea, anorexia fever, and weight loss. Without therapy, disease in immunocompetent patients is usually self-limiting and lasts for 1 to 2 weeks. Oocyst excretion starts 4 to 5 days p.i. and continues for 5 to 10 days.

Immunocompromised patients, particularly patients with AIDS and <50 CD4$^+$ T lymphocytes/mm^3 blood and those receiving immunosuppressive treatment, develop persistent, profuse, watery, cholera-like diarrhea (volumes 1 to 25 l/day) with dehydration, malabsorption, weight loss, cachexia, and wasting syndrome. Especially in patients with HIV, cryptosporidia also colonize the bile duct, causing cholangitis, cholecystitis, and pancreatitis. Cryptosporidia have also been found in the respiratory tract, usually together with other respiratory pathogens. Their origin at this site (possibly contamination or inhalation of aerosol) is unclear.

Diagnosis. The small oocysts (4 to 5 μm) can be demonstrated in stool, duodenal secretions, or bile, if necessary after concentration, by flotation using Sheather's sugar or zinc sulphate solution, by direct examination (phase contrast), or by staining (Giemsa, auramin-rhodamine, modified Ziehl-Neelsen, or Kinyoun staining or fluorescent antibody technique). Also, a "negative staining" with Carbol-fuchsin is recommended (oocysts remain unstained and contrast to other components of feces; see Fig. 4.9). Coproantigens can be demonstrated by ELISA. PCR techniques are generally very sensitive and specific. It has generally to be considered that oocyst excretion is often irregular. Thus, negative results have to be confirmed by repeated examinations.

Differential Diagnosis. Diarrheas of different etiology, exsudative gastroenteropathy, Verner-Morrison syndrome (apudoma or "pancreatic cholera"), and endocrine tumors of the gastrointestinal tract (gastrinoma or somatostatinoma) must be considered in the differential diagnosis.

Therapy. In immunocompetent patients, the infection is usually self-limiting; fluid and electrolyte levels must be restored. The scope of causative therapy measures is limited. Nitazoxanide, 500 mg twice a day, orally for 3 days is the drug of choice. Diarrhea and oocyst excretion had ceased in 90% of the patients 4 days after treatment. The effect was weaker and uncertain in HIV patients. Partial success was achieved with 500 mg twice a day for 2 weeks or 500 mg three to four times a day over 12 weeks. Paromomycin, 500 mg four times a day orally plus azithromycin, 600 mg one or two times a day orally for at least 4 weeks (thereafter, paromomycin alone) is recommended.

For symptomatic treatment of profuse diarrhea, antidiarrheic drugs (loperamide, several opiates, octreotide) are used. The best treatment of life-threatening cryptosporidiosis in HIV patients is highly active antiretroviral combination therapy (HAART).

Prophylaxis. *Cryptosporidium* spp. oocysts resist disinfectants, for example, 3% sodium hypochlorite solution, iodophores, and 5% formaldehyde. They lose their infectivity after heating to 73 °C for 1 min. Modern techniques of drinking water treatment, including ozone and UV light disinfection, inactivate *Cryptosporidium* oocysts. As shedding of oocysts still persists for approximately 2 weeks after symptoms have disappeared, cured patients should avoid public swimming pools at least for this period.

Immunosuppressed patients should avoid direct skin contact with human or animal feces or garden soil, should not swim in public baths, and should drink boiled or filtered water only.

REFERENCES

Ajjampur SSP, Sankaran P, Kang G, *Cryptosporidium* species in HIV-infected individuals in India: an overview. *Natl. Med. J. India* 21, 178–184, 2008.

Amer S et al., *Cryptosporidium* genotypes and subtypes in dairy calves in Egypt. *Vet. Parasitol.* 169, 382–386, 2010.

Betancourt WQ, Rose JB, Drinking water treatment processes for removal of *Cryptosporidium* and *Giardia*. *Vet. Parasitol.* 126, 219–234, 2004.

Cacció SM et al., Unravelling *Cryptosporidium* and *Giardia* epidemiology. *Trends Parasitol.* 21, 430–437, 2005.

Chalmers RM, Davies AP, Minireview: Clinical cryptosporidiosis. *Exp. Parasitol.* 124, 138–146, 2010.

Chalmers RM et al., Long-term *Cryptosporidium* typing reveals the aetiology and species-specific epidemiology of human cryptosporidiosis in England and Wales, 2000 to 2003. *Euro. Surveill.* 14, 19086, 2009.

Chappell CL et al., *Cryptosporidium meleagridis*. Infectivity in healthy adult volunteers. *Am. J. Trop. Med. Hyg.* 85, 238–242, 2011.

De Waele V et al., Control of cryptosporidiosis in neonatal calves: use of halofuginone lactate in two different calf rearing systems. *Prev. Vet. Med.* 96, 143–151, 2010.

Feltus DC et al., Evidence supporting zoonotic transmission of *Cryptosporidium* spp. in Wisconsin. *J. Clin. Microbiol.* 44, 4303–4308, 2006.

Feng Y, Li N, Xiao L, *Cryptosporidium* genotype and subtype distribution in raw wastewater in Shanghai, China: evidence for possible unique *Cryptosporidium hominis* transmission. *J. Clin. Microbiol.* 47, 153–157, 2009.

Hale CR et al., Estimates of enteric illness attributable to contact with animals and their environment in the United States. *Clin. Infect. Dis.* 54, Suppl. 5: S472–479, 2012.

Jagal JS et al., Seasonality of cryptosporidiosis: a meta-analysis approach. *Environ. Res.* 109, 465–478, 2009.

Kvác M et al., Prevalence and age-related infection of *Cryptosporidium suis*, *C. muris*, and *Cryptosporidium* pig genotype II in pigs on a farm complex in the Czech Republic. *Vet. Parasitol.* 160, 319–322, 2009.

Lebbad M et al., Unusual cryptosporidiosis cases in Swedish patients: extended molecular characterization of *Cryptosporidium viatorum* and *Cryptosporidium chipmunk* genotype I. *Parasitology.* 140, 1735–1740, 2013.

Lucio-Forster A et al., Minimal zoonotic risk of cryptosporidioses from pet dogs and cats. *Trends Parasitol.* 26, 174–179, 2010.

Ng JS et al., Molecular characterization of *Cryptosporidium* outbreaks in Western and South Australia. *Exp. Parasitol.* 125, 325–328, 2010.

Plutzer J, Karanis P, Genetic polymorphism in *Cryptosporidium* species: an update. *Vet. Parasitol.* 165, 187–199, 2009.

Rossignol JF, *Cryptosporidium* and *Giardia* treatment options and prospects for new drugs. *Exp. Parasitol.* 124, 45–53, 2010.

Ryan U, *Cryptosporidium* in birds, fish and amphibians. *Exp. Parasitol.* 124, 113–120, 2010.

Schnyder M et al., Prophylactic and therapeutic efficacy of nitazoxanide against *Cryptosporidium parvum* in experimentally challenged neonatal calves. *Vet. Parasitol.* 160, 149–154, 2009.

Slapeta J, Cryptosporidiosis and *Cryptosporidium* species in animals and humans: A thirty colour rainbow. *Int. J. Parasitol.* 43, 957–970, 2013.

Smith HV, Nichols RA, *Cryptosporidium*: detection in water and food. *Exp. Parasitol.* 124: 61–79, 2009.

Tzipori S, Widmer G, A hundred-year retrospective on cryptosporidiosis. *Trends Parasitol.* 24: 184–189, 2008.

Yoder JS, Beach MJ, *Cryptosporidium* surveillance and risk factors in the United States. *Exp. Parasitol.* 12, 31–39, 2010.

Xiao L, Molecular epidemiology of cryptosporidiosis: an update. *Exp. Parasitol.* 124, 80–89, 2010.

4.2.6 GIARDIASIS (LAMBLIASIS)

Giardiasis is caused by the ubiquitous flagellated protozoon *Giardia duodenalis* (syn. *G. lamblia* or *G. intestinalis*). It is a clinically highly variable disease, predominantly of the small intestine.

Etiology. *G. duodenalis* belongs to the class Mastigophora. The motile, vegetative form (trophozoite), a 10 to 20 µm long and 8 to 15 µm wide, pear-shaped flagellate with two nuclei and eight flagella (four pairs; Fig. 4.11) parasitizes the proximal part of the jejunum and occasionally the gall bladder; it fixes to the intestinal wall by a sucker-like structure. Trophozoites multiply by binary fission. Infective stages are oval-shaped, thin-walled cysts, 8 to 14 µm long and 7 to 10 µm wide, which contain two parasites (four nuclei).

G. duodenalis is a complex of eight morphologically indistinguishable genotypes (assemblages, partly divided into subassemblages), with different host specificities (see Tab. 4.4). Only genotypes A I, A II, and B III and B IV are zoonotic pathogens, in which A II seems to be

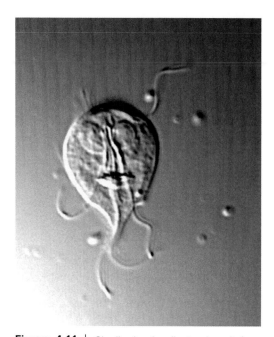

Figure 4.11 | *Giardia duodenalis*: trophozoit from feces. Interference contrast (picture: Institute of Parasitology, Zurich, Switzerland).

Table 4.4 | Genetic grouping and occurrence of *Giardia intestinalis* assemblages

ASSEMBLAGES	HOSTS
A[1]	Humans, other primates, dogs, cats, various other wild and domestic animals, including freshwater and marine fish
B[2]	Humans, other primates, dogs, some wild and domestic animals, fish
C, D	Canids
E	Cattle, other ungulates
F	Cats
G	Rats
H	Marine mammals (pinnipeds)

[1] Four subassemblages (AI to AIV); AI and AII (predominantly) found in humans; AIII and AIV isolates from various animals.
[2] Four subassemblages (BI to BIV); BI and BII: animal isolates; BIII and BIV: human isolates.

best adapted to humans. The genus *Giardia* contains five additional, morphologically distinct species in rodents, birds, and amphibia.

Occurrence. *Giardia* infections of humans are diagnosed worldwide, but considerable geographical differences exist. Recorded prevalence rates in temperate climates are 2 to 10% in adults and up to 25% in children, whereas in tropical areas, about 50 to 80% of people are carriers. The variable occurrence in distinct groups of the population is possibly related to certain nutritional conditions, that is, consumption of food rich in carbohydrates or starvation. According to WHO estimates, the incidence of symptomatic giardiasis in Asia, Africa, and Latin America is about 200 million, with some 500 000 new infections per year.

Giardia infections are common worldwide in lambs, calves (cumulative incidences up to 100%), and pigs. Zoonotic subassemblages (see Tab. 4.4) are frequently found. Clinical diseases are rare and may occur predominantly in lambs. Overall prevalence rates in dogs and cats of 2 to 15% are reported from North America with higher rates in young animals. Generally, the zoonotic assemblages A and B are found approximately two times more often in pets than assemblages C and D. Numerous species of wild animals are infected with *G. duodenalis* and harbor zoonotic types at a high percentage. A few years ago, freshwater and marine fishes have been shown to be infected with *G. duodenalis*, with an overall prevalence of 2 to 8%. Zoonotic assemblages are common, that is, fish may also be a reservoir for human infections.

Transmission. The infectious cysts of *G. duodenalis* are excreted in large numbers, often several million per day, in feces of infected persons. They may contaminate hands, drinking water, and food. Human and animal feces used as fertilizer contaminate vegetables and fruits. Flies are possible carriers of infectious cysts. Cysts may survive in cold water for several months. Ten to 100 cysts will be sufficient to cause clinical symptoms in humans. Shortcomings of the municipal drinking water treatment resulted in mass infections in recent years in industrial countries (USA, Canada, and Norway). Oral-anal contacts (anilingus) are risky.

Clinical Manifestations. Acute *Giardia* infections may occur in a clinical asymptomatic form but may also cause severe disease. The reasons of such different courses are not fully understood.

The prepatent period lasts 6 to 15 days and the incubation period lasts 7 to 21 days. The main clinical symptoms are a sudden onset of diarrhea accompanied by yellowish, foul-smelling stools without blood, mucus, or pus, abdominal cramps, vomiting, anorexia, nausea, bloating with malodorous flatulence, and sometimes malaise, headache, and chills. Acute and subacute disease may relapse for years, particularly in children 1 to 4 years old in day care centers and, less often, in schoolchildren. The chronic stage presents with periodically occurring diarrhea with malodorous stools and periods of constipation. Abdominal distension and flatulence are also typical. Anorexia, malabsorption, loss of weight, and lethargy are common. Impairment of the B cell system with hypogammaglobulinemia disposes for giardiasis, whereas HIV patients do not seem to be particularly prone.

Relatively often patients complain of a state of exhaustion and persistent gastrointestinal disorders in terms of post infectious irritable bowel syndrome even years after parasite elimination. It concerned 41% of approximately 1000 patients after 2 years after an epidemic in Norway.

Diagnosis. Giardiasis is diagnosed by antigen detection in feces and duodenal aspirates (ELISA using monoclonal antibodies to *Giardia* antigens) and by microscopy of fecal samples for cysts or (rarely seen) trophozoites (SAF and merthiolate-iodine-formaldehyde techniques; fixed smears stained with Wheatley trichrome stain or Giemsa, Heidenhain, or iron-hematoxylin stain). Microscopy (phase or interference contrast) for trophozoites must be done immediately after sampling, as these stages die and lyse rapidly. At least three stool samples should be examined on two or three consecutive days.

Serodiagnostic methods are useful in epidemiological studies. Specific IgM response develops early after infection and lasts for a few weeks. Anti-*Giardia*-IgG antibodies develop late and persist for months or years.

Differential Diagnosis. Giardiasis must be differentiated from bacterial diarrhea, amebic dysentery, salmonellosis, and viral gastroenteritis.

Therapy. The recommended therapy is with tinidazole, 2 g orally, or nitazoxanide, 500 mg twice a day orally for 3 days, or metronidazole, 250 mg three times a day orally for 5 days, or paromomycin, 25 to 35 mg in three divided doses for 5 to 10 days. Antibiotics are contraindicated, as the survival time of *Giardia* is prolonged in largely abacterial environments.

Prophylaxis. Food must be protected from contamination with *Giardia* oocysts. Good water hygiene (i.e., production, processing, and control) is essential (US: National Safety Foundation Standard 53 or Standard 58). In areas of endemicity, animal and human feces should not be used as fertilizers and drinking water should be filtered or boiled (10 min), as *Giardia* cysts resist chlorine. Avoid uncooked food (e.g., salads), in addition, fruit should be peeled.

REFERENCES

Almeida AA et al., Genotype analysis of Giardia isolated from asymptomatic children in northern Portugal. *J Eukaryot. Microbiol.* 53, (Suppl. 1), S177–S178, 2006.

Anonym, From the Ceners of Disease Control and Prevention. Prevalence of parasites in fecal material from chlorinated swimming pools – United States, 1999. *JAMA* 285, 2969, 2001.

As M et al., Temporal patterns of human and canine *Giardia* infection in the United States: 2003–2009. *Prev. Vet. Med.* 113, 249–256, 2014.

Ballweber LR et al., Giardiasis in dogs and cats: update on epidemiology and public health significance. *Trends Parasitol.* 26, 180–189, 2010.

Betancourt WQ, Rose JB, Drinking water treatment processes for removal of Cryptosporidium and Giardia. *Vet. Parasitol.* 126, 219–234, 2004.

Caccio SM et al., Unravelling *Cryptosporidium* and *Giardia* epidemiology. *Trends Parasitol.* 21, 430–437, 2005.

Craun GF, Calderon RL, Craun MF, Outbreaks associated with recreational water in the Unites States. *Int. J. Environ. Health Res.* 15, 243–262, 2005.

Dixon B et al., The potential for zoonotic transmission of *Giardia duodenalis* and *Cryptosporidium* spp. from beef and dairy cattle in Ontario, Canada. *Vet. Parasitol.* 175, 20–26, 2011.

Halliez MC, Buret AG, Extraintestinal and longterm consequences of *Giardia duodenalis* infections. *World Gastroenterol.* 19, 8974–8985, 2013.

Lengerich EJ, Addiss DG, Juranek DD, Severe giardiasis in the United States. *Clin. Infect. Dis.* 18, 760–763, 1994.

Morch K et al., High rate of fatigue and abdominal symptoms 2 years after an outbreak of giardiasis. *Trans. R. Soc. Trop. Med. Hyg.* 103, 530–532, 2009.

Morch K et al., Chronic fatigue syndrome 5 years after giardiasis: differential diagnoses, characteristics and natural course. *BMC Gastroenterol.* 13, 28, 2013.

Robertson LJ et al., Giardiasis – why do symptoms never stop. *Trends Parasitol.* 26, 75–82, 2010

Roxström-Lindquist K et al., *Giardia* immunity – an update. *Trends Parasitol.* 22, 26–31, 2006.

Ryan U, Caccio SM, Zoonotic potential of *Giardia*. *Int. J. Parasitol.* 43, 943–956, 2013.

Van der Giessen JVV et al., Genotyping of *Giardia* in Dutch patients and animals: a phylogenic analysis of human and animal isolates. *Int. J. Parasitol.* 36, 849–858, 2006.

4.2.7 LEISHMANIASIS

Leishmaniases pose a considerable health problem in many areas of the world. According to estimates of the WHO (2009), there is a risk of infection for 10% of the world population. About 12 million people in 88 countries are affected and there are 2 million new infections with 70 000 deaths yearly.

The genus *Leishmania* is closely related to *Trypanosoma* (chapter 4.2.11). Like that genus, the parasites exhibit a kinetoplast (part of the mitochondrium) and pass through stage transformations in the transition from vertebrate to invertebrate hosts and backwards. The taxonomy of the genus is still not settled. Currently, more than 30 species are distinguished by means of molecular methods and more than 20 of the species are pathogenic for humans.

The genus is divided into two subgenera, *Viannia* (V.) and *Leishmania* (L.) (Tab. 4.5), based on their different development in the insect host. The subgenus *Viannia* occurs only in Central and South America, while the subgenus *Leishmania* is distributed worldwide. The most important agents are represented by the following species/species complexes:

- *L. donovani*-complex (*L. donovani*, *L. infantum*/*L. chagasi*, *L. archibaldi*);
- *L. tropica*, *L. major*, and *L. aethiopica*;
- *L. mexicana*-complex (*L. mexicana*, *L. amazonensis*, *L. aristidesi*)
- *L. (V.) braziliensis*-complex (*L. braziliensis*, *L. peruviana*, *L. guayanensis*, *L. panamensis*).

Vectors are Phlebotominae (subfamily Psychodidae), in the Old World represented by the genus *Phlebotomus*, in the New World by *Lutzomyia* spp.

Within the vertebrate host, *Leishmania* spp. inhabit the cells of the mononuclear phagocytic system (MPS: macrophages, Langerhans cells, monocytes) as round or oval-shaped amastigote (flagellum-free) stages, 2 to 3 μm in size, containing nucleus and kinetoplast (Fig. 4.12). They reside within a parasitophorous vacuole where they multiply by binary fission. Several surface molecules and enzymes of the parasites—among others leishmanolysin (GP 63), lipophosphoglycan, and some cystein proteases—promote their incorporation by phagocytosis, obstruct innate immune defense mechanisms, and inhibit their lysis by macrophages. After completion of the multiplication, the parasites are released by disintegration of

Table 4.5 | *Leishmania* spp. causing human diseases

DISEASE	AGENT	DISTRIBUTION	VECTOR	RESERVOIR HOSTS
Visceral leishmaniases of the Old and the New World				
Kala-Azar	*L. donovani*	India, Southwest Asia, China, Nepal, East Africa	*Phlebotomus argentipes*	Humans (dogs, rodents)
Visceral leishmaniasis	*L. infantum*	Mediterranean area, the Balkans, Southwest Asia, North and East Africa, Central and Southwest Asia, China	*P. perniciosus, P. papatasi*, and others	Dogs, other canids
	L. infantum/ chagasi	Central and South America	*Lutzomyia spp. (L. intermedia, L. longipalpis)*	Dogs, other canids, rodents, opossums
Cutaneous leishmaniases of the Old world				
Oriental sore, Aleppo boil, Leishmaniasis recidivans	*L. tropica*	Eastern Mediterranean countries, South and West Asia, India	*P. sergenti*	Humans (dogs)
Cutaneous leishmaniasis	*L. major*	Central Asia, Southwest Asia, Italy, North, East and South Africa, Southwest Asia	*P. papatasi, P. perfiliewi, P. caucasicus, P. longipes*	Rodents
Cutaneous leishmaniasis, Diffuse cutaneous L.	*L. aethiopica*	Ethiopia, Kenya	*P. longipes*	Hyraxes (rodents?)
Cutaneous and mucocutaneous leishmaniases of the New World				
Espundia (MCL)	*L. (V.) braziliensis*	Brazil, eastern Andean regions, Venezuela, Paraguay	*Lutzomyia spp.*	Rodents, dogs, armadillos
Pian bois (Forest Yaw)	*L. (V.) guayanensis*	Northern South America	*L. umbratilis*	Rats, opossums
Panaman leishmaniasis	*L. (V.) panamensis*	Panama (Columbia?)	*Lutzomyia spp.*	Sloths, porcupines, marmosets, tamarins
Uta	*L. (V.) peruviana*	Peru, Bolivia, Ecuador	*Lutzomia spp.*	Dogs
Chiclero's ulcer	*L. mexicana*	Central America	*L. olmeca*	Tree-dwelling rodents
Diffuse cutaneous leishmaniasis	*L. mexicana, L. amazonensis*	Northwest Brazil, Dominican Republic, Venezuela, Amazon basin	*Lutzomyia spp.*	Cats
Amazonian leishmaniasis	*L.amazonensis*	Amazon basin, Panama, Venezuela	*L. flaviscutellata*	Small rodents, opossums, sloths

the host cell and are phagocytized by new cells. The hematophagous phlebotomines are infected by ingesting parasitized cells. The parasites are released inside the insect's midgut, change into a flagellated form (promastigote, the kinetoplast is localized in front of the nucleus; Fig. 4.12), propagate, migrate to the proboscis of the insect, and are transmitted to new hosts by the next bite.

Dependent on the *Leishmania* species, their virulence and tropism, their specific vectors and the immune response of the host, either visceral, cutaneous or mucocutaneous manifestations develop. Special variants are the post-kala-azar dermal leishmaniasis (PKDL), the recidivating leishmaniasis, leishmaniasis recidivans (RL), and the diffuse cutaneous

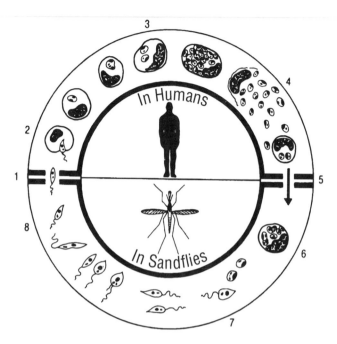

Figure 4.12 | Developmental cycle of *L. donovani*. (1) Transmission of flagellated leishmaniae by bite of bloodsucking *Phlebotomus* spp. (sand flies); (2) entrance of so-called promastigote forms into monocytes; (3) intracellular reproduction of now amastigote form leishmaniae (free of flagellae) by binary fission; (4) bursting of host cell and repeated infection of monocytes, predominantly in spleen and liver; (5) uptake of an infected host cell, containing amastigote leishmaniae, by sand flies; (6) transformation to ciliated promastigote stage and rapid multiplication by binary fission; (7) migration to proboscis of sand fly and formation of infectious metacyclic stage.

leishmaniasis (DCL). The various manifestations are traditionally attributed to certain *Leishmania* species, yet molecular biological studies have shown that such strict correlations do not apply. Thus, certain *Leishmania* species may cause different disease features and different *Leishmania* complexes may trigger corresponding clinical manifestations. In addition, mixed infections may modify clinical pictures.

Experimental studies in mice showed that the clinical course of an infection with *Leishmania* species is immunologically determined by a complex cooperation of macrophages and T cells. Whether an infection can be immunologically controlled or not depends on the T helper-cell population that dominates the reaction. A parasite induced IL-12 and Th1 response is generally associated with a suppression of the parasite's proliferation and a subsequent asymptomatic course of the infection. Whereas an activation of a Th2 dominated response early after infection, in general, fails to control the parasite's multiplication and may end with clinical disease. The mode of reaction in mice is genetically determined and recent studies in humans indicate a genetic background of the response to *Leishmania* spp. as well.

REFERENCES

Colmenares M et al., Mechanisms of pathogenesis: differences amongst *Leishmania* species. *Trans. R. Soc. Trop. Med. Hyg.* 96, Suppl. 1, 3–7, 2002.

Harms G, Schönian G, Feldmeier H, Leishmaniasis in Germany. *Emerg. Inf. Dis.* 9, 872–875, 2003.

Peacock CS et al., Genetic epidemiology of visceral leishmaniasis in northeastern Brazil. *Genet. Epidemiol.* 20, 383–396, 2001.

Schönian G, Mauricio I, Cupolillo E, Is it time to revise the nomenclature of *Leishmania*? *Trends Parasitol.* 26, 466–469, 2010.

Vladimirov V et al., Different genetic control of cutaneous and visceral disease after *Leishmania major* infection in mice. *Infect. Immun.* 71, 2041–2046, 2003.

WHO, Control of leishmaniases. Report of a WHO Expert Committee. *WHO Tech. Rep. Ser.* 793, 1990.

4.2.7.1 Visceral Leishmaniasis (Kala-Azar)

Kala-azar (named black fever due to skin hyperpigmentation) is caused by generalized human infection with species of the *Leishmania donovani* group.

Etiology. Visceral leishmaniasis is caused predominantly by species of the *L. donovani*-complex (*L. donovani* s.s., *L. infantum/L. chagasi*). The disease occurs in Africa, Southwest Asia and South America (Tab. 4.5). *L. infantum* in the Mediterranean region is largely restricted to infants; however, it affects people of all ages suffering from immunosuppressive diseases.

Occurrence. More than 90% of kala-azar cases reported worldwide occur in Bangladesh, India, Nepal, Brazil, and Sudan. Other endemic areas are parts of Myanmar, China, Central Asia, Mediterranean littoral and regions of Sub-Saharan Africa, Central and South America. The number of new cases estimated worldwide is 400 000 per year and the number of related deaths is 50 000 per year.

All age groups are susceptible, yet, the disease occurs mainly in children and adolescents up to an age of 20 years (~60% of cases). In the past, about 80% of the cases in the Mediterranean area concerned children below 5 years. Due to increasing numbers of clinical leishmanial disease in adult HIV infected people, the age related distribution has changed (see below). The disease is more common in rural areas, where living conditions of the human population and bionomics of phlebotomines fit closely together. However, rural exodus and increase of slums in bigger cities may result in the future in a higher prevalence in urban areas.

Typical for visceral leishmaniasis caused by *L. donovani* are epidemic outbreaks attributed to fluctuations in the human population and varying densities of the phlebotomes. A significant factor may also be general impairment of resistance to pathogenic agents due to malnutrition, particularly protein deficits, and helminth infections. The epidemiological type of the Mediterranean-Central Asian form of kala azar is found all over the Mediterranean basin, on the Atlantic coast of North Africa, Portugal, the Caucasus, Iraq, and the Asian countries of the former Soviet Union as well as Central Asia and northern China. Epidemics with large numbers of diseased people are not observed in the Mediterranean area; however, the frequency of *L. infantum* infections can be nonetheless relatively high. Specific antibodies could be detected in 8.2% of schoolchildren in northern Greece and in 32.8% in the region around Granada in Spain. High seroprevalences, however, must not be equalized with a high disease prevalence. For example, in a recent study in the south of France, 13% of asymptomatic blood donors showed antibodies to *Leishmania* antigens but only 1.6% reacted in a *Leishmania* specific PCR. Also, increasing seroprevalences with age suggest that most *L. donovani* infections remain clinically inapparent.

Visceral leishmaniasis has increasingly become a problem of people infected with HIV. It is estimated that in coming years, 2 to 9% of all AIDS patients will develop the disease. Already now, about 70% of all *Leishmania* cases in Europe occur in HIV-infected patients.

The prevalence of *L. donovani/L. chagasi* infections in South America is regionally variable, but altogether lower than in endemic areas in Europe and Asia. Nevertheless, the infection rate may be high in particular areas; for example, 6% of the population suffer clinical visceral leishmaniasis in a rural province in the northeast of Brazil. Epidemic and epizootic outbreaks may also be observed in relation with heaped infections in dogs and other canids.

The zoonotic relationships in visceral leishmaniasis are geographically variable. Anthroponotic forms caused by *L. donovani* s.s. are mainly found in India and East Africa. In other parts of Africa, rodents mainly act as reservoir hosts. The crucial reservoir of infections in Middle East, the Mediterranean areas, and South America are canids (dogs, jackals, foxes), in the Mediterranean areas, it is predominantly the domestic dog. Studies in stray dogs in Spain, for example, showed seroprevalences of 50 to 70% and positive PCR results in up to 90% of the animals. Correspondingly, the prevalence in vectors can be high. In highly endemic areas of Spain, up to 6.2% of sand flies are infected with *L. infantum*.

The presence of vector-competent phlebotomes is essential in the endemicity of the infection. *Phlebotomus* and *Lutzomyia* spp. are nocturnal Nematocera demanding special biotopes. Good conditions are generally found in warm temperate and subtropical zones, but phlebotomes can also occur in Central Asia up to 50°N. In daytime, the phlebotomes need dark, cool, and relatively moist places (e.g., rodent burrows, termites' nests, root systems of fallen trees) to hide. The larvae require sufficient amounts of organic material which they find for instance in rubbish dumps. Certain species dominate regionally. *Lutzomyia* spp. are vectors of *L. infantum/L. chagasi* in South America and prefer moist tropical regions (rain forests).

Transmission. Transmission is achieved by the bite of infected phlebotomes (Fig. 4.12). Only female phlebotomes are hematophagous, and not all species use humans as blood resources. Feeding usually takes place after sunset or shortly before sunrise. Some species, as the important *Leishmania*-vectors *P. papatasi* and *P. sergenti* also invade buildings (attics, latrines, stables) where they can also bite during the day. Flight activity of the phlebotomes is high only at times of calm weather and high humidity.

Alternative ways of transmission are of increasing significance. Infections have been reported after blood transfusion or organ transplantation. Drug addicts are infected by used syringes and needles. Congenital transmissions have been described several times but they seem rare.

A frequent question in practice is whether humans can be directly infected by a parasitized dog. Infected dogs may develop ulcerated disseminated skin sores in which parasites can be detected. Theoretically, they can pass on to humans by contact, for example, via skin lesions (compare vaccination methods in cutaneous leishmaniases). Yet no case was hitherto documented. Infections by excreta of dogs are implausible from a parasitological point of view.

Clinical Manifestations. The majority of infections (80 to 95%) remains asymptomatic. In some geographical regions (Kenia, Sudan, Central Asia) primary skin lesions (leishmaniomas) may develop at the biting site shortly after the bite of an infected phlebotomine, that is, an itching papule with an erythematous rim, 1 to 2 cm in size, which may necrotize and ulcerate.

In cases without leishmanioma, the incubation period ranges from 2 to 6 months but may also last for years. The beginning of the disease, especially in inhabitants of endemic areas, is often a slow process, usually without a distinct prodromal stage. Early uncharacteristic symptoms as slight, irregular increases in body temperature, headache, pain in the limbs, fatigue, gastrointestinal complaints, in children, and catarrh of the respiratory tract, are often ignored or overlooked,

Acute disease starts abruptly with sudden, high fever of 40 °C and more, rarely with chills. Remittent or intermittent fever is observed in more than 95% of cases and 2 to 3 fever attacks may happen within 24 h. Declining body temperatures are often associated with profuse perspiration. The initial fever continues for 2 to 6 weeks or longer, occasionally interrupted by short or longer remissions, not exceeding 38 to 39 °C.

In the beginning, the patients' general condition is not severely affected, but weakness, anorexia, weight loss, anemia, and a tendency to peripheral edema formation, particularly in malnourished children, are observed. Excessive eyelash growth may occur in children (Fig. 4.13).

Chronic kala-azar is characterized by fever, anemia and massive hepatosplenomegaly, generalized peripheral lymphadenopathy (Fig. 4.14), pancytopeny, hemorrhages (due to a hemophagocytic syndrome), progressive cachexia, interstitial pneumonia, diarrhea, and a subicteric,

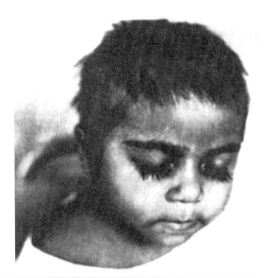

Figure 4.13 | Excessive growth of eyelashes in a child with kala-azar (Brazil).

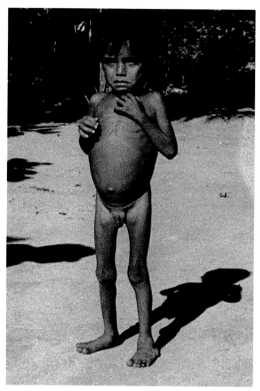

Figure 4.14 | Child with kala-azar (Brazil). Abdominal enlargement and considerable swelling of the inguinal lymph nodes are visible.

grey to dark-brown coloration of the skin (Fig. 4.14). Secondary infections, especially of the skin, of the respiratory tract, and the middle ear are frequent and prognostically unfavorable.

A fatal outcome is observed after 6 to 12 months in approximately 25% of the cases due to superinfections and gastrointestinal bleeding. The prognosis is particularly poor in children. If untreated, kala-azar is lethal in about 75% of the cases. Patients usually die after a slowly progressing course within 1.5 to 3 years after onset. In children, the prognosis is even worse, and mortality may approach 100%.

Up to 20 years after spontaneous recovery or successful therapy of leishmaniasis in the case of Indian and East African parasite strains, PKDL may appear. Cutaneous lesions, that is, hyperpigmented or erythematous macules, papules, and nodules, emerge on the face, trunk, limbs, and oral mucosa, and may persist for decades.

They contain numerous parasites, and are potential reservoirs of infection.

Diagnosis. In areas of endemicity, fever, progressive weight loss, weakness, pronounced hepatosplenomegaly, pancytopenia, hypergammaglobulinaemia, and hyperalbuminaemia, and in children, anemia is pathognomonic.

Diagnosis is proven by direct or indirect detection of the parasites. Microscopically, the parasites may be detected in Giemsa-stained blood smears or bone marrow smears and/or in spleen impression smears. The intracellular parasites may also be found scattered extracellularly after destruction of the host cell. A reliable morphologic characteristic is the side-by-side existence of a round nucleus and the rod-shaped kinetoplast (Fig. 4.15). PCR techniques clearly outmatch the microscopical methods by higher sensitivity and by allowing a species differentiation, in particular after *in vitro* cultivation of the parasites. Suitable media are Schneider's *Drosophila* Medium or NNN-Medium where the parasites transform into promastigotes within 3 to 21 days.

Various assays are available for the serodiagnosis of visceral leishmaniasis. IFA using amastigote parasites seems the most sensitive and most specific method. ELISA assays are commercially available. Well-suited for field examinations are rapid tests as for example the direct agglutination test, the fast-agglutination-screening

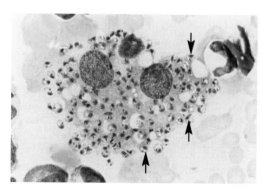

Figure 4.15 | *Leishmania donovani*: intracellular proliferation of the parasites in a macrophage (two nuclei). The amastigote stages (arrows) are characterized by a round nucleus and a rod-like kinetoplast (picture: T. Naucke, Bonn, Germany).

test, and the rK39-Dipstick test. The identification of the causative *Leishmania* species is not possible by means of antibodies. Cross-reacting antibodies are found in *Trypanosoma cruzi* and *T. gambiense/rhodesiense* infected people. Cross-reactive antibodies are also observed in cases of tuberculosis, leprosy, and malaria. Generally, in visceral leishmaniasis antibodies can be detected in 90% of cases. In HIV co-infections, the reliability of antibody tests depends on the stage of the immuno-suppression. Antibody assays are not suited to give information on the clinical status of the infection.

Differential Diagnosis. Bacterial infections, for example, typhus, typhoid fever, paratyphoid fever, brucellosis, tuberculosis, recurrent fever; viral diseases as mononucleosis, hepatitis, and rubella; parasitoses as sleeping sickness, malaria, schistosomiasis, amebiasis, and Chagas' disease; organic or systemic diseases as tropical splenomegaly and anemia, liver cirrhosis, Morbus Boeck, and rheumatic fevers must be considered.

Therapy. Hospitalization of the patient is recommended. Contact with potential vectors should be avoided by use of mosquitoe nets, repellents, and insecticides.

Pentavalent antimony compounds are highly efficient and relatively well tolerated standard drugs, which are applied for the treatment of leishmaniasis for more than 70 years. Adverse effects are general indisposition, weakness, elevated levels of liver aminotransferases, pancreatitis, arthralgia, myalgia, and prolonged QT interval. Available drugs are sodium stibogluconate (SSG, pentostam, 100 mg Sb^{5+}/ml) and N-methylglucamine-antimonate (glucantime, 85 mg Sb^{5+}/ml). The recommended dose is 10 mg of Sb^{5+}/kg twice a day, diluted, slowly i.v. or i.m. for at least 30 days, and in cases of relapse or delayed effects, for 40 days. The reported recovery rate is 90 to 95% and in AIDS patients, it is <80%. Antimony therapy is, however, now ineffective in Nepal and some regions of India, for example, in the Bihar state, which houses 90% of India's cases, that is, 40% of all kala-azar cases worldwide.

Liposomal amphotericin B (presently the only anti-kala-azar drug licensed in the US) or amphotericin B lipid complex are recommended for immunocompetent patients: 3 mg/kg/day i.v. at days 1 to 5, 14, and 21 (cumulative dose 21 mg/kg). Immunocompromised patients are treated with 4 mg/kg/day i.v. at days 1 to 5, 10, 17, 24, 31, and 38 (cumulative dose 40 mg/kg). Due to the lipid content, the substance is preferentially taken up by macrophages and it thus reaches the desired area of activity directly. Alternatively, amphotericin B in a standardized formulation, 1 mg/kg/day i.v. over 15 to 20 days is administered. Side effects are nephrotoxicity, fever, chills, and thrombophlebitis. Paromomycin, 15 to 20 mg/kg/day i.v. or i.m. for 21 days is used in India with a recovery rate of 95%; side effects are ototoxicity and nephrotoxicity.

The oral therapy with miltefosin (hexadecylphosphocholine) may lead to recovery rates of >95% by a recommended dosage of 2.5 mg/kg/day (maximum dose: 150 mg/day) for 28 days. Miltefosin is teratogenic. Hypercaloric food, rich in protein and vitamins should be provided. Blood transfusion and specific treatment of secondary bacterial infections should be applied.

There are no reliable criteria for a success of the treatment. Important signs are shrinking of enlarged lymph nodes, weight gain, improvement of pancytopenia, and regression of hepatosplenomegaly. Careful observation for 3 to 12 months is necessary. Recrudescence is frequent in patients coinfected with HIV.

Prophylaxis. Effective chemoprophylactic measures for a vaccine for humans do not exist. Individual prophylaxis against phlebotomine bites is achieved by the use of repellents (NN-diethyl-*m*-toluamide, hexamethyl-benzamide) and the use of repellent-impregnated, small meshed (0.2 mm) mosquitoe nets.

Vector control measures with insecticides, applied in the control of malaria, had some effects against phlebotomes. Spraying of their breeding and resting places, but also human dwellings, should be sufficient to control transmission. Development of larvae can be hindered or prevented by regular removal of organic waste (animal manure, refuse, foliage, and kitchen waste) from breeding places.

Animal reservoirs (infected dogs, rodents) have to be under surveillance and the number of stray dogs has to be reduced. Effective vaccines for dogs are available

REFERENCES

Abdalmaura GH et al., Human visceral leishmaniasis: a picture from Italy. *J. Infect. Public Health* 6, 465–472, 2013.

Abubakar AJ et al., Visceral leishmaniasis outbreak in South Sudan 2009-2012: epidemiological assessment and impact of a multisectoral response. *PLoS Negl. Trop. Dis.* 8, e2720, 2014.

Alexander B, Maroli M, Control of phlebotomine sandflies. *Med. Vet. Entomol.* 17, 1– 18, 2003.

Baneth G et al., Canine leishmaniosis – new concepts and insights on an expanding zoonosis – part one. *Trends Parasitol.* 24, 324–330, 2008.

Carillo E, Moreno J, Cytokine profiles in canine visceral leishmaniasis. *Vet. Immunol. Immunopathol.* 128, 67–70, 2009.

Cascio A et al., Pediatric visceral leishmaniasis in western Sicily, Italy: a retrospective analysis of 111 cases. *Eur. J. Clin. Microbiol. Infect. Dis.* 21, 227–282, 2002.

Cole RN, Reed SG, Second-generation vaccines against leishmaniasis. *Trends Parasitol.* 21, 244–249, 2005.

Costa CH et al., Asymptomatic human carriers of *Leishmania chagasi. Am. J. Trop. Med. Hyg.* 66, 334–337, 2002.

Cota GF et al., *Leishmania*-HIV-Co-infection: clinical presentations and outcomes in an urban area in Brazil. *PLoS Negl. Trop. Dis.* 8, e2816, 2014.

Dujardin JC, Risk factors in the spread of leishmaniases: towards integrated monitoring? *Trends Parasitol.* 22, 4–6, 2006.

Farkas R et al., First survey to investigate the presence of canine leishmaniasis and its phlebotomine vectors in Hungary. *Vector Borne Zoonotic Dis.* 11, 823–834, 2011.

Grech V et al., Visceral leishmaniasis in Malta – an 18 year paediatric, population based study. *Arch. Dis. Child.* 82, 381–385, 2000.

Harhay MO et al., Urban parasitology: visceral leishmaniasis in Brazil. *Trends Parasitol.* 27, 403–409, 2011.

Hodiamont JC et al., Species directed therapy for leishmaniasis in returning travelers: a comprehensive guide. *PLoS Negl.Trop. Dis.* 8, e2832, 2014.

Maroli M et al., The northward spread of leishmaniasis in Italy: evidence from retrospective and ongoing studies on the canine reservoir and phlebotomine vectors. *Trop. Med. Int. Health* 13, 256–264, 2008.

Miró G et al., Canine leishmaniosis – new concepts and insights on an expanding zoonosis – part two. *Trends Parasitol.* 24: 371–377, 2008.

Müller N et al., Occurence of *Leishmania* sp. in cutaneous lesions of horses in Central Europe. *Vet. Parasitol.* 166, 346–351, 2009.

Mohamed HS et al., Genetic susceptibility to visceral leishmaniasis in the Sudan: linkage and association with IL4 and IFNGR1. *Genes Immun.* 4, 351–355, 2003.

Reis AB et al., Immunity to Leishmania and the rational search for vaccines against canine leishmaniasis. *Trends Parasitol.* 26, 341–349, 2011.

Schönian G et al., Leishmaniases in the Mediterranean in the era of molecular epidemiology. *Trends Parasitol.* 24, 135–142, 2007.

Shaw SE, Langton DA, Hillman TJ, Canine leishmaniosis in the United Kingdom: a zoonotic disease waiting for a vector. *Vet. Parasitol.* 163, 281–285, 2009.

Werneck GL et al., The burden of *Leishmania chagasi* infection during an urban outbreak of visceral leishmaniasis in Brazil. *Acta Trop.* 83, 13–18, 2002.

Zijlstra EE et al., Postkala-azar dermal leishmaniasis. *Lancet Infect. Dis.* 3, 87–98, 2003.

4.2.7.2 Old World Cutaneous Leishmaniasis

Cutaneous Leishmaniasis of the Old World occurs as a usually benign skin disease (oriental sore, Aleppo boil) in the Mediterranean area and in vast regions of Africa and Asia.

Etiology. The disease is predominantly caused by members of the *Leishmania tropica*-complex, *L. tropica* s.s. (dry form, leishmaniasis recidivans), *L. major* (moist form), and *L. aethiopica* (chronic oriental sore, diffuse leishmaniasis of the Old World) (Tab. 4.5). However, in principle, other *Leishmania* species can cause cutaneous leishmaniases.

Occurrence. With the exception of Latin America, where *L. tropica* is not endemic, the gross geographical distribution of the disease is almost identical to that of kala-azar. However, usually only one of the leishmaniases dominates regionally. Ninety percent of cases of cutaneous leishmaniasis occur in Afghanistan, Algeria, Pakistan, Saudi Arabia, and Syria. *L. major* is present in rural regions of North Africa, southwestern and western Asia, and the Sahel. Reservoir hosts are several rodent species. *L. tropica* causes an urban anthoponosis in the Mediterranean and Central Asia. Occasional reservoir host are canids. *L. aethiopica* occurs in East Africa, mainly in mountain areas with *Hyrax* species as reservoir hosts.

Information on prevalence is variable and only reliably exists for a few regions. In Lebanon, for example, in 1993 to 1997, 0.18% and 0.41% of the population were infected in rural and urban areas, respectively. In selected regions of Iran, typical scars and active lesions were found in 0.7 to 3.2% and 0.2 to 1.3% of the population, respectively, at the end of the last century. In contrast, considerably lower prevalence of 0.13 to 7 cases per 100 000 inhabitants were reported from Israel for the years 1961 to 2000.

Transmission. *L. tropica* and *L. major* are transmitted mainly by *P. sergenti* and *P. papatasi*; *L. aethiopica* predominantly by *P. longipes* (Tab. 4.5).

Whether transmission of oriental sore occurs from person to person without an insect host is still controversial. In areas where cutaneous leishmaniasis is endemic, for example, Southwest Asia, it is common practice to deliberately inoculate young girls with material from oriental sores of sick patients to usually hidden skin parts. These girls develop a stable, lifelong immunity after natural healing of the local lesion.

Clinical Manifestations. Classical cutaneous leishmaniasis (L. tropica nodosa) is characterized by dermatological lesions at the site where promastigotes were inoculated.

The incubation period is usually 2 weeks and in rare cases, several months. After infection with *L. tropica*, a minute, itching, reddish-blue papule emerges that develops to a firm nodule of 0.5 to several cm in diameter, which eventually ulcerates after 3 to 4 months. The painless ulcer with raised borders is covered with yellowish-brown scabs, and it increases slowly in size. A patient's general condition is scarcely impaired. After 2 to some months, the ulcer heals by epithelization and, after 1 to 2 years, a radially retracted, depigmented scar has formed. The course is typical for >90% of cases and, after healing, results in lifelong immunity.

Infections with *L. major* and *L aethiopica* induce often multiple cutaneous lesions, associated with severe inflammations and exsudative "moist" ulcers, healing within several months. Scars are often distended and disfiguring. Predilection sites are usually the face, including the nose and ears, and the outer parts of the limbs.

Next to classical courses ~10% do not recover entirely but develop extensively spreading multiple cutaneous nodules and lesions in years. These relatively rare features are DCL and RL. The former is caused especially by *L. aethiopica* and numerous amastigotes are present in skin macrophages. In contrast, amastigotes are rarely found in the skin of RL cases; this form is mainly caused by *L. tropica*.

Diagnosis. For direct detection of leishmanial parasites, skin biopsy specimens are taken from the margin of the most recent lesions (only low numbers of parasites are found in older lesions). Touch preparations are Giemsa-stained and examined microscopically for amastigotes. *In vitro* cultivation can be done, for example, on NNN agar. PCR techniques are helpful. Specific antibodies are detected in only about 15% of cases with cutaneous leishmaniasis.

Differential Diagnosis. In classical forms, furunculosis, impetigo, pyoderma, erysipelas, lupus erythematodes, lupus vulgaris, tertiary syphilis, leprosy, keloid, tuberculosis verrucosa, ulcus tropicum, ulcus molle phagedaenicum, acne vulgaris, skin carcinoma, and psoriasis must be considered in the differential diagnosis. The diffuse skin leishmaniasis is to be distinguished from pityriasis rosea, erythema nodosum, syphilis, yaws, sarcoidosis, lupus vulgaris, lupus erythematodes, erysipela, onchocercosis, and streptococcal infections. Confusions with syphilis and tuberculosis are frequent.

Therapy. Cutaneous leishmaniases of the Old World usually heal spontaneously within 6 to 15 months, resulting in protective immunity. A specific therapy is recommended to prevent disfiguring scars and secondary infections; however, it should not be started before the development of ulcerations to enable the patient to develop a protecting immunity. In case of an uncomplicated course (<4 lesions, not >5 cm in diameter, no cosmetically problematic sites involved, no lesion over joints), a topical therapy with 15% paromomycin plus

15% methylbenzethonium chloride in paraffin, twice a day for 20 days is recommended. Local hypothermia or cryothermia are often effective. In cases with larger and disfiguring lesions, treatment with Sb^{5+} drugs, 20 mg/kg/day i.v. (diluted and slowly infused over 2 h) or i.m for 20 days, or fluconazole, 200 mg/d p.o. for 6 weeks is recommended. Leishmaniasis recidivans and diffuse cutaneous leishmaniasis should be systemically treated in any case.

Prophylaxis. The measures are the same as in Kala-Azar. Vaccinations against cutaneous leishmaniasis by skin-scarifications and rubbing in of material from florid lesions has already been performed hundreds of years ago in endemic areas on purely empirical basis. The aim was to induce lesions on hidden parts of the body together with a protective immunity. However, this method is problematic because of the danger of transmission of other pathogens and of fulminant leishmaniases. The development of vaccines for humans from attenuated or devitalised parasites against cutaneous leishmaniases was not successful until now.

REFERENCES

Anis E, **Leventhal A**, **ElkanY**, Cutaneous leishmaniasis in Israel in the era of changing environment. *Publ. Health Rev.* 29, 37–47, 2001.

Ashford RW, The leishmaniases as emerging and reemerging zoonoses. *Internat. J. Parasit.* 30, 1269–1281, 2000.

Choi CM, **Lerner EA**, Leishmaniasis: recognition and management with a focus on the immunocompromised patient. *Am. J. Clin. Dermatol.* 3, 91–105, 2002.

Croft SL, **Yardley V**, Chemotherapy of leishmaniasis. *Curr. Pharm. Des.* 8, 319–342, 2002.

Gamier T, **Croft SL**, Topical treatment for cutaneous leishmaniasis. *Curr. Opin. Investig. Drugs* 3, 538–544, 2002.

Larréché S et al., Cluster of zoonotic cutaneous leishmaniasis (*Leishmania major*) in European travelers returning from Turkmenistan. *J. Travel Med.* 20, 400–402, 2013.

Nuwayri-Salti N et al., The epidemiology of leishmaniasis in Lebanon. *Trans. R. Soc. Trop. Med. Hyg.* 94, 164–166, 2000.

Pearson RD, **de Queiroz Sousa A**, Clinical spectrum of leishmaniasis. *Clin. Inf. Dis.* 22, 1–11, 1996.

Vega-Lopez F, Diagnosis of cutaneous leishmaniasis. *Curr. Opin. Infect. Dis.* 16, 97–101, 2003.

4.2.7.3 American Cutaneous and Mucocutaneous Leishmaniases (Espundia and Related Forms)

New World leishmaniases occur in many tropical regions of Latin America and are known as American leishmaniasis, espundia, uta, pian bois, chicleros ulcer, and forest yaw. They are of the skin and of mucocutaneous body regions and they are diseases of considerable importance to public health.

Etiology. Cutaneous leishmaniases can be caused by all species of the *L. mexicana*-complex. The pathogens of mucocutaneous leishmaniasis are primarily members of the *L. (V.) braziliensis*-complex (mainly *L. braziliensis* s.s., *L. panamensis, L. guyanensis*), but generally all other South American *Leishmania* species can produce cutaneous disorders. They induce diverse clinical syndromes differing strongly in certain endemic areas (Tab. 4.5).

Occurrence. The endemic areas extend from southern Texas to northern Argentina, except Chile and Uruguay, and include Andean regions up to 3000 m above sea level. The New World leishmaniases predominantly affect the population of rural and forested areas. The epidemiological situation is variable and the danger of epidemic spreads—based on sporadic cases or small endemic foci—always exists when woodland biotopes are drastically impaired, for example, by land reclamations, road constructions, and settlement of larger areas. Natural infections are found, dependent on the parasite species, in various rodents, in sloths, opossums, and bats. (Tab. 4.5)

Transmission. Intermediate hosts and vectors belong to the genus *Lutzomyia* (Tab. 4.5).

Clinical Manifestations. The skin sores in cutaneous leishmaniases of the New World resemble those of the benign Old World leishmaniases. However, the recovery rates of these benign forms are generally worse, and the scarring is more extended than in the oriental sore (Fig. 4.16).

Malignant mucocutaneous forms, spreading to mucous membranes, soft tissues and cartilage

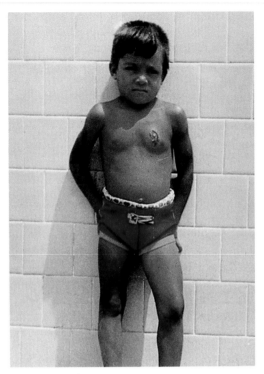

Figure 4.16 | Cutaneous leishmaniasis (Brazil).

can lead to disfiguring damage. They do not affect inner organs but tend to persist instead of healing. Several forms of the disease are distinguished.

Espundia (Breda's disease, mucocutaneous leishmaniasis): Pathogenic agents are species of the *L. (V). braziliensis*-complex. Only a subset, that is, less than 5%, of patients infected with *L. (V.) braziliensis* develop mucosal leishmaniasis months or years after a primary lesion. Occasionally, cutaneous and mucosal lesions are seen together. Usually, extensive granuloma formation begins in the nasal septum, which subsequently perforates, and extends to the hard and soft palate, the lips, cheeks, pharynx, and larynx. Tissue destruction is presumably due to excessive immune response. Lymphatic dissemination may occur, and even the genitalia may be affected. Initial symptoms are nasal stuffiness and epistaxis (nasal bleeding). One or both nostrils may be blocked by granulomatous tissue. Hoarse voice and aphonia point to laryngeal involvement. Tissue destruction may result in

dreadful mutilations, for example, loss of the cartilaginous nose or lips, and severe functional impairment. Cachexia, aspiration pneumonia, and laryngeal closure (suffocation) may result in a fatal outcome.

Pian bois (forest yaws), caused by *L. (V.) guayanensis*, is characterized by multiple cutaneous ulcers, spreading along the lymphatics. Spread to the nasopharyngeal area appears in 5% of cases.

Panaman leishmaniasis, caused by *L. (V.) panamensis*, is a relatively mild disease, and frequently only a single cutaneous lesion is observed. Occasionally, a number of flat ulcers develops along the lymphatics. Spreading and nasopharyngeal complications are rare. Nasal lesions usually develop at the inoculation site.

Uta. In contrast to the other neotropic (New World tropical) cutaneous leishmaniases, the distribution of this type of *L. (V.) braziliensis* and *L. (V.) peruviana* infections occur in the dry Andean highlands with poor vegetation (between 600 and 2000 m above sea level) and the western slopes of the Andes. The disease is benign like the oriental sore, that is, a solitary lesion without spread to the mucosa. Without treatment, scarred healing of the boils is usually observed about 1 year after infection.

Chiclero's ulcer (ulcera de los chicleros, chewing gum ulcer). Ciclero's ulcer is an occupational disease of gum (chicle) collectors and wood workers in tropical forests of Central America (Yucatan, Guatemala, and Belize), where it is caused by *L. mexicana* s.s. and in South America (Brazil, Venezuela) and Panama, where it is caused by *L. amazonensis*. This zoonosis is a mostly benign, self-limiting disease. However, depending on the immune status of the patient, protracted or chronic courses with ulcerations are observed in about 40% of the cases. Mucosal membranes are not involved. Frequently chiclero's ulcers occur on the pinna of the ear, which may be destroyed after long-standing disease. Ulcerations may also develop under the eyelid and on the upper limbs.

Leishmaniasis tegumentaria diffusa (diffuse cutaneous leishmaniasis; anergic cutaneous leishmaniasis). This type of disease is caused by *L. mexicana, L. amazonensis* and *L. venezuelensis* and it manifests itself by extended leprosy-like skin lesions that finally cover the entire skin except the hairy part of the head, the armpits, and the groin.

Diagnosis. Diagnostic measures are the same as in Old World cutaneous leishmaniases. The identification of the causing Leishmania species by PCR is important in order to exclude pathogens of the *L. (V) braziliensis*-complex. Microscopical attempts to demonstrate the parasites are unsuccessful in most cases and serological tests usually fail in case of Leishmaniasis tegumentaria diffusa.

Differential Diagnosis. Ulcus tropicum, mycoses (blastomycosis), lues, yaws, tuberculosis of the skin, and neoplasms have to be considered.

Therapy. The American leishmaniases, especially those caused by *Viannia* species, should be treated systemically, as the parasites may be disseminated to mucosal sites. In cases of mucocutaneous or diffuse cutaneous manifestations, a systemic treatment is compulsory. Antimonial drugs (pentostam, glucantime) are recommended: Sb^{5+}, 20 mg/kg/day i.v. or i.m. for 4 weeks, or liposomal amphotericin B (see therapy of visceral leishmanisis, chapter 4.2.7.1). The efficacy of miltefosin is uncertain in cases of mucocutaneous leishmanisis.

Plastic surgery is often required but should be performed at least 1 year after recovery in order to prevent the loss of the grafts by relapse.

Prophylaxis. The same prevention measures as for Kala-Azar and oriental sore are applied for the individual protection against sand fly bites and the repellents may be used.

REFERENCES

Arevalo I et al., Successful treatment of drug-resistant cutaneous leishmaniasis in humans by use of imiquimod, an immunomodulator. *Clin. Infect. Dis.* 33, 1847–1851, 2001.

Ashford RW, The leishmaniases as emerging and reemerging zoonoses. *Internat. J. Parasitol.* 30, 1269–1281, 2000.

Campbell-Lendrum D et al., Domestic and peridomestic transmission of American cutaneous leishmaniasis: changing epidemiological patterns present new control opportunities. *Mem. Inst. Oswaldo Cruz* 96, 159–162, 2001.

Da-Cruz AM et al., T-cellmediated immune responses in patients with cutaneous or mucosal leishmaniasis: long-term evaluation after therapy. *Clin. Diagn. Lab. Immunol.* 9, 251–256, 2002.

Eichner S et al., Clinical complexicity of *Leishmania (Viannia) braziliensis* infections amongst travelers. *Eur. J. Dermatol.* 23, 218–223, 2013.

Follador I et al., Epidemiologic and immunologic findings for the subclinical form of *Leishmania braziliensis* infection. *Clin. Infect. Dis.* 34, E54–58, 2002.

Gontijo CM et al., Epidemiological studies of an outbreak of cutaneous leishmaniasis in the Rio Jequitinhonha Valley, Minas Gerais, Brazil. *Acta Trop.* 81, 143–150, 2002.

Guerra JA et al., Mucosal leishmaniasis caused by *Leishmania (Viannia) braziliensis* and *Leishmania (Viannia) guayensis* in the Brazilian Amazon. *PLoS Negl. Trop. Dis.* 5, e980, 2011.

Reveiz L et al., Interventions for American cutaneous and mucocutaneous leishmaniasis: a systemic review update. *PLoS One* 8, e61843, 2013.

Rodrigues EH et al., Evaluation of PCR for diagnosis of American cutaneous leishmaniasis in an area of endemicity in northeastern Brazil. *J. Clin. Microbiol.* 40, 3572–3576, 2002.

Royer MA, Crowe CO, American cutaneous leishmaniasis. *Arch. Pathol. Lab. Med.* 126, 471–473, 2002.

Sundars S, Rai M, Advances in the treatment of leishmaniasis. *Curr. Opin. Infect. Dis.* 15, 593–598, 2002.

4.2.8 MICROSPOROSES

Microsporoses are parasitic infections caused by protozoa of the order Microsporida. Microsporida cause generalized infections, particularly in immunocompromised people, or they remain restricted to individual organs.

Etiology. Microsporida are obligately intracellular, spore-forming, primitive eucaryotes. Traditionally, they are registered as parasites but according to molecular characteristics, they are closely related to fungi. The infectious stage is the environmentally resistant, ovale, polar-tubule-bearing spore, 1 to 4 µm in size. The spore is released into the environment.

Microsporida have been identified as parasites in every major animal phylum, including mammals. More than 1200 species in approximately 140 genera have been described. To date, at least 14 species in eight genera have been recognized as pathogens in humans (Tab. 4.6).

Table 4.6 | Microsporida infecting humans

SPECIES	SITE(S) OF INFECTION	ANIMAL HOSTS
Enterozytozoon bieneusi	IC: Intestine IS: Disseminated	Vertebrates
Encephalitozoon hellem	IC: Cornea IS: Disseminated	Birds (psittacines)
Encephalitozoon intestinalis	IC: Intestine IS: Disseminated	Mammals
Encephalitozoon cuniculi[1] **Strain I**	IC: Not found IS: Disseminated	Rabbits
Encephalitozoon cuniculi[1] **Strain III**	IC: Not found IS: Disseminated	Dogs
Vittaforma corneae	IC: Cornea IS: Disseminated	Unknown
Pleistophora ronneafiei	IC: Not found IS: Skeletal muscles	Unknown[2]
Anncaliia (Brachiola) vesicularum	IC: Not found IS: Skeletal muscles, cornea	Unknown
Annacaliia (B.) connori	IC: Not found IS: Disseminated	Unknown
Annacaliia (B.) algerae	IC: Skeletal muscles, cornea IS: Skeletal muscles, cornea	Culicidae
Nosema oculorum	IC: Cornea IS: Disseminated	Unknown
Tubulinosoma sp.	IC: Not found IS: Skeletal muscles	Insects
Trachipleistophora anthropophthera	IC: Not found IS: Disseminated	Unknown
Trachipleistophora hominis	IC: Not found IS: Skeletal muscles, cornea	Unknown
Microsporidium africanum?[3]	Cornea	Unknown
Microsporidium ceylonensis?[3]	Cornea	Unknown

IC, immonocompetent person; IS, immunosuppressed person. Bold represents the most frequent species in humans.
[1] A further strain of *E. cuniculi* (Strain II) occurs in rodents and foxes, but is not yet found in humans.
[2] Members of the genus are found in fish, reptiles, amphibians, and insects.
[3] Immunological status of patients unknown.

The four most prevalent species in humans are *Enterocytozoon* (*Ent.*) *bieneusi*, *Encephalitozoon* (*E.*) *hellem*, *E. intestinalis* (Syn.: *Septata intestinalis*), and *E. cuniculi*. *Ent. bieneusi* might be a complex of species. To date, >90 genotypes have been characterized (mainly based on ITS-nucleotide sequences of rRNA), of which >30 were found until now only in humans, others (>10) were detected in humans and in one or more animal species, whereas further genotypes were only observed in animals. *E. intestinalis* was found in humans and in numerous mammalian and bird species. *E. hellem* infects humans and birds (psittacines). In the case of *E. cuniculi*, three separate strains are known; two of them (strain I from rabbits and strain III from dogs) were demonstrated in humans. Concerning the other species, which are found in humans more rarely or very rarely, no animal hosts are known, except mosquitoes in the case of *Brachiola algerae* (see Tab. 4.6).

Occurrence. Microsporida were found either exclusively or at least in the vast majority of cases in immunocompromised patients. *Ent. bieneusi* is one of the most important HIV-associated enteropathogenic agents, present in up to 50% of the patients. It is also common and disseminates in graft recipients. Some of the zoonotic genotypes are probably distributed worldwide, while others show more local distribution. *Ent. bieneusi* prevalence in farm animals is often rather high, for example, in Central Europe up to 90% of piglets and 5 to 25% of cattle are infected, usually by mixed populations of various genotypes.

Encephalitozoon spp. are found more rarely in humans. Surveys in Europe showed *E. intestinalis* in 1 to 2% of HIV infected patients. Other species occur sporadically. Clear data on animal infections are only available for strain I of *E. cuniculi*: it is obviously a cosmopolitan parasite and it was found in various rabbit stocks in

up to 80% of the animals. Pigeons, as they populate places and buildings in many cities, are widespread excretors of zoonotic Microsporida. Spores of *Ent. bieneusi* have been found in cow milk and, besides spores of other species, in oysters.

Transmission. Spores are the infective stage. Mature spores contain a tubular extrusion apparatus (tubular pore filament). At infection, the tubular polar filament is extruded, penetrates the wall of a host cell, and the infective content of the spore (sporoplasm) is injected into the cell through the tubular lumen of the polar filament (Fig. 4.17). The sporoplasm of the parasite multiplies asexually in the cytoplasm of the host cell and finally, mature spores are produced. The host cell ruptures and the infectious spores are released, where they infect further host cells or are shed with feces, urine, or sputum. They are quite resistant to the external environment and may be ingested by other hosts. Aerosolization of spores provides another route of transmission. Sexual contacts have also been considered as a possible way. *E. cuniculi* in rabbits may also be transmitted transplacentally.

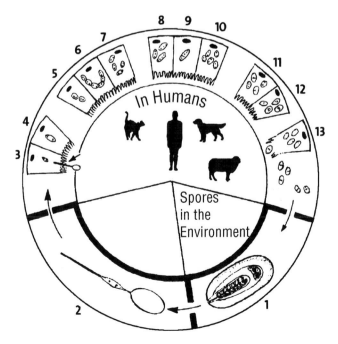

Figure 4.17 | Developmental cycle of microsporida. (1) Infectious spore; (2 and 3) extrusion of the tubular polar filament, penetration of the wall of an intestinal cell, and injection of the sporoplasm; (4 to 12) growth and asexual division via quadrinucleate stages (merogony) and finally encystment and formation of spores (sporogony); (13) rupture of host cell and liberation of infectious spores into the intestinal lumen.

Clinical Manifestations. In immunocompetent individuals, zoonotic infections with Microsporida commonly occur without symptoms; however, keratoconjunctivitis and intestinal infections with self-limiting watery, bloodless diarrhea, nausea, abdominal pain, and fever have been observed occasionally in adults and in children.

In immunocompromised patients, particularly in HIV patients, Microsporida are widely distributed. Intestinal infections with *Ent. bieneusi* and *E. intestinalis* are found in 10 to 40% of AIDS patients with chronic diarrhea, anorexia, and cachexia. Microsporida are detected after dissemination in patients with cholangitis, cholecystitis, sinusitis, and bronchiolitis. Infections with *Encephalitozoon* spp. manifest as keratoconjunctivitis, sinusitis, bronchiolitis, and pneumonia. *E. hellem* is often found in the urogenital tract in cases of interstitial nephritis, urethritis, cystitis, and prostatitis. *E. cuniculi* may infect almost all organ systems, particularly CNS and the peritoneum. Microsporida have also been found in patients with myositis (see Tab. 4.6).

Diagnosis. Depending on the localization of the disease, spores may be detected in stool specimens, duodenal, bile, or bronchial aspirates, and in biopsy specimens. In case of disseminated infections, spores are found in bronchoalveolar fluid, urine sediments, sputum, nasal secretions, conjunctival smears, corneal scrapings, biopsy specimens, and in CSF.

Smears are fixed with methanol, stained with a modified trichrome stain (Weber-Green modification), and screened microscopically [magnification, ×630 or ×1000 (oil immersion)]. Commercially available chemofluorescent stains (Calcofluor White 2 MR or Cellufluor) may also be applied.

Cytological preparations and biopsy specimens are stained with modified (Brown-Benn or Brown-Hopps) Gram, Giemsa, or silver stain (Warthin-Starry stain) or by chemofluorescent methods. These techniques are most useful for rapid and reliable detection of Microsporida spore in HIV patients. Transmission electron microscopic investigation, immunological test procedures, or molecular biological techniques, such as PCR, may also be used. Reliable serological techniques are available for *E. cuniculi* infections.

Differential Diagnosis. Depending on clinical signs and distribution of the agents in patients, diseases of different etiology must be considered in the differential diagnosis.

Therapy. Albendazole, 400 mg two times a day orally for 3 to 4 weeks is the drug of choice. In case of intestinal *Ent. bieneusi* infections, fumagillin, 20 mg three times a day orally, for 2 to 4 weeks is recommended. Infections of the eyes with *E. hellem* should be treated with albendazole/fumagillin eye drops. Topically applied fumagillin is effective in cases of keratoconjunctivitis caused by *Enzephalitozoon* spp. In HIV patients, successful antiretroviral therapy (HAART) usually leads to recovery from microsporidosis.

Prophylaxis. Because of the oral route of infection, application of a high standard of personal hygiene in handling of animals is recommended.

REFERENCES

Anane S, Attouchi H, Microsporidiosis: epidemiology, clinical data and therapy. *Gastroenterol. Clin. Biol.* 34, 450–464, 2010.

Andreu-Ballester JC et al., Microsporidia and its relation to Crohn's disease. a retrospective study. *PLoS One* 8, e62107, 2013.

Bart A et al., Frequent occurrence of human associated microsporidia in fecal droppings of urban pigeons in Amsterdam, The Netherlands. *Appl. Environ. Microbiol.* 74, 7056–7058, 2008.

Cali A, Weiss LM, Takvorian PM, A review of the development of two types of human skeletal muscle-infections from microsporidia associated with pathology in invertebrates and cold-blooded vertebrates. *Folia Parasitol. (Praha)* 52, 51–61, 2005.

Curry A et al., *Trachipleistophora hominis* infection in the myocardium and skeletal muscle of a patient with AIDS. *J. Infect.* 51, e139–144, 2005.

Franzen C, Microsporidia: how can they invade other cells? *Trends Parasitol.* 20, 275–279, 2004.

Didier ES et al., Therapeutic strategies for human microsporidia infections. *Expert. Rev. Antiinfect. Ther.* 3, 419–434, 2005.

Gosh K, Weiss LM, Molecular diagnostic tests for Microsporidia. *Interdisciplinary Perspectives on Infectious Diseases* 926521, 13. doi: 10.1155/2009/926521, 2009.

Henriques-Gil N et al., Phylogenetic approach to the variability of the microsporidian *Enterocytozoon bieneusi* and its implications for inter- and intrahost transmission. *Appl. Environ. Microbiol.* 76, 3333–3342, 2010.

Lanternier F et al., Microsporidiosis in solid organ transplant recipients: two *Enterocytozoon bieneusi* cases and review. *Transpl. Infect. Dis.* 11, 83–88, 2009.

Lin H et al., Prevalences and genetic characterization of *Cryptosporidium, Enterocytozoon, Giardia* and *Cyclospora* in diarrheal outpatients in China. *BMC Infect. Dis.* 14, p25, 2014.

Lobo ML et al., Microsporidia as emerging pathogens and the implication for public health: a 10-year study on HIV-positive and -negative patients. *Int. J. Parasitol.* 42, 197–205, 2012.

Nkinin SW et al., Microsporidian infection is prevalent in healthy people in Cameroon. *J. Clin. Microbiol.* 45, 2841–2846, 2007.

Santin M, Fayer R, *Enterocytozoon bieneusi* genotype nomenclature based on the internal transcribed spacer sequence. A consensus. *J Eukaryot. Microbiol.* 56, 34–38, 2009.

Santin M, Fayer R, *Enterocytozoon bieneusi* in domesticated and wild animals. *Res. Vet. Sci.* 90, 363–371, 2010.

Vávra J et al., Opportunistic nature of the mammalian microsporidia: experimental transmission, of *Trachipleistophora extenrec* (Fungi: Microsporidia) between mammalian and insect hosts. *Parasitol. Res.* 108, 1565–1573, 2011.

Visvesvara GS et al., Public health importance of *Brachiola algerae* (Microsporidia) – an emerging pathogen of humans. *Folia Parasitol. (Praha)*, 52, 83–94, 2005.

Wang L et al., Zoonotic *Cryptosporidium* species and *Enterocytozoon bieneusi* genotypes in HIV-positive patients on antiretroviral therapy. *J. Clin. Microbiol.* 51, 557–563, 2013.

Watts M et al., *Annacaliia algerae* microsporidiae myositis. *Emerg. Infect. Dis.* 20, 185–191, 2014.

4.2.9 MONKEY MALARIA (SIMIAN MALARIA)

Malaria is an important febrile human disease caused by various *Plasmodium* spp. (class Sporozoa). The name is derived from the Italian *mal aria*, meaning "bad air" and, depending on the causative *Plasmodium* species, summarizes a variety of clinical manifestations.

Etiology. The genus *Plasmodium* includes >170 named species of intraerythrocytic parasites that infect a wide range of mammals, birds, reptiles, and amphibians. *P. falciparum, P.vivax, P. ovale*, and *P. malariae* commonly infect humans. *P. falciparum* causes "malaria tropica," the most severe type of malaria with high lethality (if untreated 50 to 60% in patients from nonendemic areas).

P. vivax and *P. ovale* [possibly two separate (sub)species: *P. ovale curtisi* and *P. ovale wallikeri*] are the agents of the so-called "malaria tertiana"; *P. malariae* (syn. *P. rodhaini*) causes the "malaria quartana." The latter diseases are of a usually benign type. It was generally supposed that except *P. malariae*, which also occurs in chimpanzees, these species infect exclusively humans. However, as DNAs of all four species have been isolated from African anthropoid apes, which were obviously naturally infected, discussion arose on whether they are zoonotic agents as well. However, because, so far, no gamonts were found in the apes, it cannot be ruled out, therefore, they represent a "blind end" in the developmental cycle. Due to this unclear situation, *P. falciparum, P. ovale* and *P. vivax* will not be discussed in this book.

In contrast, *P. knowlesi* is certainly a zoonotic parasite, with monkeys as reservoir hosts. *P. knowlesi* is meantime termed the fifth human *Plasmodium* species. There is furthermore good evidence that neotropic primates in the Amazon rainforests are reservoirs of plasmodia that are pathogenic for humans. It is supposed that many cases, which were diagnosed as human *P. malariae* infections, in reality were caused by *P. brasilianum*, a common parasite in neotropic monkeys. Some authors even consider *P. brasilianum* a subtype of *P. malariae*. In addition, >25 *Plasmodium* spp. are known from nonhuman primates. Some of them, that is, *P. cynomolgi, P. inui, P schwetzi, P. simium, P. coatneyi*, and *P. eylesi* have been transmitted naturally, accidentally, or experimentally to humans.

Occurrence. *P. knowlesi* occurs in humans in Southeast Asia in an area that ranges from the Philippines to the Malaysian part of Borneo (Sarawak), Malaysia, and Myanmar. After discovery of the endemic zone in Sarawak in 2004, many hundreds of human cases became known, often in co-infection with classical human *Plasmodium* species. In relation to the total amount of malaria cases <5 to 70% were caused by *P. knowlesi*. Recent studies have shown that *P. knowlesi* is also responsible for 0.5 to 0.7% of human malaria cases in Thailand. Main final hosts of the parasite are various species of macaques (*Macaca fascicularis* and *M. nemestrina*).

P. malariae occurs in the tropical regions of the Old World and focally also in Central and South America. The species infects chimpanzees in Africa. *P. brasiliensis* is considered its local variant and it infects various monkey species (*Aotus* spp., *Callitrix* spp.) in Brazil, Peru, Colombia, Venezuela, and Panama.

P. cynomolgi, *P. inui*, *P. coatneyi*, and *P. eylesi* parasitize in monkeys in various tropical countries in Asia (Bangladesh, India, Philippines, Sri Lanka, and western China). *P. schwetzi* is a parasite of anthropoid primates in West Africa. *P. simium* infects howler monkeys (*Aluatta* spp.) and spider monkeys (*Brachyteles* spp.) in southern and eastern Brazil.

Except the suggested *P. brasilianum* infections in the Amazonas region and the *P. knowlesi* infections, only few cases are known where monkey plasmodia have been transmitted to humans on the natural route under field conditions. Dark figures cannot be estimated.

Personnel in scientific laboratories has become infected accidentally with plasmodia of simian origin as a result of bites by infected anopheline mosquitoes. At least 10 cases of laboratory-acquired mosquitoe-born *P. cynomolgi* infections have been reported. Altogether >150 cases are documented where monkey plasmodia were experimentally and successfully transmitted to humans

Transmission. All *Plasmodium* parasites are transmitted by female mosquitoes during the blood meal. In case of the species infecting humans, the potential vectors belong to the genus *Anopheles*. Out of 400 known *Anopheles* species (including subspecies and varieties), 60 are reported to be transmitters of malaria. It is not known in every case of simian plasmodia, however, which mosquitoe species is the natural arthropod host. In general, simian malaria is transmitted by *Anopheles* spp. feeding in the treetops (acrodendrophilic species), whereas vectors of human plasmodia generally feed at ground level or in dwellings (endophil species). In the case of *P. knowlesi*, the transmitting species belong to the *A. leucophyrus* group, which is adapted to the rainforest. This corresponds with the observation that most of the *P. knowlesi* patients stayed in the rainforest (e.g., tourists on trekking tours) or lived as farmers at its borders.

During the bite of an infected female mosquitoe, sporozoites invade the blood stream of their vertebrate (intermediate) host. After less than an hour, parasites enter hepatic parenchymal cells, where they divide and multiply intracellularly to form schizonts (preerythrocytic phase). Thousands of nucleated merozoites appear in each schizont. After the bursting of the host cell, the merozoites are released into the circulation, where they quickly invade erythrocytes and start the erythrocytic phase with a prepatency of 6 to 9 days p.i., depending on the species. Subsequently they divide, forming the species-characteristic erythrocytic schizont, which contains merozoites. After rupture of the blood schizont, the merozoites burst out and immediately invade new erythrocytes, followed again by agamic (vegetative) multiplication and the development of schizonts within 24 to 72 h. This phase of the life cycle is repeated continuously. When parasitized erythrocytes are finally disrupted and the merozoites burst out, pyrogenic metabolic products are released that activate macrophages and trigger the typical fever attacks via cytokines such as tumor necrosis factor alpha.

Besides this continuous process, some merozoites develop inside of erythrocytes into gametocytes, sexually determined stages (male microgamonts and female macrogamonts) after a predetermined period. They are the only infectious stages for the arthropod vectors and are ingested with the blood of humans or animals. In the mosquitoes, gamonts become gametes and after fertilization, zygotes are formed that develop to oocysts in the epithelial cells of the mosquito's midgut. Finally, oocysts mature and form masses of slender sporozoites, 9 to 14 μm in size. After bursting of the oocysts, sporozoites enter the vector's salivary glands of the mosquitoes to be inoculated into a vertebrate host during the next blood meal.

Clinical Manifestations. *P. knowlesi* may cause variable clinical signs in humans. After an incubation period of 9 to 15 days, the patients complain about fever, chill, headache, rigidity of limbs, indisposition, anorexia, myalgia, more rarely cough, dizziness, and stomach ache. Thrombocytopenia to various extent is an important symptom. Severe disease (according to the WHO criteria for *P. falciparum* infections) with dyspnea and renal failure develops in 5 to 10% of the cases. The severity of disease is closely related to parasitemia density, which may reach >100 000 µl blood but is usually <500 µl. The erythrocytic cycle lasts 24 h, which is shorter than in all other known species. The mortality rates if untreated amounts to 1 to 3%.

Patients who naturally acquired other simian *Plasmodium* spp. developed fever, fatigue, anorexia, nausea, and hepatosplenomegaly. Parasitemia was low, and the patients did not require therapy. However, although human malaria caused by simian plasmodia resembles a mild and benign disease, one should keep in mind that splenectomised monkeys may rapidly succumb to simian plasmodian infection. Therefore, anybody without a spleen or on immunosuppressive therapy should avoid exposure to presumably or experimentally infected mosquitoes.

The incubation period of a vector-borne *P. cynomolgi* infection is 10 days. In 55 volunteers with experimentally induced *P. cynomolgi* infections, the mean prepatent period until blood smear positivity was 19 days (range 15 to 37 days). Experimentally infected people had usually low parasitemia and remained asymptomatic or at most had a self-limiting febrile disease. The periodicity of parasitemia was 48 h (*P. cynomolgi, P. schwetzi, P. simium,* and *P. eylesi*) or 72 h (*P. inui* and *P. brasilianum*).

In their natural hosts in Asia, simian *Plasmodium* spp. cause a mild or often clinically inapparent disease. *P. knowlesi* infection in *Macaca fascicularis*, the natural host in eastern Asia, is generally asymptomatic or characterized by mild and irregular fever, while in *M. mulatta*

(Rhesus monkey) experimental infection caused a serious and fatal disease. Infections with *P. inui* and *P. cynomolgi* are even less pathogenic for the natural hosts. *P. schwetzi* causes a mild infection in chimpanzees, its natural hosts. *P. eylesi* causes high parasitemia in mandrills. *P. brasilianum* appears to be more pathogenic for its natural host. Experimental infections, especially in *Cebus* and *Ateles* spp., can produce either an acute and fatal disease or a disease with less serious symptomatology but of long duration and with relapses.

Diagnosis. Routine diagnosis for humans and monkeys is done by examination of thick and thin blood smears (Giemsa stain). The differentiation by morphological criteria of the various simian *Plasmodium* spp. from the known human pathogenic species is often difficult. Similarities between the erythrocytic stages may lead to mistaken identities between *P. knowlesi* and *P. malariae*, during early merogony also between *P. knowlesi* and *P. falciparum*, between *P. cynomolgi* and *P. vivax, P. brasilianum* and *P. malariae*, and *P. simium* and *P. malariae*. In fact, *P. kowlesi* was often and is often mistaken for *P. malariae* in field studies. Alternatively, PCR techniques can be applied for species differentiation. This implies markedly enhanced sensitivity of diagnosis whereby the plasmodial DNA may be also demonstrated with high sensitivity in sputum and urine samples. The practicability of so-called malaria rapid diagnostic tests, which allow a rapid immunological diagnosis by the application of genus-specific antigens (*Plasmodium*-LDH or aldolase), usually by dipstick techniques, has not been tested so far in simian malaria.

Therapy. Chloroquine resistance does not occur naturally in simian *Plasmodium* spp. In the case of *P. knowlesi* infections, a chloroquine-primaquine therapy is recommended: chloroquine, 10 mg (base)/kg orally; subsequently, chloroquine, 5 mg (base)/kg orally after 6, 24, and 48 h; 24 h after beginning of treatment and after exclusion of glucose-phosphate-dehydrogenase deficiency, 15 mg primaquine (base) orally are administered for 2 days. In other infections with simian plasmodia, chloroquine is recommended: one 600 mg (base) loading dose and then doses of 300 mg each after 6, 24, and 48 h; total dose, 1500 mg), or primaquine, 0.3 mg (base)/kg/day for 2 weeks.

Prophylaxis. For journeys into *P. knowlesi* endemic areas that include a stay in the rainforest, chemoprophylaxis with mefloquine is recommended [250 mg (base) per week orally; adults <45 kg and children >5 kg: 5 mg/kg/week]. In other cases, special control measures under field conditions do not seem necessary, as natural transmission is extremely rare. The same measures that are recommended for the prevention of other *Plasmodium* infections are effective. Mosquitoes bite at night, especially between dawn and dusk; therefore, it is advisable to wear bright clothing with long sleeves and long trousers or skirts from the evening until daybreak. Bare skin should be smeared with repellents. Protection by mosquitoe nets is essential. Pregnant women should not enter malaria-infested areas.

Laboratory personnel working with simian malaria should carefully adhere to rules of good laboratory practice when handling infected blood, isolated sporozoites, or infected mosquitoes.

REFERENCES

Castro Duarte AMR et al., Natural *Plasmodium* infections in Brazilian wild monkeys: reservoirs for human infections? *Acta Trop.* 107, 179–185, 2008.

Coatney RG, The simian malarias: zoonoses, anthroponoses, or both? *Am. J. Top. Med. Hyg.* 20, 795–803, 1971.

Collins WE, Jeffery GM, *Plasmodium malariae*: parasite and disease. *Clin. Microbiol. Rev.* 20, 579–592, 2007.

Cox-Singh J et al., *Plasmodium knowlesi* malaria in humans is widely distributed and potentially life threatening. *Clin. Infect. Dis.* 46, 165–171, 2008.

Daneshvar C et al., Clinical and laboratory features of human *Plasmodium knowlesi* infection. *Clin. Infect. Dis.* 49, 852–860, 2009.

Daneshvar C et al., Clinical and parasitological response to oral chloroquine and primaquine in uncomplicated human *Plasmodium knowlesi* infections. *Malar. J.* 9, 238, 2010.

Divis PC et al., A TaqMan real-time PCR assay for the detection and quantitation of *Plasmodium knowlesi*. *Malar. J.* 30, 344, 2010.

Duval L et al., African apes as reservoirs of *Plasmodium falciparum* and the origin and diversification of the Laveriana subgenus. *Proc. Natl. Acad. Sci. USA* 107, 10561–10566, 2010.

Fatih FA et al., Susceptibility of human *Plasmodium knowlesi* infections to anti-malarials. *Malar. J.* 12, 425, 2013.

Jiang N et al., Co-infection with *Plasmodium knowlesi* and other malaria parasites, Myanmar. *Emerg. Inf. Dis.* 16, 1476–1478, 2010.

Jongwutiwes S et al., *Plasmodium knowlesi* malaria in humans and maccaques, Thailand. *Emerg. Infect. Dis.* 17, 1799–1806, 2011.

Kawai S et al., Cross-reactivity in rapid diagnostic tests between human malaria and simian malaria parasite *Plasmodium knowlesi* infections. *Parasitol. Int.* 58, 300–302, 2009.

Krief S. et al., On the diversity of malaria parasites in African apes and the origin of *Plasmodium falciparum* from Bonobos. *PLoS Pathog.* 6, e1000765, 2010.

Oddoux O et al., Identification of the five human *Plasmodium* species including *P. knowlesi* by real-time polymerase chain reaction. *Eur. J. Clin. Microbiol Infect. Dis.* 30, 597–601, 2011.

Schlagenhauf P et al., The position of mefloquine as a 21st century malaria chemoprophylaxis. *Malar. J.* 9, 357, 2010.

Sing B, Daneshvar C, Human infections and detection of *Plasmodium knowlesi*. *Clin. Mictrobiol. Rev.* 26, 165–184, 2013.

Sulistyaningshi E et al., Diagnostic difficulties with *Plasmodium knowlesi* infection in humans. *Emerg. Infect. Dis.* 16, 1033–1034, 2010.

Sundararaman SA et al., *Plasmodium falciparum*-like parasites infecting wild apes in southern Cameroon do not represent a recurrent source of human malaria. *Proc. Natl. Acad. Sci. USA.* 110, 7020–7025, 2013.

Van Hong N et al., A modified seminested multiplex malaria PCR (SnM-PCR) for the identification of the five human *Plasmodium* species occurring in Southeast Asia. *Am. J. Trop. Med. Hyg.* 89, 721–723, 2013.

4.2.10 SARCOSPORIDIOSIS

Sarcosporidiosis (Sarcocystosis) is a zoonotic, predominantly intestinal disease caused by coccidian protozoa of the genus *Sarcocystis*. It occurs either as an innocent intestinal infection or with symptoms of acute food poisoning. Occasionally cyst stages are found in the cardiac or skeletal musculature.

Etiology. *Sarcocystis* spp., formerly known in humans as *Isospora hominis*, belong to the cyst forming coccidia. *Sarcocystis* development is based on predator-prey relationships. More than 100 different species of *Sarcocystis* with generally defined intermediate and final host relationships are known worldwide. Two species, *Sarcocystis bovihominis* (syn. *S. hominis*) and *S. suihominis*, infect humans as final hosts. Intermediate hosts are cattle and pigs. When cysts are found in the human musculature, humans are accidental intermediate hosts. The species, potentially involved in cyst formation in humans have not yet been defined and were summarized under the term *S. lindemanni*. However, in recent years emerging intramuscular human infections have been observed in Southeast Asia. At least the cases in Malaysia seem to be caused by *S. nesbitti*, with snakes (cobras and pytons) as final hosts.

Occurrence. Patent human *Sarcocystis* infections with shedding of oocysts are found worldwide with varying incidences, depending on the eating behavior of the local population. The prevalence in Central Europe, for example, is generally <1%, and suggested to be higher than in other industrial societies. Cattle as intermediate hosts of *S. bovihominis* are infected at a rate of 21 to 64% in Europe. The infection rate in pigs is strongly management dependent. Under good hygienic conditions, *Sarcocystis* spp. infections are rare, whereas infection rates may be almost 100% if hygiene is poor. In Germany, for example, *S. suihominis* is found in approximately 5% of pigs for slaughter.

Sarcosporidiosis of the musculature was generally estimated to be very rare. Less than 100 cases were documented, which had been discovered incidentally in asymptomatic persons. Neither the parasite species involved (mostly it was named *S. lindemanni*) nor the general clinical importance were known. There were, however, long time disregarded reports, which suggested higher prevalence rates (approximately 20%) of subclinical intramuscular infections in several areas and ethnic groups of Southeast Asia. Accordingly, 2011 and 2012 (the latter with >100 cases) clinical intramuscular infections were reported in travelers to the Tioman island, located off the east coast of peninsular Malaysia. The causal agent was probably *S. nesbitti*, a species of cobras and pythons as final hosts.

Transmission. Human intestinal infection occurs by consumption of raw or undercooked cyst-containing meat from cattle or pigs containing mature cysts with merozoites (Fig. 4.18). In humans, the definite host, sexual reproduction (gamogony) takes place in the intestinal epithelium, where oocysts with two sporocysts, each containing four sporozoites, develop. Infectious oocysts and free sporocysts are shed in the feces. Prepatent periods in humans after infections with *S. bovihominis* and *S. suihominis* last 10 to 14 days. Oocysts are shed throughout a period of 2 to 4 weeks.

After ingestion of such stages by intermediate host and gut penetration, repeated asexual multiplications occur in vascular endothelial cells (schizogony, formation of merozoites). Hematogenous dissemination of merozoites leads to invasion of cardiac and skeletal muscle cells, where segmented cysts (sarcocysts) develop. The cycle is completed, when muscle cysts are eaten by an appropriate definitive host. Humans may be incidental intermediate hosts when food or water contaminated with oocysts/sporocysts are ingested.

Clinical Manifestations. Ingestion of heavily infested meat of cattle or pigs by immunocompetent persons resulted rapidly, after 3 to 24 h, sometimes also later, in nausea, dizziness, abdominal pain, flatulence, and diarrhea. Symptoms persist for 1 to 3 days and cease without any treatment. In cases of heavy infections with *S. suihominis* by meat of experimentally infected pigs, severe diarrhea with dehydration and even collapse have been reported. However, it seems questionable that a corresponding intensity of infection may occur under natural conditions.

If humans are infected with fecal oocysts/sporocysts they may develop tissue cysts in cardiac and skeletal muscles. Albeit most infections in the past seem to have taken an asymptomatic course, the recent *S. nesbitti* cases in Malaysia were generally associated with prominent musculo-skeletal complaints. Patients experienced myalgia, arthralgia, asthenia, headache, cough, often fever, and diarrhea, and showed eosinophilia, and increased serum CPK levels.

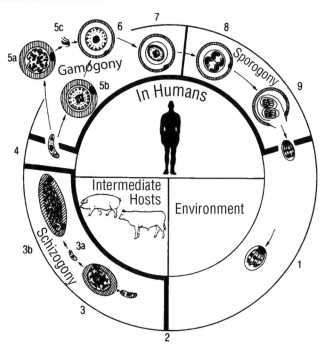

Figure 4.18 | Developmental cycle of *Sarcocystis* spp. with *Homo sapiens* as the definitive host. (1) Sporocyst with four infectious sporozoites, found in feces; (2) oral ingestion of sporocysts by intermediate hosts and liberation of sporozoites; (3) development of two generations of schizonts with 50 to 90 merozoites each by endopolygeny (multiple divisions) in endothelial cells of blood vessels (intestine, liver, kidney, lung, and other organs); (3a) free motile merozoite (second generation) entering a striated muscle cell; (3b) mature cyst (approximately 3 months p.i.) with cystozoites in skeletal muscle cells after a further schizogony (resting stages with thousands of cyst merozoites); (4) free cystozoite, after ingestion of a muscle cyst by the final host, entering cell of lamina propria; (5a) microgamont (male); (5b) macrogamont (female) in lamina propria (21 h p.i.); (5c) flagellated male microgamete; (6) macrogamete; (7) zygote (in intestinal epithelial cell); (8) sporogony within intestinal epithelial cell (formation of sporocysts); (9) sporulated oocyst (7 days p.i.) with two sporocysts, each containing four sporozoites, inside host cell.

Histological findings were myositis and myocyte degenerations; however, not every case had muscular cysts.

Diagnosis. Oocysts/sporocysts may be detected in feces, beginning 5 to 14 days after infection, by concentration techniques, for example, flotation with zinc chloride or zinc sulphate-NaCl, or by the merthiolate-iodine-formaldehyde technique and in biopsy specimens of intestinal mucosa. Sporocysts in feces measure approximately 9×15 µm. Serology and PCR reactions may be used in patients with suspected muscle infections.

Differential Diagnosis. Gastrointestinal diseases of bacterial, viral, or other parasitic etiology must be ruled out in the differential diagnosis of intestinal sarcosporidiosis. In cases of muscle infestation, trichinosis has to be considered.

Therapy. There is no specific therapy for human sarcosporidiosis. Treatment is symptomatic.

Prophylaxis. Raw beef and pork should not be consumed. Deep-freezing (−20 °C, 24 h) or heating (>65 °C) inactivates the parasites. Human feces should not be used as fertilizer for pasture grounds. Employees in livestock farming must avoid consumption of raw meat products in order not to become secretors of sporocysts. Caution and strict personal hygiene is recommended after handling of dead or live snakes (possible contamination with oocysts/ sporocysts of *S. nesbitti*).

REFERENCES

AbuBakar T et al., Outbreak of human infection with *Sarcocystis nesbitti*, Malaysia, 2012. *Emerg. Infect. Dis.* 19, 1989–1991, 2013.

Arness MK et al., An outbrake of acute eosinophilic myositis attributed to human *Sarcocystis* parasitism. *Am. J. Trop. Med. Hyg.* 61, 548–553, 1999.

Fayer R, *Sarcocystis* spp. in human infections. *Clin. Microbiol. Rev.* 17, 894–902, 2004.

Chen XW, Zuo YX, Hu JJ, Experimental *Sarcocystis hominis* infection in a water buffalo (*Bubalus bubalis*). *J. Parasitol.* 89, 393–394, 2003.

Thomas V, Dissanaike AS, Antibodies to *Sarcocystis* in Malaysians. *Trans. R. Soc. Trop. Med. Hyg.* 72, 303–306, 1978.

Vangeel L et al., Molecular-based identification of *Sarcocystis hominis* in Belgian minced beef. *J. Food Prot.* 70, 1523–1526, 2007.

Velásquez JN et al., Systemic sarcocystosis in a patient with acquired immune deficiency syndrome. *Hum. Pathol.* 39, 1263–1267, 2008.

Xin Wen C, Yang Xian Z, Wei Wei Z, Observation on the clinical symptoms and sporocyst excretion in human volunteers experimentally infected with *Sarcocystis hominis*. *Clin. J. Parasitol. Parasit. Dis.* 17, 25–27, 1999.

4.2.11 SLEEPING SICKNESS (AFRICAN TRYPANOSOMIASIS)

African trypanosomiasis is a disease of humans (also known as sleeping sickness or *maladie du sommeil*) in tropical Africa and is caused by parasites of the flagellate family Trypanosomatidae, which are transmitted by the bite of tsetse flies. If left untreated in humans, African trypanosomiasis (HAT) is 100% fatal.

Etiology. The morphologically identical parasites, *Trypanosoma brucei gambiense* and *T. brucei rhodesiense* (Fig. 4.19), are leaf-like or spindle-like in shape with a central nucleus, a kinetoplast (part of the mitochondrion; in blood stages near the posterior extremity), and a single flagellum that is attached to the body of the organism by an undulating membrane. Based on morphology and life cycle (continuous multiplication in the mammalian host, development in the tsetse vector by multiplication in the

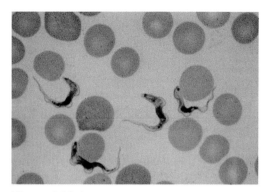

Figure 4.19 | *T. brucei rhodesiense* in blood smear (Giemsa stain).

midgut, migration to the salivary gland of the insect, and transmission by insect bite to the host) both subspecies belong to the *T. brucei* (salivaria) group. Differentiation can be made predominantly by epidemiological and clinical aspects and also on the basis of differences in virulence and pathogenicity. A third subspecies, *T. brucei brucei*, causes lethal infections in horses, and is pathogenic in ruminants but does not infect humans. In addition, a variety of other *Trypanosoma* species may infect domesticated animals. They are, for example, etiologic agents of the lethal Nagana in cattle (*T. vivax* and *T. congolense*) and may cause severe diseases in other animals but generally not in humans (for exceptions see chapter 4.13).

Occurrence. Areas of endemicity cover more than 40 Sub-Saharan African countries between 14°N and 20°S and from the Atlantic Ocean to the Indian Ocean. *T. brucei gambiense*, which occurs in West and Central Africa, infects primarily humans; infections of wild and domestic animals are less important. *T. brucei rhodesiense*, which occurs in East Africa, is mainly a parasite of wild and domestic animals and may be transmitted to humans incidentally. Usually, animals (cattle, sheep, goats, dogs, buffaloes, various antelopes, lions, hyenas, and others) are latently infected. The main reservoir of *T. brucei rhodesiense* are antelopes.

HAT occurs predominantly in rural, remote areas without a sufficient medical supply. Sixty million people are at risk of infection in an area of approximately 7 million km². There are about 250 known definable, focally distributed endemic regions. More than 95% of HAT cases are caused by *T. brucei gambiense*; 25 000 new cases of HAT were notified in 2002; in 2006, approximately 11 400 and 500 new *T.brucei gambiense* and *T. brucei rhodesiense* cases were reported, respectively. Front-runners were the Republic of Angola, The Democratic Republic of Congo, and Sudan with 1000 new HAT cases each, followed by the Republic of Chad, the Central African Republic, the Republic of the Congo (Congo-Brazzaville), and the Republic of Uganda, each with 100 to 1000 new infections per year. Realistic estimates suggest approximately 70 000 new infections annually. The occurrence of HAT coincides with occurrence of tsetse flies (in the so-called "tsetse-belt").

Transmission. The obligatory vectors and arthropod hosts of African trypanosomes are tsetse flies (family Glossinidae). The >20 species of the genus *Glossina* (the only genus of the family) are divided into three main groups, that is, *Glossina palpalis* (in wetlands along with rivers and lakes), *G. morsitans* (in savanna areas), and *G. fusca* (in rain forests). *T. brucei gambiense* is mainly transmitted by the *G. palpalis* group with the species *G. palpalis, G. tachynoides,* and *G. fuscipes*; *T. brucei rhodesiense* vectors are mainly species of the second group, *G. morsitans, G. pallidipes,* and *G. swynnertoni*, but also *G. fuscipes*.

In the vertebrate host, African trypanosomes live extracellularly in blood, tissue fluid, and CSF. In phases of increasing parasitemia, long, slender, spindle-shaped trypomastigte forms (15 to 40 µm) with a free-ending flagella detected, which replicate by binary, longitudinal fission. Later on, in phases of decreasing parasitemia, short blunt (stumpy) forms (12 to 15 µm) appear. These stages do not replicate in the vertebrate host but are infectious for tsetse flies and are taken up by the fly in the course of a blood meal. Within the arthropod, they undergo a complex development and stage-transformation, multiply, accumulate after 15 to 35 days in the salivary glands of the insect as infective stages for the vertebrate host, and are transmitted during the next blood meal. The developmental cycle is shown in Fig. 4.20.

Clinical Manifestations. The pathogenesis of HAT is complex. The primary, localized

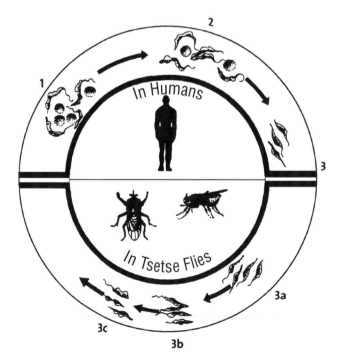

Figure 4.20 | Developmental cycle of salivary trypanosomes. (1) Trypanosomes (trypomastigote form) in peripheral blood after bite by tsetse fly (*Glossina* spp.). (2) Trypanosomes in stage of reproduction (peripheral blood); infection of CNS. (3) Development in the tsetse fly: (a) in stomach and crop; (b) epimastigote form in intestine in constant reproduction (binary fission); (c) metacyclic (trypomastigote) infectious form in salivary gland.

inflammatory lesion at the site of the parasites' inoculation is followed by intensive local multiplication of the trypanosomes and dissemination via lymphatics and blood to regional lymph nodes, internal organs, and the CNS. They induce a generalized lymphadenopathy, splenomegaly, increased vascular permeability, edema, hemostasis, intravascular coagulopathy, anemia, tissue hypoxia, formation of immune complexes, and finally immunosuppression.

The clinical course of an infection with *T. brucei rhodesiense* is more rapid and severe than that of an infection with *T. brucei gambiense*, which in areas of endemicity, tends to be chronic. Nevertheless, in both types of diseases different phases are distinguished.

Primary lesion (trypanosomal chancre). At first, the trypanosomes that were injected by the biting tsetse fly multiply at the inoculation site in the subcutaneous tissue. After days or up to 2 weeks p.i., an inflammatory, tender nodule develops, often with a centrally located pustule that extends to a diameter of several cm, and heals after 2 to 3 weeks. In *T. brucei gambiense*-infected patients, the trypanosomal chancre is observed in >5% of Africans and in about 20% of Europeans, but it occurs in 50% of *T. brucei rhodesiense*-infected patients.

Stage I (hemolymphatic stage). After 2 to 3 weeks (*T. brucei gambiense*) or 1 to 2 weeks (*T. brucei rhodesiense*) p.i., the parasites are disseminated via lymphatics and blood. In *T. brucei gambiense* infected patients, parasitemia is low and intermittent; in *T. brucei rhodesiense*-infected patients, it is high and often persistent. Bouts of high temperature lasting for some days alternate with afebrile periods. In people from nonendemic areas (travelers), the first symptoms are usually fever and chills.

The undulating time courses of parasite density in the blood and temperatures are due to an immune evasion strategy of the parasites. African trypanosomes are covered by a 10 to 15 nm-thick surface coat, which is built by a single, highly antigenic glycoprotein [variant surface glycoprotein (VSG)]. The host develops IgM antibodies that eliminate the trypanosomes; however, part of the parasite population changes the VSG and gives rise to a new wave of parasitemia. This process continues, as the repertoire of VSGs are very large, if not endless, with 10 to 15% of the parasite genome encoding VSGs exclusively. The host responds with a continuous synthesis of new IgM antibodies.

Lymphadenopathy is a prominent sign in *T. brucei gambiense*-infected patients: supraclavicular, cervical, and nuchal nodes (Winterbottom's sign) are enlarged, discrete, movable, and nontender. Additional symptoms are headache, malaise, arthralgias, myalgias, hepatosplenomegaly, edema of the face and limbs, weight loss, congestive heart failure, and tachycardia or cardiac arrhythmias due to myocarditis (particularly in *T. brucei rhodesiense*-infected patients), endocrinological disorders (e.g., impotence and amenorrhea caused by lesions in the endocrine glands), anemia, thrombocytopenia, and disseminated coagulopathy. Pruritus and an erythematous rash, 5 to 10 cm in diameter with clean centers may occur on the shoulders, trunk, buttocks, and thighs. Symptoms may be mild or even absent in *T. brucei gambiense* infection until the CNS is invaded, whereas in *T. brucei rhodesiense* infection, death may occur within weeks or months, frequently before the CNS is invaded.

Stage II (meningoencephalitic stage). *T. brucei gambiense* invades the CNS within 4 to 6 month p.i., or even years later, whereas in *T. brucei rhodesiense* CNS invasion takes place after a few weeks to months. Meningoencephalitic signs and symptoms may progress over months and >6 years, but final stages with coma and death may occur within a few days to weeks, especially in the case of *T. brucei rhodesiense* infections.

Signs and symptoms are persistent headache, memory loss, progressive apathy, mask-like face, faltering and indistinct speech, ataxia, tremors, seizures, depression, sleep disturbances with daytime somnolence and nocturnal insomnia, impaired vision up to total blindness, and finally coma and death.

In general, if untreated, patients with *T. brucei rhodesiense* succumb to the infection within 6 to 9 months; those infected with *T. brucei gambiense* succumb within 2 to 6 years.

Diagnosis. The patient's geographical origin and clinical symptoms, such as fever, headache, and enlargement of cervical lymphnodes, should arouse suspicion. Definitive diagnosis is based on microscopic identification of trypanosomes in the fluid expressed from trypanosomal chancre, in lymph node aspirate, peripheral blood, bone marrow aspirate, or CSF (sediment). Lumbar puncture is mandatory in all patients with confirmed or suspected African trypanosomiasis.

Trypanosomes may be seen in wet preparations (highly motile parasites) or Giemsa-stained smears. Due to higher parasitemia, trypanosomes are more readily detected in fluids from patients infected with *T. brucei rhodesiense* than in *T. brucei gambiense*-infected patients. Repeated examinations are indicated. Parasites may be more easily detected by examining thick blood smears, buffy coat (hematocrit capillary tube centrifugation), or eluate of an anion exchange column (Lanham technique, mini anion exchange centrifugation technique, and cAECT).

Trypanosomes can be cultivated in liquid media. T. *brucei rhodesiense* rather than *T. brucei gambiense* proliferates in rodents after i.p. injection and induces parasitemia. Increased white cell counts, elevated protein contents, high levels of IgM, and/or the presence of Mott cells (plasma cells with eosinophilic inclusions that contain Ig proteins) in CSF suggest a turn to stage II of the disease.

Serologic assays [card agglutination test for trypanosomiasis (*T. brucei gambiense*), latex agglutination tests, IHA, IFA, and ELISA) are available. Increased IgM levels in serum (3.5 to 4 times the normal concentrations) and CSF (>10% of total proteins) support a serologic diagnosis. Suitable primers for molecular biological techniques (PCR and loop-mediated isothermal amplification as a more simple method) are published.

Differential Diagnosis. Malaria, kala-azar, oriental sore, tuberculosis, brucellosis, and lymphoma during the early phase, and neurosyphilis, brain tumors, and viral meningoencephalitis during the late phase must be considered in the differential diagnosis.

Therapy. Effective drugs are suramin (Germanin), pentamidine diisethionate, melarsoprol, and eflornithine. These drugs are toxic, and treatment should be carried out under supervision of a physician, preferable in a hospital. Side effects are fever, nausea, vomiting, nephropathy, seizures, and shock (suramin); nausea, vomiting, and nephropathy (pentamidine); diarrhea, anemia, and seizures (eflornithine); and fever, headache, encephalopathy with speech disorders, tremor, seizures, coma, and death in 5 to 10% of treated patients (melarsoprol). The choice of drugs depends on the stage of infection and the *Trypanosoma* species involved.

- Infections with *T. brucei gambiense*, stage I: Pentamidine diisethionate, 4 mg/kg/day i.m. or i.v. for 10 days; or suramin, 100 mg, i.v. (test dosis to exclude hypersensitivity), thereafter, 1 g/day (children 20 mg/kg/day, max. 1 g/day), slow i.v. infusion at days 1, 3, 7, 14, and 21;

- Infections with *T. brucei gambiense*, stage II: Eflornithine, 100 mg/kg four times a day i.v. for 2 weeks, or (better) 200 mg/kg twice a day i.v. for 7 days plus nifurtimox, 5 mg/kg three times a day orally for 10 days. Alternatively: melarsoprol, 2.2 mg/kg/day applied in three i.v. infusions per day, for 10 days, or (better) melarsoprol plus nifurtimox. Melarsoprol should be combined with prednisolon, 1 mg/kg/day orally (max. 40 mg/day) 1 to 2 days before first melarsoprol application until the last application;

- Infections with *T. brucei rhodesiense*, stage I: Suramin, 100 mg i.v. (test dosis) and subsequently 1 g/day slow i.v. infusion at days 1, 3, 7, 14, and 21;

- Infection with *T. brucei rhodesiense*, stage II: Melarsoprol 2 to 3.6 mg/kg applied in three i.v. infusions/day for 3 days. After an interval of 1 week, a second series, and after another 10 to 21 days, a third series of infusions are given. For children the total dosage is 18 to 25 mg/kg, given during a period of 1 month. As recommended in case of *T. brucei gambiense* infections, melarsoprol treatment should be combined with prednisolon applications.

Any patient treated for African trypanosomiasis should be monitored at intervals of 3 to 6 months for 2 to 3 years after completion of therapy. About 2% of individuals treated for sleeping thickness with CNS involvement relapse.

Prophylaxis. Humans should avoid areas of endemicity. Tsetse flies show diurnal activity. Humans should wear light-colored clothes and use insect repellents. An individual prophylaxis with pentamidine diisethionate (3 mg/kg i.m. every 6 months) is possible but not recommended for tourists because of toxicity. Infected humans and animals should be treated. Presumably, infected game should be kept away from human dwellings. Tsetse fly populations should be reduced by traps and screens, provided with attractants, and by clearing breeding places, for example, brush vegetation near riverbanks and around settlements.

REFERENCES

Chappius F et al., Options for field diagnosis of human African trypanosomiasis. Clin. Microbiol. Rev. 18, 133–146, 2005.

Checkley AM et al., Human African trypanosomiasis: diagnosis, relapse and survival after severe melarsoprol-induced encephalopathy. Trans. R. Soc. Trop. Med. Hyg. 101, 523–526, 2007.

De Clare Bronsvoort BM et al., No gold standard estimation of the sensitivity and specifity of two molecular diagnostic protocols for *Trypanosoma brucei* spp. in Western Kenia. *PLoS One* 5, e8628, 2010.

Fèvre EM et al., Human African trypanosomiasis: epidemiology and control. Adv. Parasitol. 61, 167–221, 2006.

Fèvre EM et al., The burden of human African trypanosomiasis. *PLoS Negl. Trop. Dis.* 2, e333, 2008.

Franco JR et al., The journey towards the elimination of gambiense human trypanosomiasis: not far, nor easy. *Parasitology* 141, 748–760, 2014.

Hargrove JW et al., Insecticide-treated cattle for tsetse control: the power and the problems. *Med. Vet. Entomol.* 14, 123–130, 2000.

Hide G, Tait A, Molecular epidemiology of African sleeping sickness. *Parasitology* 136, 1491–1500, 2009.

Ilemobade AA, Tsetse and trypanosomiasis in Africa: the challenges and the opportunities. *Onderstepoort J. Vet. Res.* 76, 35–40, 2009.

Kennedy PG, Diagnostic and neuropathogenesis issues in human African trypanosomiasis. *Int. J. Parasitol.* 36, 505–512, 2006.

MacLean LM et al., Focus-specific clinical profiles in human African trypanosomiasis caused by *Trypsonosoma brucei rhodesiense*. *PLoS Negl. Trop. Dis.* 4, e906, 2010.

Mogk S et al., Clinical appearance of African trypanosomes in the cerebrospinal fluid: new insights in how trypanosomes enter the CNS. *PLoS One* 9, e91372, 2014.

Palmer JJ et al., A mixed methods study of health worker training intervention to increase syndromic referral for gambiense human African trypanosomiasis in South Sudan. *PLoS Negl. Trop. Dis.* 8, e2742, 2014.

Picozzi K, Carrington M, Welburn SC, A multiplex PCR that discriminates between *Trypanosoma brucei brucei* and zoonotic *T. b. rhodesiense*. *Exp. Parasitol.* 118, 41–46, 2008.

Simarro PP et al., Estimating and mapping the population at risk of sleeping sickness. *PloS Negl. Trop. Dis.* 5, e1007, 2012.

Sternberg JM, Human African trypanosomiasis: clinical presentation and immune response. *Parasite Immunol.* 26, 469–476, 2004.

Wastling SL et al., LAMP for African trypanosomiasis: a comparative study of detection formats. *PLoS Negl. Trop. Dis.* 4, e865, 2010.

4.2.12 TOXOPLASMOSIS

Toxoplasmosis is a systemic disease occurring worldwide in humans and animals after infection with *Toxoplasma gondii*. It is especially problematic in children after congenital transmission and in opportunistic infections in immunocompromised people.

Etiology. The parasite is the only species in the genus *Toxoplasma* and belongs to the class Coccidea (order Eimeriida). Although considered as one species, *T. gondii* shows a distinctly clonal structure in its population with different genotypes occurring worldwide. According to the currently accepted typing system on the bases of isoenzyme, PCR-RFLP, and microsatellite analyses, three dominating clonal populations are found in Europe and North America, termed as types I, II, and III. A similar situation seems to exist in Africa and Asia. The three types differ genetically only by approximately 1%, but inter alia they vary in the virulence in mice (only type I is highly virulent) and the prevalence in humans. The situation in South America appears to be different. Parasites isolated there often differ from the types I to III and overall are genetically much more multifaceted. Cross-breeding between the types occurs under natural conditions in cats in the course of sexual propagation and may result in altered virulence of the progeny.

The question, however, of whether the various types display different pathogenic implications in humans, is so far not definitely answered. The developmental cycle of *T. gondii* is optionally heterogenetic (see Fig. 4.21). Developmental stages are:

i. sporozoites, formed in the environment (sporulation) within oocysts (12 µm in diameter), which are excreted in the feces by infected felids as final hosts (Fig. 4.22);

ii. merozoites, intracellular, half-moon-shaped stages of multiplication, 6 by 3 µm in size;

occurring as tachyzoites in so-called pseudocysts or as bradyzoites (resting stages) in tissue cysts (up to 400 µm in size; Fig. 4.23) in various tissues of intermediate hosts (and also final hosts);

iii. gamonts/gametes in enterocytes of felines as sexually determined stages, which lead to the formation of oocysts.

Occurrence. *T. gondii* is highly prevalent in humans, in domestic, game and other wild animals worldwide. The host spectrum is extremely broad and includes all warm-blooded animals.

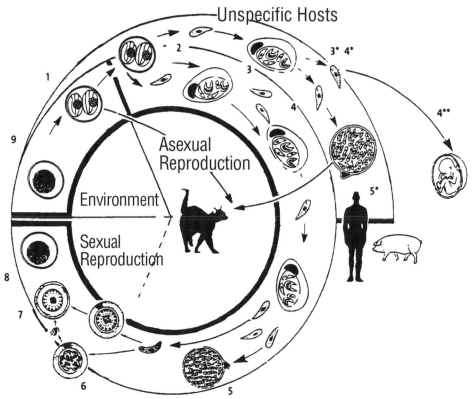

Figure 4.21 | Developmental cycle and transmission of *T. gondii*. (1) Sporulated oocyst or tissue cyst (5) is ingested orally by final host (cat) or unspecific (intermediate) host (mammals, birds, or humans). (2) Sporozoites and/or merozoites are set free in the gut and invade all types of nucleated cells. (3) Parasites multiply inside the cells by quick fissions (asexual reproduction: schizogony by endodyogeny); "pseudocysts" which contain numerous merozoites (tachyzoites) are formed. (4) Schizogony is repeated several times until the immune response of the host increases. (A) Diaplacental transmission is possible during this phase, leading to congenital toxoplasmosis. (5) Tissue cysts are formed under immune pressure with slowly multiplying merozoites (bradyzoites). (6) In cats, part of the merozoites reinvades epithelial cells of the gut and undergoes sexual differentiation. After fertilization (7), oocysts are formed (8). (9) Oocysts sporulate in the environment.

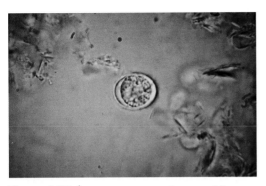

Figure 4.22 | *Toxoplasma gondii*: oocyst (diameter 12 μm) in feces of a cat (picture: Institute for Parasitology, Giessen, Germany).

It is estimated on the basis of seroepidemiological studies that up to one-third of the world's human population is exposed to *T. gondii*. The prevalence in humans varies in different geographical areas, even within one country, and among different ethnic groups. Seroprevalences in women of childbearing age have declined in recent decades, for example, in France, from 84% (1960) to 44% (2003), in Switzerland from 39% (1996) to 23% (2006). In the United States, the seroprevalence in the same group is between 3% and 35%, whereas seroprevalences in west African countries or in Latin America may reach >70%. The prevalence in human populations increases with age. In Europe and in North America type II is the major *T. gondii* type in humans, types I and III occur more rarely.

Domestic cats and other felines, predominantly kittens, are the sole animals to shed

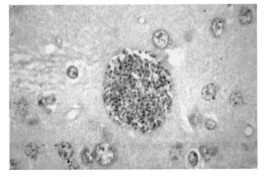

Figure 4.23 | *Toxoplasma gondii*: tissue cyst in the brain (mouse). Hematoxilin-eosin-staining (picture: Institute for Parasitology, Giessen, Germany).

oocysts, that is, are the sole final hosts. Based on seroepidemiological studies, the prevalence of infection with *T. gondii* in cats ranges between 10% and 80%. In Central Europe 0.1 to 6% of domestic cats excrete oocysts. After primary infection, cats shed large numbers of oocysts, that is, 10^6/g of feces, during a period of 1 to 14 days. Immunocompetent cats develop immunity that reduces or even prevents shedding of oocysts after reinfection.

Pigs may be intermediate hosts and contain cysts as a source for human infections. They were considered the main origin of human infections in Europe and the United States, but risks of human infection via pigs have decreased due to improved pig production management and measures of hygiene (no cats in piggeries!). In the 1970s, 10 to 55% of slaughtered pigs were infected; now, the prevalence is <1%. However, it should not be overlooked that some new trends in animal husbandry may again increase the risks. Organic free-range breeding of pigs in the Netherlands, for example, was associated with an increase of *T. gondii* in pigs by the factor 15.

Latent *Toxoplasma* infections in ruminants are widespread. In Europe, the prevalence in sheep is between 20% and 90%. *T. gondii* infections are important causes of abortion in small ruminants. In cattle, the bradyzoites in the cysts survive only for a short time. Tissue cysts are therefore rarely found in beef. Infections result from feeding on pastures contaminated by cat feces. Game is frequently infected. In the United States, up to 60% of wild ruminants are seropositive. Rabbits may develop clinically overt toxoplasmosis with high mortality within a few days after infection with sporulated oocysts. Poultry was often disregarded as a source of human infection. The risk may be small in case of intensive poultry management but in case of free-range poultry farming 30 to 40% of the animals showed antibodies to *T. gondii*.

Transmission. Transmission of *T. gondii* to humans occurs by occasional oral ingestion of sporulated oocysts or by consumption of cyst-containing raw or undercooked meat.

Cats and true felines are the sole final hosts of *T. gondii*, and therefore, play a central role in transmission (see Fig. 4.21). Infected animals shed oocysts with zygotes in the feces (Fig. 4.22). Dependent on the environmental temperature the oocysts sporulate, that is, the zygote develops to two sporocysts, containing four sporozoites each and becomes infectious. Sporulated oocysts are infectious after oral ingestion for both cats as final hosts and intermediate hosts. In both cases, sporozoites hatch in the small intestine, disseminate and invade all kinds of nucleated cells where tachyzoites multiply rapidly by endodyogeny (schizogeny) forming "pseudocysts," with crescent-shaped, so-called tachyzoites, 4 to 7 by 2 to 4 µm in size. Schizogeny is repeated several times. The cycles of rapid endodyogeny are terminated after 10 to 14 days by the immune response, which induces the formation of intracellular cysts (Fig. 4.23), 100 µm or more in diameter, and containing numerous, slowly multiplying bradyzoites (stage conversion). Exclusively in cats and other felids, however, part of the tachyzoites does not undergo this conversion but migrates back to intestinal epithelial cells and starts a sexual multiplication, which again results in the production of oocysts that are shed in the feces.

When cysts in the tissue of intermediate hosts are ingested by felids the corresponding development takes place, that is, bradyzoites induce the formation of tachyzoites and pseudocysts, followed by subsequent stage conversion to bradyzoites in tissue cysts as well as sexual multiplication in the intestine and oocyst excretion. Likewise, when cysts in intermediate hosts are ingested by nonfelids, tachyzoite multiplication results in the formation of tissue cysts without sexual reproduction.

Humans become infected with *T. gondii* by accidental oral ingestion of sporulated oocysts or by ingestion of cyst-containing, raw or undercooked tissue of infected nonfelid animals, that is, intermediate hosts. The question, which route of infection is more important in human toxoplasmosis, was, and is, intensely discussed, but there is probably no axiomatic answer, because many factors may be of influence as general way of living, eating habits, and personal hygiene. However, according to a recent study, at least in North America, the unrecognized ingestion of sporulated *T. gondii* oocysts seems to be the prevailing route of infection (the authors determined antibodies to a particular sporozoite specific antigen that are not created in merozoite- (i.e., cyst-) induced infections infected people.

Infection with *T. gondii* by accidental ingestion of sporulated oocysts is favored by the extreme resistance to environmental influences of these stages. In moist soil (cats cover their feces with earth) and low temperatures, they remain infectious for several years. Human infections via drinking water contaminated with oocysts have been described, such as in 1995, where 112 people fell ill with toxoplasmosis in Vancouver, Canada.

Infection by tissue cysts in general results from ingestion of raw or undercooked lamb or pork, and possibly poultry. Beef was suggested to be a less important source of infection, because of a relatively short survival time of cysts in cattle. Recent studies in the Netherlands, however, have revised this risk assessment. In addition, sources of infection may vary in populations with different living conditions and eating habits. Inuit in Canada suffered from *T. gondii* infections after the skinning of furbearing animals and eating raw caribou meat, dried seal meat, and seal liver. Raw kangaroo meat (in Australia) and raw pig liver and spleen (in Korea) have also been identified as major sources of human infection.

Oral infections of humans by tachyzoites (e.g., in goat milk) have been described, furthermore, raw eggs can also be a possible source of human infection, although the infection mode is unclear. In contrast to bradyzoites, tachyzoites are usually killed in the course of a stomach passage; it is therefore supposed that these stages invade by mucosal lesions in the mouth. Iatrogenic transmission of *T. gondii* from human-to-human has been observed; tachyzoites may be transmitted by donated blood and tissue for grafts.

During primary infection, followed by proliferation and dissemination in pregnant women, tachyzoits may invade the placenta, where they multiply, enter the fetal circulation, and infect the fetus. Congenital infection may cause abortion and stillbirth in humans, sheep, goats, and pigs, as well as congenital fetopathy. In cases of reinfection to immunocompetent intermediate hosts, as in humans, the parasites do not proliferate. In immunocompetent women, congenital *Toxoplasma* infection is therefore limited to primary infections, acquired shortly before or in the course of pregnancy.

Clinical Manifestations. Acute *T. gondii* infection in immunocompetent adult persons: 80 to 90% of all *T. gondii* infections are clinically inapparent. Symptoms of a manifest disease are localized, mostly cervical, or generalized lymphadenopathy, low fever, headache, general weakness, and myalgia. Encephalopathy, chorioretinitis, pneumonia, and myocarditis are rare. Most symptoms abate within a few weeks. Lymphadenopathy may persist for months. The *T. gondii* infection causes an effective, protective immunity to challenge infections.

Toxoplasmosis in immunocompromised adults: In over 90% of cases, toxoplasmosis results from a reactivated (recrudescent), previously acquired, latent *T. gondii* infection by activation of tissue cysts. It is rarely a new infection. The disease is manifested mainly in the CNS with lesions in the brainstem and basal ganglia, exceptionally in the eyes, lungs, heart, and other organs, with focal or generalized disorders. Symptoms are personality changes, apathy, confusion, ataxia, aphasia, seizures, and, according to organ manifestation, visual disorders, dyspnea, and diarrhea. *T. gondii* encephalitis develops in up to 40% of patients with AIDS.

Ocular toxoplasmosis: The disease is mostly based on congenital infection with *T. gondii* and rarely with acquired infections. It manifests as iridocyclitis, chorioretinitis, and uveitis. Damage of the eye develop in approximately 70% of congenital infections. According to a Swiss study, 10% are recognized within the first month of life, the others within a period of up to the age of 13 years (mean 6.3 years). *T. gondii* infections are counted among the major causes of chorioretinitis. Symptoms of ocular toxoplasmosis are blurred vision, scotoma, photophobia, ophthalmodynia, and loss of central vision. Foci in ocular muscles cause strabismus.

Toxoplasmosis in pregnancy and congenital toxoplasmosis: Toxoplasmosis in pregnancy in immunocompetent women is exclusively due to a primary infection with *T. gondii*. During gestation, immunocompetent pregnant women have relatively and absolutely decreased numbers of CD4 helper cells (reduction of the T cell mediated immune response appears useful, as is the risk of graft rejection, that is, fetal abortion due to immune reaction against paternal antigens is reduced). Due to the physiological immunodeficiency during gestation, pregnant women have an increased risk of infections, particularly with obligately intracellular bacteria, viruses, and parasites, the control of which depends on an effective and intact T cell activity.

The probability of primary *T. gondii* infections in the aforementioned seronegative women in the course of pregnancy accounts for 0.5 to 0.7%. The risk of a resulting fetal infection depends on the time of primary maternal infection in the course of gestation. If maternal infection was acquired ≥6 months before conception, fetuses are generally not affected. The risk of fetal infection increases, however, with the shortness of the time interval between infection and conception. During the first trimester, the risk of fetal infection by infection of the mother is approximately 15%, but fetal disease is more severe than that subsequent to infection during the third trimester. During this time, the risk of transmission is about 65%, but children infected in the last trimester experience sequelae that are less severe or are even asymptomatic. Referring to the number of all live births, the risk of congenital toxoplasmosis in Central Europe is 0.01 to 0.03%.

Toxoplasmosis in pregnancy may induce abortion, stillbirth (in about 10% of infected fetuses), or preterm delivery. Congenital infection may be manifested either immediately postpartum or many years later. Approximately, 10 to 20% of infected newborns show clinical symptoms. Classical signs are hydrocephalus, intracranial calcifications, and chorioretinitis (found in one-tenth of the cases). Others show a florid inflammation with lymphadenopathy, anemia, jaundice, hepatosplenomegaly, seizures, and fever. The mortality rate in these children is 10 to 15%. In 50% of the remaining congenitally infected newborns, late deficits are observed during the first 2 decades of life, predominatly ocular lesions, but also psychomotor and mental retardation, deafness, and learning difficulties.

In addition to all these implications of *T. gondii* infections, the parasite is suspected of being a cause for various psychiatric disorders in humans, including schizophrenia. Individuals with schizophrenia show increased prevalence of antibodies to *T. gondii* when compared with controls. There is also evidence that the parasites may modulate several neuronal functions, either directly or indirectly; however, the exact pathophysiological mechanisms are unclear.

Diagnosis. Toxoplasmosis is mainly diagnosed by serology, that is, detection of specific IgM and IgG antibodies and the determination of the avidity of specific IgG antibodies. High specific IgM antibody levels in immunocompetent patients indicate floride infection. IgM titers peak approximately 8 weeks after infection and disappear usually after 6 to 9 months. IgG antibodies are detected 2 to 3 weeks p.i. and reach a maximum approximately 6 to 8 weeks after infection. Subsequently, they decrease slowly and possibly persist at some level for life. Antibody titers should be reexamined after 3 to 4 weeks to get information on the status of the infection (fresh or older infection) by changes of the IgM and IgG antibody levels. Several kinds of assays are applied, for example, ELISA, EIA, and IFA; other test systems, such as the Sabin-Feldman dye test and the CF test, have lost their previous importance. Additional insights may be obtained by determining the avidity of specific IgG antibodies. IgG antibodies "mature" during ongoing confrontation with the antigen, that is, they increase in avidity to the inducing antigen.

In ocular toxoplasmosis, typical lesions and positive IgG titers are proof of the infection. In fresh infections, locally synthetized IgG antibodies can be demonstrated in the aqueous fluid.

For immunodeficient patients, serodiagnostic results should be interpreted cautiously. An IgM response often fails to appear, and IgG titers may originate from a former infection. CT and magnetic resonance tomography (MRT) may lead to diagnosis. In biopsy specimens, *T. gondii* DNA can be amplified by PCR.

Prenatal demonstration of *T. gondii* in the amnion fluid, predominantly by PCR, is in principal possible, but the sensitivity is low (40 to 70%). Considering the general risk of amniocentesis, the value of this procedure is seen rather critically. In most cases, the diagnosis of congenital *T. gondii* infection in newborns is based on a combined examination for specific IgM and IgA antibodies (no transplacental transmission to the fetus), which increase approximately until 2 weeks after delivery. Immunological identification or demonstration by PCR of tachyzoites in lymph node biopsy specimens may lead to diagnosis. However, the etiologic evaluation may be difficult in particular cases.

T. gondii may be detected by i.p. inoculation of blood biopsy material, or CSF into mice. After 1 week, the parasites are found in the blood; after 4 to 6 weeks, they are found in the brain, and at the same time specific antibodies are detectable.

Differential Diagnosis. For immunocompetent patients, cat scratch disease, infectious mononucleosis, lymphoma, CMV infection, and tuberculosis must be ruled out. In immunosuppressed patients, HIV encephalopathy, CNS cryptococcosis, lymphoma, and brain tumors must be excluded. In case of congenital toxoplasmosis, syphilis, listeriosis, rubella, and CMV infection must be considered.

Therapy. Acute toxoplasmosis in immunocompetent patients is treated in severe cases (meningoencephalitis and chorioretinitis) or in cases with persisting symptoms. Adults and children (≥6 years old) receive a combination of pyrimethamine, 200 mg orally on day 1, and then 50 to 75 mg per day plus sulfadiazine, 1 to 1.5

g four times a day orally for 3 to 6 weeks or 1 to 2 weeks when symptoms have disappeared. Patients with meningoencephalitis and chorioretinitis are additionally treated with prednisolon (1 mg/kg/day in 2 doses) until the protein concentration in the liquor has normalized and chorioretinitis has subsided. To prevent bone marrow toxicity, folic acid, 20 mg three times a week, is given orally until 1 week after the last pyrimethamine application.

Toxoplasmosis in pregnancy is treated in the first trimester with spiramycin, 1 g three times a day, if necessary until delivery. From the 4th month of pregnancy, therapy may consist of pyrimethamine, 50 mg twice a day on days 1 and 2 and then 50 mg/day plus sulfadiazine, 75 mg/kg on day 1, subsequently 50 mg/kg twice a day plus folic acid, 10 to 20 mg/day. The efficacy of prenatal treatment of the mother in prevention of transmission of *T. gondii* to the fetus and in reduction of the morbidity rate of the newborn are not really proven.

Congenitally infected newborns and children are treated with pyrimethamine, 2 mg/kg/day on days 1 and 2, then 1 mg/kg/day for 2 to 6 months, and then three times a week 1 mg/kg/day plus sulfadiazine, 50 mg twice a day, plus folic acid, 10 mg three times per week for at least 12 months. In cases of active chorioretinitis, prednisolone is given in addition, with 1 mg/kg/day in 2 doses. Effects of these treatments are doubted too. None of the drugs kills tissue cysts.

AIDS patients with cerebral toxoplasmosis are treated with pyrimethamine, 200 mg on the first day and then at a dosage of 75 mg/day, plus sulfadiazine, 1 to 1.5 g four times a day, plus folic acid, 10 to 20 mg/day for at least until 6 weeks after symptoms have disappeared or, if necessary, indefinitely as suppressive therapy (see below). Combined antiretroviral therapy (HAART) reduces the risk of activation of latent *Toxoplasma* infections.

Suppressive *T. gondii* therapy after cerebral toxoplasmosis uses pyrimethamine, 25 to 50 mg/day, plus sulfadiazine, 2 to 4 g/d in 2 to 4 doses, plus folic acid, 10 to 25 mg/day. Instead of sulfadiazine, clindamycin, three times 600 mg/day, or atovaquone, 2 to 3 times 750 mg/day. Treatment is continued until the number of CD4-cells has increased to >200/µl for at least 3 months.

In patients with sulfadiazine intolerance, the therapy may consist of pyrimethamine plus folic acid plus, alternatively, clindamycin, 600 mg four times a day orally, or cotrimoxazole, TMP/SMX, 5/25 mg/kg twice a day orally or intravenously for 30 days, or atovaquone, 750 mg four times a day orally or intravenously until at least 6 weeks after the disappearance of symptoms.

Prophylaxis. Preventive measures are indicated in seronegative pregnant women and immunodeficient people. Meat should never be eaten raw or undercooked. By heating (56 °C for 10 min) or freezing (−20 °C for 3 days), cysts are killed. According to most of the relevant studies, pickling and smoking kill the parasites within a few days. Short-time smoking at high temperatures (e.g., preparation of "smoked pork chop") is not always effective. Parasites are usually killed in few days in orderly prepared "raw sausages" whereas "barely seasoned raw sausages" are risky.

Utmost caution is required when cat feces or soil contaminated by cat feces (e.g., sandboxes or garden soil) is handled; single-use gloves should be worn. During pregnancy, clinically most inapparent *T. gondii* infection is detected by serological tests, and patients should be treated immediately.

Toxoplasmosis is a notifiable disease in most European countries. Some European countries have established a monitoring program that aims to protect pregnant women and newborns by early chemotherapy after early stage diagnosis. However, these programs are up for discussion; for example, Denmark stopped it in 2007 because of insufficient efficacies.

A primary prophylaxis in *T. gondii* infected AIDS patients (antibody-positive, CD4-T cells <100/ml) is recommended by treatment with trimethoprim-sulfamethoxazole or atovaquone, 750 mg twice a day.

Cats should be fed only canned or cooked food, never raw meat or slaughter waste; they also should be prevented from hunting potential intermediate hosts (mice, rats, birds). An often asked question is of whether a particular cat may represent an actual risk in the surroundings of a family or, especially, seronegative pregnant women. To minimize the risk, the cat should be kept indoors, fed canned or cooked food, and investigated by fecal examination for shedding of oocysts for 36 days (maximum prepatent period in cats). If the animal remains coproscopically negative throughout this period, the risk is small, provided it is still kept indoors and fed as specified.

REFERENCES

Accorinti M et al., Toxoplasmic retinochorioditis in an Italian referral center. *Eur. J. Ophthalmol.* 19, 824–830, 2009.

Bénard A et al., Survey of European programmes for the epidemiological surveillance of congenital toxoplasmosis. *Euro Surveill.* 13, pii:18834, 2008.

Bobic B et al. Comparative evaluation of three commercial *Toxoplasma*-specific IgG antibody avidity tests and significance in different clinical settings. *J. Med. Microbiol.* 58, 358–364, 2009.

Boyer KM et al., Unrecognized ingestion of *Toxoplasma gondii* oocysts leads to congenital toxoplasmosis and causes epidemics in North America. *Clin. Infect. Dis.* 53, 1081–1089, 2011.

Commodaro AG et al., Ocular toxoplasmosis: an update and review of the literature. *Mem. Inst. Oswaldo Cruz* 104, 345–350, 2009.

Dubey JP et al., New *Toxoplasma gondii* genotypes isolated from free-range chickens from the Fernando de Noranha, Brazil: unexpected findings. *J. Parasitol.* 96, 709–712, 2010.

Fekuda A, Shibre T, Claere AJ, Toxoplasmosis as a cause for behaviour disorders – overview of evidence and mechanisms. *Folia Parasitol.* 57, 105–113, 2010.

Flori P et al., Reliability of immunoglobulin G antitoxoplasma avidity test and effects of treatment on avidity indexes of infants and pregnant women. *Clin. Diagn. Lab. Immunol.* 112, 669–674, 2004.

Fond G et al., *Toxoplasma gondii* - a potential role in the genesis of psychiatric disorders. *Encephale* 39, 38–43, 2013.

Fuller EF, Yolken RH, *Toxoplasma* oocysts as a public health problem. *Trends Parasitol.* 29, 380–384, 2013.

Garcia-Méric P et al., Prise en charge de la toxoplasmosis congénitale en France: données actuelles. *Press Med.* 39, 530–538, 2010.

Garweg JG et al., Congenital ocular toxoplasmosis - ocular manifestations and prognosis after early diagnosis of infection. *Klin. Monbl. Augenheilkd.* 222, 721–727, 2005.

Garweg JG, Scherrer JN, Halberstadt M, Recurrence characteristics in European patients with ocular toxoplasmosis. *Br. J. Ophthalmol.* 92, 1253–1256, 2008.

Jones JL, Dubey JP, Waterborne toxoplasmosis – recent developments. *Exp. Parasitol.* 124, 10–25, 2010.

Kijlstra A, Jongert E, *Toxoplasma*-safe meat: close to reality? *Trends Parasitol.* 25, 18–22, 2008.

McLeod R et al., Prematurity and severity are associated with *Toxoplasma gondii* alleles (NCCCTS, 1981-2009). *Clin. Infect. Dis.* 54, 1595–1605, 2012.

Melamed J et al., Ocular manifestations of congenital toxoplasmosis. *Eye* 24, 528–534, 2010.

Pereira-Chioccola VL, Vidal JE, Su C, *Toxoplasma gondii* infection and cerebral toxoplasmosis in HIV-infected patients. *Future Microbiol.* 4, 1363–1379, 2009.

Röser D et al., Congenital toxoplasmosis – a report on the Denish screening programme 1999-2007. *J. Inherit. Metab. Dis.* 33 (Suppl. 2), 241–247, 2010.

Romand S et al., Prenatal diagnosis using polymerase chain reaction on amnionic fluid for congenital toxoplasmosis. *Obstet. Gynecol.* 97, 296–300, 2001.

Rudin C et al., Toxoplasmosis during pregnancy and infancy. A new approach for Switzerland. *Swiss Med. Wkly* 138 (Suppl. 168), 1–8, 2008.

Sibley LD et al., Genetic diversity of *Toxoplasma gondii* in man and animals. *Philos. Trans. R. Soc. Lond. B Biol. Sci.* 364, 2749–2761, 2009.

Sousa S et al., Serotyping of naturally *Toxoplasma gondii* infected meat-producing animals. *Vet. Parasitol.* 169, 24–28, 2010.

Velmuruga GV, Dubey JP, Su C, Genotyping studies of *Toxoplasma gondii* isolates from Africa revealed that the archetypal clonal lineages predominate as in North Amderica and Europe. *Vet. Parasitol.* 155, 314–318, 2008.

Villena I et al., Congenital toxoplasmosis in France in 2007: first results from a national surveillance system. *Euro Surveill.* 15, pii.19600, 2010.

Yolken RH, Dickerson FB, Fuller Torrey E, *Toxoplasma* and schizophrenia. *Parasite Immunol.* 31, 706–715, 2009.

4.2.13 OTHER ZOONOTIC PROTOZOAL INFECTIONS

Occasionally, infections in humans with animal-specific trypanosomes have been observed, for example, with *Trypanosoma lewisi* or *T. lewisi*-like trypanosomes (according to molecular analyses). *T. lewisi* is a cosmopolitan parasite of rats of low pathogenicity. The species belongs to the Stercoraria group (see chapter 4.2.4) and it is transmitted by the oral ingestion of infected fleas—fleas are intermediate hosts—or the feces of these fleas. All human patients were febrile but recovered within weeks by self-healing, except one case with intense clinical symptoms and trypanosomes in the CSF. The patient was cured by treatment with melarsoprol.

According to sporadic reports, humans can also be infected with *Trypanosoma congolense* (causing Nagana in cattle in Africa, south of the Sahara) and *T. brucei evansi* [highly pathogenic in horses and camelids, causing Surra; mechanically transmitted by blood-sucking flies (gadflies)]. In case of *T. brucei evansi*, a particular mutation in the gene encoding the apolipoprotein L1 (ApoL1) seems to be the precondition. ApoL1 promotes trypanosoma lysis by forming pores in lysosomal membranes and is responsible for the resistance of humans against *T. brucei brucei* (pathogenic for horses and camelids) and some other animal-specific trypanosomes. The human *T. brucei evansi* infections took a chronic course with fever episodes for months but they were successfully treated with suramin.

REFERENCES

Lun ZR et al., Atypical human trypanosomiasis: a neglected disease or just an unlucky accident? *Trends Parasitol.* 25, 107–108, 2009.

Powar RM et al., A rare case of human trypanosomiasis caused by *Trypanosoma evansi. Indian j. Med. Microbiol.* 24, 72–74, 2006.

Sarataphan N et al., Diagnosis of a *Trypenosoma lewisi*-like (*Herpetosoma*) infection in a sick infant from Thailand. *J. Med. Microbiol.* 56, 1118–1121, 2007.

Shegokar VR et al., Short report: human trypanosomiasis caused by *Trypanosoma evansi* in a village in India: preliminary serologic survey of the local population. *Am. J. Trop. Med. Hyg.* 75, 869–870, 2006.

Truc P et al., Atypical human infections by animal trypanosomes. *PloS Negl.Trop. Dis.* 7, e2256, 2013.

Vanhollebeke B et al., Human *Trypanosoma evansi* infection linked to a lack of apolipoprotein L-I. *N. Engl. J. Med.* 355, 2752–2756, 2006.

4.3 Zoonoses Caused by Trematodes

Parasites causing the zoonoses discussed in the chapters 4.3 to 4.6 are Metazoa and are generally summarized under the term Helminthes (helminths). It includes the zoological Phyla, Plathelminths, Nematoda, and Acanthocephala. Plathelminths, amongst others, include two classes of important parasites, the Trematoda (flukes) and the Cestoda (tapeworms).

Trematodes of interest (subclass Digenea) are in general dorsoventrally flattened flukes that measure from <1 mm up to several cm in length. They are enclosed by a tegument, a metabolically active surface structure, which in turn is closely connected with an internal system of muscles. Two suckers (acetabula)—an oral sucker and a ventral sucker (its position varies)—are used as organs of attachment. Digenic flukes possess an intestine that opens with the oral sucker and usually divides into two blind caeca.

Except the Schistosomatidae (chapters 4.3.1 and 4.3.9), digenetic trematodes are hermaphrodite. Eggs in general contain a zygote and variable amounts of yolk cells. As a first larval stage, a miracidium develops in the egg. All species of parasitic flukes develop in an indirect cycle with one or two intermediate hosts. The first intermediate host is in all cases a (water or land) snail, which either ingests the miracidium with the egg or it is actively invaded by the larva. In the course of several asexual reproduction steps, cercariae develop in the snail. They leave the snail and (i) invade actively their final hosts (e.g., schistosomes) or (ii) invade a specific second intermediate host (e.g., *Clonorchis*), where they transform to metacercariae, which is the infective stage for the final host. As a third way, for example, in case of *Fasciola*, the cercariae attach to (water)plants and transform to metacercariae, which are resistant to environmental influences.

4.3.1 CERCARIAL DERMATITIS

Cercarial dermatitis arises after repeated invasions of humans by cercariae of several species of the family Schistosomatidae, which can invade the skin but cannot accomplish their development in humans. Other names of the disease are "swimmer's itch," "lake itch," "duck itch," "rice paddy itch," and "clam digger's itch." In North America, terms such as "duck worms," "duck rash," "duck lice," "beaver lice," or, in Brazil, "lagoas da coceira" are used. In Australia, it is called "pelican itch," in Japan "kubure" or "kobanyo," "sawah" in Malaysia, and "hoi con" in Thailand.

Etiology. Causative agents are cercariae of several species of animal-specific schistosomatids, for example, of the genera *Austrobilharzia, Trichobilharzia, Gigantobilharzia* or *Schistosomaticum.* Waterfowl, and in some cases mammals, are the final natural hosts. Cercariae are released from intermediate hosts, which are mainly freshwater snails. In Central Europe, the disease is often caused by cercariae of the duck-specific parasites *Trichobilharzia ocellata* (*szidati*) and *Trichobilharzia franki* n.sp. The cercariae are fork-tailed and 600 to 800 µm in length. The fresh water snails *Lymnaea* spp. and *Radix* spp. are the species-specific intermediate hosts, respectively. The adult worms live in the intestinal veins of ducks. Lately, *T. regenti* was detected in Central Europe and Iceland, which, in its adult stage, inhabits the nasal mucosa of waterfowl. Obviously, the parasite reaches this site by a particular migratory route through the CNS. The parasite has not yet been observed in humans. In North America, cercarial dermatitis is encountered especially in the upper Midwest, caused by *Trichobilharzia* spp. and lymnaeid snails as intermediate hosts. Recently outbreaks of cercarial dermatitis took place also in southern United States. In coastal areas of the United States (including Hawaii), *Austrobilharzia variglandis* causes swimmer's itch. Final hosts are sea swallows and ducks, with marine snails (*Nassa* spp., *Littorina* spp.) as intermediate hosts. Cercarial dermatitis of workers in rice fields in Southeast Asia and Iran is apparently caused by the ruminant schistosomes *Schistosoma spindale*, and *Orientobilharzia turkestanicum.* Infection of snails occurs via buffaloes and cattle, which defecate during plowing of rice fields.

Occurrence. Cercarial dermatitis is an infectious disease occurring worldwide except in Antarctic areas. Locally, it may attain epidemic dimensions.

Transmission. In Central Europe, the infection is acquired by swimming or bathing in lakes or ponds populated by snails. Repeat infections of water in aquariums were reported in which snails were kept that had been taken from natural water bodies.

The development of the worms corresponds with that of *Schistosoma* spp. (chapter 4.3.8). Eggs of the parasites in feces of infected animals reach surface water. Hatched miracidia invade snails as intermediate hosts (for the developmental cycle of schistosomatidae see Fig. 4.32). After asexual propagation, masses of cercariae are released. On their search for specific final hosts, usually waterfowl or other animals, they also enter the skin of bathing or working humans as accidental hosts. In the skin, they migrate a few millimeters parallel to the surface (Fig. 4.24) but usually die within a few hours (although some schistosomula migrated up to the lungs after experimental infections of monkeys). Cercarial antigens can sensitize the host: reinfections lead to allergic reactions.

Clinical Manifestations. Primary infections are usually clinically almost inapparent. Patients may experience a prickling sensation; the parasites are eliminated without significant inflammatory reactions. Reinfections, however, lead to considerable clinical signs. The patients react with itching, which decreases after about 1 hour,

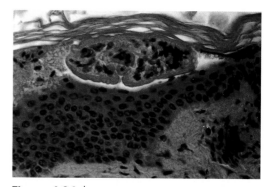

Figure 4.24 | Cercarial dermatitis: Cercaria of *Trichobilharzia* sp. after invasion of the skin. Hematoxilin-eosin-staining (picture: P. Kimmig, Hohemheim, Germany).

and reddish spots several mm in diameter at the sites where the parasites entered the skin. After 5 to 7 h, strong itching develops again. Papules or lumps several millimeters in diameter, surrounded by erythema, appear (Fig. 4.25) and itching increases within the following 1 to 2 days. Reactions vanish after 7 to 10 days. Patients sometimes show fever and fatigue. Repeated infections can result in threatening anaphylactic reactions. Secondary bacterial infections due to scratching are common in children.

Diagnosis. Important anamnestic hints are bathing in natural water bodies, especially in lakes and ponds in wooded areas, bathing and wading in shallows in coastal regions, and working in flooded rice fields.

A direct detection of the pathogen in patients is not possible. Provided schistosomiasis can be excluded, an intradermal test with *Schistosoma* skin-test antigen can be applied. Later, 3 to 10 days after the contact with cercariae, antibodies against cercariae may be detected in the serum of patients by the "Zerkarienhüllen-Reaktion" (cercarial envelope reaction) or by IFA. Species determination is possible in part of the agents by PCR. A PCR-product of the gene locus ToSAU3 allows the differentiation of *T. ocellata*, *T. franki* and *T. regenti*.

Differential Diagnosis. Skin lesions are similar to dermatologic reactions developing in schistosomiasis patients.

Therapy. Therapy consists of local application of antiphlogistic and antipruritic powders or lotions. The skin must be kept clean to avoid secondary infections after scratching.

Prophylaxis. Intermediate host snails are usually found near the banks of natural water bodies. Some ecological measures such as elimination of littoral weeds or plowing the mud at the banks may reduce the snail population. Ducks and other waterfowl should consequently be kept away from lakes used for bathing (no bird feeding). In cases of heavy contamination, bathing and swimming must be prohibited by the authorities.

Some unguents or lotions that act as repellents against jellyfishes may also protect from cercarial invasion. Niclosamide at a concentration of 0.05% in waterproof sunscreen was also reported to act as repellent.

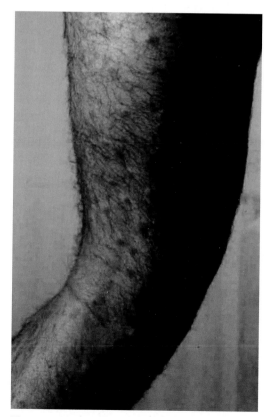

Figure 4.25 | Cercarial dermatitis: maculopapulous exanthema 24 h after infection (picture: P. Kimmig, Hohenheim, Stuttgart, Germany).

REFERENCES

Brant SV, Loker ES, Schistosomes in the southwest United States and their potential for causing cercarial dermatitis or "swimmers itch". *J.Helminth.* 83, 191–198, 2009.

Bastert J et al., Aquarium dermatitis: cercarial dermatitis in an aquarist. *Dermatol.* 197, 84–86, 1998.

CDC, Parasites–Cercarial dermatitis (also known as swimmers itch) *CDC* 24/7, 2012.

Cort WW, Schistosome dermatitis in the United States. *Michigan J. Am. Med. Assoc.* 90, 1027–1029, 1928.

de Gentile L et al., Cercarial dermatitis in Europe: a new public health problem? *Bull. WHO* 74, 159–163, 1996.

Jouet D et al., Final hosts and variability of *Trichobilharzia regenti* under natural conditions. *Parasitol. Res.* 10, 923–930, 2010.

Hertel J et al., Detection of bird schistosomes in lakes by PCR and filter-hybridization . *Exp. Parasitol.* 101, 57–63, 2002.

Hradlikova K, Horak P, Neurotropic behaviour of *Trichobilharzia regenti* in ducks and mice. *J. Helminthol.* 76, 137–141, 2002.

Kimmig P, Meier M, Parasitologic studies, diagnosis and clinical aspects of cercarial dermatitis – public health significance for bathing waters in temperate zones. *Zentralbl. Bacteriol. Microbiol. Hyg B.* 181, 390–408, 1985.

Kolarova L, Sykora J, Bah BA, Serodiagnosis of cercarial dermatitis with antigens of *Trichobilharzia szidati* and *Schistosoma mansoni. Cent Eur J Public Health* 2, 19–22, 1994.

Müller V, Kimmig P, *Trichobilharzia franki* n.sp.- a causative agent of swimmer`s itch in south-western Germany. *Appl. Parasitol.* 35, 12–31, 1994.

Narain K, Rajguru SK, Mahanta J, Incrimination of *Schistosoma spindale* as a causative agent of farmer's dermatitis in Assam with a note on liver pathology in mice. *J. Commun. Dis.* 30, 1–6, 1998.

Wulff C, Haeberlin S, Haas W, Cream formulations protecting against cercarial dermatitis by *Trichobilharzia. Parasitol. Res.* 101, 91–97, 2007.

4.3.2 CLONORCHIASIS

Clonorchiasis, a liver disease in Asian countries, is caused by the Chinese liver fluke. This trematode parasitizes primarily the bile duct system.

Etiology. The lancet-shaped, transparent (in the living stage, pink) parasite *Clonorchis sinensis* is 3 to 5 mm by 8 to 15 mm in size. It is characterized by paired, ramified testes in the posterior part of the body.

Occurrence. *C. sinensis* occurs in Asian countries, from Indochina to Japan, and in the Russian Far East. About 600 million people live at risk of infection and approximately 35 million are probably infected by the trematode. Besides humans, cats, dogs, pigs, various small carnivores like martens, and rats are affected. These reservoirs are difficult to control. Areas where *C. sinensis* is endemic are Korea, Socialistic Republic of Vietnam, Republic of China (Taiwan), and the People's Republic of China, with prevalence rates of up to 50%.

Transmission. Final hosts are infected by ingesting raw or insufficiently cooked freshwater fish, predominantly carps, which serve as second intermediate hosts of the parasite.

Feces of infected vertebrates containing worm eggs contaminate surface water. Eggs with larvae (miracidia) are ingested by snails (*Bulinus* and *Parafossarulus* spp.). In these first intermediate hosts, the parasites undergo several stages of asexual development and multiplication. Finally, cercariae are released by the snails and they invade actively small freshwater fishes, predominantly members of the family Cyprinidae, where they encyst in the muscles and develop into metacercariae. In humans, the young flukes hatch in the duodenum and migrate via the common bile duct into the distal bile ducts. There, they adhere to epithelial cells, mature to adult flukes, and start egg production after 2 to 4 weeks. The parasites may live 20 to 25 years in the final hosts. The developmental cycle is shown in Fig. 4.26.

Clinical Manifestations. *C. sinensis* causes inflammatory and proliferative alterations in the bile ducts. The severity depends on the number of flukes and the duration of their persistence. First signs of infection are fatigue, loss of appetite, and gastrointestinal disturbances, such as diarrhea and meteorism. Massive infections cause pain in the right upper abdomen, hepatomegaly, fever, icterus, and occasionally, urticaria. A massive worm load after repeated infections (more than 1000 flukes per patient have been found) leads to general health disturbances, with dizziness, tremor, convulsions, and loss of weight as well as developmental anomalies in children. Persisting infections are accompanied by liver cirrhosis, edema, and ascites.

Colonization of pancreatic ducts induces pancreatitis. Biliary stones are common. Bacterial superinfections (mostly by *Escherichia coli*) and cholecystitis may occur. Clonorchiasis provides a predisposition for cholangiocarcinoma. The parasite is classified as carcinogenic (Group 1) by the International Agency for Research on Cancer (IARC) of WHO.

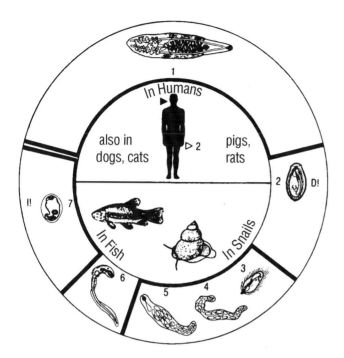

Figure 4.26 | Developmental cycle of *C. sinensis*. (1) Adult fluke (8 to 15 mm) in bile duct; (2) *C. sinensis* egg with miracidium (0.017 to 0.030 mm) excreted with feces (D, diagnostic phase); (3) miracidium (0.03 mm) hatched from egg within intestine of first intermediate host (freshwater snail, e.g., *Parafossarulus manchuricus*); (4) sporocyst (1.2 to 1.8 mm); (5) redia (>0.75 mm) in first intermediate host; (6) cercaria (about 0.5 mm) swimming actively in water; (7) metacercaria (≤0.285 mm; I, infectious stage) in second intermediate host (freshwater fish, e.g., a species of the Cyprinidae).

Diagnosis. Eggs can be detected in feces and duodenal secretions by microscopic examination. They resemble those of *Opisthorchis* and *Heterophyes* spp., are 17 by 30 μm in size, have a yellowish tinge, and an operculum. Excretion of eggs may start as early as 14 days p.i. Because of their small size, they are often overlooked in fecal samples. For that reason, concentration techniques, for example, formol-ether sedimentation, are recommended.

Serological procedures are also used for diagnosis. Eosinophilia may be observed in the acute state of infection.

Differential Diagnosis. Depending on stage and severity of the infection, liver cirrhosis of other origin has to be considered in the differential diagnosis. Symptoms resemble those of infections with *Opisthorchis* and *Dicrocoelium*.

Therapy. Effective treatment is achieved by praziquantel, 25 mg/kg three times a day orally for 2 days, or albendazole, 10 mg/kg per day for 7 days. Eggs disappear from feces and duodenal chyme within a few days after treatment with praziquantel.

Prophylaxis. The most important prophylactic measure in areas of endemicity is cooking or frying fish carefully. As changing traditional eating habits like eating raw fish is not accomplished easily in Asian countries, gamma radiation (0.15 kGy) of fish is employed to kill the metacercariae. Introduction of human or pig feces into fish waters must be avoided to prevent infection of snails with eggs. With progress in aquaculture techniques, hazard analysis critical control point (HACCP) are introduced to enhance the safety of this type of fish production.

REFERENCES

Chen D et al., Epidemiological investigations of *Clonorchis sinensis* infection in freshwater fishes in the Pearl River Delta. *Parasitol. Res.* 107, 835–839, 2010.

Choi D, Hong ST, Imaging diagnosis of clonorchiasis. *Korean J. Parasitol.* 45, 77–85, 2007.

Dorny P et al., Emerging food-borne parasites. *Vet. Parasitol.* 163, 196–206, 2009.

Fried B, Reddy A, Mayer D, Helminths in human carcinogenesis. *Cancer Lett.* 305, 239–249, 2011.

Hun NM, Madsen H, Fried B, Global status of fish-borne zoonotic trematodiasis in humans. *Acta Parasitol.* 58, 231–258, 2013.

Kaiser J, Utzinger J, Food-borne trematodiasis. *Clin. Microbiol. Rev.* 22, 466–483, 2009.

Kim YJ et al., Performance of an enzyme-linked immunosorbent assay for detection of *Clonorchis sinensis* infestation in high- and low-risk groups. *J. Clin. Microbiol.* 48, 2365–2367, 2010.

Kim EM et al., Detection of *Clonorchis sinensis* in stool samples using real-time PCR. *Ann. Trop. Med. Parasitol.* 103, 513–518, 2009.

Li K et al., Risk of fishborne zoonotic trematodes in tilapia production systems in Guangdong province, China. *Vet. Parasitol.* 198, 223–229, 2013.

Lin R et al., Investigations on the epidemiological factors of *Clonorchis sinensis* infection in an area of south China. *Southeast Asian J. Trop. Med. Public Health* 36, 1114–1117, 2005.

Nguyen TL et al., Prevalence and risks for fishborne zoonotic trematode infections in domestic animals in a highly endemic area in North Vietnam. *Acta Trop.* 112, 198–203, 2009.

Phan VT et al., Fish-borne zoonotic trematodes in cultured and wild-caught freshwater fish from the Red River Delta, Vietnam. *Vector Borne Zioonotic Dis.* 10, 861–866, 2010.

Rim HJ, Clonorchiasis: an update. *J. Helminthol.* 79, 269–281, 2005.

Shin HR et al., Descriptive epidemiology of cholangiocarcinoma and clonorchiasis in Korea. *J. Korean Med. Sci.* 25, 1011–1016, 2010.

Tantrawatpan C et al., Development of a PCR assay and pyrosequencing for identification of important human fish-borne trematodes and its potential use for detection in fecal specimens. *Parasite Vectors* 7, 88. doi: 10.1186/1756-3305-7-88, 2014.

Vennervald BJ, Polman K, Helminths and malingnacy. *Parasite Immunol.* 31, 686–696, 2009.

WHO Report Series Number: RS/2002/GE/40 (VTN), 2002.

4.3.3 DICROCOELIAIS (DISTOMATOSIS)

Dicrocoeliasis is a chronic liver disease that is rare in humans. It is caused by flukes parasitizing predominantly the bile duct system.

Etiology. The etiologic agents are the small or lancet liver flukes *Dicrocoelium dendriticum* and *D. hospes*, both 2 mm by 5 to 12 mm in size.

Occurrence. *D. dendriticum* occurs in the temperate zones of the Northern Hemisphere. Usually infections are confined to distinct areas, because the parasite depends on the simultaneous occurrence of two intermediate hosts, that is, land snails and certain ant species. The final hosts are various mammals, for example, ruminants and rabbits. High prevalence in domestic ruminants are observed in Southern Europe. The occurrence of *D. hospes* is limited to Eastern and Central Africa. Human infections are known from all endemic areas; however, incidences accumulate in certain regions, for example, the Arabian area and Central Asia. According to postmortem examinations, average prevalence rates in Uzbekistan reach 0.28%, and 1.8% of Kirghiz schoolchildren shed *D. dendriticum* eggs with the feces.

Transmission. Infection occurs by accidental oral uptake of parasite-infected second intermediate hosts, distinct ant species such as *Formica* spp. (*D. dendriticum*) and *Camponotus* spp. (*D. hospes*).

Dicrocoelium spp. have an unusual developmental cycle. Eggs containing larvae are shed with the feces of final hosts into the environment. They are ingested by land snails such as *Helicella* spp., *Zebrina* spp., and *Cionella* spp. (*D. dendriticum*), and *Limocolaria* spp. (*D. hospes*). In the snails, cercariae develop through several stages and asexual multiplication. They are released by the snails in mucous balls, which are taken up by ants, the second intermediate hosts; the parasites develop to metacercariae within the perigastrium of the ants. In addition, one cercaria invades the suboesophageal ganglion of the ant, resulting in a significant change of behavior of the insect. Whereas uninfected ants return to their burrows when the temperature is declining in the evening, infected ants cling to and remain on plants, and are ingested by grazing animals, the final hosts, or are accidentally ingested by humans. The young flukes are released in the duodenum and they migrate via the common bile duct into small bile ducts. There they reach sexual maturity and start egg production after 9 to 10 weeks.

Clinical Manifestations. Clinical symptoms depend on the fluke load. The colonization of the bile ducts results in acute and later chronic cholangitis. Late sequelae are periportal cirrhotic lesions.

In severe infections, the patients complain of continuous pain in the right upper abdomen, icterus, enlargement of the liver and spleen, alternations between diarrhea and constipation, flatulence, dizziness, vomiting, headache, and, in advanced cases, anemia.

Diagnosis. In patent infection, diagnosis is achieved by detection of the small (25 by 40 μm), dark brown, operculated eggs in the feces. Fecal examination should be repeated to exclude possible passenger eggs accidentally present in the intestine by ingestion of an infected liver.

Differential Diagnosis. Cholangitis and cholestasis of other etiology must be ruled out.

Therapy. Praziquantel (three 25 mg/kg doses in 1 day) is the drug of choice.

Prophylaxis. Watch for ants if eating fallen fruits or plants from natural habitat. Do not chew on grass blades.

REFERENCES

Cabezza-Berrera I et al., *Dicrocoelium dendriticum*: an emerging spurious infection in a geographical area with a high level of immigration. *Ann. Trop. Med. Parasitol.* 105, 403–406, 2011.

Jeandron A et al., Human infections with *Dicrocoelium dendriticum* in Kyrgyztan: the top of the iceberg? *J. Parasitol.* 97, 1170–1172, 2011.

Drabick JJ et al., Dicrocoeliasis (lancet fluke disease) in an HJV seropositive man. *JAMA* 259, 567–568, 1988.

Karadag B et al., An unusual case of biliary obstruction caused by *Dicrocoelium dendriticum*. *Scand. J. Infect. Dis.* 37, 385–388, 2005.

Magi F et al., *Dicrocoelium dendriticum*: a true infection? *Infez. Med.* 17, 115–116, 2009.

Manga-González MY, González-Lanza C, Field and experimental studies on *Dicrocoelium dendriticum* and dicrocoeliasis in northern *Spain*. *J. Helminthol.* 79, 291–302, 2005.

Otranto D, Traversa D, Dicrocoeliasis of ruminants: a little known fluke disease. *Trend Parasitol.* 19, 12–15, 2003.

Romig T, Lucius R, Frank W, Cerebral larvae in the second intermediate host of *Dicrocoelium dendriticum* (Rudolphi, 1819) and *Dicrocoelium hospes* Loos, 1907 (Trematodes, Dicrocoeliidae). *Z. Parasitenkd.* 63, 277–286, 1980.

Schweiger F, Kuhn M, *Dicrocoelium dentriticum* infection in a patient with Crohn's disease. *Can. J. Gastroenterol.* 22, 571–573, 2008.

Soyer T et al., Rare gallbladder parasitosis mimicking cholelithiasis: *Dicrocoelium dentriticum*. *Eur. J. Pediatr. Surg.* 18, 280–281, 2008.

4.3.4 DWARF FLUKE INFECTIONS (INTESTINAL DWARF FLUKE INFECTIONS)

Dwarf flukes represent a large group of small (maximum length approximately 2 mm) flukes of several families, which infest the intestine. They cause clinically mostly inapparent infections; however, occasionally, patients show intestinal symptoms, and rarely, extraintestinal signs. According to the agents, infections are known as echinostomiasis, heterophyiasis, or gymnophalloidiasis.

Etiology. The agents belong to a broad spectrum of small trematodes (0.5 to 2 mm in length) in >10 families in five orders. Particularly species-rich and widespread are the families Echinostomatidae (approximately 20 species in eight genera: *Echinostoma*, *Echinochasmus*, *Acanthoparyphium*, *Hypoderaeum*, and others) and Heterophyidae (about 30 species in nine genera: *Metagonymus*, *Haplorchis*, *Centrocestus*, *Heterophyes*, *Heterophyopsis*, *Pygidiopsis*, *Stellantchasmus*, *Stictodora*, and others). Also important are Plagiorchidae (*Plagiorchis* spp.), Lecithodendriidae (*Phaneropsulus* spp., *Prosthodendrium molenkampi*), and Gymnophallidae (*Gymnophalloides seoi*).

Occurrence. Most of the species found in humans are limited to Southeast and East Asia with marked differences in the local distributions. Some species are found in Europe, North Africa, and in the Near East [*Echinochasmus perfoliatus*, *Echinostoma echinatum* (syn. *E. lindoense*)], while others are cosmopolitans (*Echinostoma revolutum*, *Isthmiophora melis*, *Metagonimus yokogawai*). The natural spectra of final hosts are in general broad and include (domestic) aquatic birds and various mammals (rats, dogs, cats, pigs).

Human infections are common in rural areas of endemic regions. Prevalence rates sometimes amount to >70% and individual fluke burdens may come up to tens of thousands. In Europe, only a few cases have been reported.

Transmission. The life cycles of dwarf flukes are complicated with two intermediate hosts. Eggs are released with the feces and they must reach surface water. Miracidia develop in the eggs within a few weeks, hatch and invade freshwater or brackwater snails, where they are transformed to cercariae in the course of several asexual multiplications. Cercariae leave the snails, invade second intermediate hosts and encyst to metacercariae. Usually this stage is not very host specific; again, snails or amphibia (frogs, tadpoles) and fish may be considered, but some species are nevertheless specialized. Thus, Lecithodendriidae develop in dragonflies or in their larvae, which are consumed by humans in some ethnic groups; *Gymnophalloides seoi* shows a marine cycle and uses the Pacific oyster (*Crassostrea gigas*) as an intermediate host. Several hundred metacercariae may be found in one particular oyster.

Humans become infected by the ingestion of raw or undercooked second intermediate hosts. The young flukes attach to the intestinal mucosa and reach sexual maturity within 1 to 3 weeks, dependent on the species.

Clinical Manifestations. In most cases, the infection is inapparent. When the parasites adhere to the mucosa, a local catarrhal inflammation develops, which in massive infestations may cause clinical symptoms, such as diarrhea, flatulence, and abdominal pain.

Diagnosis. Diagnosis is done by microscopic detection of the operculated eggs in the feces. Eggs are mostly brownish but variable in size. In case of echinostomatids they measure 60 by 80 μm up to 90 by 130 μm; in some other species they are much smaller (e.g., 15 by 30 μm). The smallness of these eggs and the low reproductivity of the flukes hamper the diagnosis.

Differential Diagnosis. Enteritis of other genesis, gastric and duodenal ulcers must be considered in the differential diagnosis.

Therapy. Treatment uses praziquantel, three times 25 mg/kg for 1 day orally.

Prophylaxis. In endemic areas, consumption of raw or undercooked fish or suspicious, specific local food should be avoided.

REFERENCES

Abou-Basha LM et al., Epidemiological study of heterophyiasis among humans in an area of Egypt. *East Mediterr. Health J.* 6, 932–938, 2000.

Anh NT et al., Poultry as reservoir for fishborne zoonotic trematodes in Vietnamese fish farms. *Vet. Parasitol.* 169, 391–394, 2010.

Belizario YY et al., Intestinal heterophyiasis: an emerging food-borne parasitic zoonosis in southern Philippines. *S.E. Asian J. Trop. Med. Public Health* 32, Suppl. 2, 36–42, 2011.

Boerlage AS et al., Survival of heterophyid metacercariae in common carp (*Cyprinus carpio*). *Parasitol. Res.* 112, 2759–2762, 2013.

Carney WP, Echinostomiasis – a snail-borne intestinal trematode zoonosis. *Southeast Asian J. Trop. Med Public Health.* 22, pS206–S211, 1991.

Chai JY et al., High prevalence of *Haplorchis taichui*, *Prosthodendrium molenkampi*, and other helminth infections among people in Khammouane Province, Lao PDR. *Korean J. Parasitol.* 47, 243–247, 2009.

Fried B, Graczyk TK, Tamang L, Food-borne intestinal trematodiasis in humans. *Parasitol. Res.* 93, 159–170, 2004.

Graczyk TK, Fried B, Echinostomiasis: a common but forgotten food-borne disease. *Am. J. Trop. Med. Hyg.* 58, 501–504, 1998.

Hong SJ et al., Infection status of dragonflies with *Plagiorchis muris* metacercariae in Korea. *Korean J. Parasitol.* 37, 65–70, 1999.

Lee SH, Chai JY, A review of *Gymnophalloides seoi* (Digena: Gymnophallidae) and human infections in the Republic of Korea. *Korean J. Parasitol.* 39, 85–118, 2001.

Li K et al., Risk for fishborne zoonotic trematodes in tylapia production systems in Guangdong province, China. *Vet. Parasitol.* 58, 231–258, 2013.

Saijuntha W, Duenngai K, Tantrawatpan C, Zoonotic echinostome infections in free-grazing ducks in Thailand. *Korean J. Parasitol.* 51, 663–667, 2013.

WHO, Report Joint WHO/FAO workshop on food-borne trematode infections in Asia. Report Series Number: RS/2002/GE/40(VTN), 2002.

4.3.5 FASCIOLIASIS

Fascioliasis is an acute or chronic disease of the liver caused by infection of humans with liver flukes.

Etiology. Humans are infected mainly by the large liver fluke, *Fasciola hepatica* (14 by 30 mm in size) (Fig. 4.27). Human infections with the giant liver fluke, *Fasciola gigantica* (~70 mm in its natural host), are rare and limited to distinct geographical areas.

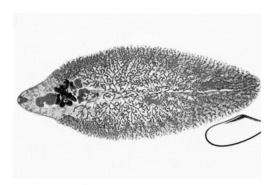

Figure 4.27 | Large liver fluke (*Fasciola hepatica*); original size: 2 cm). Carmin staining (picture: Institute for Parasitology, Giessen, Germany).

Occurrence. *F. hepatica* is distributed world-wide and it is especially common in moist regions with high rainfall that favor the development of the amphibious snails of the genus *Lymnaea* that serve as intermediate hosts. The main final hosts are domestic and wild ruminants, especially sheep; infections also occur in other herbivores and omnivores. In domestic ruminants, clinically and economically important diseases are common and often occur in epidemic dimensions.

F. gigantica is found in tropical zones of Asia and Africa, in Southeast Asia, and in countries of the Pacific area, often together with *F. hepatica*. In these regions, the latter parasite is usually found at higher altitudes. However, hybrid types may also have developed. Separate areas of distribution of *F. gigantica* are found in the Near East and the southern republics of the former Soviet Union. The host spectrum is identical to that of *F. hepatica*. Intermediate hosts are lymnaeid snails. In Egypt, the planorbid species *Biomphalaria alexandrina* has also been found naturally infected.

Human infections with *F. hepatica* occur worldwide, but a positive correlation between prevalence in humans and domestic animals does not necessarily exist. Considerable problems in humans are found in high-altitude regions of South America, mainly in Bolivia and Peru, and likely Ecuador. In the northern Altiplano of Bolivia, the prevalence may be 70%. In the Cusco (Cajamarca) area in Peru, >10% of schoolchildren are infected, and even in the urban hinterland of the capital Lima >25% of the inhabitants are carriers of *F. hepatica*. The highest prevalence rates are generally found in the age group of <15 years.

In the hyperendemic Andean regions, animal reservoirs are of minor importance. In other South American areas, the situation varies; 11.9% of schoolchildren in rural areas of Argentina showed antibodies to *F. hepatica*. A high prevalence is also reported from the Caribbean. Only a few cases of human fascioliasis are known from North America, Oceania, and Asia, except a high level of endemicity in the Asian former Soviet republics (mainly Uzbekistan and Tajikistan) and Iran. In Africa, frequent infections (a prevalence of 2 to 17%) have been found mainly in Egypt (Nile delta) where both *Fasciola* species coexist. In Europe, France, northern Portugal, and northern Spain are regarded as problematic zones. In France, about 400 cases a year were documented with regional accumulation in the years of 1970 to 1982, but the incidence has decreased in recent years. Altogether, a considerable number of undetected cases may exist in rural areas worldwide.

Transmission. Humans and animals are infected by ingestion of metacercariae adhering to plants (Fig. 4.28), for example, watercress and other vegetables raised in water. Careless chewing of such plants is sufficient for infection. Drinking water containing floating metacercariae also leads to infection (common in the Andean region of South America). Also in South America, consumption of "emolientes," a beverage of plant extracts that can be consumed cold or hot, is supposed to be medicative, but it is a risk factor. In addition, ingestion of raw liver, containing immature flukes may lead to infection.

Eggs of adult flukes in bile ducts are released through the common bile duct into the duodenum and are shed in feces into the environment. For further development, they must reach surface water, where miracidiae (ciliated larvae) develop within 1 to 2 weeks. They hatch from eggs and search actively for snails as intermediate hosts. After several asexual developmental steps, cercariae develop that leave the

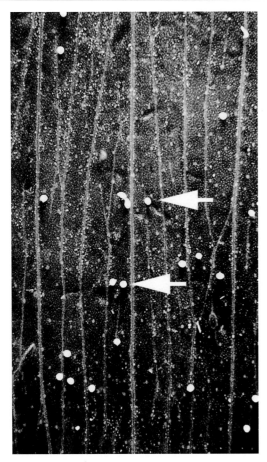

Figure 4.28 | Encysted metacercariae of *Fasciola hepatica*, attached to a blade of grass (picture: Institute for Parasitology, Giessen, Germany).

intermediate hosts, swim actively through the water, and finally adhere to plants, where they encyst to form metacercariae, which is the infective stage (Fig. 4.28). Under moist conditions, these remain viable and infectious for several months.

After oral ingestion of metacercariae, young flukes hatch in the duodenum, penetrate the intestinal wall, and enter the liver from the peritoneal cavity. After 6 to 8 weeks of migration through the liver parenchyma, the flukes penetrate the bile ducts, and reach their final destination. In ruminants, sexual maturity is reached about 10 weeks p.i.; in humans, patency is delayed by at least one month (prepatent period 3 to 4 months). The parasite can survive for more

than 10 years in ruminants and humans. The developmental cycle of *F. hepatica* is shown in Fig. 4.29.

Clinical Manifestations. In humans, the number of attacking flukes is usually low. As a result, infections, especially in the prepatent period, are often clinically inapparent. In the early stage (beginning about 2 weeks p.i.), perihepatitis resulting from migrating flukes develops, with general symptoms, for example, fever, fatigue, and anorexia. Usually leukocytosis, eosinophilia, and increased levels of IgE are found.

After adult parasites have settled in the bile duct, these become inflamed, eventually resulting in fibrosis and calcification. Anemia develops by continuous withdrawal of blood by the flukes. Besides intermittent fever, patients suffer from anorexia, weight loss, pruritus, and pain, usually localized under the right costal arch. Obstruction of bile ducts due to migrating flukes leads to recurrent episodes of icterus. Occasionally, parasites are ectopically localized in connective tissue, CNS, and eyes.

Diagnosis. During the prepatent period (3 months or more) serological tests, using excretory-secretory antigens of adult *F. hepatica*, may be used for diagnosis (crude antigens may cross-react with antibodies to other trematodes, i.e., *Opisthorchis* or *Schistosoma* spp.). After the beginning of patency, the typical operculated eggs of *F. hepatica* (90 by 150 µm) or *F. gigantica* (90 by 190 µm) may be detected in feces.

The simple sedimentation technique using tap water (cup sedimentation) has shown to be superior to other concentration techniques (merthiolate-iodine-formaldehyde or formaldehyde-ether concentration) and also to the Kato-Katz thick-smear method.

As eggs are not shed continuously, repeated examinations are necessary, and examinations may fail despite the presence of flukes. A single positive result is no proof either, as eggs and liver flukes within contaminated beef liver (sausages) may pass the intestinal tract of the host without morphological alterations. As an alternative to microscopical fecal examination, excretory-

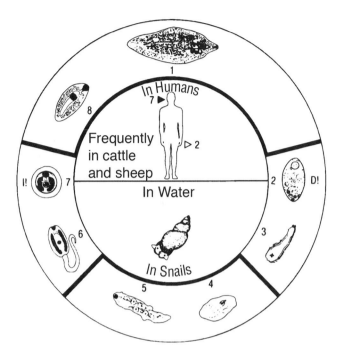

Figure 4.29 | Developmental cycle of *F. hepatica*. (1) Adult liver fluke (15 to 20 mm) in bile duct; (2) egg of liver fluke (0.09 to 0.15 mm) with zygote and nutrition cells (D, diagnostic stage); (3) miracidium (about 0.15 mm), hatched from egg and swimming in water; (4) sporocyst (0.3 to 0.5 mm) within snail (intermediate host, e.g., *Lymnaea truncatula*); (5) redia (1.5 to 2.5 mm) in a snail; (6) cercaria (0.67 to 1.45 mm), swimming in water; (7) metacercaria (encysted cercaria) (about 0.25 mm), adhering to a plant (I, infectious stage); (8) liver fluke (5 to 6 mm) in liver tissue, about 20 days old.

secretory antigens of *F. hepatica* can be demonstrated in feces by ELISA. This technique is especially suitable to confirm success of chemotherapeutic measures (negative results >15 days after successful treatment). In addition, CT scans, MRI, and X-rays may be used for diagnosis. Anemia is an important sign in chronic fascioliasis.

Differential Diagnosis. In the acute stage of the disease, perihepatitis of other etiology must be considered in differential diagnosis. In the chronic stage, cholestasis of different genesis and bile stones must be excluded.

Therapy. Patients are treated with one dose of triclabendazole, 10 mg/kg orally. Also nitazoxanide, 500 mg twice a day for 7 days, and bithionol, 20 to 30 mg/kg (maximum 2 g per day) every second day, altogether 10–15 applications are recommended. Resistance of *F. hepatica* to triclabendazole is spreading worldwide.

Prophylaxis. Plants on moist ground in grazing areas and near waters with temporary flooding may be contaminated with metacercariae. Do not chew on such plants and avoid consumption of watercress from natural habitats in these areas; do not drink unboiled or unfiltered surface water.

REFERENCES

Aksoy DY et al., *Fasciola hepatica* infection: clinical and computerized tomographic findings in ten patients. *Turk. J. Gastroenterol.* 17, 40–45, 2006.

Behar JM, Winston JS, Borgstein R, Hepatic fascioliasis at a London hospital – the importance of recognising typical radiological features to avoid a delay in diagnosis. *Br. J. Radiol.* 82, 189–193, 2009.

Cantisani V et al., Diagnostic imaging in the study of human hepatobiliary fascioliasis. *Radiol. Med.* 115, 83–92, 2010.

Dauchy FA et al., Distomatose à *Fasciola hepatica*: etude retrospective sur 23 ans au CHU de Bordeaux. *Presse Med.* 36, 1545–1549, 2007.

Espinoza JR et al., Evaluation of Fas2-Elisa for the serological detection of Fasciola hepatica infection in humans. *A. J. Trop. Med. Hyg.* 76, 977–982, 2007.

Espinoza JR et al., [Human and animal fascioliasis in Peru: impact in the economy of endemic zones; *article in Spanish*]. *Rev.Peru Med. Exp. Salud Publica* 27, 604–612, 2010.

Hammami H, Hamed N, Ayadi A, Epidemiological studies on *Fasciola hepatica* in Gafsa Oases (south west of Tunesia). *Parasite* 14, 261–264, 2007.

Le TH et al., Human fascioliasis and the presence of hybrid/introgressed forms of *Fasciola hepatica* and *Fasciola gigantica* in Vietnam. *Int. J. Parasitol.* 38, 725–730, 2008.

Lopez M, White AC Jr, Cabada MM, Burden of *Fasciola hepatica* infection among children in Cusco, Peru. *Am. J. Trop. Med. Hyg.* 86, 481–485, 2012.

Mailles A et al., Commercial watercress as a emerging source of fascioliasis in Northern France in 2002: results from an outbrake investigation. *Epidemiol. Infect.* 134, 942–945, 2006.

Marcos L et al., Risk factors for *Fasciola hepatica* infection in children: a case-control study. *Trans. R. Soc. Trop. Med. Hyg.* 100, 158–166, 2006.

Marcos A et al., Natural history, clinicoradiologic correlates, and response to triclabendazole in acute massive fascioliasis. *Am. J. Trop. Med. Hyg.* 78, 222–227, 2008.

Mas-Coma S, Agramunt VH, Valero MA, Neurological and ocular fascioliasis in humans. *Adv. Parasit.* 84, 27–149, 2014.

Mas-Coma S, Valero MA, Bargues MD, *Fasciola*, lymnaeids and human fascioliasis, with a global overview on disease transmission, epidemiology, evolutinary genetics, molecular epidemiology and control. *Adv. Parasitol.* 69, 41–146, 2009.

Parkinson M, O'Neill SM, Dalton JP, Endemic human fasciolosis in the Bolivian Altiplano. *Epidemiol. Infect.* 135, 669–674, 2007.

Ubeira FM et al., MM3-ELISA detection of *Fasciola hepatica* coproantigens in preserved human stool samples. *Am. J. Trop. Med. Hyg.* 81, 156–162, 2009.

Yilmaz H, Gödekmerkan A, Human fascioliasis in Van province, Turkey. *Acta Trop.* 92, 161–162, 2004.

Ying M, Xiaosu H, Wang B, A case of ectopic parasitism: *Fasciola hepatica* larvae burrow through a human brain and mimic cerebral aneurysm. *Trans. R. Soc. Trop. Med. Hyg.* 101, 1051–1052, 2007.

Zhou L et al., Multiple brain hemorrhages and hematomas associated with ectopic fascioliasis in brain and eye. *Surg. Neurol.* 69, 516–521, 2008.

4.3.6 FASCIOLOPSIASIS

Fasciolopsiasis is a clinically variable inflammatory-ulcerous disease of the intestine due to an infection with the giant intestinal fluke.

Etiology. The causative agent is *Fasciolopsis buski*, one of the largest parasitic trematodes with a size of 2 to 3 by 7 to 10 cm.

Occurrence. *F. buski* occurs in southeastern and eastern Asia. Its natural final hosts are humans and pigs. Prevalence rates vary regionally. Areas of endemicity are large parts of the People's Republic of China and the Republic of China (Taiwan), India, Bangladesh, Indonesia, Thailand, and Vietnam. Especially in children, prevalence rates may reach 70%.

Transmission. Infection occurs by oral ingestion of metacercariae adhering to water plants and their fruits. Epidemiologically important are water nuts and walnuts (fruits of *Trapa natans, T. bicornis*, and *Elocharis tuberosa*), which are cultivated with manure as fertilizer and are eaten by humans and are utilized as pig food.

After a maturation period of several weeks in a moist environment, miracida hatch from eggs in feces of infected hosts. They invade snails of the genera *Planorbis* and *Segmentina*, propagate asexually, and develop into cercariae, which are released from the snails and they encyst on water plants. Metacercariae are sensitive to dryness and infectivity is usually reduced during transport of contaminated water fruits to regional markets.

After cracking of contaminated nuts with the teeth, metacercariae reach the oral cavity, where they are swallowed. Young flukes are liberated in the duodenum, attach to the duodenal mucosa, and reach sexual maturity within 3 months.

Clinical Manifestations. The flukes cause inflammatory and ulcerous lesions. After an incubation period of 1 to 2 months, epigastric and hypogastric pain and pasty feces or diarrhea, occasionally alternating with constipation, may develop. In severe cases, loss of weight, anemia, edema, and ascites are found. Cachexia follows, possibly caused by toxic action of metabolic products of the flukes, and death may occur.

Diagnosis. After the end of the prepatent period, diagnosis is made by fecal examination and demonstration of operculated eggs (80 to 130 μm) filled with yolk material. However, these eggs are easily mistaken for eggs of *F. hepatica* or Echinostomatidae (see chapter 4.3.4).

Differential Diagnosis. Signs of this disease are nonspecific; however, the predominantly intestinal symptoms allow differentiation from *F. hepatica* infestations. Enteritis and intestinal ulcers of other etiology must be considered.

Therapy. Patients are treated with praziquantel, three 25 mg/kg doses in 1 day.

Prophylaxis. Avoid cracking water nuts and chestnuts with your teeth. Treatment of nuts with scalding water kills metacercariae of *F. buski*. Hands may become contaminated while handling contaminated fruit. Human or pig feces should not get into surface water without decontamination (lime and storage) and should not be used as fertilizer for production of water fruit.

REFERENCES

Bhattacharjee HK,Yadav D, Bagga D, Fasciolopsiasis presenting as intestinal perforation: case report. *Trop. Gastroenterol.* 30, 40–41, 2009.

Graczy, K, Gilman RH, Fried B, Fasciolopsiasis: is it a controllable food-borne disease? *Parasitol. Res.* 87, 80–83, 2001.

Le TH et al., Case report: unusual presentation of *Fasciolopsis buski* in a Vietnamese child. *Trans. R. Soc. Trop. Med. Hyg.* 98, 193–194, 2004.

Mas-Coma S, Bargues MD, Valero MA,Fascioliasis and otherplant-borne trematode zoonoses. *Int. J. Parasitol.* 35, 1255–1278, 2005.

Plaut AG, Kampanart-Sanyakorn C, Manning GS, A clinical study of *Fasciolopsis buski* infection in Thailand. *Trans. R. Soc. Trop. Med. Hyg.* 63, 470–478, 1969.

Sing UC et al., Small bowel stricture and perforation: an unusual presentation of *Fasciolopsis buski*. *Trop. Gastroenterol.* 32, 320–322, 2011.

Sripa B et al., Food –borne trematodiases in Southeast Asia: epidemiology, pathology, clinical manifestation and control. *Adv. Parasitol.* 72, 305–350, 2010.

Wiwanitkit V, Suwansaksri J, Chalyakhun Y, High prevalence of *Fasciolopsis buski* in an endemic area of liver fluke infection.MedGenMed. 4, 6, 2002.

4.3.7 OPISTHORCHIASIS

Opisthorchiasis is a liver disease, predominantly of the bile duct system.

Etiology. Etiologic agents are the liver flukes of cats: *Opisthorchis felineus* (7 to 12 mm by 2 to 3 mm in size) and *O. viverrini* (6 to 16 by 1 to 2 mm).

Occurrence. *O. felineus* occurs in Eastern Europe, including eastern Brandenburg (Germany) and Southern Europe, and the Asiatic part of the former Soviet Union, including Siberia, especially along big rivers. *O. viverrini* is found in Southeast Asia, predominantly in northeastern Thailand and in Laos as well as in East Asia. Animal hosts are piscivorous mammals, mainly felines and canines. A predominantly anthroponotic cycle occurs in the case of *O. viverrini*.

Human infections occur throughout the above mentioned areas but prevalence rates vary extremely. Cases in Europe are rare although eight outbreaks with >200 cases were observed in central Italy between 2003 and 2011; all patients had eaten tench (*Tinca tinca*) caught in two north Italian lakes. Otherwise, in areas of endemicity, more than 80% of the population may be infected, for example, with *O. felineus* in western Siberia and with *O. viverrini* in northern Thailand. In zones of hyperendemicity, parasites are transmitted without involvement of animal reservoir hosts.

Closely related zoonotic agents are *Metorchis albidus* and *Pseudoamphistomum truncatum*, which live in bile ducts of piscivorous carnivores (cats, dogs, otters) in North America and Europe.

Transmission. Infection occurs by ingestion of raw or insufficiently cooked freshwater fish (mostly cyprinids), containing metacercariae within the intramuscular connective tissue.

Eggs released with the feces of infected hosts contain larvae (miracidia) and must reach water for further development. They are ingested by water snails of the genus *Codiella* (*O. felineus*) or *Bythinia* (*O. viverrini*). Several steps of asexual multiplication in these intermediate hosts result in the production of so-called pipe head cercariae, which leave the snails and enter fishes (second intermediate hosts). There they encyst to 0.2 mm diameter metacercariae. The cycle closes when the metacercariae are ingested by suitable hosts. Young flukes are released in the duodenum, migrate through the common bile duct to small bile ducts, and mature into adult, egg-producing flukes within 3 to 4 weeks. Parasites survive in humans for 10 years or more.

Clinical Manifestations. Pathogenesis and clinical symptoms of the disease resemble that of clonorchiasis: cholangitis and, in late stages, liver cirrhosis and pancreatitis ensue. For *O. viverrini*, a close causal relation exists between the infection and the occurrence of cholangiocarcinoma (according to IARC/WHO Type 1-carcinogen). Cholangiocarcinoma morbidity rate in the North East of Thailand (Khon Kaen area), a hyperendemic zone with *O. viverrini* prevalence of 30 to 50%, reaches up to 60 cases per 100 000 inhabitants.

Diagnosis. Diagnosis is achieved by microscopic detection of the operculated, yellow-brownish eggs of *O. viverrini* (15 by 27 µm) or *O. felineus* (15 by 35 µm) in fecal samples. Alternatively, specific DNA sequences can be demonstrated by PCR. Suitable serological tools are also available.

Differential Diagnosis. Besides infections with other hepatotropic trematodes, diseases of the bile duct and liver due to other causes must be considered.

Therapy. The drug of choice is praziquantel, three 25 mg/kg doses per day for 2 days. Dependent on the extent of damage to organs, supporting therapeutic measures are required.

Prophylaxis. Infection is prevented if fish is eaten when properly cooked (see also "Clonorchiasis" above).

REFERENCES

Andrews RH, Sithithavorn P, Petney TN, *Opisthorchis viverini: an underestimated parasite in world health. Trends Parasitol.* 4, 497–501, 2008.

Armignacco O et al., Human illnesses caused by *Opisthorchis felineus* fluke, Italy. *Emerg. Infect. Dis.* 14, 1902–1905, 2008.

Enes JE et al., Prevalence of *Opithorchis viverrini* infection in canine and feline hosts in three villages, Khon Kaen Province, northeastern Thailand. *Southeast Asian J. Trop. Med. Public Health* 41, 36–42, 2010.

Ewald PW, An evolutionary perspective on parasitism as a cause of cancer. *Adv. Parasitol.* 68, 21–43, 2009.

Intapan PM et al., Rapid molecular detection of *Opisthorchis viverrini* in human fecal samples by real-time polymerase chain reaction. *Am. J. Trop.Med. Hyg.* 81, 917–920. 2009.

Lima dos Santos C, Hazard analysis critical control point and aquaculture. In: *Public, animal, and environmental aquacultures health issues.* (eds. ML Jahncke, ES Garrett, A. Reilly, R.E. Martin, E. Cole), Wiley-Interscience Inc., Chichester, pp. 103–119, 2002.

Lovis I et al., PCR diagnosis of *Opisthorchis viverrini* and *Haplorchis taichui* infections in a Lao community in an
area of endemicity and comparison of diagnostic methods for parasitological field surveys. *J. Clin. Microbiol.* 47, 1517–1523, 2009.

Petney TN et al., The zoonotic fish-borne liver flukes *Clonorchis sinensis, Opisthorchis felineus* and *Opisthorchis viverrini. Int. J. Parasitol.* 43, 1031–1046, 2013.

Pitaksakulerat O et al., A cross-sectional study on the potential transmission of the carcinogenic liver fluke *Opithorchis viverrini* and other fishborne zoonotic trematodes by aquaculture fish. *Foodborn Pathog. Dis.* 10, 35–41, 2013.

Pozio E et al., *Opisthorchis felineus*, an emerging infection in Italy and its implication for the European Union. *Acta Trop.* 126, 54–62, 2013.

Schuster RK, Opisthorchiidosis – a review. *Infect. Disord. Drug Targets* 10, 402–415, 2010.

Touch S et al., Discovery of *Opisthorchis viverrini* metacercariae in freshwater fish in southern Cambodia. *Acta Trop.* 111, 108–113, 2009.

WHO Report Series Number: RS/y2002/GE/40(VTN), 2002.

Yossepowitch O et al., Opisthorchiasis from imported raw fish. *Emerg. Infect. Dis.* 10, 2122–2126, 2004.

4.3.8 PARAGONIMIASIS (PULMONARY DISTOMATOSIS)

Paragonimiasis is a mostly chronic, pulmonary disease that is a consequence of infection with lung flukes. These parasites may also produce ectopic infections of other organs, for example, the CNS.

Etiology. Human lung flukes are members of the genus *Paragonimus*. The most common species is *P. westermani*. At least eight further species/subspecies attack humans. The reddish-brown, oval parasites carrying surface spines reach a size of 4 to 8 by 8 to 16 mm.

Occurrence. The various species are distinguished zoogeographically. *P. westermani* and *P. ohirai* are prevalent predominantly in Central, Southeast and East Asia. *P. skrjabini* occurs mainly in the mountainous region of China, *P. myazakii* is present predominantly in Japan, and *P. heterotremus* occurs preponderantly in southern China, Thailand, and Laos. Furthermore, *P kellicotti* is found mainly in North America, *P. mexicana* (a synonym for several formerly used species names) occurs mainly in Central and South America, and *P africanus* and *P. uterobilateralis* are present in tropical Africa (particularly in Cameroon and Nigeria). However, the biodiversity is probably higher than stated.

The main hosts are various mammals that eat crustaceans, that is, canids, felids, small beasts of prey, and omnivores. Prevalence in humans may be >10% and is generally highest in mountainous areas. In some regions, for example, Thailand and Korea, prevalence has decreased in recent years, whereas increased prevalence has been observed in some parts of China. Due to different nutrition habits, only 10 to 15 cases are known from the United States. About 20 million humans may be infected worldwide.

Transmission. Transmission usually occurs by ingestion of undercooked meat of freshwater crabs and other crustaceans. Raw freshwater crabs are often eaten in Asia soaked with soybean sauce, liquor or rice wine ("drunken crabs"). Ingestion of underdone meat of infected hosts harboring immature stages of the parasites in their tissues, for example, pigs, may also lead to infection.

Adult parasites often live in pairs in cysts within lung connective tissue. Eggs are expectorated or are swallowed and excreted with the feces. They must reach water for further development. In water, miracidia develop within weeks, hatch, and enter first intermediate hosts, which are amphibic or aquatic operculated snails (*Melania* spp. and *Ampullaria* sp.). After asexual multiplication at several stages, cercariae develop, which leave the snails and enter their second intermediate hosts, crustaceans. There they encyst in muscles and inner organs to metacercariae.

After oral ingestion of second intermediate hosts by the final hosts, young flukes are liberated in the gut, penetrate the intestinal wall, and migrate within 3 weeks through the peritoneal cavity and the diaphragm into the parenchyma of the lungs. The parasites become encapsulated by connective tissue and they start laying eggs within 6 to 7 weeks p.i. Ectopic invasion of other organs, for example, the liver or the CNS, may occur.

Clinical Manifestations. Migrating parasites cause inflammation with eosinophilic infiltration of the peritoneum, pleura, and lungs. Clinical signs during the prepatent period depend on the number of invading lungs flukes; in the lungs, focal infiltrations develop. Patent infections are associated with chest pain, cough, dyspnea, and fever. The sputum is viscous and often rusty-brown. Ectopic localization of the parasites is common in humans and accompanied by organ-specific symptoms. Severe disease occurs if flukes migrate into the brain or spinal cord where they are encapsulated by granulomatous tissue. First signs of disease are cramps, headache, dizziness, vomiting, and fever. Migrating subcutaneous nodes with young flukes are common in *P. skrjabini* infection.

Diagnosis. The operculated eggs of *Paragonimus* spp. have a size of 60 by 90 μm and are detected beginning 12 weeks p.i. in bloody sputum, or occasionally, in feces.

Ziehl-Neelsen staining destroys *Paragonimus* eggs and may therefore interfere with lung fluke diagnosis. It is recommended, particularly in cases with low fluke loads, to collect expectorated sputum of 24 h, to liquefy it with 3% sodium hydroxide solution, and to concentrate the eggs by centrifugation.

Auscultation and percussion as well as X-ray and tomographic examination of the thorax are diagnostically important. However, the findings are not pathognomonic. Cysts containing parasites measure 5 to 30 mm in diameter. In sputum-negative ("closed") *Paragonimus* infections, serodiagnostic methods are helpful for diagnosis. Serologic cross-reactions between the various *Paragonimus* species allow a group-specific diagnosis.

Differential Diagnosis. Pulmonary tuberculosis, bronchopneumonia, bronchitis of other etiology, histoplasmosis, and lung tumors must be excluded if eggs are not detected. Symptoms of cerebral paragonimiasis resemble those of toxoplasmosis, cysticercosis, and viral and bacterial infections, as well as brain tumors. In the case of migrating subdermal nodes (*P. skrjabini*), spargana (see chapter 4.5.4) and

Gnathostomum infections (chapter 4.5.8) must be considered.

Therapy. Drugs of choice are praziquantel, 25 mg/kg three times per day orally for 2 days, or bithionol, 30 to 50 mg/kg (maximum 2 g/day) every second day, 10 to 15 applications. In addition to drug therapy, surgical treatment may be indicated in special cases.

Prophylaxis. Do not consume undercooked crustaceans. Pickled crustacean meat may still be infectious. In addition, meat of other animals should not be consumed uncooked in areas of endemicity as it could contain infectious, immature stages.

REFERENCES

Aka NA et al., Human paragonimiasis in Africa. *Ann. Afr. Med.* 7, 153–162, 2008.

Blair D et al., *Paragonimus skjabini* Chen, 1959 (Digenea: Paragonimidae) and related species in eastern Asia: a combined molecular and morphological approach to identification and taxonomy. *Syst. Parasitol.* 60, 1–21, 2005.

Calvopina M et al., Comparison of two single-day regimens of triclabendazole for the treatment of human pulmonary paragonimiasis. *Trans. R. Soc. Trop. Med. Hyg.* 97, 451–454, 2003.

Cha SH et al., Cerebral paragonimiasis in early active stage: CT and MR features. *Am. J. Roentgenol.* 162, 141–145, 1994.

Choo JD et al., Chronic cerebral paragonimiasis combined with aneurysmalsubarachnoid hemorrhage. *Am J. Trop. Med. Hyg.* 69, 466–469, 2003.

Diaz JH Paragonimiasis acquired in the United States: native and nonnative species. *Clin Microbiol. Rev.* 26, 493–504, 2013.

Fischer PU et al., Serological diagnosis of North American paragonimiasis by Western blot using *Paragonimus kellicotti* adult worm antigen. *Am. J. Trop. Med. Hyg.* 88, 1035–1040, 2013.

Kuroki M et al., High resolution computed tomography findings on *P. westermani. J. Thorac Imaging* 20, 210–213, 2005.

Lane MA et al., *Paragonimus kellicotti* in Missouri, USA. *Emerg. Infect. Dis.* 18, 1263–1267, 2012.

Liu Q et al. Paragonimiasis: an important food-borne zoonosis in China. *Trends Parasitol.* 24, 318–323, 2008.

Nikouawa A et al., Paragonimiasis in Cameroon: molecular identification, serodiagnosis and clinical manifestation. *Trans. R. Soc.Trop.Med. Hyg.* 103, 255–261, 2009.

Niu JF, Lin LH, Advances in clinical therapeutics of paragonimiasis, *Endemic Dis. Bulletin* 16, 101–102, 2001.

Procop GW, North American paragonimiasis (caused by *Paragonimus kellicotti*) in the context of global paragonimiasis.*Clin Microbiol. Rev.* 22, 415–446, 2009.

Sim YS et al., *Paragonimus westermani* found in the tip of a little finger. *Intern. Med.* 49, 1645–1648, 2010.

Vidamali S et al., Paragonimiasis: a common cause of persistent pleural effusion in Lao PDR. *Trans. R. Soc. Trop. Med. Hyg.* 103, 1019–1023, 2009.

4.3.9 SCHISTOSOMIASIS (BILHARZIOSIS)

Schistosomiasis, caused by *Schistosoma* spp., is common in tropical and subtropical areas. The area affected is dependent on the parasite species, and is predominantly the intestinal tract and liver, or the urogenital tract.

Etiology. The most important schistosomes in humans are *Schistosoma mansoni*, which causes intestinal schistosomiasis; *S. haematobium*, which causes schistosomiasis of the urinary bladder, and *S. japonicum*, which causes Asian intestinal schistosomiasis. Additional species, occurring in humans are *S. mekongi, S. intercalatum, S. malayensis*, more rarely *S. bovis, S. matheei, S. magrebowiei*, and *S. rodhaini* (see Tab. 4.7). Hybridization between species is known, particularly between *S. haematobium* and *S. intercalatum*, as well as between *S. mansoni* and *S. rodhaini*.

Schistosomes are 7 to 20 mm (males) and 8 to 28 mm (females) in length and <1 mm in diameter. They live in blood vessels in permanent copulation (Fig. 4.28).

Occurrence. *S. haematobium* is highly prevalent in North Africa but is present throughout Africa and in the Middle East. According to recent observations (2011 to 2013), the parasite was introduced to the south of the island of Corsica. *S. mansoni* occurs in Egypt and East, Central and West Africa, in the Middle East, in northern and western South America, and on the Caribbean islands. *S. japonicum* is limited to Southeast and East Asia. *S. mekongi* is prevalent in Laos and the Mekong valley of Cambodia (population at risk approximately 150 000), and *S. malayensis* locally in Sarawak (Malaysia). The other species occur in tropical Africa.

Table 4.7 | *Schistosoma* spp. found in humans; geographical distribution, major final, and intermediate hosts

SPECIES	GEOGRAPHICAL DISTRIBUTION	MAJOR FINAL HOSTS	INTERMEDIATE HOSTS
S. mansoni	Africa, Middle East, Central and South America	Humans, other primates, rodents	*Biomphalaria* spp.
S. haematobium	Africa, Middle East	Humans, other primates rodents	*Bulinus* spp.
S. japonicum	Southeast and East Asia	Humans, ruminants[1], dogs[2], rats, other rodents	*Oncomelania* spp.
S. mekongi	Laos, Cambodia	Humans, dogs, rodents	*Neotrichura aperta*
S. malayensis	Malaysia (local)	Humans	*Robertiella* sp.
S. intercalatum	Central Africa	Humans (sheep, rodents)	*Bulinus* spp.
S. magrebowiei	West and Central Africa	Waterbucks (humans)	*Bulinus* spp.
S. matthei	South and Southeast Africa	Waterbucks, cattle (humans)	*Bulinus* spp.
S. bovis	Africa (north 10°N)	Cattle, other ruminants (humans)	*Bulinus* spp.
S. rodhaini	East Africa	Rodents, dogs (humans)	*Biomphalaria* spp.

[1] Lowlands.
[2] Hilly areas, Philippines.

The WHO suggests that 650 million people currently live at risk of infections with schistosomes and that 190 to 200 million are infected. Most infected people (165 million) live in Africa, south the Sahara (Nigeria: 26 million; Ghana: 12 million; Mozambique: 11 million); 19 million infected people reside in the Near East and the Mediterranean area (Egypt: 10 million), 7.4 million in Central and South America (Brazil: 7 million), and 1.7 million in Asia.

Humans are the main hosts for *S. haematobium*, *S.mansoni*, and *S. japonicum*. The role of animal reservoirs seems of minor importance in the case of *S. haematobium*, but baboons and other monkey species, pigs and various rodents may be involved. Various monkey and rodent species act as reservoir hosts for *S. mansoni*. Zoonotic relationships are most pronounced with *S. japonicum*. Reservoir hosts are domestic ruminants (water buffaloes and cattle), in the hilly areas of China and on the Philippines they are predominantly dogs but also rats (*Rattus r. mindanensis*). The main reservoir for *S. mekongi* are dogs. The other species infective for humans, *S. intercalatum*, *S. bovis*, *S. magrebowiei*, and *S. mattheei*, occur in various domestic and free-living ruminants; *S. rodhaini* is primarily a rodent parasite.

Transmission. The infectious stages of schistosomes consists of cercariae swimming in water (Fig. 4.30) and invading the final host percutaneously.

Schistosoma eggs are excreted with feces or urine by infected final hosts. They contain ciliated larvae (miracidia) that hatch when the eggs come into water and invade aquatic snails as intermediate hosts, predominantly in shallow water zones: *S. mansoni* invades *Biomphalaria* spp., *S. haematobium* invades *Bulinus* spp., and *S.japonicum* invades *Oncomelania* spp. Within the intermediate host, cercariae develop in the course of several asexual multiplications and

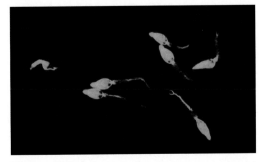

Figure 4.30 | Cercariae of *Schistosoma mansoni*: demonstrated by immunofluorscent staining (picture: Institute for Parasitology, Giessen, Germany).

leave the snails actively. They swim close to the water surface until they meet suitable hosts (cercariae may survive in the water for about 2 days) (Fig. 4.31). They adhere to the skin, shed their tail, and penetrate the skin within minutes with the aid of secreted enzymes. During invasion, they transform to schistosomula, which then are already adapted to a life in a mammalian host. They reach the lungs through lymph and blood vessels and from there the portal vein, where they develop to sexually mature trematodes. Subsequently, they migrate to their final destination, that is, the mesenteric veins (*S. mansoni, S. japonicum*) or the veins of the urinary bladder (*S. haematobium*). Five weeks p.i., the first eggs may be found in feces or urine. Egg production is between 200 and 3000 eggs per pair of worms per day. Worms may survive for 30 years.

The mechanism of egg excretion is complicated. The spined eggs reach the capillaries of the mucosa of the intestinal tract or urinary bladder against the blood stream; meanwhile, the miracidia develop in the eggs. The eggs finally get stuck in the capillaries, where they induce granulomatous reactions. If this process occurs close to the mucosal surface, eggs break through into the lumen of the organ. Otherwise, the miracidia die within 3 to 4 weeks and the granulomas are organized by connective tissue. By the continuing egg production, severe irreversible lesions develop. Eggs transported to other organs, for example, the liver, by blood circulation induce corresponding granulomatous

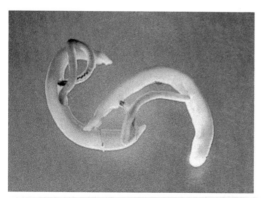

Figure 4.31 | Adult *Schistosoma* flukes (female and male in copulation), isolated from a mesenteric vein.

reactions. The developmental cycle of *S mansoni* is shown in Fig. 4.32.

Clinical Manifestations. Acute schistosomiasis (toxemic phase, Katayama syndrome): Invading cercariae cause itching papules (in particular in case of reinfections) at the invasion site that persist for 2 to 4 days. Subsequently, within 2 weeks until approximately 3 months after heavy infection, a complex of severe symptoms with fever, anorexia, headache, generalized pains, dizziness, vomiting, diarrhea, hepatosplenomegaly may develop, which is immunologically associated with proinflammatory, Th1-dominated reactions. The symptoms may persist for some weeks, sometimes for 2 to 3 months, until Th2-determined reactions start to reduce inflammatory responses and lead over to a more chronic status of the disease.

Chronic schistosomiasis. Schistosomiasis of the bladder: 10 to 12 weeks after infection with *S. haematobium*, hematuria, strangury, and increased frequency of miction develop due to the continuous deposition of eggs in the wall of the urinary bladder. As only part of the eggs reaches the lumen of the bladder and many eggs remain in the wall, fibrotic changes with calcification occur during chronic schistosomiasis and result in obstructive uropathy. Secondary bacterial urinary tract infections are frequently observed. The urinary cancer rate is increased in *S. haematobium* infection. Ureters and female genitalia are often involved in the disease process. Ectopically localized eggs are found in the liver, lungs, and CNS.

Schistosomiasis of the intestinal tract: Colicky pain and severe bloody diarrhea, alternating with constipation, occur after beginning of patency in heavy infections. Infections with fewer parasites may take an inapparent course. Prolonged disease results in fibrosis of the intestinal wall and colonic polyposis.

Other sequelae of schistosomal infections: Many eggs are swept downstream to the liver, where they elicit intense granuloma formation; subsequently, these granulomas are replaced by fibrous tissue. Portal blood flow is blocked, giving rise to portal hypertension and

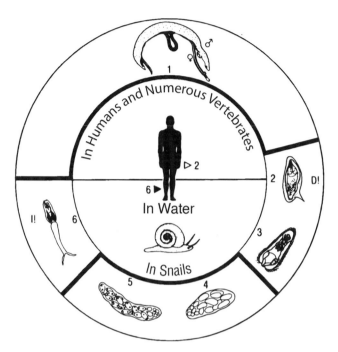

Figure 4.32 | Developmental cycle of *S. mansoni*. (1) Adult *S. mansoni* fluke (male, 6 to 10 mm; female, 7 to 15 mm) in intestinal and mesenterial veins or in the portal vein system (female fluke within the canalis gynaecophorus of the male); (2) *S. mansoni* egg (0.05 to 0.15 mm) shed with feces, with miracidium ready to hatch (D, diagnostic stage); (3) miracidium (ca. 0.13 mm), swimming in water; (4 and 5) mother sporocyst (4) and daughter sporocyst (5) in snail (intermediate host, e.g., *Biomphalaria glabrata*); (6) furcocercous cercaria ("furcocercaria") (about 0.375 to 0.590 mm), swimming in water (I, infectious stage).

portosystemic, collateral circulation with splenomegaly and esophageal varices, which may bleed profusely. In addition, viral infections and malnutrition may accelerate the disease process, which finally results in liver cirrhosis and organ failure.

Portosystemic circulatory shunt favors schistosomal eggs to bypass the liver. They may be swept into the pulmonary capillaries. Here, too, blood flow is blocked by granulomas, thus, inducing pulmonary hypertension. Particularly in *S. japonicum*, infections eggs are swept into the CNS and the granulomas may cause localized cerebral lesions or generalized encephalopathy with, for example, seizures.

Diagnosis. In patent infections, schistosomal eggs are detected in urine or feces. Eggs of *S. haematobium*, 50 by 150 μm in size, with a terminal spine, are generally found in endstream urine after sedimentation. Eggs of *S. mansoni*, 50 by 150 μm in size and equipped with a lateral spine, and eggs of *S. japonicum*, 55 by 90 μm in size with only a small terminal spine, are detected in feces after concentration, for example, by the formaldehyde-ether or other procedure.

Because of irregular egg excretion in light of chronic infections, several samples have to be examined for a positive result. Rectal biopsies are no more sensitive than repeated fecal examinations. If only few eggs are excreted, the miracium-hatching test may be employed.

Serological investigations are particularly helpful in cases of travelers returning from areas of endemicity, while for residents in such areas, who are constantly exposed to infections, they may fail. Various techniques (IHA, ELISA, and IFA) are available. Purified reagents such as microsomal antigens from adult flukes or (soluble) egg antigens (SEA) may be used, whereby, their species specificity allows differentiation by immunoblotting. Antibodies (IgG and IgM) persist for years after therapy and, therefore, they cannot be used to control therapeutic success.

An alternative is demonstrating circulating antigens, especially of the genus-specific circulating anodic antigen (CAA) and of the circulating cathodic antigen (CCA). They can be demonstrated in serum (predominantly CAA) or urine (mainly CCA) by ELISA applying monoclonal antibodies. These techniques detect even moderate infections 4 to 5 weeks p.i., and antigen levels are correlated with the number of living flukes. The assays are therefore suitable for therapy control. Ultrasonography is useful for detection of *Schistosoma*-induced organ lesions.

Differential Diagnosis. In the toxemic phase, other infections have to be excluded. In cases of intestinal schistosomiasis, infections with other enteropathogens, as well as hepatosplenomegaly of other etiology, for example, chronic viral hepatitis, liver cirrhosis, and miliary tuberculosis, must be considered. Hematuria, as in *S. haematobium* infections, may also be due to bacterial cystitis, urogenital tuberculosis, and renal cell carcinoma.

Therapy. Praziquantel is the drug of choice. Patients infected with *S. mansoni* or *S. haematobium* are treated with two doses of 20 mg/kg orally in 1 day; those infected with *S. japonicum* or *S. mekongi* with three doses of 20 mg/kg orally, given 4 h apart, in 1 day. Oxamniquine, one dose of 15 mg/kg orally, is active against *S. mansoni*; patients in North and East Africa are treated with 20 mg/kg/day, orally, for 3 days. Metrifonate, active against *S. haematobium*, is given orally in a dose of 7.5 to 10 mg/kg, to be repeated twice at 2 week intervals.

Prophylaxis. Avoid contact with surface water in zones of endemicity. Infected snails may be found occasionally in cisterns and other water reservoirs. It is important to avoid contamination of any kind of surface waters by feces and urine of humans suffering from schistosomiasis. In clearly defined regions, use of molluscicides to destroy the intermediate hosts of schistosomes (snails) has been successful. Alternatively, biological control measures are applied, for example, the release of snail species that are able to supersede the transmitter population. In China, mass treatment against *S. japonicum* in connection with control measures has considerably reduced the pressure and prevalence of infection (1 million currently infected humans versus 30 million in previously). However, reinfections must be expected constantly. Currently, vaccines against *S. japonicum* for domestic animals are in development to reduce animal reservoirs.

REFERENCES

Amarir F et al., National serologic survey of haematobium schistosomiasis in Morocco: evidence for elimination. *Am. J. Trop. Med. Hyg.* 84, 15–19, 2011.

Attwood SW et al., The distribution of Mekong schistosomiasis, past and future: preliminary indications from an analysis of genetic variation in the intermediate host. *Parasitol. Int.* 57, 256–270, 2008.

Attwood SW et al., The phylogeography of Asian *Schistosoma* (Trematoda: Schistosomatidae). *Parasitology* 125, 99–112, 2002.

Burke ML et al., Immunopathogenesis of human schistosomiasis. *Parasite Immunol.* 31, 163–176, 2009.

Chen YY et al., New integrated strategy emphasizing infection source control to curb schistosomiasis japonica in a marshland area of Hubai province, China: findings, from an eight-year longitudinal study. *PloS One* 9, e89779, 2014.

Chitsulo L et al., The global status of schistosomiasis and its control. *Acta Trop.* 77, 41–51, 2000.

Chuah C et al., Cellular and chemokine-mediated regulation in schistosome-induced hepatic pathology. *Trends Parasitol.* 30, 141–150, 2014.

Duus LM et al., The *Schistosoma*-specific antibody response after treatment in non-immune travellers. *Scand. J. Infect. Dis.* 41, 285–290, 2009.

Gray DJ et al., A cluster-randomised intervention trial against *Schistosoma japonicum* in the Peoples' Republic of China: bovine and human transmission. *PLoS One* 4, e5900, 2009.

Holtfreter M et al., *Schistosoma haematobium* infections acquired in Corsica, France, August 2013. *Euro Surveill.* 19, pii. 20821, 2014.

Hotez PJ, Fenwick A, Schistosomiasis in Africa: an emerging tragedy in our new global health decade. *PLoS Negl. Trop. Dis.* 3, e485, 2009.

Jauréguiberry S, Paris L, Caumes L, Acute schistosomiasis, a diagnostic and therapeutic challenge. *Clin. Microbiol. Infect.* 16, 225–231, 2010.

Kato-Hayashi N et al., Identification and differentiation of human schistosomes by polymerase chain reaction. *Exp. Parasitol.* 124, 325–329, 2010.

Lieshout van L et al., Immunodiagnosis of schistosomiasis by determination of the circulating antigens CAA and CCA, in particular in individuals with recent or light infections. *Acta Trop.* 77, 69–80, 2000.

McManus DP, Loukas A, Current status of vaccines for schistosomiasis. *Clin. Microbiol. Rev.* 21, 225–242, 2008.

Mo AX et al., Schistosomiasis eliminationn strategies and potential role of vaccine in achieving global health goals. *Am. J. Trop. Med. Hyg.* 90, 54–60, 2014.

Muth S et al., *Schistosoma mekongi* in Cambodia and Lao People Democratic Republic. *Adv. Parasitol.* 72, 179–203, 2010.

Nascimento-Cavalho CM, Moreno-Cavalho OA, Neuroschistosomiasis due to *Schistosoma mansoni*: a review of pathogenesis, clinical syndromes and diagnostic approaches. *Rev. Inst. Trop. Sao Paulo* 47, 179–184, 2005.

Nlenga SM et al., Once a year school-based deworming with praziquantel and albendazole combination may not be adequate for control of urogenital schistosomiasis and hookworm infection in Matuga district, Kwale County, Kenya. *Parasite Vectors* 7, 74, 2014.

Pinto-Silva RA et al., Ultrasound in schistosomiasis mansoni. *Mem. Inst. Oswaldo Cruz* 105, 479–484, 2010.

Ross AG et al., Katayama syndrome. *Lancet Infect. Dis.* 7, 218–224, 2007.

Rudge JW et al., Population genetics of *Schistosoma japonicum* within the Philippines suggest high transmission between humans and dogs. *PLoS Negl. Trop. Dis.* 2, e340, 2008.

Rudge JW et al., Parasite genetic differentiation by habitat type and host species: molecular epidemiology of *Schistosoma japonicum* in hilly and marshland areas of Anhui Province, *China. Mol. Ecol.* 18, 2134–2147, 2009.

Sagin DD et al., Schistosomiasis malayense-like infection among the Penan and other interior tribes (Orang Ulu) in upper Rejang River Basin, Sarawak, Malaysia. *Southeast Asian J. Trop. Med. Public Health* 32, 27–32, 2001.

Shiff C et al., Non-invasive methods to detect *Schistosoma*-based bladder cancer: is the association sufficient for epidemiological use. *Trans. R. Soc. Trop. Med. Hyg.* 104, 3–5, 2010.

Standley CJ et al., Confirmed infection with intestinal schistosomiasis in semi-captive wild-borne chimpanzees on Ngamba Island, Uganda. *Vector Borne Zoonotic Dis.* 11, 169–176, 2011.

Steinauer ML et al., Introgressive hybridization of human and rodent schistosome parasites in western Kenia. *Mol. Evol.* 17, 5062–5074, 2008.

Wolmarans CT et al., An experimental *Schistosoma mattheei* infection in man. *Onderstepoort J. Vet. Res.* 57, 211–214, 1990.

4.3.10 OTHER ZOONOTIC TREMATODE INFECTIONS

Eurytrema pancreaticum is occasionally found in the pancreatic duct of humans in China. The main hosts are ruminants. Transmission occurs by oral ingestion of metacercariae in crickets or grasshoppers, serving as second intermediate hosts. Like *D. dendriticum*, *E. pancreaticum* is a member of the family Dicrocoeliidae [see "Dicrocoeliasis (Distomatosis)"; chapter 4.3.3], and its developmental cycle is similar to that of *D. dendriticum*. The parasite causes an inflammation of the pancreatic duct. In ruminants, eosinophilic granulomas develop, caused by eggs penetrating the wall of the pancreatic duct. In patent infections (prepatent period in ruminants, 3 months), the small eggs (45 by 30 μm) of the parasite can be detected in feces. Therapy may be achieved with praziquantel.

Gastrodiscoides hominis (family Gastrodiscidae) is found in the caecum of humans and in the colon of pigs and various other animals in Asia. Development occurs in aquatic snails, the intermediate hosts. The infection is transmitted by vegetables and waterfruit contaminated with metacercariae. The parasites adhere to the intestinal wall by their ventral sucker and cause enteritis with continuous and often viscous diarrhea. The infection is successfully treated with praziquantel (15 mg/kg). Prophylactic measures correspond with those of fasciolopsiasis (see "Fasciolopsiasis"; chapter 4.3.5).

Nanophyetus salmincola is an intestinal fluke prevalent in the Pacific area, in the northwestern United States, and in Siberia. Its host spectrum is rather broad and includes canids, felids, mustelids, piscivorous birds, and humans. In the United States, the main hosts are raccoons and skunks. Its developmental cycle resembles that of *Opisthorchis felineus* (see "Opisthorchiasis" above). The infection is transmitted by fish, predominately salmonids, contaminated by metacercariae. The flukes adhere with their ventral suckers to the intestinal mucosa and, in severe infections, may cause hemorrhagic enteritis. For veterinary medicine, it is important that this parasite is able to transmit *Neorickettsia helminthoeca*, a ricketsial agent causing "salmon poisoning," a deadly disease in canids. For therapy of humans, praziquantel, three doses of 20 mg/kg orally in 1 day, is recommended. As prophylaxis, fish must be sufficiently cooked before consumption.

The genus *Alaria* (order Strigeatida, family Diplostomidae) is widely distributed as an intestinal parasite of canids in Eurasia (*Alaria alata*), North America (*A. americana* and others), and South America. The prevalence of *A. alata* in European foxes, for example, comes up to 30%. Eggs are excreted in the feces. Miracidia are formed in the environment within the eggs, hatch and invade planorbid freshwater snails. They develop to cercariae, leave the snail and invade frogs and tadpoles as second intermediate hosts, where they form so-called mesocercariae. These larvae have to be ingested by final hosts, where they migrate with the blood stream to the lungs and via the trachea to the small intestine and reach sexual maturity. Mesocercariae, which are ingested by paratenic hosts (amphibia, reptiles, mammals) accumulate in various organs and persist. Mesocercariae of *A. alata* are occasionally found in muscles of wild boars (*Agamodistomum suis*; Dunker's muscle fluke). Transmission to other paratenic hosts is possible. Human infections were caused in North America by *A. americana* (seven reported cases), mostly by ingestion of under-cooked frog meat. The parasites were found in the eye (four cases), in the lungs, and the subcutaneous tissue. Treatment was done by surgery. One patient died 8 days after a massive disseminated infection.

REFERENCES

Butcher AR et al., Locally acquired *Brachylaima* sp. (Digena: Brachylaimidae) intestinal fluke infections in two South Australian infants. *Med. J. Australia* 164, 475–478, 1996.

Chai JY et al., Foodborne intestinal flukes in Southeast Asia. *Korean J. Parasitol.* 47, Suppl. S69–S102, 2009.

Freeman RS et al., Fatal human infection with mesocercariae of the trematode *Alaria americana*. *Am. J. Trop. Med. Hyg.* 25, 803–807, 1976.

González-Fuentes H et al., Tenacity of *Alaria alata* mesocercariae in homemade German meat products. *Int. J. Food Microbiol.* 176, 9–14, 2014.

Gupta A et al., *Gastrodiscoides hominis* infestation of colon: endoscopic appearance. *Gastrointest. Endosc.* 79, 549–550, 2014.

Kramer MH, Eberhard ML, Blankenberg TA, Respiratory symptoms and subcutaneous granulomas caused by mesocercariae: a case report. *Am. J. Trop. Med. Hyg.* 55, 447–448, 1996.

McDonald HR et al., Two cases of intraocular infection with *Alaria* mesocercariae (Trematoda) *Am. J. Ophthalmol.* 117, 447–455, 1994.

Möhl K et al., Biology of *Alaria* spp. and human exposition risk to *Alaria* mesocercariae – a review. *Parasitol. Res.* 105, 1–15, 2009.

4.4 Zoonoses Caused by Cestodes

Tapeworms are hermaphrodite endoparasites, usually dwelling in the small intestine of their final hosts. They consist of a head (scolex) and a flat elongated body, the strobila, which is assembled of a number of segments or proglottids. Each proglottid contains one or two sets of reproductive organs. Proglottids are formed in a growth region behind the scolex and with the growth of the tapeworm, they are pushed away from the scolex. In the course of this development, they mature and finally become packed with eggs. The body of tapeworms are covered by a tegument that resembles that of trematodes. Cestodes lack an alimentary channel and nutrients are resorbed by the tegument. Cestodes have indirect lifecycles (for a quasi-exception see chapter 4.4.5: hymenolepiasis). Two orders of cestodes must be considered that differ morphologically and by their developmental cycles: Pseudophyllida and Cyclophyllida.

Pseudophyllida (see chapters 4.4.2 and 4.4.6) are phyllogenetically older than Cyclophillida and still resemble trematodes in some ways. Eggs shed in proglottids are immature and the first larva, the ciliated coracidium, develops in the environment in water. The parasites have to pass two intermediate hosts, whereby the coracidium is ingested by small copepods and it develops to a second larval stage, the procercoid. Second intermediate hosts are fish, and in other cases amphibia, ingest infected copepodes and allow the development of plerocercoids; the infective stages for the final hosts (see Fig. 4.33, developmental cycle of *D. latum*).

In the case of Cyclophyllida, the eggs contain fully developed first larvae, the oncospheres, when they are shed in proglottids with the feces. Except the genus *Mesocestoides* (see chapter 4.4.9.1), cyclophyllid tapeworms affecting humans involve only one intermediate host. Various types of metacestodes (larval stages) develop in these intermediate hosts. Tapeworms transmitted by arthropods, for example, *Dipylidium caninum*, develop through so-called cysticercoids. The corresponding stage in vertebrates, caused by members of the genus *Taenia*, is the cycsticercus, where a single scolex invaginated into itself lies in a fluid-containing bladder. In some species of the genus (e.g., *T. multiceps*), a coenurus develops in the intermediate host instead, that is, a large fluid-containing bladder with a number of invaginated scolices attached to the inner side of the wall, is formed. The genus *Echinococcus* finally develops bladder-like hydatids (echinococcus hydatidosus) or a so-called alveolar echinococcus, which both produce many protoscolices and are usually pathogenic to the intermediate host due to their size or an infiltrative growth.

4.4.1 COENUROSIS

Coenurosis is a rare disease in humans caused by a particular type of metacestodes, a coenurus, in the CNS or connective tissue.

Etiology. Cerebral coenurosis is caused by *Taenia multiceps*. Metacestodes of *T. brauni* and *T. serialis* (possibly also *T. glomerata*) reside in connective tissue. However, reported cases have not always addressed the etiology.

Occurrence. *T. multiceps* and *T. serialis* occur worldwide. *T. brauni* is found in tropical and Southern Africa. *T. glomerata* is limited to West Africa. Final hosts are canids. Dogs, in particular sheepdogs, which played an important role in transmission of *T. multiceps* in Europe, are currently only rarely infected. However, foxes may carry the parasites more often. For example, 2.3 and 3.3% of foxes in Germany were found infected with *T. serialis* and *T. multiceps*, respectively. Other wild living carnivores may be infected more often. For example, approximately 30 and 50% of wolves in the northwest of Spain and in Lithuania carried *T. multiceps*, respectively. The latter parasite is a common parasite of coyotes in North America. Intermediate hosts under natural conditions are herbivorous animals (in case of *T. multiceps* predominantly sheep) and small mammals.

Human infections are rare nowadays. Six cases are altogether known from North America. Previously, coenurosis was suggested as a work-related disease in European shepherds.

Transmission. Humans are intermediate hosts in the case of coenurosis. Infection occurs by accidental oral ingestion of tapeworm eggs, for example, on contaminated vegetables.

Mature tapeworms are 40 to 100 cm in length and inhabit the small intestine of their final hosts. Eggs are shed in proglottids with the feces and are ingested by intermediate hosts, allowing the oncophores to hatch in the intestine. In case of *T. multiceps* the larva is neurotropic, migrates to the brain and spinal cord, and develops into the coenurus. In the other species, the coenuri inhabit predominantly connective (subcutaneous) tissue. The coenurus is a unilocular, transparent cyst or bladderworm 5 cm or more in diameter. The fluid-containing cyst holds numerous, single tapeworm heads (protoscolices) attached to its inner wall.

Final hosts become infected by the ingestion of infected intermediate hosts (in case of *T. multiceps*, the brain is infested). The often-heavy infections of final hosts are explained by the large numbers of protoscolices in a coenurus.

Clinical Manifestations. Heavy *T. multiceps* infections may cause an acute meningoencephalitis. Chronic infections with few metacestodes are more common, where the growth of the coenurus results in pressure-induced atrophy of the surrounding CNS tissue. Symptoms are severe headache, nausea, vomiting, seizure, paraplegia, hemiplagia, aphasia, or eye symptoms. Deaths due to coenurosis have been reported.

Symptoms in infected sheep are referred to as "gid" or "staggers." Clinical symptoms due to coenuri in connective tissue are rare and vary with the localization of the metacestodes.

Diagnosis. Coenuri in the brain can be demonstrated by imaging techniques.

Differential Diagnosis. Cysticercosis and tumors have to be considered.

Therapy. Coenuri must be surgically removed. Praziquantel kills the metacestodes, but this is accompanied with heavy inflammatory reactions around the parasites.

Prophylaxis. Vegetables harvested from natural locations (e.g., corn salad or sorrel) should be washed carefully. The most important preventive measures are parasitological examination and deworming of dogs. Dogs should not be fed with waste from slaughtering.

REFERENCES

Achenef M et al., Coenurus cerebralis infection in Ethiopian highland sheep: incidence and observations on pathogenesis and clinical signs. *Trop. Anim. Health Prod.* 31, 15–24, 1999.

Ambekar S et al., MRS findings in cerebral coenurosis due to *Taenia multiceps. J. Neuroimaging* 23, 149–150, 2013.

Avcioglu H et al., Prevalence and molecular characterization of bovine coenurosis from Eastern Anatolian region of Turkey. *Vet. Parasitol.* 176, 59–64, 2011.

Bagrade G et al., Helminth parasites of the wolf *Canis lupus* from Latvia. *J. Helminthol.* 83, 63–68, 2009.

Benger A et al., A human coenurus infection in Canada. *Am. J. Trop. Med. Hyg.* 30, 638–644, 1981.

Benifla M et al., Huge hemispheric intraparenchymal cyst caused by *Taenia multiceps* in a child. Case report. *J. Neurosurg.* 107, 6 Suppl. 511–514, 2007.

Collomb J et al., Contribution of NADH dehydrogenase subunit I and cytochrome C oxidase subunit I towards identifying a case of human coenuriasis in France. *J. Parasitol.* 93, 934–937, 2007.

El-On J et al., *Taenia multiceps*: a rare human cestode infection in Israel. *Vet. Ital.* 44, 621–631, 2008.

Fain A, Coenurosis in man and animals caused by *Taenia brauni setti* in Belgian Congo and Ruanda-Urundi. II. Report of 8 human cases. *Ann. Soc. Belg. Med. Trop.* 36, 679–696, 1956.

Ing MB, Schantz PM, Turner JA, Human coenurus in North America. Case report and review. *Clin. Infect. Dis.* 27, 519–523, 1998.

Oryan A et al., Pathological, molecular, and biochemical characterization of Coenurus gaigeri in Iranian native goats. *J. Parasitol.* 96, 961–967, 2010.

Pau A et al., Long-term follow-up of the surgical treatment of intracranial coenurosis. *Br. J. Neurosurg.* 4, 39–43, 1990.

Varcasia A et al., Molecular characterization of subcutaneous and muscular coenurosis in goats in United Arab Emirates. *Vet. Parasitol.* 190, 604–607, 2012.

4.4.2 DIPHYLLOBOTHRIASIS (BROAD TAPEWORM INFECTION)

Diphyllobothriasis is a disease caused by an infection with "broad tapeworms" or "fish tapeworms." Often the infections take an asymptomatic course. Symptoms may be abdominal discomfort and, in severe cases, megaloblastic anemia and neurological disorders.

Etiology. Causative agents are members of the order Pseudophyllida that differ by morphology and development from the phylogenetically younger Cyclophyllida (see chapters 4.4.3 to 4.4.5, 4.4.7, and 4.4.8). Their spoon-shaped scolex has two long grooves (bothria or sucking organs) to fix to the intestinal wall. They are different from Cyclophyllida and their genital pore is on the ventral side of the proglottids. These parasites usually measure 5 to 10 m in length but occasionally may reach 25 m.

More than 15 species of the genera *Diphyllobothrium* (D.) and *Diplogonoporus* were found in humans. *D. latum* is the most common species and the largest cestode of humans. The most important species including their final and second intermediate hosts, as well as their geographical distribution are listed in Tab. 4.8.

Occurrence. *D. latum* is predominantly a parasite of temperate and subarctic areas of the Northern Hemisphere. Major hosts besides humans are cats, dogs, and pigs, but all other fish-eating mammals may become infected. Areas of endemicity with human infections are states around the Baltic Sea, Ireland, France, Italy, the delta of the river Danube, Siberia and other northern areas of Russia, Alaska, North America (lake areas), and northern China. *D. latum* occurs focally in other areas of China and sporadically in Japan. *D. dendriticum* is usually found north of *D. latum* in fish-eating birds, predominantly sea gulls, and mammals. *D. dalliae* and *D. alascense* occur in dogs, the Arctic fox, and occasionally in humans in North America and Alaska. *D. nihonkaiense* inhabits the brown bear and humans in the coastal regions of the North Pacific. In South America, where *D. pacificum* dominates in the coastal regions, Chile and Peru are concerned. Sea lions and related species are the main hosts. *D. stemmacephalum* and *Diplogonoporus balaenoptera* (syn. *D. grandis*) are parasites of marine mammals in circumpolar regions.

According to WHO estimates, 15 to 20 million humans may be infected by pseudophyllid cestodes worldwide. Prevalence in humans,

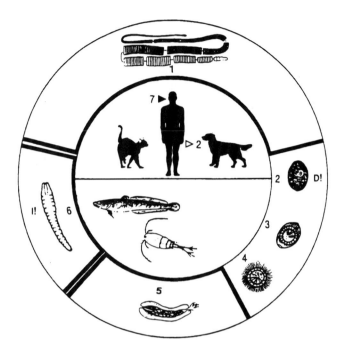

Figure 4.33 | Developmental cycle of *D. latum*. (1) Mature tapeworm (5 to >10 m in length) in the small intestine of humans and fish-eating mammals; (2) *D. latum* egg (0.045 by 0.070 mm) excreted with feces, with zygote and yolk cells (D, diagnostic stage); (3) egg with coracidium in water; (4) hatched motile coracidium (0.04 to 0.05 mm) swimming in water; (5) procercoid (0.5 to 0.6 mm; second larval stage) developed in a cyclopid copepod after ingestion of the coracidium; (6) plerocercoid (up to 50 mm; third larval stage developed in freshwater fish [second intermediate host] after ingestion of an infected copepod [I, infective stage]).

previously estimated for *D. latum* in some regions above 20%, has decreased in recent decades. Otherwise, diphyllobothriasis is considered an emerging disease in particular areas, such as the sub-Alpine region in Europe. Several hundred cases were observed during the recent two decades in Italy, France, and Switzerland, around Lake Geneva and the Lago Maggiore. There is no reliable information on the occurrence of diphyllobothrial cestodes in Australia and Africa.

Transmission. Humans become infected after eating raw or insufficiently cooked fish, which are the second intermediate hosts. Pseudophyllida develop differently from Cyclophillida, the order to which most of the other cestodes found in humans belong (e.g., see chapters on taeniases, 4.4.7 and 4.4.8). Their cycle includes two intermediate hosts. Infected final hosts shed eggs with the feces that must come into water, where a larva, the ciliated, swimming coracidium, develops within 2 weeks. It is ingested

Table 4.8 | Pseudophyllidea found in humans

SPECIES	MAJOR FINAL HOSTS	OCCURRENCE
Diphyllobothrium latum	Humans, terrestrial mammals	Europe, North America
D. dendriticum	Fish-eating birds (humans)	Circumpolar (north the area of *D. latum*)
D. dalliae	Dogs, arctic foxes (humans)	North America, Alaska
D. alascense[1]	Dogs, orcas (humans)	North America, Alaska
D. nihonkaiense[1]	Brown bear, humans	North Pacific Region
D. pacificum[2]	Sea lion, humans	Coastal regions of South America, Japan
D. stemnacephalum[2]	Tumblers, dolphins (humans)	Circumpolar areas
Diplogonoporus balaenopterae[2]	Whales (humans)	Circumpolar areas

[1] Andromous species.
[2] Marine species.

by small copepods (*Cyclops* spp., *Diatomus* spp. and others), where it develops to a procercoid. When infected copepods are ingested by fish, the procercoids settle in their tissues and become 4 to 5 mm long plerocercoids, which is the infectious stage for the final host.

If these fish are ingested by other fish, the plerocercoids establish themselves in the latter (paratenic) host. Thus, the spectrum of potentially transmitting hosts is correspondingly large; nevertheless, it depends on the general habitat of the parasites. So-called freshwater types (*D. latum, D. dendriticum,* and *D. dalliae*) are usually transmitted by predatory fishes (perch, pike, walleye, burbot) or trout and *Dallia* spp. The incidence in these fish may be high. For example, >10% of perch caught in 2003 to 2006 in Lake Geneva were infected with plerocercoids of *D. latum*. *D. nihonkaiense* and *D. pacificum* are so-called anadromous species. They use anadromous fish species (i.e., species that are born in freshwater, spend most of their life in saltwater and return to freshwater to spawn, like salmonids and whitefish) as second intermediate hosts. The so-called marine types (*D. stemmacephalum, Diplogonoporus balaenopterae,* and others) develop in marine fish of a hardly known spectrum.

Human infection is supported by eating increasingly popular dishes with raw fish in many countries: in Europe many kinds of "carpaccio" (thin slices of raw, flavored fish) are eaten; "gefilte fish," eaten in the Jewish populations, "ceviche," (marinated raw fishes) in South America, or "sushi" or "sashimi" in Japan are likewise risky dishes.

If infected fish is ingested raw or undercooked, the plerocercoid hatches in the small intestine and grows to the adult stage that starts egg production approximately 3 weeks after infection. The adult parasite can survive for 35 years. The developmental cycle is shown in Fig. 4.33.

Clinical Manifestations. In most cases, the infection remains asymptomatic (~80%). General symptoms are weakness and dizziness; abdominal pains, intestinal obstruction, and diarrhea may occur. In severe cases, neurological disorders (paresthesia, vision disorders, and ataxia) are observed. Approximately 2% of the patients develop a megaloblastic anemia as the parasite competes with the host for vitamin B_{12}. Symptoms disappear after elimination of the tapeworm.

Diagnosis. Diagnosis is made by demonstration of eggs in the feces. Eggs have thick shells and an operculum and measure 45 by 70 µm. Species differentiation can be performed by PCR.

Differential Diagnosis. If applicable, pernicious anemia must be considered.

Therapy. Drugs of choice are praziquantel (5 to 10 mg/kg orally) or niclosamide (one 2 g dose orally). Vitamin B_{12} deficiency should be treated parenterally (cyanocobalamine, 1 mg i. m. weekly until normalization of the blood picture).

Prophylaxis. Fish-derived food should be sufficiently heated (55 °C, 5 min). Smoking does not assuredly kill the parasites. Frozen fish (−20 °C, 24 h) is safe. Consequently, the EU regulates by law, that fish scheduled for being eaten raw, may only be marketed if they have been frozen before [VO (EG) Nr. 853/2004 Annex III]. The US Food and Drug Administration recommends blast freezing to −35 °C or below for 15 h or freezing to −20 °C or below for 7 days.

REFERENCES

Beldsoe GE, Oria MP, Potential hazards in cold-smoked fish. *J. Food Sci.* 66 (Suppl), S1100–1103, 2001.

Dupouy-Camet J, Perduzzi R, Current situation of human diphyllobothriasis in Europe. *Euro Surveill.* 9, 31–35, 2004.

Jackson Y et al., *Diphyllobothrium latum* outbrake from marinated raw perche, Lake Geneva, Switzerland. *Emerg. Infect. Dis.* 13, 2007–2008, 2007.

Kuchta R et al., Tapeworm *Diphyllobothrium dentriticum* (Cestoda) - neglected or emerging human parasite. *PLoS Negl. Trop. Dis.* 7, e2535, 2013.

Sager H et al., Coprological study on intestinal helminths in Swiss dogs: temporal aspects of anthelminthic treatment. *Parasitol. Res.* 98, 333–338, 2006.

Shimizu H et al., Diphyllobothriasis nihonkaiense: possibly acquired in Switzerland from imported Pacific salmon. *Intern. Med.* 47, 1359–1362, 2008.

Wicht B et al., Multiplex PCR for a differential identification of broad tapeworms (Cestoda: *Diphyllobothrium*) infecting humans. *J. Clin.Microbiol.* 48, 3111–3116, 2010.

4.4.3 DIPYLIDIOSIS

Dipylidiosis is a human infection caused by a common tapeworm of dogs and cats. It is in general, clinically inapparent.

Etiology. Dipylidiosis is caused by *Dipylidium caninum*, a tapeworm 20 to 40 cm in length.

Occurrence. *D. caninum* is distributed worldwide in canids and felids with prevalence rates in dogs of 0.5 to 5%. Human infections are rare but are found worldwide, predominantly in children.

Transmission. Humans become infected by accidental ingestion of cysticercoids or infected fleas. The tapeworm lives in the small intestine of dogs and cats and releases proglottids with eggs (Fig. 4.34). Eggs occur in egg capsules with 8 to 15 eggs and contain larvae. Larval stages of fleas ingest eggs; the infective stage for the final host, the cysticercoid, develops in the flea's body cavity during its pupal stage. When the final host swallows the flea along with the cysticercoid, this intermediate stage develops into an adult in the definite host's small intestine within 3 weeks.

Humans usually become infected by cysticercoids when the hand is licked by dogs still harboring the infective stage in their oral cavity.

Clinical Manifestations. The infection is usually asymptomatic. Heavy infections with more than 100 worms cause abdominal discomfort, bloody mucous diarrhea, pruritus ani, and loss of weight.

Diagnosis. Proglottids are voided in the feces. They measure 7 to 12 mm by 2 to 3 mm, show two lateral genital pores (Fig. 4.34), resemble in shape cucumber seeds, are pink to reddish in color, and contain egg capsules with eggs of 40 µm in size. There are no uterine structures detectable in the proglottids as in taeniid tapeworms. Egg capsules may be also found free in the feces.

Differential Diagnosis. Other intestinal disorders must be considered. Proglottids are sometimes misdiagnosed as pinworms.

Therapy. Effective drugs are niclosamide (one 2 g dose; for children, one-half or one-fourth that) and praziquantel (one 10 mg/kg dose).

Prophylaxis. Licking of the hands by dogs or cats should be avoided, or at least hands should be thoroughly washed after being licked. Pets should be subjected to parasitological examination and anthelmintic treatment. Flea control is a preventive measure.

REFERENCES

Chappell CL, Enos JP, Penn HM, *Dipylidium caninum*, an underrecognized infection in infants and children. *Ped. Inf. Dis.* 9, 745–747, 1990.

Molina CP, Ogburn J, Adegboyega P, Infection by *Dipylidium caninum* in an infant. *Arch. Pathol. Lab. Med.* 127, 157–159, 2003.

Narasimhan MV et al., *Dipylidium caninum* infection in a child: a rare case report. *Indian J. Med. Microbiol.* 31, 82–84, 2013.

Raitiere CR, Dog tapeworm (*Dipylidium caninum*) infestation in a 6-months old infant. *J. Fam. Practice* 34, 101–102, 1992.

Reid CJ, Perry EM, Evans N, *Dipylidium caninum* in an infant. *Eur. J. Pediatr.* 151, 502–503, 1992.

Samkari, A. et al., *Dipylidium caninum* mimicking recurrent *Enterobius vermicularis* (pinworm) infection. *Clin.Pediatr. (Phila)* 47, 397–399, 2008.

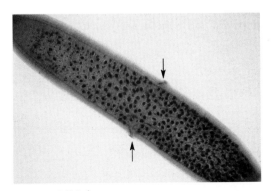

Figure 4.34 | Proglottid of *Dipylidium caninum*. Each proglottid contains two sets of genital organs and two genital pori (arrows): Giemsa staining (picture: Institute for Parasitology, Giessen, Germany).

Taylor T, Zitzmann MB, *Dipylidium caninum* in a 4-month old male. *Clin. Lab. Sci.* 24: 212–214, 2011.

Wijesundera MD, The use opf praziquantel in human infections with *Dipylidium*. *Trans. R. Soc. Trop. Med. Hyg.* 83, 383, 1989.

4.4.4 ECHINOCOCCOSIS

Echinococcosis is a chronic disease of humans with a severe prognosis. It is caused by metacestodes (echinococci) of the genus *Echinococcus*. The long-lasting discussion on the taxonomy of the genus is not yet finalized, but there is a consent that *Echinococcus granulosus* is a species complex (see Tab. 4.8). However, as many questions on the epidemiology and pathogenicity of the species are still unsolved, the name *E. granulosus* (sensu lato) will be used for the whole complex in the following text.

Depending on the species (*E. multilocularis* or *E. granulosus*), an alveolar or a cystic echinococcosis develops. *E. vogeli* and *E. oligarthra* in Central and South America cause an intermediate type (polycystic echinoccosis; Tab. 4.9) with low prevalences in humans (<40 and two cases, respectively). *E. shiquicus*, a parasite of wild and domestic canids in the Tibetan area, has not been found in humans so far.

REFERENCES

D'Alessandro A, Polycystic echinococcosis in tropical America: *Echinococcus vogeli* and *E. oligarthrus*. *Acta Trop.* 67, 43–65, 1997.

Deplazes P et al., Role of pets and cats in the transmission of helminth zoonoses in Europe, with a focus on echinococcosis and toxocarosis. *Vet. Parasitol.* 182, 42–52, 2011.

Eckert J, Deplazes P, Kern P, Alveolar echinococcosis (*Echinococcus multilocularis*) and neotropical forms of echinococcosis (*Echinococcus vogeli, Echinococcus oligarthus*). In: Brown D, Palmers S, Torgerson PR, Soulsby EJL (eds.): *Zoonoses*. 2nd ed. Oxford University Press, Oxford, 2011.

Mcmanus DP et al., Echinococcosis. *Lancet* 362, 1295–1304, 2003.

Nakao M et al., Phylogenetic systematics of the genus *Echinococcus* (Cestoda: Taeniidae). *Int. J. Parasitol.* 43, 1017–1029, 2013.

Saarma U et al., A novel phylogeny for the genus *Echinococcus*, based on nuclear data, challenges relationships based on mitochondrial evidence. *Parasitology* 136, 317–328, 2009.

Thompson RC, The taxonomy, phylogeny and transmission of *Echinococcus*. *Exp. Parasitol.* 119, 439–446, 2008.

Thompson RC, McManus DP, Towards a taxonomic revision of the genus *Echinococcus*. *Trends Parasitol.* 18, 452–457, 2002.

4.4.4.1 Alveolar echinococcosis

Alveolar echinococcosis is a chronic, destructive disease, preferentially of the liver by an echinococcus that spreads infiltratively and metastazises. The mortality rate in untreated patients is high.

Etiology. The disease is caused by metacestodes of the small (maximum length 4.5 mm; only five proglottids) tapeworm *Echinococcus multilocularis*.

Occurrence. *E. multilocularis* is found in the Northern Hemisphere in three major geographic regions (see Fig. 4.35). North America: Alaska, some regions of Canada and the northern and central United States. Eurasia: Turkey, and northern and eastern Asia (including Siberia,

Table 4.9 | Agents of alveolar and polycystic Echinococcosis

SPECIES	DEFINITIVE HOSTS	INTERMEDIATE HOSTS	DISEASE	DISTRIBUTION
E. multilocularis	Red fox and other wild canids, dog, cat	Rodents: common vole, water vole, muskrat, lemmings, deer mice	Alveolar echinococcosis	Northern Hemisphere
E. shiquicus	Tibetan sand fox (*Vulpes ferrilata*)	Pikas (*Ochotona* spp.)	(not in humans)	Tibet
E. oligarthra	Wild felids	Pacas and other rodents	Polycystic echinococcosis	Latin America
E. vogeli	Bush dog, dog	Pacas and other rodents	Polycystic echinococcosis	Latin America

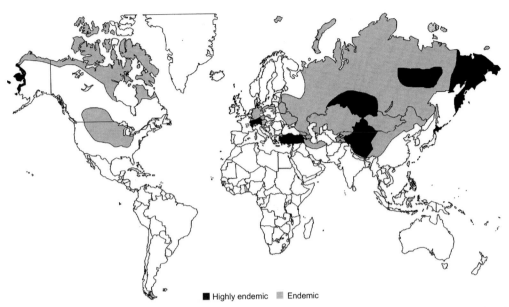

Figure 4.35 | Approximate geographic distribution of *E. multilocularis* as of 1999. Shaded areas indicate that the organism is highly endemic (black) or endemic (gray). (Source: J. Eckert, F. Grimm, and H. Bucklar [Institute of Parasitology, University of Zürich, Zürich, Switzerland]. Reprinted from Eckert et al., 2000.)

northern China, and northern Japan). Central Europe: central and southern France, the Benelux, Germany, Switzerland, Austria, Czech Republic, Poland, Estonia, Belarus and the Ukraine, recently also detected in Sweden. Ireland, the UK, Finland, and Norway are supposed to be free of *E. multilocularis.*

Natural final hosts are the red fox and the arctic fox. In endemic regions of Germany and Switzerland, up to >50% of the foxes are infected. Considering the short life span (2 to 5 months) of *E. multilocularis*, the foxes may become infected several times during their life. The intensity of infection varies: studies in Central Europe showed massive infections (>10 000 worms), particularly in young foxes, while older animals often contain only a few parasites. In the North American tundra, prevalence of 40 to 100% are found in arctic foxes.

Other canids are also affected (dogs, coyotes, wolves, raccoon dogs, and also cats). The prevalence in dogs in France may be as high as 5%. More than 10% of the dogs were found to be infected in particular areas of Alaska. A similar prevalence in dogs was reported from some Chinese provinces. Up to 35% of the coyotes in North America are infected. The raccoon dog (*Nyctereutes procyonoides*), invading from the East into Central Europe since the middle of the 20th century, is a suitable host for *E. multilocularis* and will probably play a potential role in the epidemiology of the disease in future. Prevalence rates of 12% were found in eastern Germany. Cats seem to be less susceptible than dogs but may be particularly predisposed for the infection by eating rodents. The parasite occurs in 0.5 to 2.9% of cats in southern Germany.

Intermediate hosts under field conditions are rodents: in Central Europe, several vole species, mainly the common vole (*Microtus arvalis*) and muskrats (*Ondatra zibethicus*), in Alaska the northern vole (*Microtus oeconomus*) and the brown lemming (*Lemmus sibiricus*), and in central North America next to *Microtus* spp. also deer mouse (*Peromyscus maniculatus*). The prevalence in rodents varies but is usually seldom higher than 1%. An exceptional situation seems to exist in the tundra region of North America, where >50% of the rodents were found to be infected. Prevalence of >40% were also detected locally in the city of Zurich (Switzerland).

Probably the larval tissue of the tapeworm can develop in all mammals, but is often not fertile or dies off at an early stage. Human infections occur throughout all areas of endemicity. In the endemic parts of Switzerland and France, one clinically and pathologically proven case is expected per 1 million inhabitants per year. The incidence in some regions of Alaska and Central Asia is much higher: for example, 7 to 98 new cases per 100 000 inhabitants per year were observed on St Lawrence Islands (USA) between 1947 and 1990.

In Western Europe, an increased risk of infection seems to exist in people engaged in farming. Alveolar echinococcosis is recognized as an occupational disease in these persons. In Alaska, a significant correlation exists between risk of infection and keeping dogs.

Transmission. Humans become infected by ingestion of *Echinococcus* eggs that are shed with segments (proglottids) in the feces by the final hosts. Modes of infection are ingestion via contaminated food or hand and swallowing of eggs that are aerolized. In Europe and Japan, the increase of fox populations in urban areas may be of epidemiological importance.

Provided there is sufficient humidity, the eggs of *E. multilocularis* can survive in the environment for months. Their resistance to cold temperatures is of particular importance. They survive storage at −18 °C for at least 8 months; definitive killing requires −70 °C (4 days) or −80 °C (2 days). Dryness or high environmental temperatures are not tolerated by the eggs. Proglottids or eggs of *E. multilocularis* may adhere to hairs of infected definitive hosts, that is, hunters may be in danger of contaminating their hands when skinning foxes without wearing gloves. This also holds true when infected dogs or cats are handled.

Final hosts are infected by ingestion of infected intermediate hosts. As the metacestode, the echinococcus, often contains masses of protoscolices, each representing a source of a tapeworm, they may acquire masses of parasites. The protoscolices penetrate between the intestinal villi, reach sexual maturity within 26 to 35

days and release proglottids that contain 200 to 300 eggs each. Shedding is highest in the first weeks of patency (up to 100 000 eggs per gram of feces were found) and lasts for up to 4 months. Eggs are released by mazeration of the proglottids, which already happens in the intestine. Eggs contain a larval stage (oncosphere), that is, are infective when they are released.

After ingestion of eggs by intermediate hosts or humans, the oncosphere hatches, invades the intestinal mucosa and is transported to the liver via lymph or blood vessels (98% of the parasites settle there) but can spread throughout the whole body. The larva develops to the metacestode by infiltrating the host tissue with solid tracks of cells, which subsequently dilate to tubes or vesicles. The protoscolices are generated on the inner wall of these vesicles (in humans, the echinococcus often lacks protoscolices). In this way, a sponge-like echinococcus develops, which in cross sections shows an alveolar picture often with central cavities of decay (Fig. 4.36). The echinococcus in general expands by continuous growth of protrusions into the surrounding tissue. These protrusions are usually macroscopically undetectable because of their small diameter.

Clinical Manifestations. The initial disease is characterized by a long asymptomatic incubation period of 5 to 15 years, during which the *Echinococcus* grows slowly. In humans as

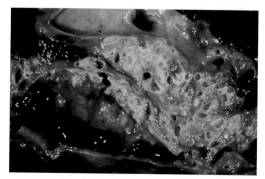

Figure 4.36 | Alveolar echinococcosis (*Echinococcus multilocularis*) in the liver: human case. The tissue of the larva grows infiltratively and metastasizes. The cross section shows a sponge-like structure (picture: Parasitology, Hohenheim Germany)

accidental hosts, it can degenerate or die off by immune attacks in the course of this time. Serological data suggest that more than 90% of the *Echinococcus* infections heal spontaneously. Otherwise, a symptomatic (progressive) phase develops.

The mean patient's age at which the first symptoms are recognized is about 50 years. The time course of the disease is not predictable. In some cases, the echinococcus hardly increases for years; in other cases, it increases rapidly and metastasizes. Clinical signs develop in general in an advanced stage and involve the right upper abdomen. Icterus is common (one-third of cases), likewise abdominal pain (one-third of cases). In other cases, only unspecific symptoms, such as tiredness or loss of weight, are observed. The primary localization of the parasites is generally the liver, particularly its right lobe. From there, the larval tissue infiltrates or metastasizes into other organs (diaphragm, kidney, lung, spleen, brain). In an advanced phase, hepatomegaly develops; bile ducts and blood vessels become infiltrated and congested, which is associated with icterus and ascites. The status of the disease is assessed according to WHO PNM criteria (P = parasite mass in liver; N = involvement of neighboring organs; M = metastases).

Alveolar echinococcosis is life threatening. The prognosis depends on the stage of the disease, the extent of metastasis, and the time point at which the disease is diagnosed. Mortality in untreated patients is high, but the expectancy of life has markedly increased in recent decades due to advanced stage-specific treatment measures. Thus, the expected life span after diagnosis in Europe was only 3 years in 1970 and is expanded to approximately 20 years today.

Diagnosis. The diagnosis of alveolar echinococcosis is based on the combination of imaging techniques (sonography, CT scanning, MR imaging) and serology. Sonography in early stages shows a coexistence of echo-rich and echo-poor areas with unclear demarcations. Minute calcifications are regarded as characteristic. In later stages, cystic structures without echo are found and pseudocystic changes occur due to decaying cavities.

Biopsy was generally suggested to be contraindicated, as it supports metastases. However, sonography-guided fine-needle biopsy is acceptable. The aspirate can be investigated in native form for protoscolex hooks, or immunohistologically or by molecular methods (PCR). Demonstration of mRNA gives information on the viability of the parasite.

For immunodiagnosis, the combined application of at least two serological tests is recommended. For IFA, freeze-sections of the *E. multilocularis* protoscolices are used (due to cross-reactions between the *Echinococcus* species, also commercial assays with protoscolices of *E. granulosus* as antigen can be employed). The assay is very sensitive. The *E. multilocularis* antigens EM2 and II/3-10 are preferentially used for ELISA (commercially available as a combination test: Em2plus ELISA) with a species-specificity of up to 95%. Commercial immunoblot assays seem similarly reliable. Immunodiagnostic procedures are of particular importance in early diagnosis needed for successful surgical intervention.

Differential Diagnoses. Liver tumors, liver cirrhosis, cystic echinococcosis, and amoebic abscess must be considered.

Therapy. The therapy of choice, if it is possible, is the extensive surgical resection followed by mandatory treatment with albendazole, 400 mg twice a day orally (together with a meal). It should be started 10 weeks before planned surgical treatment and continued for at least 2 years. Albendazole levels in plasma may vary from patient to patient; it is therefore recommended to monitor the level individually (optimum levels: 0.5 to 1.6 µg/ml). Continuous treatment over many years is mandatory in cases when the parasite was only partly removed by surgery or in inoperable patients as the drug acts parasitostatic rather than parasitocidal.

Orthotopic liver transplantation were not considered a useful option for a long time in alveolar echinococcosis, as it requires immunosuppressive measures that may support residues of the parasite. According to recent retrospective analyses, however, it may be approved under certain conditions in life-threatening cases under certain precautionary conditions. Preoperative albendazole treatment is mandatory in these cases.

Prophylaxis. Wild-grown berries and mushrooms from areas of endemicity should not be eaten raw or unwashed. *Echinococcus* eggs must be frozen at least at −70 °C to kill the oncospheres. Heating the eggs to >60 °C kills the larvae within 5 min. Disinfectants (based on aldehydes, ethanol, or derivatives of phenol) are usually not effective. Sodium hypochlorite kills the eggs within 10 min at a minimum concentration of 3.75% (!).

Care should to be taken with captured or dead foxes. Gloves are necessary for skinning. Bodies of foxes must be destroyed. If bodies of foxes or other potentially infected animals are to be necropsied, they should be frozen at −80 °C before necropsy to protect the staff.

In Germany, Switzerland, and other countries, it was tested in field studies whether treatment of wild foxes with praziquantel, offered in baits, can reduce the prevalence in these animals. Although the results were promising, area-wide measures were not performed because of the cost. Dogs and cats that have access to wild rodents in endemic areas should be treated prophylactically in 3-week intervals with praziquantel, 5 mg/kg orally (prepatent period of *E. multilocularis*: 26 to 35 days).

Diagnosis in the final host is difficult and uncertain as the proglottids and eggs are shed discontinuously and often only in small amounts. In addition, proglottids are very fragile and small (1 mm in length), and eggs of *Echinococcus* spp. cannot be distinguished from those of other taeniid tapeworms of carnivores. The detection of coproantigens (secretory-excretory antigens discharged by the worms and excreted with the feces; commercial ELISA) seems helpful, although, it is unreliable when the animals harbor less than 100 worms. A nested PCR with feces is more sensitive and able to differentiate *E. multilocularis* and *E. granulosus*. People suspected to be infected should be controlled serologically. Some countries in Europe, supposed to be free of *E. multilocularis*, do not allow the importation of dogs from endemic areas without certification of treatment with praziquantel.

REFERENCES

Bresson-Hadni S et al., A twenty-year history of alveolar echinococcosis: analysis of a series of 117 patiens from eastern France. *Eur.J. Gastroenterol. Hepatol.* 12, 327–336, 2000.

Ciftcioglu MA et al., Fine needle aspiration biopsy in hepatic *Echinococcus multilocularis*. *Acta Cytol.* 41, 649–652, 1997.

Deplazes P, Eckert J, Diagnosis of the *Echinococcus multilocularis* infection in final hosts. *Appl. Parasitol.* 37, 245–252, 1996.

Deplazes P et al., Wilderness in the city: the urbanization of *Echinococcus multilocularis*. *Trends Parasitol.* 20, 77–84, 2004.

Dyachenko V et al., *Echinococcus multilocularis* infections in domestic dogs and cats in Germany and other European countries. *Vet. Parasitol.* 157, 244–253, 2008.

Godot V et al., Resistance/susceptibility to *Echinococcus multilocularis* infection and cytokin profile in humans. Influence of the HLA B8, DR3, DQ2 haplotype. *Clin. Exp. Immunol.* 121, 491–498, 2000.

Jenkins DJ, Romig T, Thompson RCA, Emergence/re-emergence of *Echinococcus* spp. – a global update . *Int. J. Parasitol.* 35, 1205–1219, 2005.

Kadry Z et al., Surgical is better than conservative therapy in alveolar echinococcosis: Long term follow-up in 90 consecutive patients. *J. Gastrointest. Surg.* 7, 287, 2003.

Kantarci M et al., A rare reason for liver transplantation: hepatic alveolar echinococcosis. *Transplant. Infect. Dis.* 16, 480–482, 2014.

Koch S et al., Experience of liver transplantation for incurable alveolar echinococcosis: a 45 case European collaborative report. *Transplantation* 75, 856–863, 2003.

Konyaer SV et al., Genetic diversity of *Echinococcus* species in Russia. *Parasitology* 140, 1637–1647, 2013.

Liccioli S et al., Spatial heterogeneity and temporal variations in *Echinococcus multilocularis* infections in wild hosts in North American urban setting. *Int. J. Parasitol.* 44, 457–465, 2014.

Overgaauw PAM et al., Zoonotic parasites in fecal samples and fur from dogs and cats in The Netherlands. *Vet. Parasitol.* 163, 115–122, 2009.

Romig T, Dinkel A, Mackenstedt U, The present situation of echinococcosis in Europe. *Parasitol. Intern.* 55, 187–191, 2006.

Romig T et al., Impact of praziquantel baiting on intestinal helminths of foxes in southwestern Germany. *Helminthologia* 44, 206–213, 2007.

Santos GB et al., Rapid detection of *Echinococcus* species by a high-resolution melting approach. *Parasit Vectors* 6, 327, 2013.

Schürer JM et al., *Echinococcus multilocularis* and *Echinococcus canadensis* in wolves from Western Canada. *Parasitology* 141, 159–163, 2014.

Süld K et al., An invasive vector of zoonotic disease sustained by anthropogenic resources: the raccoon dog in northern Europe. *PLoS One* 22, e96358, 2014.

Thompson RC et al., Comparative development of *Echinococcus multilocularis* in its definitive hosts. *Parasitology* 132, 709–716, 2006.

Torgerson PR, Dogs, vaccines and *Echinococcus*. *Trends Parasitol.* 25, 57–58, 2009.

Veit P et al., Influence of environmental factors on the infectivity of *Echinococcus multilocularis* eggs. *Parasitology* 110, 79–86, 1995.

4.4.4.2 Cystic Echinococcosis (Hydatidosis)

Cystic echinococcosis is a chronic disease caused by expansive growth of *Echinococcus* cysts (metacestodes).

Etiology. The disease is caused by metacestodes (echinococcus cysticus) of the small dog tapeworm, *E. granulosus* s.l. Several strains, differing in biology, host preferences, biochemistry, and genetics are known. Some of them are considered as valid species (see Tab. 4.10).

Occurrence. *E. granulosus* occurs worldwide and is found as an adult tapeworm in dogs,

other canids and some large cats (lions, leopards) but rarely in domestic cats. Endemic and hyperendemic areas (see Fig. 4.37) are the countries adjoining to the Mediterranean Sea, the Middle East, the western states of the former Soviet Union, China, particularly the western parts of the country, India, South Australia, large parts of the southern areas of South America (mainly Chile and Uruguay), as well as Central, South and East Africa (Ethiopia, Kenia). *E. granulosus* is endemic in Canada, the United States, and some regions of Central America. Major zoonotic problems occur in regions of extensive sheep farming.

The prevalence in final hosts vary with geographic areas. In some highly endemic regions, such as the Mediterranean area, up to 50% of the dogs are infected. The prevalence in Central Europe is less than 1%. Accordingly, the frequency of infection varies in the intermediate hosts.

The prevalence in humans in highly endemic areas, for example, in parts of East Africa, South America and China, may reach 5% and more. In

Table 4.10 | Strains/species of *Echinococcus granulosus*, major intermediate and final hosts, infectivity for humans, and geographical distribution

STRAIN	MOLECULAR TAXONOMY	FINAL HOSTS	INTERMEDIATE HOSTS	INFECTIVITY (HUMANS)	SUPPOSED GEOGRAPHICAL DISTRIBUTION
Sheep strain (G1)	*E. granulosus* sensu stricto	Dog, several wild canids	Sheep + other ruminants, pig, camel, kanguroos	Yes	Global
Tasmanian sheep strain (G2)	*E. granulosus* sensu stricto	Dogs, foxes	Sheep	Yes	Tasmania, Argentina
Buffalo strain (G3)	*E. granulosus* sensu stricto	Dogs	Buffalos, cattle (?)	Yes	Asia, South Europe
Horse strain (G4)	*E. equinus*	Dogs	Horses, other equids	Low/no	Worldwide except Australia (?)
Camel strain (G6)	*E. canadensis*	Dogs	Camel, goats, cattle (?)	Yes	Middle East, Africa, China, Argentinia
Cervid strain (G8)	*E. canadensis*	Wolves, dogs	Cervids	Yes	Eurasia, North America
Fennoscandinavian cervid strain (G10)	*E. canadensis*	Wolves, dogs	Cervids	?	Eurasia, North America
Lion strain	*E. felidis*	Lions	Wild African ruminants, hippos	?	Sub-Saharan Africa

G1 to G 10, genotypes 1 to 10.

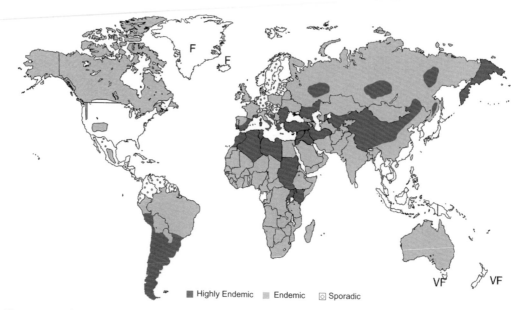

Figure 4.37 | Approximate geographic distribution of *E. granulosus* as of 1999. F, free; PF, provisionally free. (Source: J. Eckert, F. Grimm, and H. Bucklar [Institute of Parasitology, University of Zürich]. Reprinted from Eckert et al., 2000.)

some countries, where governmental control measures fell off, such as Bulgaria and Kasakhstan, infections of humans have increased considerably in recent years.

Transmission. Humans and intermediate hosts become infected by ingestion of *E. granulosus* eggs that are excreted within the progottids in the feces of final hosts, for instance, in infected dogs. It may take place via contaminated food or hands contaminated with egg-containing soil or sand (e.g., of playgrounds). Proglottids may stick to the hairs of infected dogs as a source of contamination. Eggs remain infective in cool, moist climates for months. They tolerate low temperatures similar to *E. multilocularis* eggs and are sensitive to dryness.

As in the case of *E. multilocularis*, the oncospheres hatch in the intestine, invade the intestinal wall and are spread to the liver or other organs. Differences in predilection sites of the metacestodes are known for the various strains/species. While usually the liver becomes predominantly infested, the camel and the pig strain often settle in the lungs. The ingestion of

proglottids with their hundreds of eggs leads to multiple infections.

The oncosphere develops to a cyst (echinococcus cysticus) that slowly increases in size. It is surrounded by connective tissue of the intermediate host and shows an outer laminated layer and an inner germinative membrane from which brood capsules, which contain protoscolices, develop. Brood capsules may become detached from the germinative membrane and may develop daughter cysts inside. Detached protoscolices, remnants of eventually ruptured daughter cysts, and small calcar bodies constitute the so-called hydatid sand.

The final host is infected by oral ingestion of cysts, for instance, with waste of slaughtering. Cysts may contain large amounts of protoscolices, and thus, may lead to heavy infections with sometimes more than 10 000 adult tapeworms. However, under stable endemic conditions with high prevalence, generally, infections with smaller numbers are found. The small tapeworm, only 3 to 6 mm in length, produces about 500 eggs per week. Thus, infected dogs represent a potentially dangerous

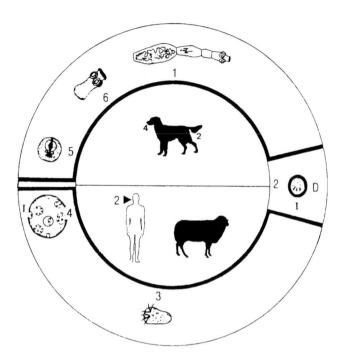

Figure 4.38 | Developmental cycle of *E. granulosus*. (1) Mature tapeworm (3 to 6 mm) in the small intestine of a dog; (2) *E. granulosus* egg (0.032 by 0.036 mm) containing the oncosphere, passed in the feces either free or still included in the proglottid (D, diagnostic stage in the dog; I, infective stage for intermediate hosts, including humans); (3) free oncosphere (0.022 to 0.028 mm) in intermediate host; (4) hydatid cyst (echinococcus cysticus) (walnut to orange sized, sometimes even bigger) in liver, lung, or other organs of the intermediate host (I, infectious stage for the dog); (5) protoscolex (0.12 to 0.20 mm) liberated from the cyst in the intestine of the dog; (6) evaginated, maturing young tapeworm in the intestine of the dog.

source of infection. The life cycle is shown in Fig. 4.38.

Clinical Manifestations. The consequences of an *E. granulosus* infection differ from those of an infection with *E. multilocularis*. The cyst grows slowly and expansively but does not infiltrate the tissue. It does not develop metastases except when the cyst is destroyed. In Western Europe and Australia, in 50 to 70% of cases, the liver becomes involved (Fig. 4.39), in 30 to 50%, the lungs are affected, and in 3 to 8%, the spleen and the peritoneum are involved; more rarely, all other parenchymatous organs and the brain may be affected. Multiple infections may occur. The cysts can grow to a fist size and bigger (Fig. 4.40). The mean age of patients when clinical signs begin is around 50 years.

Infestation of the liver with small cysts often remains asymptomatic or it is associated with nonspecific disorders of the upper abdomen. Clinical symptoms develop when growing cysts compress the bile ducts or blood vessels and lead to icterus and ascites (Fig. 4.40). Nonspecific signs may develop when cysts are located elsewhere. The growth of the cysts may vary markedly from patient to patient (1 to 50 mm per year), or the size even may decline. The reasons are unknown. Spontaneous rupture of cysts or accidental damage during surgery can cause severe anaphylaxis by the release of hydatid fluid (the infection is generally accompanied by high levels of specific IgE antibodies).

Diagnosis. Cysts can be detected by various imaging techniques. The basic diagnostic

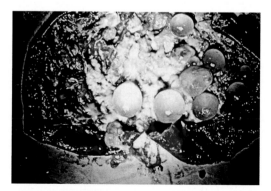

Figure 4.39 | Multiple hydatid cysts (*Echinococcus granulosus*) in the liver: human case (picture: Media, Royal Tropical Institute Amsterdam, The Netherlands).

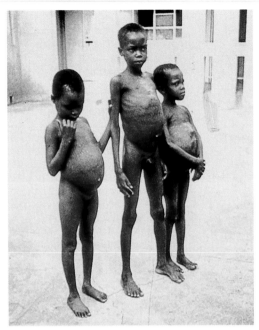

Figure 4.40 | Clinical picture of cystic echinococcosis (picture: I. Mann, Nairobi, Kenya).

method is sonography. CT and MRI are indicated in cases of special localization and for particular evaluations prior to surgical measures. *E. granulosus* cysts show more often calcifications demonstrable by X-rays than alveolar echinococci.

Serological examinations with hydatid fluid as antigen (IHA, ELISA) or with protoscolices (IFA) show cross reactions primarily with *E. multilocularis* and *T. solium*. High specificity (99%) is achieved by employing the "antigen B" of hydatid fluid (also commercially available as recombinant protein). However, serologic assays often fail, as the encapsulation of the cyst restrains the release of antigens. Thus, the sensitivity of tests is 85 to 98% in the case of liver cysts but only 50 to 60% in the case of exclusive infestations of the lungs. CNS infestations usually result in poor antibody responses.

Differential Diagnosis. Tumors, abscesses, and other tissue cysts must be considered.

Therapy. Therapeutic measures are based on the international classification of cystic echinococcosis (WHO-IGWE Ultrasound Classification of Echinococcal Cysts) according to clinical and diagnostic criteria (imaging methods, serology).

Surgical excision of the cyst is the optimal treatment. Chemoprophylaxis with albendazole is recommended, starting 1 month before and lasting up to 1 to 3 months after surgery The aim is to reduce the turgor, and by this, prevent the rupture of the cyst. The effect of an albendazole treatment could be significantly enhanced by combination with praziquantel. In the cases of inoperable cysts, in cases where cysts could be only partially removed, or after cyst rupture, chemotherapy (albendazole, 400 mg twice a day orally for 3 to 6 months) is essential, in the latter case to prevent the development of secondary cysts. The parasites are completely eliminated by chemotherapy relatively often. In most cases, at least an involution of the cyst and clinical improvement were observed. However, the prognosis is not always predictable. Particularly in cases of large, well-encapsulated cysts, treatment may fail. Albendazole is administered over cycles of 4 weeks interrupted by 2-week rest periods. Drug levels should be monitored as in alveolar echinococcosis. Inoperable cases and cases with incomplete resection of cysts need long-term surveillance. Relapses have been observed after more than 10 years. In case of a cyst rupture, treatment should start immediately and it should be extended over 2 to 3 cycles.

An alternative to surgical cyst removal and in inoperable patients, the WHO recommends the puncture-aspiration-injection-reaspiration technique, in which cysts are punctured under sonographic control and cyst fluid is aspirated, followed by an injection of 20 to 30% sodium chloride solution or 95% ethanol into the cyst. This is sucked off after 20 min, followed by a lavage with saline. Recovery is achieved in >90% of the cases. The procedure should be accompanied by albendazole treatment (see above).

Prophylaxis. In most cases, dogs that were fed raw, cyst containing organs from slaughtered animals are the source of human infections. In principle, this cycle is easy to interrupt; however, it must be considered that small cysts, particularly in the lungs, may be overlooked during meat inspection. The protoscolices can be killed by cooking or freezing (−20 °C for 2 days).

The diagnosis of *E. granulosus* infections in final hosts is uncertain according to *E. multilocularis* infections. Proglottids are released in irregular intervals and may be overlooked due to their small size. They are motile and migrate quickly away from the feces. The detection of coproantigens or parasite DNA by nested PCR, including species differentiation, can be helpful. Diagnostic deworming with arecolin derivatives is possible (dogs defecate within 2 h and shed proglottids if infected). Therapeutic treatment of infected final hosts uses praziquantel. The feces excreted by the animals within 2 days after treatment must be destroyed as they contain viable eggs.

REFERENCES

Alvarez Rojas CA, Romig T, Lighttowlers MW, *Echinococcus granulosus* sensu lato genotypes infecting humans - review of current knowledge. *Int. J. Parasitol.* 44, 9–18, 2014.

Brunetti E, Kern P, Vuitton DA, Writing Panel for the WHO-IWGE: Expert consensus for diagnosis and treatment of cystic and alveolar echinococcosis in humans. *Acta Trop.* 114, 1–16, 2010.

Carmena D, Cardona GA, *Echinococcus* in wild carnivorous species: epidemiology, genotypic diversity, and implications for veterinary public health. *Vet. Parasitol.* 202, 69–94, 2014.

Cobo F et al., Albendazole plus praziquantel versus albendazole alone as a pre-operative treatment in intraabdominal hydatidosis caused by *Echinococcus granulosus*. *Trop. Med. Int. Health* 3, 462–466, 1998.

Dakak M et al., Surgical treatment for pulmonary hydatidosis (a review of 422 cases). *J. R. Coll. Surg. Edinb.* 47, 689–692, 2002.

Dinkel A et al., Detection of *Echinococcus multilocularis* in the definitive host: coprodiagnosis by PCR as an alternative to necropsy. *J. Clin. Microbiol.* 36, 1871–1876, 1998.

El-On J, Benzimidazole treatment of cystic echinococcosis. *Acta Trop.* 85, 243–252, 2003.

Franchi C, Di Vico B, Teggi A, Long-term evaluation of patients with hydatidosis treated with benzimidazole carbamates. *Clin. Infect. Dis.* 29, 304–309, 1999.

Ito A et al., Cystic echinococcosis in Mongolia: molecular identification, serology and risk factors. *PLoS Negl. Trop. Dis.* 19, e2937, 2014.

Singh BB et al., Economic losses due to cystic echinococcosis in India. Need for urgent action to control the disease. *Prev. Vet. Med.* 113, 1–12, 2014.

Skuhaka T et al., Albendazole sulphoxide concentrations in plasma and hydatid cyst and prediction of parasitological and clinical outcomes in patients with liver hydatodosis caused by *Echinococcus granulosus*. *Croat. Med. J.* 55, 146–155, 2014.

Seimenis A, Overview of the epidemiological situation on echinococcosis in the Mediterranean region. *Acta Trop.* 85, 191–195, 2003.

Torgerson PR et al., The emerging epidemic of echinococcosis in Kazakhstan. *Trans. R. Soc. Trop. Med. Hyg.* 96, 124–128, 2002.

WHO/OIE, Manual on echinococcosis in humans and animals. Eds.: Eckert J, Gemmell MA, Meslin FX, Pawlowski Z. PAM3, Office International des Epizooties, 2001.

WHO Informal Working Group, International classification of ultrasound images in cystic echinococcosis for application in clinical and field epidemiological settings. *Acta Trop.* 85, 253–261, 2003.

4.4.5 HYMENOLEPIASIS (DWARF TAPEWORM INFECTION)

Hymenolepiasis is an intestinal infection by dwarf tapeworms.

Etiology. In most cases infections are caused by *Hymenolepis nana* (*H. fraterna*), the smallest human tapeworm with a length of 8 to 9 cm. Human infections with *H. diminuta* are rare. This parasite reaches a length of >30 cm and is mainly found in rats.

Occurrence. Both species are found worldwide. Natural hosts of *H. nana* are rodents, most often mice, but also golden hamsters, for example, if kept as pets. Human infections are found predominantly in children. Infections are more common in rural than in urban areas and occur frequently under conditions of poor hygiene. A high prevalence (10 to 20%) is reported from Southern Europe, North and Central Africa, the Near and Far East, and Central America.

Transmission. Human infections with *H. nana* occur by ingestion of egg or rarely by infected intermediate hosts (insects, predominantly flour beetles, and other pests), which contain the infective stages, the cysticercoid, in their body cavity. *H. nana* is the only human tapeworm that does not require an intermediate host. It may be acquired by ingestion of cysticercoids in intermediate hosts but also by eggs transmitted from person-to-person and by autoinfection. In the direct cycle where eggs are ingested, the development, which otherwise takes place in

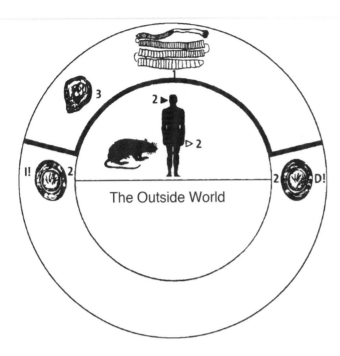

Figure 4.41 | Developmental cycle of *H. nana* (direct cycle). (1) Adult tapeworm (10 to 90 mm) in the small intestine of rodents and humans; (2) *H. nana* egg (0.040 to 0.050 mm) with oncosphere passed with feces (D, diagnostic stage; I, infective stage); (3) cysticercoid (0.050 to 0.135 mm) in an intestinal villus.

the intermediate host, occurs in the villi of the small intestine of vertebrate hosts. The oncospheres ingested with the eggs hatch, penetrate the villi, and develop to cysticercoids within 5 days. They emerge from the tissue, develop into adult tapeworms, and start to release proglottids with infective eggs 15 to 17 days after infection. Autoinfections via contaminated hands seem frequent in humans. In addition, in constipated individuals, larvae hatch in the intestine and repeat the cycle without leaving the host. After autoinfections the cysticercoids persist in the villi until the adult worms are excreted (these live only for about 2 months) or are eliminated after chemotherapy. Long-lasting infections may result.

The eggs are not resistant to environmental influences. Thus, infections from soiling occur more frequently than infections via contaminated food. The infection is relatively common in nurseries, probably as a result of fecal contamination of hands. The life cycle of *H. nana* is shown in Fig. 4.41.

H. diminuta, a parasite of rats and mice, requires an obligatory arthropod intermediate host (beetles and myriapods). Humans become infected by accidental ingestion of these arthropods containing cysticercoids. It is, therefore, a rare infection in humans.

Clinical Manifestations. The clinical picture depends on the number of worms and the duration of the infection. Weak infections do usually not cause symptoms. Heavy infections (>100 worms) result in atrophy of the villi and mucosal inflammation with abdominal pain, pulpy feces, and diarrhea. Patients are weak, fretful, and often have headache. Loss of weight was observed in cases where infections lasted for years. Hymenolepiasis may be an opportunistic infection in immunosuppressed patients.

Diagnosis. The proglottids are macerated in the intestine. Diagnosis is therefore based on the demonstration of the colorless eggs that contain the oncospheres and measure 40 by 50 μm in the case of *H. nana*. The eggs of *H. diminuta* are bigger (60 by 70 μm) and differ in eggshell structure from those of *H. nana*.

Differential Diagnosis. Enteritis of other etiology must be considered.

Therapy. The drug of choice is praziquantel, one 25 mg/kg dose is given orally. It eliminates the adult worms and kills cysticercoids in the intestinal villi.

Prophylaxis. Rodents and insects must be kept away from foods. Good personal hygiene is an important measure, especially for infected people, including cleanliness of the environment (toilets). Nurseries must be strictly surveyed for hygiene conditions.

REFERENCES

Chhakda T et al., Intestinal parasites in school-aged children in villages bordering Tonle Sap Lake, Cambodia. *Southeast Asian J. Trop. Med. Public Health* 37, 859–864, 2006.

Gupta A et al., Chronic diarrhea caused by *Hymenolepis nana* in a renal transplant recipient. *Clin. Exp. Nephrol.* 13, 185–186, 2009.

Karuna T, Khasanga S, A case of *Hymenolepis diminuta* in a young male in Odisha. *Trop. Parasitol.* 3, 145–147, 2013.

Marangi M et al., *Hymenolepis diminuta* infection in a child living in the urban area of Rome, Italy. *J. Clin. Microbiol.* 41, 3994–3995, 2003.

Mehraj V et al., Prevalence and factors associated with intestinal parasitic infections among children in an urban slum of Karachi. *PLoS One* 3, e3680, 2008.

Patamia I et al., A human case of *Hymenolepis diminuta* in a child from eastern Sicily. *Korean J. Parasitol.* 48, 167–169, 2010.

Steinmann P et al., Rapid appraisal of human intestinal helminth infections among school children in Oshoblast, Kyrgyzstan. *Acta Trop.* 116, 178–184, 2010.

Taha HA, Soliman MI, Banjar SA, Intestinal parasitic infections among expatriate workers in Al-Madina Al-Munawarah, Kingdom of Saudi Arabia. *Trop. Biomed.* 30, 78–88, 2013.

Worku N et al., Malnutrition and intestinal parasitic infections in school children of Gondar, North West Ethiopia. *Ethiop. Med. J.* 47, 9–16, 2009.

4.4.6 SPARGANOSIS

Sparganosis is a rare disease caused by tapeworm larvae of the order Pseudophyllida (see chapter 4.4.2; "Diphyllobothriasis"), which invade humans as accidental hosts and persist as so-called spargana for some time in various tissues.

Etiology. Spargana belong predominantly to the genus *Spirometra*. Detailed classification of the parasite is often impossible. Thus, the whole spectrum of sparganosis-inducing parasites is unknown. Spargana are usually at the stage of plerocercoids. They are string-like and show a head with two lateral grooves that resembles the head of adult tapeworms. Spargana measure up to 30 cm in length. *Sparganum proliferum* is an etiologically unclear form, which may divide by budding and spreads in the body.

Occurrence. *Spirometra mansoni*, *S. mansonoides*, and *S. erinaceieuropaei* occur in Asia, North America, and Eurasia, respectively, and infect dogs, cats, and wild carnivores. Spargana are found in humans worldwide. Most cases were reported from Asia (China, Korea, in the latter country, seroprevalences up to 8%) and the USA.

Transmission. Humans become infected by the ingestion of the larvae in intermediate or paratenic hosts. The adult pseudophyllids live in the small intestine of their specific final mammalian hosts. The life cycle is waterbound and includes two intermediate hosts. It resembles that of *D. latum* (see chapter 4.4.2; "Diphyllobothriais"). A ciliated coracidium emerges from the egg and is ingested by a small copepod (e.g., *Cyclops* spp.), where it develops to a procercoid. Infected copepods are swallowed by second intermediate hosts (fish, amphibians, such as frogs, and reptiles), and develop into plerocercoids.

Spargana develop in humans as accidental hosts after accidental ingestion of copepid crustaceans carrying procercoids, for example, with drinking water, or by consumption of undercooked second intermediate hosts or paratenic hosts that contain plerocercoids. Procercoids and plerocercoids migrate through the intestinal wall and invade various tissues, often the subcutaneous tissue. Another route of infection is related to traditional healing techniques: in the Far East, raw, chopped meat of frogs is put on wounds, ulcers, or the eyes; plerocercoids in the frogs may then actively invade the patients.

Clinical Manifestations. Larvae may persist for years in knobs, 1 to 2 cm in size, without noticeable reactions; however, most patients are affected by slowly growing, tender, often painful, subcutaneous nodules that may migrate. After the death of the larvae, severe local inflammation may develop around the parasite.

Spargana near the eye induce edema, ophthalmodynia, lacrimation, and ptosis. Invasion of the brain results in headache, seizures, and other disorders, dependent on the number, localization, and migration route of the larvae.

Diagnosis. Diagnosis depends on the demonstration and localization of the larvae; in cases of infestations of the brain, CT and MRT can be applied.

Differential Diagnosis. Infections with *Gnathostoma spinigerum* and, in CNS infestation, other space-occupying processes must be ruled out. Serological techniques may be helpful.

Therapy. Larvae are removed by surgery. Effective drugs are not available.

Prophylaxis. Potentially contaminated water should not be used for drinking. Meat of frogs, snails, and fish should be sufficiently cooked before consumption, particularly in Southeast Asia.

REFERENCES

Bao XY, Ding XH, Lu YC, Sparganosis presenting as radicu-lalgia at the conus medullaris. *Clin Neurol Neurosurg.* 110, 843–846, 2008.

Gong C et al., Cerebral sparganosis in children : epidemiological, clinical and MR imaging characteristics. *BMC Pediatr.* 12, 155, 2012.

Hong D et al., Cerebral sparganosis in mainland Chinese patients. *J. Clin. Neurosci.* 20, 1514–1519, 2013.

Iwatani K et al., Sparganum mansoni parasitic infection in the lungs showing a nodule. *Pathol. Int.* 56, 674–677, 2006.

Kim HJ et al., Intramuscular and subcutaneous sparganosis: sonographic findings. *J. Clin. Ultrasound* 36, 570–572, 2008.

Li MW et al., Enzootic sparganosis in Guangdong, People's Republic of China. *Emerg. Infect. Dis.* 15, 1317–1318, 2009.

Meric R et al., Disseminated infection caused by Sparganum proliferum in an AIDS patient. *Histopathology* 56, 824–828, 2010.

Pampiglione S, Fiovaranti ML, Rivasi F, Human sparganosis in Italy. Case report and review of the European cases. *APMIS* 111, 349–354, 2003.

Rengarajan S et al., Cerebral sparganosis: a diagnostic challenge. *Br. J. Neurosurg.* 22, 784–786, 2008.

Song T et al., CT and MR characteristics of cerebral sparganosis. *Am. J. Neuroradiol.* 28, 1700–1705, 2008.

Ye H et al., Clinical features of 8 cases of orbital sparganosis in southern China. *Can. J. Ophthalmol.* 47, 453–457, 2012.

4.4.7 TAENIASIS SAGINATA (INCLUDING TAENIASIS ASIATICA)

Taeniasis saginata is the human infection with adult tapeworms derived from cysticerci in cattle. Taeniasis asiatica is caused by the related species *T. asiatica*. Humans are the sole final hosts.

Etiology. Taeniasis saginata is caused by *Taenia saginata*, an intestinal tapeworm, 4 to 12 m long. The head (scolex) carries four suckers that allow the parasite to attach to the intestinal mucosa. The scolex lacks a rostellum or hooks, a trait that distinguishes it from *T. solium*. The larval or cysticercus stage (Cysticercus inermis) occurs in cattle after ingestion of the egg containing the oncosphere.

T. asiatica occurs in Southeast Asia. It is morphologically and genetically very close to *T. saginata* but differs from this species with regard to the intermediate host. Its cysticerci (Cysticercus viscerotropicus) are found predominantly in pigs.

Occurrence. *T. saginata* is a cosmopolitan parasite, especially common in countries with high beef consumption, particularly where beef is eaten raw or undercooked. Forty million people are assumed to be infected with *T. saginata* worldwide. Prevalence rates of 0.1 to 10% are supposed for Europe; a similar situation is assumed for North America. A much higher prevalence must be expected in parts of Africa.

The intermediate hosts of *T. saginata* are cattle, where the cysticerci are found in skeletal muscles and the heart. The prevalence in cattle as determined in industrial countries by meat inspection is in general 1 to 1.5%, but may vary between regions, even between individual abattoirs, from 0.01 to 7%. However, a substantially higher prevalence is observed in areas of high endemicity such as East Africa.

T. asiatica is found in Southeast Asia and China. Up to 20% of the inhabitants of rural areas are infected. The spectrum of intermediate

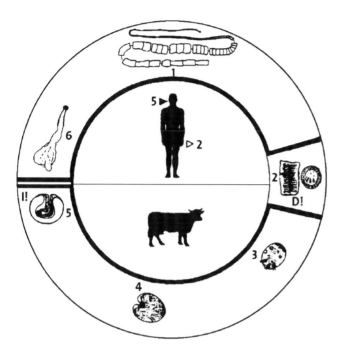

Figure 4.42 | Developmental cycle of *T. saginata*. (1) Adult tapeworm (4 to 12 m) in the small intestine of a human; (2) mature proglottid (ca. 16 to 20 mm) passed with feces or actively emigrated, and egg (0.03 to 0.04 mm) of *T. saginata* with an oncosphere, in the feces (D, diagnostic stage); (3) free oncosphere (ca. 0.02 mm) in intestine and blood vessels of the intermediate host (cattle); (4) formation of the cysticercus (*Cysticercus bovis*) in striated muscle of the intermediate host; (5) mature *C. bovis* (5 to 8 mm) in striated muscle of cattle (I, infectious stage); (6) evaginated *C. bovis* in the human small intestine.

hosts is broader than that of *T. saginata* and includes several species (pigs, ruminants, and monkeys). Pigs are the major intermediate hosts containing most of the cysticerci in the liver.

Transmission. *T. saginata* is transmitted by the consumption of raw or undercooked beef that contains the cysticerci. Eggs of *T. saginata* are shed in mature segments (proglottids; up to 100 000 eggs per proglottid) with the human feces. Four to nine mature proglottids are produced daily. Eggs are liberated into the environment by maceration of the proglottids and must be ingested by the intermediate host. This may happen when pastures are directly contaminated with human feces, when wastewater is used to fertilize pastures, or insufficiently purified wastewater is spread on pastures, for example, by floods (eggs can pass through sewage treatment plants). Spreading of eggs by arthropods or birds is also possible. Eggs may survive on pastures for months. The larvae (oncospheres) hatch from the eggs in the intestine of cattle, penetrate the intestinal wall, are hematogenously disseminated, and settle in the striated musculature (sites of predilection: diaphragm, heart, and masseters). They develop

into infective cysticerci within 3 months. Cysticerci are thin-walled, fluid-containing, small bladders, 5 by 8 mm, with a single tapeworm scolex inside.

After ingestion of a cysticercus by a human, the scolex is everted, attaches to the mucosa of the upper small intestine and starts formation of segments (proglottids). First mature proglottids are shed 12 weeks after infection (end of prepatent period). A single *T. saginata* worm can survive in humans for 30 to 40 years. The developmental cycle is shown in Fig. 4.42.

Cysticerci of *T. asiatica* are predominantly found in the liver and other peritoneal organs of the intermediate hosts. Consumption of such raw or undercooked organs can cause infection.

Clinical Manifestations. Infection with adult tapeworms may persist for years without clear symptoms. Otherwise, anorexia alternating with ravenous appetite, nausea, feeling of intestinal pressure, epigastric colic, malabsorption, and weight loss have been reported associated with the infection. Most commonly, the patients describe the discomfort and embarrassment by proglottids crawling from the anus. Reactive arthritis due to *T. saginata* infection is discussed.

The broad intermediate host spectrum of the Asiatic *Taenia* in combination with the predominant invasion of organs suggested that *T. asiatica* might develop to cysticerci in humans. There is, however, no evidence for this.

Diagnosis. Direct demonstration of eggs in the feces is rarely possible. The eggs are round, 30 to 40 µm in size, and enclosed by a thick shell that shows radial striation. Usually, yellowish proglottids, 10 to 20 mm by 4 to 8 mm in size, which resemble flat noodles and contain eggs are passed. Proglottids may be found in the underwear, as they may emerge from the anus without the patient noticing. In most cases, they are found as single segments; segments sticking together suggest *T. solium* infection.

Squeeze-preparations of native or stained (acidic carmine solution) mature *T. saginata* segments show (under 2- to 5-fold magnification) the uterine stem and 10 to 30 lateral branches. Proglottids that are dried up must be soaked in water before fixation and staining.

T. saginata and *T. asiatica* on the one hand and *T. solium* on the other hand coexist in some areas and they must be differentiated because of the complex of problems in the case of the latter infection (cysticercosis). *T. solium* proglottids usually only show 10 to 12 lateral branches. The presence (*T. saginata*) or absence (*T. solium*) of a vaginal sphincter muscle allows clear differentiation of the proglottids of the two species. *T. solium* but not *T. saginata* is provided with a rostellum and hooks at the scolex. Mixed infections have been reported. Noteworthy are increased serum IgE levels in infested patients.

Differential Diagnosis. Infestations with other tapeworms must be considered.

Therapy. Niclosamide, one 2 g dose orally and praziquantel, one 20 mg/kg dose orally are effective and well-tolerated anthelmintics. The cestodes are digested within the intestine after praziquantel treatment.

Prophylaxis. Raw or undercooked beef should not be eaten. Mincing of beef does not necessarily destroy the cysticerci. Pickling and smoking may also be ineffective in this respect. Frozen beef (kept at −10 °C for at least 8 days) is safe. In areas endemic for *T. asiatica*, raw or undercooked organs and meat of pigs and other animals should not be consumed.

Meat inspection reduces the risk of infection. However, the common procedures [incisions in specified muscles; obligatory EU regulation (RL 95/23 EG)] are not very sensitive (<15%) and fail to identify low-grade infections. Thus, in spite of all costly and laborious measures of meat inspection, the risk of infection with *T. saginata* has not changed in recent decades.

REFERENCES

Abusei S et al., Visual diagnosis of *Taenia saginata* cysticercosis during meat inspection: is it unequivocal? *Parasitol. Res.* 99, 405–409, 2006.

Ale A et al., Epidemiology and genetic diversity of *Taenia asiatica*. A systematic review. *Parasit. Vectors* 7, 45, 2014.

Anantaphruti MT et al., Sympatric occurrence of *Taenia solium*, *T. saginata*, and *T. asiatica*, Thailand. *Emerg. Infect. Dis.* 13, 1413–1416, 2007.

Boone I et al., Distribution and risk factors of bovine cysticercosis in Belgian dairy and mixed herds. *Prev. Vet. Med.* 82, 1–11, 2007.

Cabaret J et al., The use of urban sewage sludge on pastures: the cysticercosis threat. *Vet. Res.* 33, 575–597, 2002.

Dias AK et al., *Taenia solium* and *Taenia saginata*: identification of sequence characterized amplified region (SCAR) markers. *Exp. Parasitol.* 117, 9–12, 2007.

Dorny P, Praet N, *Taenia saginata* in Europe. *Vet. Parasitol.* 149, 2–24, 2007.

Eom KS, Jeo HK, Rim HJ, Geographical distribution of *Taenia asiatica* and related species. *Korean J. Parasitol.* 47, S115–S124, 2009.

Flütsch F et al., Case-control study to identify risk factors for bovine cysticercosis on farms in Switzerland. *Parasitology* 135, 641–646, 2008.

Galán-Puchades MT, Fuentes MV, Lights, shadows in the *Taenia asiatica* life cycle, pathogenicity . *Trop. Parasitol.* 3, 114–119, 2013.

Geysen D et al., Validation of meat inspection results for *Taenia saginata* cysticercosis by PCR-restriction fragment length polymorphism. *J. Food Prot.* 70, 236–240, 2007.

Jenkins DJ, Brown GK, Traub RJ, "Cysticercosis storm" in feedlot cattle in north-west New South Wales. *Austr. Vet. J.* 91, 89–91, 2013.

Kebede N, Tilahun G, Hailu A, Current status of bovine cysticercosis of slaughtered cattle in Addis Ababa abattoir, Ethiopia. *Trop. Anim. Health Prod.* 41, 291–294, 2009.

Koul PA et al., Praziquantel in niclosamid-resistant *Taenia saginata* infection. *Scand. J. Infect. Dis.* 31, 603–604, 1999.

Kyvsgaard NC et al., A case-control study of rist factors in light *Taenia saginata* cysticercosis in Danish cattle. *Acta Vet. Scand.* 32, 243–252, 1991.

Lightowlers MW, Cestode vaccines: origins, current status and future prospects. *Parasitology* 133, S27–S42, 2006.

Ogunremi O, Benjamin J, Development and field evaluation of a new serological test for *Taenia saginata* cysticercosis. *Vet Parasitol.* 169, 93–101, 2010.

Parija SC, Ponnamborth DK, Laboratory diagnosis of *Taenia asiatica* in humans and animals. *Trop. Parasitol.* 3, 120–124, 2023.

Pearse BH et al., Prevalence of Cycticercus bovis in Australian cattle. *Aust. Vet. J.* 88, 260–262, 2010.

Scandrett B et al. Distribution of *Taenia saginata* cysticerci in tissues of experimentally infected cattle. *Vet. Parasitol.* 164, 223–231, 2009.

4.4.8 TAENIASIS SOLIUM AND CYSTICERCOSIS

Etiology. The causative agent is the cestode *Taenia solium*. The parasite reaches a length of 1.5 to 8 m. The scolex shows a rostellum with hooks. The metacestode is called Cysticercus cellulosae.

Occurrence. The adult *T. solium* is found only in humans, whereas the larval stage is not host specific. The predominant intermediate host, however, is the pig. Endemic occurrence is limited to areas where the cycle can involve both humans and pigs, for example, where consumption of pork is not banned by religious rules.

Areas of endemicity are Central and South America, Central and Southern Africa, Southeast Asia, and Southern and Eastern Europe. Recent studies in a hyperendemic area in Laos (Lao PDR) showed excretion of proglottids in 28% of the population and seroprevalences of cysticercosis of >50%. In some rural areas in South America, serological surveys suggest a prevalence of cysticercosis of approximately 10%. On the basis of only patients with neurological disorders, the prevalence in these areas is distinctly higher (>20%). The prevalence of *T. solium* in pigs reflects that in humans and may amount to 50% in these geographical regions. Taeniasis and cysticercosis in the United States are generally imported by immigrants from Latin America, but people infected with the adult tapeworm may also be a source of infection. Approximately 1000 new cases are expected each year. The seroprevalence of *T. solium* in Latin American people in the southern United States is currently 2 to 3%.

In industrial areas, the infection became almost eliminated due to meat inspection and measures that prevent or minimize the access of pigs to human feces, such as generally increased hygiene standards and modified conditions of pig production (housing).

Transmission. The adult *T. solium* worms develop in humans after oral ingestion of cysticerci (cysticercus cellulosae) in raw or undercooked pork or other tissues of pigs. In pigs, the larvae are found predominantly in the musculature and the brain. In some regions where dogs are eaten by humans, these are probably also transmitters.

The cysticerci are freed from surrounding tissues by digestion. The preformed scolex evaginates, attaches to the mucosa, and starts the formation of proglottids. The first gravid (egg-containing) proglottids are found in the feces 9 to 10 weeks after infection. The adult parasite may survive in its host for many (25) years.

Cysticercosis develops after oral ingestion of *T. solium* eggs. Carriers of adult *T. solium* are not only a source of infection of pigs as intermediate hosts but also a risk for themselves by autoinfections and for other people. Considering that approximately 250 000 eggs per day are released with the proglottids by an infected person, these risks are high. Autoinfection may be a consequence of insufficient personal hygiene and usually occurs by egg-contaminated hands. The often-observed coincidence of infections with adult *T. solium* and cysticerci illustrates the importance of autoinfections. Transmission from human-to-human occurs when human feces that contain *T. solium* eggs, contaminate food, for example, vegetables by top fertilization or under poor hygienic conditions.

The eggs contain infective larvae, the oncospheres, which hatch in the intestine, penetrate the mucosa, are spread via blood vessels, and invade actively various organs, for example, the CNS, muscles, or subcutaneous tissue. In humans, they are distinctly neurotropic, invading the hemispheres of the brain; the eyes are another site of predilection. Within 2 to 3 months, they develop to cysticerci, bladder-like larvae of 6 by 9 mm, which contain a preformed scolex. The intact cysticercus causes hardly any inflammation of the surrounding tissue, as it releases immunomodulatory and anti-inflammatory compounds (proteases, e.g., taeniastatin). Dying or dead cysticerci leaking antigenic material, however, provoke an inflammatory reaction responsible for tissue damage and clinical symptoms. Finally, they are replaced by connective tissues and calcifications.

Clinical Manifestations. Adult *T. solium* are generally not associated with severe clinical symptoms. Similar to patients infected with *T. saginata*, tapeworm carriers may show vague signs and symptoms of the abdomen, hunger pains, diarrhea, indigestion or constipation, and low-grade eosinophilia, and increased IgE may be present.

Cysticerci outside the CNS are usually not associated with severe clinical consequences. Cerebral cysticerci may cause variable clinical symptoms dependent on their numbers and localizations. Viable cysts within the parenchyma are often tolerated without severe symptoms for years unless the parasite dies and perifocal, often intense inflammatory reactions with predominantly lymphocytic, to a lesser degree neutrophilic/eosinophilic infiltrates emerge. Seizures, focal or generalized sensomotoric disorders, reduced consciousness, and personality changes may evolve. The inflammatory reactions are finally replaced by fibrotic tissue and calcification.

Intraventricular cysts or cysts localized in the ependymal position or in the basal cysternae cause earlier symptoms: increased spinal fluid production and disorders in the CSF circulation result in increased intracerebral pressure (with nausea and vomiting) up to occlusive hydrocephalus. Chronic meningitis is accompanied by headache and neck stiffness. Vasculitis of subarachnoidal blood vessels may cause cerebral infarcts. Neuritis may result in dysfunction of one or more cranial nerves.

Infestation of the spinal cord causes segmental deficiencies, most often paresis. Myocarditis may develop with cysticerci in the cardiac muscle. Infestation of the eye (vitreous humor or retina) is followed by impaired vision or even blindness. Muscle cysts lead to myalgia and palpable nodules, which are also found when the skin or the subcutaneous tissue are infested.

Multiple cerebral infestation may cause death. Occasionally, thin-walled, ramified bladders without protoscolices (so-called cysticercus racemosus) are found in the subarachnoidal space and in the ventricles, resulting in mental deterioration, coma, and death.

Diagnosis. Taeniasis due to *T. solium* is diagnosed by the demonstration of proglottids, 7 by 20 mm in size. Often three or more unseparated proglottids are shed. Proglottids contain a relatively short uterus with 7 to 16 lateral branches, that is, generally less than in *T. saginata*. However, the numbers of lateral uterine branches are only uncertain characteristics of the two species. An unambitious differentiation needs the investigation of stained proglottids for the presence or absence of a vaginal sphincter. *T. solium* proglottids lack this sphincter. In addition, PCR techniques allow the differentiation between the species. In endemic areas, assays are used to determine and differentiate antigens or parasite DNA as indicators of active infections in the feces.

Cerebral cysticercosis is diagnosed by X-ray (calcification), CT scan, MRI, and by demonstration of specific antibodies. MRI is superior to CT, particularly in cases of racemous forms of cysticercosis and small intraparenchymatous lesions. However, films in most cases are not pathognomonic, and apart from the clinical picture and analysis of history (exposition), serological techniques must be applied. Serology was improved in recent years. Highly specific antigens are affinity-purified *T. solium* glycoproteins, which are recommended for immunoblotting. This technique is the method of choice according to the WHO and the Pan-American Health Organization. Commercial test kits are available. However, the test does not detect infections with single cysticerci, and, of course, recognizes cysticerci localized in tissue other than the CNS or infections with adult *T. solium*. More recently, new promising tests have been developed to detect parasite antigens in serum, CSF, and urine.

Subcutaneously localized cysticerci are usually detectable as sliding, lentil-sized structures.

Differential Diagnosis. In the case of taeniasis, infection with other tapeworms has to be considered. In case of cysticercosis, infection with coenuri (see chapter 4.4.1; "Coenurosis"), tumors, and meningitis tuberculosa should be excluded.

Therapy. Treatment of *T. solium* taeniasis should be started immediately after diagnosis; patients with this diagnosis represent a hazard. Niclosamide (one 2 g dose orally) and praziquantel (one 5 to 10 mg/kg dose orally) are effective but do not kill the oncospheres in the eggs. Therefore, the anthelmintic treatment should be combined with application of an antiemetic to prevent retroinfections due to regurgitation. Tapeworm patients should be isolated after treatment for several days. Released tapeworms or parts of them, as well as the feces, must be destroyed. The success of treatment should be regularly controlled over a period of 2 months by investigating the feces for proglottids.

Convulsive neurocysticercosis patients usually respond to anticonvulsives, typically for 1 to 2 years. Specific drugs are albendazole and praziquantel. Albendazole, patients >60 kg bodyweight: 400 mg orally twice a day with meals; <60 kg bodyweight: 15 mg/kg/day, given in divided doses twice a day with meals (maximum dose: 800 mg/day) for up to 30 days. Praziquantel, 100 mg/day divided in three doses orally for 30 days. Both drugs must be combined with dexamethasone, 0.1 mg/kg/day to reduce exacerbations by dying parasites (cave: cerebral edema). The clinical benefit of an antiparasitic treatment was under discussion for a long time, but recent studies suggest an earlier regression of foci and fewer seizures in patients given anthelmintics. In cases of hydrocephalus after infestation of ventricles or the subarachnoidal space, a ventriculoperitoneal shunt is recommended for CSF drainage. Failures (e.g., shunt obstruction) can be minimized by antiparasitic treatment and/or the application of corticosteroids. Surgical decompression by aspiration of cyst fluid may be necessary in cases of large cysticerci in the subarachnoidal space (cysticercus racemosus). Ocular cysticercosis requires surgical treatment to prevent persistent lesions.

Prophylaxis. To avoid taeniasis, raw or undercooked pork should not be consumed, at least in areas of endemicity. Cooking should result in a core temperature of at least 60 °C. Pickling and smoking do not always kill the cysticerci. The risk of infection is reduced by meat inspection. For cysticercosis, general hygienic rules should be observed. Vegetables and fruits should be thoroughly cleaned or peeled before they are eaten. Vaccination of pigs against *T. solium* seems a realistic preventive measure in endemic areas.

REFERENCES

Alexander AM et al., Long-term clinical evaluation of asymptomatic subjects positive for circulating *Taenia solium* antigens. *Trans. R. Soc. Trop. Med. Hyg.* 104, 809–810, 2010.

Catey PT et al., Neglected parasitic infections in the United States: cysticercosis. *Am. J. Trop. Med. Hyg.* 90, 805–809, 2014.

Ciampi de Andrade D et al., Cognitive impairment and dementia in neurocysticercosis: a cross-sectional controlled study. *Neurology* 74, 1288–1295, 2010.

Coral-Almeida M et al., Incidence of *Taenia solium* larval infection in an Ecuadorian endemic area: implications for disease burden assessment and control. *PLoS Negl. Trop. Dis.* 5, e2887, 2014.

Deckers N, Dorny P, Immunodiagnosis of *Taenia solium* taeniosis/cysticercosis. *Trends Parasitol.* 26, 137–144, 2010.

De Souza A et al., Natural history of solitary cerebral cysticercosis on serial magnetic resonance imaging and the effect of albendazole therapy on its evolution. *J. Neurol. Sci.* 288, 135–141, 2010.

Fleury A et al., Neurocysticercosis, a persisting health problem in Mexico. *PLoS Negl. Trop. Dis.* 4, e805, 2010.

Goel D et al., Natural history of solitary cerebral cysticercosis cases after albendazole therapy: a longitudinal follow-up study from India. *Acta Neurol. Scand.* 121, 204–208, 2010.

Huerta M et al., Parasite contamination of soil in households of a Mexican rural community endemic for neurocysticercosis. *Trans. R. Soc. Trop. Med. Hyg.* 102, 374–379, 2008.

Kamuyu G Exposure to multiple parasites is associated with the prevalence of active convulsive epilepsy in sub-Saharan Africa. *PLoS Negl. Trop. Dis.* 8, e2908, 2014.

Kim SW et al., Racemose cysticercosis in the cerebellar hemisphere. *J. Korean Neurosurg. Soc.* 48, 59–61, 2010.

Lightowlers MW, Eradication of *Taenia solium* cysticercosis: a role for vaccination of pigs. *Int. J. Parasitol.* 40, 1183–1192, 2010.

Matthaiou DK et al., Albendazole versus praziquantel in the treatment of neurocysticercosis: a meta-analysis of comparative trials. *PLoS Negl. Trop. Dis.* 12, e194, 2008.

Mazumdar M, Pandharipande P, Poduri A, Does albendazole affect seizure remission and computed tomography response in children with neurocysticercosis? A systematic review and meta-analysis. *J. Child Neurol.* 22, 135–142, 2007.

Okello A et al., Investigating a hyperendemic focus of *Taenia solium* in northern Lao PDR. *Parasites & Vectors* 7, 134, 2014.

Rath S et al., Orbital cysticercosis: clinical manifestations, diagnosis, management, and outcome. *Ophthalmology* 117, 600–605, 2010.

Rottbeck R, High prevalence of cysticercosis in people with epilepsy in southern Ruanda. *PLoS Negl. Trop. Dis.* 7, e2558, 2013.

Sciutto E et al., The immune response in *Taenia solium* cysticercosis: protection and injury. *Parasite Immunol.* 29, 621–636, 2007.

Sikasunge CS et al., *Taenia solium* porcine cysticercosis: viability of cysticerci and persistency of antibodies and cysticercal antigens after treatment with oxfendazole. *Vet. Parasitol.* 158, 57–66, 2008.

Willingham AL, Engels D, Control of *Taenia solium* cysticercosis/taeniosis. *Adv. Parasitol.* 61, 509–566, 2006.

4.4.9 OTHER ZOONOTIC CESTODE INFECTIONS

4.4.9.1 Intestinal Infestation: Etiology, Occurrence, and Transmission

- Infections with *Bertiella* spp. Agents are the species *Bertiella studeri* and *B. mucromata*. They are up to 30 cm long and are found in nonhuman primates. Human infections, predominantly in children, are found in Africa, Asia, and South America. Infection occurs by accidental ingestion of infected intermediate hosts [free-living mites (Oribatidae)];

- Infections with *Raillietina* spp. Several species of the genus (*Raillietina dermerariensis*, *R. asiatica*, and others) infect humans. The parasites reach lengths of 60 cm. They are found worldwide in rodents, mainly rats, and primates. Intermediate hosts are insects (flour beetles and corn beetles, e.g., *Tribolium* spp.) and cockroaches;

- Infections with *Inermicapsifer madagascariensis* (*I. cubensis*). These cestodes reach lengths of 50 cm and occur in small rodents in tropical areas. Free-living mites are probably the intermediate hosts. Human infections are known from Africa, Madagascar, and the Caribbean area;

- Infections with *Mesocestoides* spp., *Mesocestoides variabilis*, and *M. lineatus* are found in humans; however, the taxonomy of the genus is controversial. Cases are known from Africa, Asia, and North and South America. Carnivorous animals are the natural final hosts where the parasites reach a length of up to 2.5 m. The complex developmental cycle is not completely known. Free-living oribatid mites are the first intermediate hosts. Obligate second intermediate hosts are various mammals, predominantly rodents, birds, amphibians, and reptiles. The parasites develop in their body cavities to so-called tetrathyridia [developmental stages provided with four suckers (acetabula), 2 to 70 mm in length, which multiply by fission]. These are the infective stages for the final hosts, that is, humans, and must be ingested with raw or undercooked intermediate hosts or their viscera;

- Infection with *Diplogonoporus grandis*. The parasite *D. grandis* belongs to the same order as *D. latum* (chapter 4.4.2) and develops similarly. Marine mammals, especially whales, are final hosts; plerocercoids are found in various saltwater fishes. Human infections (approximately 200 known cases) were reported from Japan and they occur by ingestion of raw or undercooked saltwater fishes. The parasite may reach a length of 6 m.

Clinical Manifestations. The tapeworms settle in the small intestine. Clinical symptoms are rare in humans. Heavy infestation (occasionally in *Mesocestoides* spp. infections) may cause abdominal pain, diarrhea, and nausea.

Diagnosis. Proglottids of a size of a rice grain are shed with the feces. In case of *D. grandis*, eggs are found in the feces, as with *D. latum*.

Therapy. Praziquantel, one 10 to 15 mg/kg dose, and niclosamide, adults one 2 g dose and children one dose of 0.5 to 1 g, are effective.

Prophylaxis. Vegetable food must be carefully cleaned. Potential secondary intermediate hosts should not be consumed raw or undercooked.

4.4.9.2 Extraintestinal Infestation: Infection with Taenia crassiceps

The tapeworm is frequently found in foxes but more rarely in dogs. Intermediate hosts are rodents, which ingest the *Taenia* eggs from the feces of final hosts and develop metacestodes (cysticerci) in their connective tissue and body cavities. In contrast to *T. saginata* or *T. solium*, the cysticerci of *T. crassiceps* proliferate by budding; excessive accumulation of metacestodes may therefore occur in the tissues of the intermediate hosts.

Humans become infected by accidental ingestion of *T. crassiceps* eggs. In most of the known >10 human cases, massive, extended accumulations of whitish metacestodes, 2 to 3 mm in size, were found in the connective tissue, accompanied by edematous swellings and often distinct hemorrhages into the tissue, causing a picture of extended hematomas. Patients were HIV-infected or immunosuppressed by respective treatment, except one case, where the parasites were found in the eyes.

Surgical measures followed by antiparasitic treatment with praziquantel, 1 g twice a day orally plus albendazole, 400 mg per day orally for 28 days achieved healing. Several further reports deal with the occurrence of tetrathyridia in human CNS and parenchymas; however, they did not clear up the infection etiologically.

REFERENCES

Arizono N et al., Diplogonoporiasis in Japan: genetic analysis of five clinical isolates. *Parasitol. Int.* 57, 212–216, 2008.

Bhagwant S, Human *Bertiella studeri* (Family Anoplocephalidae) infection of probable Southeast Asian origin in Mauretanian children and an adult. *Am. J. Trop. Med. Hyg.* 70, 225–228, 2004.

Clavel A et al., Diplogonoporiasis presumably introduced into Spain: first confirmed case of human infection acquired outside the Far East. *Am. J. Trop. Med. Hyg.* 57, 317–320, 1997.

Chuck RS et al., Surgical removal of subretinal proliferating cysticercus of *Taenia crassiceps*. *Arch. Ophthalmol.* 115, 562–563, 1997.

Fuentes MV, Galán-Puchade MT, Malone JB, A new case report of human *Mesocestoides* infection in the United States. *Am. J. Trop. Med. Hyg.* 68, 566–567, 2003.

Garin YJF et al., Case report: human brain abscess due to a tetra-acetabulate plerocercoid metacestode (Cyclophyllidea). *Am. J. Trop. Med. Hyg.* 72, 513–517, 2005.

Gonzalez Nunez I, Diaz Jidy M, Nunez Fernández F, Infection by *Inermicapsifer madagascariensis* (Davaine, 1870); Baer, 1956. A report of two cases. *Rev. Cubana Med. Trop.* 48, 224–226, 1996.

Heldwein K et al., Subcutaneous *Taenia crassiceps* infection in a patient with Non-Hodgkin's Lymphoma. *Am. J. Trop. Med. Hyg.* 75, 108–111, 2006.

Kino H et al., A mass occurrence of human infection with *Diplogonoporus grandis* (Cestoda: Diphyllobothriidae) in Shizuoka Prefecture, Central Japan. *Parasitol. Int.* 51, 73–79, 2002.

Maillard H et al., *Taenia crassiceps* cystocercosis and AIDS. *AIDS* 12, 1551–1552, 1998.

Malik S, Shrivastava VK, Samantharay JC, Human bertiellosis from North India. *Indian J. Pediatr.* 80, 258–260, 2013.

Ntkouas V et al., Cerebellar cysticercosis caused by larval *Taenia crassiceps* tapeworm in immunocompetent women, Germany. *Emerg. Infect. Dis.* 19, 2008–2011, 2013.

Xin S et al., *Bertiella studeri* infection, China. *Emerg. Infect. Dis.* 12, 176–177, 2006.

Yamasaki H, Ohmae H, Kuramochi T, Complete mitochondrial genome of *Diplogonoporus balaenopterae* and *Diplogonoporus grandis* (Cestoda: Diphyllobothriidae) and clarification of theit taxonomic relationships. *Parasitol. Int.* 61, 260–266, 2012.

4.5 Zoonoses Caused by Nematodes

Nematodes are free-living or endoparasitic metazoan organisms. The body is unsegmented, usually cylindrical, and elongated. They possess an alimentary canal and the sexes are generally separate. Nematodes are enclosed by a cuticle that continues to the orifices of the body (mouth, anus, genital openings).

Adult female nematodes may be oviparous or larviparous (e.g., filariae or *Trichinella* spp.). The development may be either direct or indirect including various types of intermediate hosts. Nematodes have to pass four larval stages (larva 1 to larva 4) to reach a preadult (5th) stage, which subsequently develops to the adult male or female worm. In the course of the larval development, the larvae molt to the next stage by stripping the old cuticula. The third stage larva represents the infective stage for the final host (either acquired directly or transmitted by an intermediate host). Exceptions are the members of the order Enoplida (*Trichinella* spp., *Capillaria* spp.), which are transmitted as first larvae.

Parasitic nematodes inhabit various organs and tissues, for example, the intestinal tract, the lungs, body cavities, and parenchymas, and partly take excessive migratory routes to reach their final destinations.

4.5.1 ANGIOSTRONGYLIASIS

4.5.1.1 Cerebral Angiostrongyliasis (Eosinophilic Meningoencephalitis or Eosinophilic Meningitis)

Larvae of the rat lungworm *Angiostrongylus cantonensis* may infect humans (which are accidental hosts) and cause eosinophilic meningitis. The infection often remains clinically inapparent, but patients sometimes die.

Etiology. Agents are larvae of *A. cantonensis*, a rat lungworm.

Occurrence. *A. cantonensis* is found in various species of rats in Australia, China, India, vast areas of Southeast Asia, and Pacific and Indian Ocean islands. It is also found in Egypt, West Africa, the Caribbean area, and the southern United States. The prevalence in rats may be high. For example, >70% of rats (*Rattus norvegicus*) caught in Rio de Janeiro were found infected. Human infections are known from all areas of endemicity.

Transmission. Humans are infected by oral ingestion of raw or undercooked terrestrial snails that serve as intermediate hosts (giant snails: *Achatina fulica*; apple snails: *Pomacea* spp., *Pila* spp.; slugs, and aquatic snails) and a variety of paratenic hosts (e.g., crabs, frogs, monitor lizards, also fish), or free (emerged from intermediate hosts) larvae.

Mature worms live in the pulmonary arteries of rats. Larvae in deposited eggs hatch, and penetrate through the alveoli, are coughed up, and passed with the feces. They invade snails and develop to infective larvae. Final hosts become infected by ingestion of intermediate or paratenic hosts or free larvae that may survive in water for several days.

Larvae invade the intestinal wall of the host, are spread hematogenously, reach the brain within 4 to 6 days, and moult to fourth-stage larvae. These invade the subarachnoid space, and in the final host, migrate via the venous system to the pulmonary artery and the right heart. In humans, the larvae are 1 to 2 mm in size, they become enclosed by granulomas in the brain and die in either the parenchyma or the subarachnoid space within weeks.

Clinical Manifestations. Clinical signs depend on the number of larvae. Cerebral symptoms develop in approximately 10% of the cases after an incubation period of 1 to 5 weeks. Major signs are severe headache, vomiting, stiffness of the neck, convulsions, facial paralysis, paresthesia, sleep disturbances, hearing disorders, speech impediments, and occasionally, paresis. Fever is a common symptom. A characteristic sign is a heavy accumulation of eosinophils in the CSF (>10%), accompanied by increased CSF pressure. Occasionally larvae are found in the eye. Symptoms may persist for days up to months in untreated cases. Lethal outcomes occur.

Diagnosis. Diagnosis is based predominantly on clinical signs and anamnesis, considering the high number of eosinophils in the CSF and increased CSF pressure. Attempts to demonstrate larvae in the CSF in most cases fail. Serological tests are only available in a few laboratories and are not always reliable.

Differential Diagnosis. Other kinds of meningoencephalitis, cerebral cysticercosis, and visceral larva migrans must be considered.

Therapy. In many cases, the patients recover spontaneously. Corticosteroids and a careful reduction of CSF pressure, for example, by repeated CSF puncture, may be beneficial. Albendazole, 400 mg/kg once to twice a day for 3 weeks is larvicidal, but may temporarily enhance neurological symptoms. In case of infestation of the eye, treatment by laser technology is recommended.

Prophylaxis. Raw or undercooked snails, crabs, prawns, or crayfish should not be consumed in areas of endemicity. Vegetables must be cleaned, particularly of adhering snails. Surface water must be boiled before drinking or other use. Raw or undercooked inner organs (e.g., liver) of slaughtered animals should not be ingested.

REFERENCES

Bärtschi E et al., Eosinophilic meningitis due to *Angiostrongylus cantonensis* in Switzerland. *Infection* 32, 116–118, 2004.

Chotmongkol V et al., Comparison of prednisolone plus albendazole with prednisolone alone for treatment of patients with eosinophilic meningitis. *Am. J. Trop. Med. Hyg.* 81, 443–445, 2009.

Cowie RH, Pathways for transmission of angiostrongyliasis and the risk of disease associated with them. *Hawaii J. Med. Public Health* 72 (6 Suppl. 2), 70–74, 2013.

Diaz JH, Recognizing and reducing the risks of helminthic eosinophilic meningitis in travellers: differential diagnosis, disease management, prevention, and control. *J. Travel Med.* 16, 267–275, 2009.

Hollyer JR, Telling consumers, gardeners, and farmers about the possible risk of rat lungworm in the local food supply in Hawaii. *Hawaii J. Med. Public Health*. 72 (6 Suppl. 2), 82, 2013.

Jin E et al., MRI findings of eosinophilic myelomeningoencephalitis due to *Angiostrongylus cantonensis*. *Clin. Radiol.* 60, 242–250, 2005.

Jitpimolmard S et al., Albendazole therapy for eosinophilic meningitis caused by *Angiostrongylus cantonensis*. *Parasitol. Res.* 100, 1293–1296, 2007.

Li H et al., A severe eosinophilic meningitis caused by infection of *Angiostrongylus cantonensis*. *Am. J. Trop. Med. Hyg.* 79, 568–570, 2008.

Lv S et al., Emerging angiostrongyliasis in Mainland China. *Emerg. Infect. Dis.* 14, 161–164, 2008.

Lv S et al., Helminth infections of the central nervous system occurring in Southeast Asia and the Far East. *Adv. Parasitol.* 72, 351–408, 2010.

Morton MJ et al., Severe hemorrhagic meningoencephalitis due to *Angiostrongylus cantonensis* among young children in Sidney, Australia. *Clin. Infect. Dis.* 57, 1158–1161, 2013.

Oehler EF et al., *Angiostrongylus cantonensis* eosinophilic meningitis: a clinical study of 42 consecutive cases in French Polynesia. *Parasitol. Int.* 63, 544–549, 2014.

Sawanyawisuth K et al., Intraocular angiostrongyliasis: clinical findings, treatments and outcomes. *Trans. R. Soc. Trop. Med.Hyg.* 101, 497–501, 2007.

Sawanyawisuth K, Sawanyawisuth K, Treatment of angiostrongyliasis. *Trans. R. Soc. Trop. Med. Hyg.* 102, 990–996, 2008.

Simoes RO et al., A longitudinal study of *Angiostrongylus cantonensis* in an urban population of *Rattus norvegicus* in Brazil: the influence of seasonality and host features on the pattern of infection. *Parasit. Vectors* 7, 100, 2014.

Tsai HAT et al., Outbreak of eosinophilic meningitis associated with drinking of raw vegetable juice in southern Taiwan. *Am. J. Trop. Med. Hyg.* 71, 222–226, 2004.

Wang QP et al., Human angiostrongyliasis. *Lancet Infect. Dis.* 8, 621–630, 2008.

Wang J et al., An outbrake of angiostrongyliasis cantonensis in Beijing. *J. Parasitol.* 96, 377–381, 2010.

Wilkins PP et al., The current status of laboratory diagnosis of *Angiostrongylus cantonensis* infections in humans using serologic and molecular methods. *Hawaii J. Med. Publ. Health* 72 (6 Suppl. 2), 55–57, 2013.

4.5.1.2 Intestinal Angiostrongyliasis

Intestinal angiostrongyliasis is a severe, sometimes fatal disease caused by infection with *Angiostrongylus costaricensis*. It is characterized by iliocecal eosinophilic granulomas.

Etiology. The agent causing intestinal angiostrongyliasis is *A. costaricensis*, a nematode 2 cm (males) to 4 cm (females) in length that dwells in the intestinal arteries. The worms cause inflammatory lesions in the bowel wall in human hosts.

Occurrence. *A. costaricensis* is found in rodents. Cotton rats (*Sigmodon hispidus*), which are common in Central America and the southern United States represent a major reservoir. Up to 50% may be infected with *A. costaricensis*.

Human infections were first reported from Costa Rica. Since then, infections have been identified throughout the whole area between Mexico and Argentina. Children were predominantly found to be infected. One case of human infection was reported from Africa (Democratic Republic of Congo).

Transmission. Humans become infected by ingestion of infected paratenic or intermediate hosts. The complete spectrum of potential transmitters is unknown; however, it may correspond with that of *A. cantonensis* (see above). Direct uptake of infectious larvae is also possible, as they may egress from infected intermediate hosts (snails). Infective larvae were also found in mucous tracks of infected snails.

Ingested larvae invade the intestinal wall and develop in mesenteric lymph nodes and lymphatic vessels to preadult worms. They migrate to their final locus, the intestinal arteries and small blood vessels, where they arrive approximately 10 days p.i. The worms become sexually mature in humans (in rodents, maturity is reached 18 days after infection). Eggs released by the female worms accumulate in blood capillaries of the intestinal wall, where first-stage larvae develop. They hatch, migrate into the intestinal lumen, and are shed with the feces.

Clinical Manifestations. Parasites are found predominantly in the arteries of the appendix, the cecum, and the ascending colon, and more rarely in those of the ileum and other parts of the intestine. They induce granulomatous, eosinophilic, partly necrotic alterations, often >5 cm in size.

The disease resembles an "acute abdomen" with pains localized in the right hypogastrium, abdominal guarding, anorexia, vomitus, occasionally diarrhea, and more rarely constipation, with fever in most cases. Patients show leukocytosis and eosinophilia. Severity and course of the disease are proportional to the number of parasites. Deaths are not uncommon in heavy infections.

Diagnosis. Demonstration of the larvae in the feces (by the Baerman technique) may fail. In most cases, the infection is diagnosed by histopathological examination of tissue samples taken by biopsy or surgery. Granulomas may also be demonstrated by X-rays. Serological tests (in part commercially available kits) are used in areas of endemicity.

Differential Diagnosis. Appendicitis, enteral yersiniosis, and Crohn's disease must be excluded.

Therapy. Surgical resection of the pseudotumor is the method of choice. Also recommended is the application of mebendazole (200 to 400 mg three times a day orally for 10 days) or thiabendazole (75 mg/kg/day, divided in two doses for 3 days; maximum dose: 3 g/day). The effect is controversial.

Prophylaxis. Prophylactic measures are the same as those for cerebral angiostrongyliasis (see above).

REFERENCES

Eamsobhana P et al., Molecular differentiation and phylogenic relationships of three *Angiostrongylus* species and *Angiostrongylus cantonensis* geographical isolates based on a 66-kDa protein gene of *A. cantonensis* (Nematoda: Angiostrongylidae). *Exp. Parasitol.* 126, 564–569, 2010.

Graeff-Teixeira C, Expansion of *Achatina fulica* in Brasil and potential increased risk for angiostrongyliasis. *Trans. R. Soc. Trop. Med. Hyg.* 101, 743–744, 2007.

Graeff-Teixeira C et al., Longitudinal clinical and serological survey of abdominal angiostrongyliasis in Guaporé, southern Brazil, from 1955–1999. *Rev. Soc. Bras. Med. Trop.* 38, 310–315, 2005.

Mentz MB, Graeff-Teixeira C, Garrido CT, Treatment of mebendazole is not associated with distal migration of adult *Angiostrongylus costaricensis* in the murine experimental infection. *Rev. Inst. Med. Trop. Sao Paulo* 46, 73–75, 2004.

Miller CL et al., Endemic infections of *Parastrongylus* (=*Angiostrongylus*) *costaricensis* in two species of nonhuman primates, raccoons, and an opossum from Miami, Florida. *J. Parasitol* 92, 406–408, 2006.

Palominos PE et al., Individual serological follow-up, of patients with suspected or confirmed abdominal angiostrongyliasis. *Mem. Inst. Oswaldo Cruz* 103, 93–97, 2008.

Quirós JL et al., Abdominal angiostrongyliasis with involvement of liver histopathologically confirmed: a case report. *Rev. Inst. Med. Trop. Sao Paulo* 53, 219–222, 2011.

Rodriguez R et al., Abdominal angiostrongyliasis: report of two cases with different clinical presentations. *Rev. Inst. Med. Trop. Sao Paulo* 50, 539–541, 2008.

4.5.2 ANISAKIASIS (HERRING WORM DISEASE)

Herring worm disease is a fish zoonosis, caused by larvae of several nematode species, which in humans induce eosinophilic granulomas, several cm in size, or ulcers in the intestinal tract.

Etiology. The disease is caused by larvae of anisakids, a nematode family that is related to ascarids. The larvae invade the walls of the stomach or the small intestine and cause granulomas or ulcers. Allergic reactions are common and may be induced by the ingestion of killed larvae. Humans are accidental hosts, and the larvae do not develop further.

Anisakis spp. and *Pseudoterranova decipiens* (codworm) are the most important parasites.

Anisakis larvae have been categorized morphologically in two groupings, Type I and Type II. Genetic analyses attributed the species *A. simplex* s.s., *A. pegreffii, A. simplex C, A. typica, A. ziphidarum,* and *A. nascettii* to Group I. *A. physiterius, A. brevispiculata,* and *A. paggiae* belong to Type II. *A. pegreffii* is the major species in the Mediterranean Sea, and, together with *A. simplex* s.s., probably also in the North Pacific region. *Anisakis* larvae are in most cases 15 to 20 mm long, whitish parasites, whereas *Pseudoterranova* larvae are generally larger (20 to 40 mm in length), more burly, and red to brown in color. In addition, larvae of two other genera, *Contracaecum* and *Hysterothylacium,* are found.

Occurrence. The parasites are cosmopolitan. Cases of human anisakiasis are predominantly known from Japan, in Europe from Spain, France, the Netherlands, and Germany, and from North America. In several regions of Spain, for example, the seroprevalence amounts to 10%. However, in principle all continents are concerned, although only a few cases were observed in China and Taiwan. Infections with *Pseudoterranova* spp. are generally limited to the northern Pacific area. The regional accumulation of infections may depend on regional eating habits.

Transmission. Final hosts of *Anisakis* spp. are predominantly whales and dolphins, as well as several species of seals; adult *Pseudoterranova* spp. are found exclusively in seals. Parasites live in the stomach of the animals, and their eggs are shed with the feces (life cycle see Fig. 4.43). The (probably) third larval stage develops in the egg, hatches and it must be ingested by small saltwater crustaceans (Amphipoda, Decapoda, or Euphausiacea). The infected crustaceans become ingested by fish and squids that serve as paratenic hosts (they are useful in the cycle but not essential). Additional accumulation of infective larvae may occur in predatory fish that ingest infected fish. Final hosts are usually infected by ingestion of infected paratenic hosts.

Humans are infected by ingestions of raw or undercooked saltwater fish and squid (Fig. 4.43) that contain the parasites in their body cavities, the muscles, or other tissues. The list of potential transmitters is large (>160 species are known in Japan) and include many fish commonly eaten by humans, such as herring, mackerel, cod, and flounder. Prevalence in such

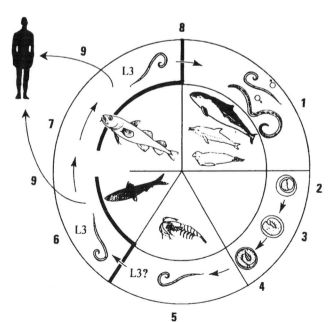

Figure 4.43 | Developmental cycle of marine anisakids. (1) Adult anisakids in the gastrointestinal tract of marine mammals produce eggs; (2) eggs excreted with feces; (3 and 4) development of first- and second-stage larvae (L1 and L2) in floating eggs, which are ingested by copepods (intermediate hosts); (5) development of third-stage larva (L3) in copepods; (6) ingestion of infected copepods by saltwater fishes (numerous species) and encapsulation of third-stage larvae in various organs (fishes serve as paratenic hosts, i.e., larvae do not develop further); (7) ingestion of infected fishes by predatory fishes may lead to accumulation of infective larvae in these fishes; (8 and 9) final hosts (8) and humans (9) are infected by ingestion of infected fishes.

fishes may be 100%, accompanied with high intensities (older fish may contain several hundreds of larvae). In addition, fish grown in aquaculture may be infested. Locally, particular fish may be of special importance, depending in local eating habits [e.g., in Western Europe the herring ("white herring") or anchovy in Spain, several fish species in "ceviche" in South America, or "Sushi" in Japan].

In humans, the larvae invade the wall of the intestinal tract (oesophagus down to the rectum; *Pseudoterranova* spp. favor the stomach wall). If at all, a fourth stage larva develops in humans.

Clinical Manifestations. In principal, two different clinical manifestations have to be considered in human anisakiasis: the tissue reaction to invading larvae and hypersensitivity reactions to larval allergens.

The incubation period lasts from a few hours up to several days. Patients display severe epigastric pains, nausea, and vomiting. Blood is often seen in the gastric juice or in the feces due to ulcerative lesions in the mucosa. Invasion of the small intestine may cause stenosis leading to ileus early in the course of infection by marked edema and later by granulomatous reactions. Intestinal perforation may occur. Egression of the larvae into extragastrointestinal tissue is observed. Usually single, very rarely many larvae are observed, but the number of larvae does not necessarily determine the clinical picture. Superinfections may enhance the tissue reactions. Patients are usually afebrile and they often show leukocytosis; eosinophilia is not a common sign.

Anisakiasis is usually a self-limiting disease as the larvae survive hardly longer than 1 week. Symptoms in general cease after 1 week, although the degenerative and later regenerative alterations may persist for a longer period.

Infections with anisakids induce allergic sensitization. Immediate-type hypersensitivity reactions with pruritus and urticaria up to generalized anaphylaxis may occur in sensitized patients hours after ingestion of fish and independent of gastrointestinal symptoms. Usually reactions pass within 24 h. They can also be induced by dead larvae, for example, in frozen or cooked fish (several thermostable allergens have been described in *A. simplex*). Allergic reactions have even been triggered by meat of chicken fed with fishmeal.

Diagnosis. The history has to consider recent ingestion of saltwater fish. Presumptive diagnosis should be verified by endoscopic demonstration of the larvae or the examination of biopsy specimens, the latter particularly to discriminate from malign tumors. Laboratory analyses and imaging techniques can only show the alterations without specifying them. Serology (ELISA, immunoblotting) is a helpful tool in chronic cases. Purified or recombinant secretory-excretory antigens (e.g., the allergen Ani s 7) give reliable results.

Hypersensitivity reactions may be specified retrospectively by demonstration of specific IgE antibodies in a 4-week time course.

Differential Diagnosis. Food poisoning, acute appendicitis, tumors, and ulcers due to other causes, Crohn's disease, eosinophilic enteritis, and infections with *Gongylonema* spp. must be excluded in the differential diagnosis. Infections with *A. costaricensis* (see chapter 4.5.1.2) should be considered in Central and South America.

Therapy. The extraction of the larvae under endoscopic control is recommended. Albendazole has been shown to be effective. When considering surgery, one should keep in mind that symptoms usually improve spontaneously within 1 week. In case of severe anaphylactic reactions, shock therapy may be required.

Prophylaxis. Fresh raw saltwater fish should not be consumed. When fish is cooked, a core temperature of 60 °C should be guaranteed. Larvae in frozen fish are killed if a core temperature of −20 °C persists for at least 24 h. Smoking and marinating does not kill anisakid larvae with any degree of certainty. Also, in the case of pickling, salt concentrations and storing times are often insufficient to kill the larvae. In the European Union, a fish hygiene edict defines particular prophylactic measures. However, it should not be overlooked that anaphylactic reactions in sensitized persons may be induced also by killed larvae. Hygiene measures of the fish industries (transillumination of freshly caught fish already on the trawlers at sea) are suitable to reduce the contamination rate of marketed saltwater fish in general

REFERENCES

Anadón AM et al., The *Anisakis simplex* Ani s 7 major allergen as an indicator of true Anisakis infections. *Clin. Exp. Immunol.* 156, 471–478, 2009.

Arai T et al., Molecular and epidemiological data on *Anisakis* spp. (Nematoda: Anisakidae) in commercial fish caught of northern Sardinia (western Mediterranian Sea). *Vet. Parasitol.* 199, 59–72, 2014.

Armantia A et al., *Anisakis* allergy after eating chicken meat. *J. Investig. Allergol. Clin. Immunol.* 16, 258–263, 2006.

Audicana MT, Kennedy MW, *Anisakis simplex*: from obscure infectious worm to inducer of immune hypersensitivity. *Clin. Microbiol. Rev.* 21, 360–379, 2008.

Choi SJ et al., The clinical characteristics of Anisakiasis allergy in Korea. *Korean J. Intren. Med.* 24, 160–163, 2009.

Daschner A et al., Gastroallergic anisakiasis: borderline between food allergy and parasitic disease – clinical and allergologic evaluation of 20 patients with confirmed acute parasitism by *Anisakis simplex*. *J. Allergy Clin. Immunol.* 105, 176–181, 2000.

Daschner A, Pascual CY, *Anisakis simplex*: sensitization and clinical allergy. *Curr. Opin. Allergy Clin. Immunol.* 5, 281–285, 2005.

Gonzalez-Muboz M, Rodriguez-Mahillo AI, Moneo I, Different Th1/Th2 responses to *Anisakis simplex* are related to distinct clinical manifestations in sensitized patient. *Parasite Immunol.* 32, 67–73, 2010.

Mattinci S et al., Anisakiasis and gastroallergic reactions associated with *Anisakis pegreffii* infection, Italy. *Emerg. Inf. Dis.* 19, 64–69, 2013.

Pravettoni V, Primavesi L, Piantamida M, *Anisakis simplex*: current knowledge. *Eur. Ann. Allergy Clin. Immunol.* 44, 150–156, 2012.

Rello FJ et al., The fishing area as a possible indicator of the infection by anisakids in anchovies (*Engraulis encrasicolus*) from southwestern Europe. *Int. J. Food Microbiol.* 129, 277–281, 2009.

Rodriguez-Mahillo AI et al., Quantification of Anisakis simplex allergens in fresh, long-term frozen, and cooked fish muscle. *Foodborne Pathog. Dis.* 7, 967–973, 2010.

Shibata E et al., CT findings of gastric and intestinal anisakiasis. *Abdom. Imaging* 39, 257–61, 2014.

Shih HH, Ku CC, Wang CS, *Anisakis simplex* (Nematoda: Anisakidae) third-stage larval infections in marine cage cultured cobia, *Rachycentron canadum* L., in Taiwan. *Vet. Parasitol.* 171, 277–285, 2010.

Suzuki J et al., Risk factors for human Anisakis infection and association between the geographic origins of *Scomber japonicus* and anisakid nematodes. *Int. J. Food. Microbiol.* 137, 88–93, 2010.

Vidacek S et al., Antigenicity and viability of *Anisakis* larvae infesting hake heated at different time-temperature conditions. *J. Food. Prot.* 73, 662–68, 2010.

4.5.3 CAPILLARIASES

4.5.3.1 Hepatic Capillariasis

Hepatic capillariasis is a rare disease caused by liver-specific roundworms. In heavy infections, severe consequences may occur.

Etiology. The agent is *Capillaria hepatica* (syn. *Calodium hepaticum*); a hair-thin nematode that reaches a length of up to 10 cm and specifically invades the liver parenchyma.

Occurrence. Rodents, predominantly rats, are the principal hosts of this cosmopolitan parasite. The prevalence in rat populations can be >80%. Human infections are rare. Altogether, approximately 70 proven cases from North and South America, Africa, Asia and Central Europe have been registered; in reality, however, the infection rate may be higher.

Transmission. Humans become infected by the accidental ingestion of embryonated eggs (eggs containing infective larvae) from the soil.

C. hepatica is a liver-dwelling parasite. Migrating through the hepatic parenchyma, the female parasites deposit typical thick-shelled eggs with a transparent plug at either pole in the locomotion trails. The eggs are enclosed by a tubular granuloma that is replaced by connective tissue. They are set free after the death of the host by decomposition or by a predator; in rats, cannibalism also plays a role. Free eggs in the environment need weeks to embryonate and become infective but persist for >1 year in the soil. After accidental oral ingestion, the larva hatches in the intestine, invades the intestinal wall, and reaches the liver via the portal system. The first eggs are produced 3 to 4 weeks after infection.

Clinical Manifestations. The clinical picture depends on the intensity of infection. Light infections, occasionally observed in post mortem examinations, are apparently asymptomatic.

Heavy infections may cause acute symptoms due to extended liver cell damage and hepatitis. Extrahepatic symptoms, for example, disease of the lungs, have been reported but are pathogenetically unclear. Heavy infections may cause death in children. Moderate infections are accompanied by uncharacteristic epigastric complaints, hepatosplenomegaly, leukocytosis, eosinophilia, and hypergammaglobulinemia.

Diagnosis. Encapsulated worms and eggs are often localized under the liver capsule and may be found by laparoscopy. Diagnosis can be confirmed by liver biopsy and demonstration of the typical eggs with a size of 30 by 50 μm. Reliable serologic assays are not available.

Differential Diagnosis. Focal or disseminated damage of the liver parenchyma due to viral or toxic etiology should be considered.

Therapy. Mebendazole and albendazole have been shown to be effective in experimental rodent infections.

Prophylaxis. Avoid potentially contaminated food and keep children away from areas where rats occur. In geographical regions, such as Central Africa, where rodents (*Cricetomys* spp. and others) are consumed by humans, the livers of these animals should be destroyed and contaminated kitchen utensils must be carefully cleaned.

REFERENCES

Camargo LM et al., Capillariasis (Trichurida, Trichinellidae, *Capillaria hepatica*) in the Brazilian Amazone: low pathogenicity, low infectivity and a novel mode of transmission. *Parasit. Vectors* 2, 3–17, 2010.

Klenzak J et al., Hepatic capillariasis in Maine presenting as a hepatic mass. *Am. J. Trop. Med. Hyg.* 72, 651–653, 2005.

Li CD, Yang HL, Wang Y, *Capillaria hepatica* in China. *World J. Gastroenterol.* 16, 698–702, 2010.

Nabi F et al., *Capillaria hepatica* infestation. *Indian Pediatr.* 44, 781–782, 2007.

Pereira VG, Mattosinho Franca LC, Successful treatment of *Capillaria hepatica* infection in an acutely ill adult. *Am. J. Trop. Med. Hyg.* 32, 1272–1274, 1983.

Sawamura R et al., Hepatic capillariasis in children: report of three cases in Brazil. *Am. J. Trop. Med. Hyg.* 61, 642–647, 1999.

Scandola P et al., Prevalence of *Capillaria hepatica* in noncommensal rodents from a forest area near Dijon, France. *Parasitol. Res.* 112, 2741–2744, 2013.

Tesana S, Puapairoj A, Saeseow O, Granulomatous, hepatolithiasis and hepatomegaly caused by *Capillaria hepatica* infection: first case report of Thailand. *Southeast Asian J. Trop. Med. Public Health* 38, 636–640, 2007.

4.5.3.2 Intestinal Capillariasis

Intestinal capillariasis is a severe disease, often lethal in untreated cases, which was first observed in 1963. It occurs often endemically and it is caused by the nematode *Capillaria philippinensis*.

Etiology. *Capillaria philippinensis* is a small (length: males, 3 mm; females, 4 mm) nematode that predominantly settles in the small intestine.

Occurrence. Its occurrence initially seemed to be limited to the Philippines; however, the parasite is obviously present in many regions of Southeast Asia and the Western Pacific area. Infections have also been observed sporadically in Iran, Egypt, India, and South America. Piscivorous birds are reported to be the natural (reservoir) hosts.

Transmission. Humans are infected by the ingestion of raw or undercooked freshwater or brackish-water fish that contain infective larvae in their intestine. The whole spectrum of potential transmitters (intermediate hosts and paratenic hosts?) is not known. The life cycle of *C. philippinensis* is unusual. Direct development, that is, infection by ingestion of embryonated eggs, is apparently not possible. However, obviously autoinfections occur, as in addition to females that produce thick-shelled eggs, larviparous females are found, with the larvae leading to autoinfection. These seem to be a substantial part of the life cycle in humans that is responsible for the sometimes extremely high worm counts in patients.

Clinical Manifestations. Symptoms are variable. Presumably, by autoinfection severe disease may develop in patients, who although infected, had remained asymptomatic for months. Patients with slight cases of disease show abdominal pain, anorexia, and occasionally, diarrhea and weakness; severe infections result in vomiting, weight loss, malabsorption, diarrhea with electrolyte and protein imbalance (edemas), muscle wasting, abdominal distension, and pneumonia. Postmortem examinations of patients with fulminant disease revealed as many as 100 000 larvae and adults of *C. philippinensis* in the lumen, walls, and glands of the intestine.

Diagnosis. Bipolar, thick-shelled eggs are detected by fecal examination. They can be discriminated from *Trichuris* eggs by their cask-like shape. Besides these eggs, thin-shelled eggs, larvae, and adult parasites may be found in the feces.

Differential Diagnosis. Infections with other pathogens causing diarrhea and malabsorption should be considered.

Therapy. Mebendazole (200 mg twice a day orally for 20 days) or albendazole (200 mg twice a day orally for 10 days) are effective therapies. Relapses may occur.

Prophylaxis. Raw or undercooked fish or crustaceans should not be consumed in areas of endemicity.

REFERENCES

Ahmed L et al., *Capillaria philippinensis*: an emerging parasite causing severe diarrhoea in Egypt. *J. Egypt. Soc. Parasitol.* 29, 483–493, 1999.

Attia R A et al., *Capillaria philippinensis* in Upper Egypt: has it become endemic? *Am. J. Trop. Med. Hyg.* 86, 126–133, 2012.

Bair MJ et al., Clinical features of human intestinal capillariasis in Taiwan. *World J. Gastroenterol.* 10, 2391–2393, 2004.

Cross JH, Intestinal capillariasis. *Clin. Microbiol. Rev.* 5 120–129, 1992.

Cross JH, Basaca-Sevilla V, Experimental transmission of *Capillaria philippinensis* to birds. *Trans. R. Soc. Trop. Med. Hyg.* 77 511–514, 1983.

Jung WT et al., An indigenous case of intestinal capillariasis with protein-losing enteropathy in Korea. *Korean J. Parasitol.* 50, 333–337, 2012.

El-Dib NA et al., Evaluation of *Capillaria philippinensis* coproantigen in the diagnosis of infection. *J. Egypt. Soc. Parasitol.* 34, 97–106, 2004.

El-Karaksy H et al., *Capillaria philippinensis*: a cause of fatal diarrhea in one of two infected Egyptian sisters. *J. Trop. Pediatr.* 50, 57–60, 2004.

Fan Z et al., Serious diarrhea with weight loss, caused by *Capillaria philippinensis* acquired in China: a case report. *BMC Res. Notes* 5, 554, 2012.

Jung, W T et al., An indigenous case of intestinal capillariasis with protein-losing enteropathy in Korea. *Korean J. Parasitol.* 50, 333–337, 2012.

Lu LH et al., Human intestinal capillariasis (*Capillaria philippinnensis*) in Taiwan. *Am. J. Trop. Med. Hyg.* 74, 810–813, 2006.

Saichua P, Nithikathkul C, Kaewpitoon N, Human intestinal capillariasis in Thailand. *World J. Gastroenterol.* 28, 506–510, 2008.

4.5.3.3 Pulmonary Capillariasis

Pulmonary capillariasis is a rare human disease (<20 reported cases) due to infection of the lung by the lung hairworm.

Etiology. The parasite is *Capillaria aerophila* (syn. *Eucoleus aerophilus*), a nematode 15 mm (males) or 20 mm (females) in length, which parasitizes the trachea and the bronchi.

Occurrence. *C. aerophila* is a cosmopolitan parasite of dogs and cats, wild and farmed fur-bearing predaceous animals, hedgehogs, and opossums.

Transmission. Humans become infected by oral ingestion of embryonated eggs of *C. aerophila*. Eggs are deposited in the bronchi by the female worms and are brought up by the ciliated epithelium or by coughing and are swallowed and excreted with the feces. Infective larvae develop within the eggs in the environment. After ingestion, the larva hatches, invades the intestinal wall, migrates via lymph and blood vessels in 7 to 10 days into the lung, and settles in the trachea or the bronchi. The prepatent period ends 6 weeks after infection in the case of carnivorous animals.

Clinical Manifestations. Infection is followed by bronchitis, coughing, production of bloody sputum, and dyspnea.

Diagnosis. Diagnosis is confirmed by the demonstration of the brownish, thick-shelled eggs with a plug on either pole in the feces. Lung biopsies may show granulomas with worm sections and eggs.

Differential Diagnosis. Bronchitis due to other etiology and infection with lung flukes must be considered.

Therapy. Thiabendazole (25 mg/kg/day orally for 3 days) is effective therapy. Experimental data also suggest the efficacy of mebendazole and albendazole.

Prophylaxis. Eggs of *C. aerophila* are found in and on the soil. Food polluted with soil should be washed. Children should be kept away from areas polluted with animal feces.

REFERENCES

Lalosevic D et al., Pulmonary capillariasis miming bronchial carcinoma. *Am. J. Trop. Med. Hyg.* 78, 14–16, 2008.

Traversa D et al., Infection by *Eucoleus aerophilus* in dogs and cats: is another extraintestinal parasitic nematode of pets emerging in Italy? *Res. Vet. Sci.* 87 270–272, 2009.

Traversa D, Di Cesare A, Conboy G, Canine and feline cardiopulmonary parasitic nematodes in Europe: emerging and underestimated. *Parasite Vectors* 3, 62, 2010.

Villela JM, Desmaret MC, Rouault R, Capillariose à *Capillaria aerophila* chez un adulte? *Méd. Malad. Infect.* 1, 35–36, 1986.

4.5.4 DIOCTOPHYMIASIS

Dioctophymiasis is a renal disease due to infection with the giant kidney worm.

Etiology. The agent, *Dioctophyma renale*, is a nematode that belongs to the order Enoplida and may reach lengths of 45 cm (males) and 100 cm (females).

Occurrence. *D. renale* parasitization occurs in mustelids, dogs, foxes, raccoons, cats, and pigs. It is found in North and South America, Asia, and Europe. Human infections are rare (~20 cases).

Transmission. Eggs of *D. renale* are shed with the urine and have to be passed into surface water. In a matter of months, the first stage larva develops in the egg, which is ingested by aquatic oligochaetes [annelid worms (*Lumbriculus variegates*)], as intermediate hosts. Infection of final hosts occurs by oral ingestion of infected intermediate or paratenic (frogs and fishes) hosts

that feed on these worms. In the final mammalian host, the parasites migrate via the peritoneal cavity to the kidneys where they settle in the parenchyma or in the renal pelvis. In mustelids, the prepatent period lasts for 5 months.

Clinical Manifestations. The infection may be inapparent. Otherwise, renal colic and hematuria are observed. Ureteral obstruction may cause hydronephrosis. Aberrant (subcutaneous) localization was reported.

Diagnosis. Diagnosis is made by the clinical picture and is proved by the demonstration of the eggs (40 by 70 µm, brown, with two polar plugs) in the urine.

Differential Diagnosis. Hydronephrosis, renal colics, and hematuria due to other causes must be considered.

Therapy. Surgical excision of the worms is the therapy of choice.

Prophylaxis. Raw or undercooked frogs or fish should not be consumed in areas of endemicity. Surface water should be boiled or filtered before drinking.

REFERENCES

Katafogoitis I et al., A rare case of a 39 year old male with a parasite called *Dioctophyma renale* mimicking renal cancer at the computed tomography of the right kidney. A case report. *Parasitol. Int.* 62, 459–460, 2013.

Li G et al., Fatal bilateral dioctophymatosis. *J. Parasitol.* 96, 1152–1154, 2010.

Narváez JA, Turell LP, Serra J, Hyperdense renal cystic lesions caused by *Dioctophyma renale*. *Am. J. Roentgenol.* 163, 997–998, 2010.

Vladimova MG et al., [A case of dioctophymosis (*Dioctophyma renale*) in a girl from Arkhangelsk] (Russian). *Med. Parazitol. (Mosk)* 4, 48–50, 2002.

4.5.5 DRACUNCULIASIS (GUINEA WORM INFECTION)

Dracunculiasis is characterized by inflammation and cutaneous ulcers in the distal limbs due to the guinea worm in the subcutaneous tissue.

Etiology. The agent, *Dracunculus medinensis* (the guinea worm), is a nematode that reaches lengths of 4 cm (males) or 120 cm (females).

Occurrence. Until recently, dracunculiasis was one of the most widespread diseases on the planet and afflicted many millions of people in the arid zones of Asia and Africa. The situation has changed remarkably, since the WHO started an eradication program in 1986. Control measures resulted in a convincing decrease of reported cases to approximately 79 000 cases in 1998 and 3185 cases in 2009. The disease is still currently observed in four countries (Chad, South Sudan, Mali, and Ethiopia). A total of 542 cases (96.1% of them in South Sudan) were reported worldwide in 2012.

Previous suggestions considered dogs as the major reservoir for human infections. This was disputed in recent years, when the zoonotic character of dracunculiasis was doubted. Recent epidemiological and genetic studies in Mali, however, seem to confirm the earlier opinion.

Transmission. Infection occurs by oral accidental ingestion of *Cyclops* spp., small crustaceans, who serve as intermediate hosts and may be swallowed in drinking water.

The larviparous adult females live in the connective tissue of the distal parts of the limbs, mainly the legs and feet. They induce a blister that opens under water, allowing the release of large numbers of larvae into the water. The larvae must be ingested by *Cyclops* within 6 days and develop to infective stages. When infected, *Cyclops* are swallowed by definite hosts, the larvae penetrate the intestinal wall and migrate to the subcutaneous and retroperitoneal tissue where they become sexually mature and copulate. The males die, whereas the females migrate to the subcutaneous tissue of the distal limbs and induce the blisters in the skin 10 to 12 months p.i.

Clinical Manifestations. The infection is asymptomatic until the female worms reach their final destination in the skin after 10 to 12 months. Patients complain of local pains and impaired general condition, pruritus, fever,

and nausea before a papule, and subsequently, a blister, develops. The blister reaches a size of up to 2 cm, ruptures when exposed to water, and forms a painful ulcer. The worm discharges a milky larva-rich fluid intermittently on exposure to water. The lesions persist for about 4 weeks. The adult worm becomes resorbed or rejected but may also be encapsulated and calcified. If the skin is not perforated, extended sterile abscesses may develop.

Secondary infections are common, particularly if attempts to extract the parasite fail because the worm disrupts and remnants stay in the subcutaneous tissue. Severe complications may develop in these cases.

The disease occurs seasonally, that is, only during the raining season.

Diagnosis. Clinical diagnosis is made after penetration of the skin. If the worm is invisible, sprinkling the ulcer with cold water may cause the emergence of the 550 to 750 μm long larvae, which can be microscopically detected.

The worm is sometimes palpable in the subcutaneous tissue 2 months before penetration. Calcified parasites are detected by X-rays.

Differential Diagnosis. The diagnosis is undoubted after penetration of the skin, but occasionally maggots of flies (myiasis) are misidentified as guinea worms.

Therapy. The common treatment is the careful extraction of the parasite after the release of most of the larvae after stimulation by repeated wetting. The anterior end of the worm (the end visible in the ulcus) is coiled around a small stick, and the parasite is extruded by continuous turning. One or two weeks are needed for complete removal. Care must be taken to avoid the rupture of the worm, as the remaining part of the worm may cause severe inflammation. These may also happen after killing the worm with mebendazole (400 to 800 mg/d orally for 6 days).

Metronidazole (20 mg three times a day orally) or niridazole (12.5 mg/kg/day orally for 10 days) usually does not kill the worm but facilitates extrusion. Analgetics and conventional wound care are recommended. The surgical excision of the worm under local anesthesia is also practiced.

Prophylaxis. Drinking water in areas of endemicity should be boiled or filtered. These measures almost completely prevent infections in areas of endemicity within a few years. Water supplies are treated with the chemical temephos (1 ppm) every 4 or 6 weeks during the rainy season.

REFERENCES

Anonym, Progress toward global eradication of dracunculiasis, January 2009 – June 2010. *MMWR Morb. Motal. Wkly. Rep.* 59, 1239–1242, 2010.

Bimi L et al., Differentiating *Dracunculus medinensis* from *D. insignis*, by the sequence analysis of the 18S rRNA gene. *Ann. Trop. Med. Parasitol.* 99, 511–517, 2005.

Cairncross S, Tayeh A, Korkor AS, Why is dracunculiasis eradication taking so long?. *Trends Parasitol.* 28, 25–230, 2012.

CDC, Progress toward global eradication of dracunculiasis – January 2012 – June 2013. *MMWR Morb. Mortal. Wkly. Rep.* 62, 829–833, 2013.

Eberhard ML, Ruiz-Thiben E, Hopkins DR, The peculiar epidemiology of dracunculiasis in Chad. *Am. J. Trop. Med. Hyg.* 90, 61–70, 2014.

Enserink M, Infectious diseases. Guinea worm eradication at risk in south Sudanese war. *Science* 343, (6168), 236, 2014.

Hours M, Cairncross S, Long-term disability due to guinea worm disease. *Trans. R. Soc. Trop. Med. Hyg.* 88, 559–560, 1994.

Kaul SM et al., Outbrake of drancontiasis in the Bhiwandi town of Maharashtra: a report. *J. Commun. Dis.* 23, 22–28, 1992.

Muller R, Guinea worm disease – the final chapter? *Trends Parasitol.* 21, 521–524, 2005.

Sankar V et al., Dracunculiasis in a South Indian Bonnet monkey. *Primates* 41, 89–92, 2000.

4.5.6 EOSINOPHILIC ENTERITIS

Eosinophilic enteritis is a rare obstructive intestinal disease in humans and animals with massive, mainly focal eosinophilic infiltrations. In humans, it became associated with atopic disturbances and food allergies but it is mostly categorized as an idiopathic disease. It is, however, at least in one type of manifestation, the consequence of hypersensitivity reactions to *Ancylostoma caninum*, a dog hookworm.

Etiology. The etiology of this particular type of disease was clarified only 20 years ago. It is caused by the common dog hookworm *Ancylostoma caninum*, which may be found in the gut of the patient. The worms are always few in number, small in size (length up to 8 mm), and mature but infertile.

Occurrence. *A. caninum* is common in all tropical and subtropical regions but is also found in areas with a temperate climate. Predominantly young dogs show patent infections. Human infections, except a few cases elsewhere, are limited to northeastern Australia, where several hundred cases were reported.

Transmission. Infected dogs shed eggs in feces. Infective, third stage larvae hatch from the eggs dependent on the environmental temperature after 1 to 2 weeks. In humans, the disease probably only emerges after oral ingestion of infective larvae, that is, not after infection on the percutaneous route, which prevails in *A. caninum* transmission and may result in Larva Migrans Cutanea (see chapter 4.5.11). Oral infection in dogs results in a temporary stay of the larvae in the intestinal wall, shortened development, and in an abbreviated prepatent period of 5 to 10 days (after percutaneous invasion the larvae take a more complicated migration route via heart and lungs and reach sexual maturity after 2 to 3 weeks).

Clinical Manifestations. Most human infections may take a clinically inapparent course. Clinical manifestations are due to an intense focal response to the worm, inducing local inflammation, ulcerations, and strictures in the distal ileum up to a length of 1 m. Patients suffer from recurrent epigastric colic, nausea, vomiting, and diarrhea. In severe cases, the clinical picture resembles an acute abdomen. Leukocytosis, eosinophilia, increased IgE levels, and antibodies against hookworm antigens are found in most patients. X-ray examinations show intestinal strictures and thickened intestinal walls. The reasons for the different clinical pictures are not understood. Previously, it was assumed that the disease develops preferentially after continuous exposure and infection. Experimental studies in humans, however, revealed that even a single oral infection might be sufficient to induce eosinophilic enteritis.

Diagnosis. Diagnosis is difficult and is based on the clinical picture. It may be supported by the demonstration of antibodies (ELISA, immunoblotting) to secretory-excretory antigens of *A. caninum*, although antibody levels and severity of the disease are not correlated in all cases. An important hint is a rapid clinical improvement (within 24 h) after anthelmintic treatment.

Differential Diagnosis. Appendicitis and Crohn's disease must be considered.

Therapy. Treatment uses mebendazole, 100 mg twice a day orally for 3 days or a single, oral dose of 400 mg albendazole.

Prophylaxis. Strict hygiene; avoid grounds polluted with dog feces. Dogs should be anthelmintically treated.

REFERENCES

Alamo Martinez JM et al., Intestinal obstruction by eosinophilic jejunitis. *Rev. Esp. Enferm. Dig.* 96, 279–283, 2004.

Bowman DD et al., Hookworms of dogs and cats as agents of cutaneous larva migrans. *Trends Parasitol.* 26, 162–167, 2010.

Landman JK, Prociv P, Experimental human infection with the dog hookworm. *Ancylostoma caninum. Med. J. Aust.* 20, 69–71, 2003.

Martinez-Ubieto F et al., [Acute abdomen caused by eosinophilic enteritis: six observations]. (Spanish). *Cir. Cir.* 81, 237–241, 2013.

4.5.7 FILARIASES

Filariasis is caused by infections with nematodes of the superfamily Filarioidea. All filarial species are viviparous, that is, female parasites release larvae (microfilariae) that circulate in the blood or are skin dwelling. They are transmitted by particular blood-sucking arthropods that ingest the microfilariae during the blood meal. After maturing to third-stage (metacyclic) larvae, they are transmitted to new hosts in the course of a further bloodmeal.

Apart from a few species, filariae contain intracellular bacteria of the genus *Wolbachia*, which are also common in arthropods. *Wolbachia* are passed vertically by the filariae and are regarded as endosymbionts, although the exact mutual reactions with the filariae are not clearly determined. Effects on the reproduction and on molting processes of the filariae are discussed. *Wolbachia* are susceptible to tetracycline. This observation opened new ways of therapy of filarial infections, for example, by the therapeutic application of doxycycline. Predominantly, infections with *Brugia malayi, B. timori. Dirofilaria immitis*, and several other *Dirofilaria* spp. are regarded as zoonoses.

Other animal-specific filariae are only rarely observed in humans. Thus, infections were detected (<20 cases worldwide) in Europe and North America by the species *Onchocerca lienalis* and *O. gutturosa* (filariae of ruminants). In Japan by *O. dewittei* (found in wild boars), in Europe by a taxonomically yet unidentified species (possibly *O. lupi* from dogs: the parasite is found in approximately 8% of the dogs in Portugal and Spain), and *O. yakutensis* (from red deer). The parasites inhabit painless, subcutaneous, or in case of *O. lupi*, subconjunctival knots. They are transmitted by Simuliidae (black flies).

In addition, infections with animal-specific *Brugia* spp. are rare in humans, irrespective of *B. malayi* and *B. timori*. These parasites have frequently not been properly identified. Most cases were reported from the northeastern US. The following species have to be considered: in North America, *B. beaveri*, a parasite of raccoons and bobcats, possibly also *B. lepori* (from rabbits), and in South America *B. guyanensis* (occurring in coatis and grisons (*Galictis* sp.), animals related to polecats. In Sri Lanka, human infections were reported with *B. ceylonensis* from dogs. Recently, human infections with *B. pahangi* from cats were described in Malaysia. Furthermore, etiologically unclear *Brugia* spp. have been found in humans in Africa. *Brugia* spp. are transmitted by mosquitoes and they inhabit lymph nodes and lymph vessels, predominantly in the groin and neck region, leading to painless swellings that usually contain only one immature worm.

In Central Africa, *Meningonema peruzzii* was occasionally found in the human subarachnoid space. The same localization is inhabited by the parasite in monkeys. Occasionally, worms were observed in the human ocular chamber, which were identified as *Molina (Dipetalonema) sprenti* (from beavers), *M. arbuta* (from porcupines), and *Pelecitus* sp. from birds.

Other filarial parasites, such as *Onchocerca volvulus, Wuchereria bancrofti, Dipetalonema perstans, D. streptocerca,* and *Mansonella ozzardi,* are human parasites for which primates may act, at most and without any epidemiologic role, as reservoir hosts. In the case of *Loa loa,* two strains are believed to exist in humans and in primates. They may be transmitted from nonhuman primates to humans and vice versa, but this is prevented under natural conditions by ecological differences between the particular intermediate hosts, two different *Chrysops* spp.

The etiology in cases of "tropical eosinophilia"—a chronic disease with eosinophilic granulomas and infiltrations in the lungs, which, according to serologic data, is related to filarial infections—is unsolved. It either may be caused by animal-specific filariae or it represents a particular type of reaction to infections with *Brugia* spp. or *W. bancrofti.* The geographical distributions of the latter parasites correspond with the occurrence of the disease.

REFERENCES

Bain O et al., Human intraocular filariasis caused by *Pelecitus* sp. nematode, Brazil. *Emerg. Infect. Dis.* 17, 867–869, 2011.

Dissanaike AS et al., Recovery of a species of *Brugia*, probably *B. ceylonensis*, from the conjunctiva of a patient in Sri Lanka. *Ann. Trop. Med. Parasitol.* 94, 83–86, 2000.

Eberhard ML et al., Zoonotic *Onchocerca lupi* infection in a 22-month-old child in Arizona: first report in the United States and review of the literature. *Am. J. Trop. Med. Hyg.* 88, 601–605, 2013.

Hira PR et al., Zoonotic filariasis in the Arabian Peninsula: autochthonous onchocerciasis and dirofilariasis. *Am. J. Trop. Med. Hyg.* 79, 739–741, 2008.

Hoerauf A et al., Filariasis: new drugs and new opportunities for lymphatic filariasis and onchocerciasis. *Curr. Opin. Infect. Dis.* 21, 673–681, 2008.

Koehsler M et al., *Onchocerca jakutensis* filariasis in humans. *Emerg. Infect. Dis.* 13, 1749–1752, 2007.

Ngure RM et al., Biochemical changes in cerebrospinal fluid of *Chlorocebus aethiops* naturally infected with zoonotic *Meningonema peruzzii. J. Med. Primatol* 37, 210–214, 2008.

Pampiglione S et al., Subconjunctival zoonotic *Onchocerca* in an Albanian man. *Ann. Trop. Med. Parasitol.* 95, 827–832, 2001.

Paniz-Mondolfi AE et al., Zoonotic filariasis caused by novel *Brugia* sp. nematode, United States, 2011 [letter]. *Emerg. Infect. Dis.* 20, [Internet] 2014 Jul [date cited], 2014.

Sallo F et al., Zoonotic intravitreal *Onchocerca* in Hungary. *Ophthalmology* 11, 502–504, 2005.

Schlesinger JJ, Dubois JG, Beaver PC, *Brugia*-like filarial infections acquired in the United States. *Am. J. Trop. Med. Hyg.* 26, 204–207, 1977.

Sréter T, Széll Z, Onchocerciasis. A newly recognized disease in dogs. *Vet. Parasitol.* 151, 1–13, 2008.

Sréter T et al., Subconjunctival zoonotic onchocerciasis in man: aberrant infection with *Onchocerca lupi? Trop. Med. Parasitol.* 96, 497–502, 2002.

Takaoka H et al., An *Onchocerca* species of wild boar found in the subcutaneous nodule of a resident of Oita, Japan. *Parasitol. Int.* 54, 91–93, 2005.

Takaoka H et al., Human infection with *Onchocerca dewittei japonica*, a parasite from wild boar in Oita, Japan. *Parasite* 8, 261–263, 2001.

Tan LH et al., Zoonotic *Brugia pahangi* filariasis in a suburbia of Kuala Lumpur City, Malaysia. *Parasitol. Int.* 60, 111–113, 2011.

Uni S et al., Zoonotic filariasis caused by *Onchocerca dewittei japonica* in a resident of Hiroshima, Honshu, Japan. *Parasitol. Int.* 59, 477–480, 2010.

Vijayan VK, Tropical pulmonary eosinophilia: pathogenesis, diagnosis and management. *Curr. Opin. Pulm. Med.* 13, 428–433, 2007.

4.5.7.1 *Brugia Filariasis (Lymphatic Filariasis)*

Brugia filariasis is often asymptomatic but may also be associated with severe, obstructive alterations of the lymphatic system and elephantiasis.

Etiology. The agents of lymphatic filariasis are *Wuchereria bancrofti, Brugia malayi* and *B. timori.* Only the *Brugia* spp., 3 cm (males) and 6 cm (females) long, hair-thin worms, are zoonotic agents.

Occurrence. *B. malayi* is endemic in South, Southeast, and East Asia. It is widely distributed in India, Burma, Thailand, Vietnam, and the Philippines.

Two strains of *B. malayi* are known for which animal reservoirs are of different importance. A nocturnally periodic strain (microfilariae are found in the peripheral blood only at night; during the day they accumulate in the lung capillaries) develops in various animals (dogs, cats, and others) but transmission occurs usually from human-to-human. Intermediate hosts are night-active mosquitoes of the genera *Aedes* and *Mansonia*. This *Brugia* strain is found predominantly in open plains that are extensively used for farming. In contrast, the subperiodic strain of *B. malayi* (microfilariae can be detected in the peripheral blood without remarkable periodicity), which is found in the rainforest areas of Southeast Asia, and is transmitted by day and night active mosquitoes, predominantly *Mansonia* spp., is zoonotic. Reservoirs are dogs, cats, and wild felids.

B. timori is found in the southeast of Indonesia. Felids and pangolins are reservoir hosts. Transmission occurs predominantly by *Anopheles* spp. The prevalence of *Brugia* spp. in humans vary regionally but can be high (>50%).

Transmission. Humans and other hosts are infected by bites of infected mosquitoes that transmit the infective, third-stage larvae. The adult parasites live in lymph vessels and lymph nodes. Females are viviparous and release first-stage larvae, the microfilaria, which circulate in the blood, are taken up by the mosquitoes during blood sucking, and they develop to third-stage larvae. After transmission in the course of a further blood meal, they migrate to their localization and develop to adult worms within >3 months. Microfilariae are first found in the blood 3 to 12 months after infection.

Clinical Manifestations. The clinical picture varies from inconspicuousness to acute fever attacks, associated with lymphangitis/lymphadenitis, edema, mostly in one extremity, to finally obstructive alterations (elephantiasis) of the limb. It is associated with complicated immunomodulatory effects, which are probably important in the sequela of the disease but are not yet completely understood.

The infection remains asymptomatic in many cases for years, although microfilariae are circulating in the blood. During this phase, patients show a mostly filariae-specific T cell suppression. Months or years after infection lymphangitis and lymphadenitis, mostly in the legs and groin, often with episodes of fever, headache, and backache, local edema and thrombophlebitis may develop. After relapsing episodes, often for years, chronic filariasis develops with extended lymphatic obstructions, elephantiasis, and hyperkeratosis (Fig. 4.44). The skin may become fissured and extravasations occur. Secondary infections are common. *B. timori* infections cause more severe alterations than *B. malayi* infections. In contrast to the early asymptomatic stage, patients with chronic, obstructive filariasis are usually free of circulating microfilaria and their T cells are hyperreactive to filarial antigens.

Diagnosis. The ensheathed microfilariae measure 220 μm in length and are 5 μm thick. They

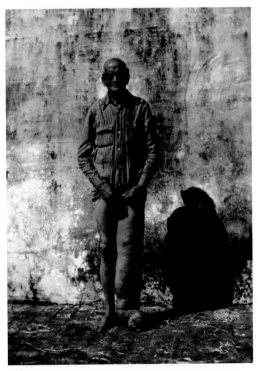

Figure 4.44 | Lymphatic filariasis: elephantiasis (picture: H. Zahner, Giessen, Germany).

can be demonstrated in Giemsa-stained blood smears, provided periodicity is considered. In cases with low microfilaremia, concentration techniques must be used, for example, filtration of the hemolyzed blood through membranes. Attempts to demonstrate filarial DNA by PCR are usually more sensitive. Symptomatic patients are often amicrofilaremic. Serologic examinations should particularly consider IgG4 antibodies. The use of serology, however, is limited in patients from endemic areas, as inhabitants of these regions often show high humoral antibody levels independent of their clinical and/or parasitological status. An alternative is the demonstration of circulating filarial antigens. Such assays are regarded as a "gold standard" by the WHO in the case of *W. bancrofti* infections (commercial test kits). Adult worms may be detected in lymph nodes and lymph vessels by sonography due to their mobility ("filarial dance sign").

Differential Diagnosis. Bacterial infections have to be excluded in cases of filarial fever. In cases of tropical eosinophilia, tuberculosis, aspergillosis, and helminth infections (*Strongyloides* spp., hookworms, and visceral larva migrans), as well as bronchial asthma have to be considered. Differentiation of *Brugia* and *Wuchereria* microfilariae is based on morphological criteria.

Therapy. Asymptomatic, subclinical, and acute cases are treated with diethylcarbamazine (DEC) as follows: day 1, 50 mg; day 2, three 50 mg doses; day 3, three 100 mg doses; days 4 to 21, 2 mg/kg three time a day orally. DEC acts against adult filariae and microfilariae. Due to the death of microfilariae and the associated release of particular microfilarial components, severe, sometimes shock-like side effects may occur. Starting with low doses, with a later increase in dose, attempts to avoid them. Albendazole, 400 mg twice a day orally for 21 days is also recommended.

The combination of DEC or DEC plus albendazole with doxycyline, 100 to 200 mg per day for 6 weeks enhances microfilaricidal efficacy and reduces adverse effects of chemotherapy.

Furthermore, ivermectin is recommended at a single dose of 100 to 400 µg/kg orally. The drug is used successfully in *W. bancrofti* infections, causes a long-lasting reduction of parasitaemia and generally only weak side effects. A combination of single doses of 200 to 400 µg/ kg ivermectin and 400 mg albendazole is currently favored.

Current attempts of the WHO aim for the global eradication of lymphatic filariasis and their agents, *W. bancrofti* and *Brugia* spp., by yearly mass treatments with 400 mg albendazole plus 200 µg of ivermectin/kg. It is supposed that transmission can be stopped within 4 to 6 years by these measures. Alternatively, the population may be supplied for 6 to 12 months with DEC-medicated sodium chloride, as successfully done in the People's Republic of China.

Prophylaxis. Repellents and mosquitoe nets should be used to prevent insect bites.

REFERENCES

Adjobimey T, Hoerauf A, Induction of immunoglobulin G4 in human filariasis: an indicator of immunoregulation. *Ann. Trop Med. Parasitol.* 10, 455–464, 2010.

Freedman DO, Immune dynamics in the pathogenesis of human lymphatic filariasis. *Parasitol. Today* 14, 229–234, 1998.

Hoerauf A, Filariasis: new drugs and new opportunities for lymphatic filariasis and onchocerciasis. *Curr. Opin. Infect. Dis.* 21, 673–681, 2008.

Huppatz C et al., Lessons from the Pacific programme to eliminate lymphatic filariasis: a case study of 5 countries. *BMC Infect. Dis.* 9, 92, 2009.

Lalitha P et al., Development of antigen detection ELISA fort he diagnosis of brugian and bancroftian filariasis using antibodies to recombinant filarial antigens Bm-SXP-1 and Wb-SXP-1. *Microbiol. Immunol.* 46, 327–332, 2002.

Michael E et al., Global eradication of lymphatic filariasis: the value of chronic disease control in parasite elimination programme. *PLoS One* 3, e2936, 2008.

Mullerpatan JB Udwadia ZF, Udwadia FE, Tropical pulmonary eosinophilia - a review. *Indian J. Med. Res.* 38, 295–302, 2013.

Nagampalli RS et al., A structural biology approach to understand lymphatic filariasis infections. *PloS Negl. Trop. Dis.* 8, e2662, 2014.

Ottesen EA, Lymphatic filariasis: treatment, control and elimination. *Adv. Parasitol.* 61, 395–441, 2006.

Pilotte N et al., A TaqMan-based multiplex realtime PCR assay for simultaneous detection of *Wuchereria bancrofti* and *Brugia malayi*. *Mol. Biochem. Parasitol.* 189, 33–37, 2013.

Pfarr KM et al., Filariasis and lymphoedema. *Parasite Immunol.* 31, 664–672, 2009.

Rao RU et al., Detection of *Brugia* parasite DNA in human blood by real-time PCR. *J. Clin. Microbiol.* 44, 3887–3893, 2006.

Simons JE, Gray CA, Lawrence RA, Absence of regulatory IL-10 enhances innate protection against filarial parasites by neutrophil-independent mechanism. *Parasite Immunol.* 32, 473–478, 2010.

Supali T et al., Doxycycline treatment of *Brugia malayi*-infected persons reduces microfilaremia and adverse reactions after diethylcarbamazine and albendazole treatment. *Clin. Infect. Dis.* 46, 1385–1393, 2008.

Taylor MJ, Wolbachia in the inflammatory pathogenesis of human filariasis. *Ann. N. Y. Acad. Sci.* 990, 444–447, 2003.

Wammes LJ et al., Regulatory T cells in human lymphatic filariasis : stronger functional activity in microfilaremics. *PloS Negl. Trop. Dis.* 6, e1655, 2012.

Wattal S et al., Evaluation of Og4C3 antigen ELISA as a tool for the detection of bancroftian filariasis under lymphatic filariasis elimination programme. *J. Commun, Dis.* 39, 75–84, 2007.

Weil GJ, Ramzy RMR, Diagnostic tools for filariasis elimination programs. *Trends Parasitol.* 23, 78–82, 2006.

4.5.7.2 Dirofilariasis

Dirofilariasis is a disease of the lungs or the subcutaneous tissue due to an infection with *Dirofilaria* spp. Clinically, it is usually unproblematic.

Etiology. The agents are *Dirofilaria immitis*, the heartworm of the dog, the connective tissue dwelling filariae *D. repens* and *D. tenuis*, and, occasionally, *D. ursi* and *D. striata*.

Occurrence. *D. immitis* is found worldwide in areas with warm climates, particularly in the southern United States, in Central and South America, in some countries of East Asia, and in the Mediterranian area, for example, Spain and the region around the river Po in Italy. Climatic conditions that are sufficient for the development of the parasite in its intermediate hosts are found in Europe northwards until the 50th latitude. Final hosts are canids and cats. *D. repens* occurs in the Old World with a similar distribution as *D. immitis*. *D. tenuis* develops in raccoons in the southern Unites States. The other species are found in bears and lynxes in the United States (*D. ursi*) and in felids in North and South America (*D. striata*).

Human infections are relatively seldom diagnosed. However, many cases may be unrecognized: specific antibodies to *Dirofilaria* are found in up to 20% of inhabitants of regions of endemicity.

Transmission. The parasites are transmitted as third-stage larvae during blood sucking by infected mosquitoes or (*D. ursi*) simulia (blackflies). Adult *D. immitis* are found in the right heart and the pulmonary artery of their definitive, final hosts. Microfilariae circulate in the blood and they are taken up by the intermediate host with the blood meal. They develop to third-stage (infective) larvae that can be transmitted to a new host. The parasites reach their final destination and sexual maturity in dogs within 3 months. The other species settle in the subcutaneous tissue.

In humans, *D. immitis* usually inhabits the parenchyma of the lungs. The connective tissue dwelling species develop subcutaneously. *D. repens* may sometimes be found in the lungs. Microfilariae are usually not observed in humans.

Clinical Manifestations. *D. immitis* infections in humans are in most cases (3/4) asymptomatic. Occasionally localized vasculitis and pulmonary infarcts are found and granulomas of several centimeters in size develop around the worm. Clinical signs are chest pains, coughing, and hemoptysis. *D. repens* and the other species settle in the subcutaneous tissue and cause nodules that are sometimes painful and itching. All *Dirofilaria* spp. may invade the human eye.

Diagnosis. The alterations may be observed by X-ray or as small nodules in the subcutaneous tissue. Excision and demonstration of the worms verify the diagnosis. Serologic assays can be applied if other filarial infections can be excluded.

Differential Diagnosis. Lung tumors and tuberculosis must be considered in the case of *D. immitis*. In the cases of subcutaneous localization of the parasites, neoplasms and, for example, subcutaneous coenurus must be excluded.

Therapy. Therapy consists of surgical excision of the parasites.

Prophylaxis. Repellents may be used to protect from biting insects.

REFERENCES

Angeli L et al., Human dirofilariasis: 10 new cases in Piedmont, Itali. *Int. J. Dermatol.* 46, 844–847, 2007.

Dantas-Torres F, Otranto D, Dirofilariasis in the Americas: a more virulent *Dirofilaria immitis*? *Parasit Vectors* 6, 288, 2013.

Fodor E et al., Recently recognized cases of ophthalmofilariasis in Hungary. *Eur. J. Ophthalmol.* 19, 675–678, 2009.

Genchi C et al., Climate and *Dirofilaria* infection in Europe. *Vet. Parasitol.* 163, 286–292, 2009.

Harizanov RN, Jordanova DP, Bikov IS, Some aspects of epidemiology, clinical manifestations, and diagnosis of human dirofilariasis caused by *Dirofilaria repens. Parasitol. Res.* 113, 1571–1579, 2014.

Lee ACY et al., Public health issues concerning the widespread distribution of canine heartworm disease. *Trends Parasitol.* 26, 168–173, 2010.

Miliaras D et al., Human pulmonary dirofilariasis: one more case in Greece suggests that *Dirofilaria* is a rather common cause of coin lesions in the lungs in endemic areas of Euope. *Int. J. Immunopathol. Pharmacol.* 23, 345–348, 2010.

Morchón R et al., Zoonotic *Dirofilaria immitis* infections in a province of Northern Spain. *Epidemiol. Infect.* 138, 380–383, 2010.

Poppert S et al., *Dirofilaria repens* infection and concomitant meningoencephalitis. *Emerg. Infect. Dis.* 15, 1844–1846, 2009.

Pozgain Z et al., Life *Dirofilaria immitis* found during coronary artery bypass grafting procedure. *Eur. J. Cardiothorac. Surg.* 44, 1–3, 2013.

Szénási Z et al., Human dirofilariasis in Hungary: an emerging zoonosis in central Europe. *Wien. Klin. Wochenschr.* 120, 96–102, 2008.

4.5.8 GNATHOSTOMIASIS

Gnathostomiasis is caused by migrating nematode larvae. It is associated with painful swelling in the subcutaneous tissue or, in its visceral form, with inflammation in inner organs.

Etiology. The disease is usually caused by larvae of *Gnathostoma spinigerum* and, more rarely, by other species of the genus (*G. hispidum, G. doloresi, G. binucleatum*, and G. *nipponicum*).

Occurrence. *G. spinigerum* is found in humans and animals predominantly in Southeast Asia, but also in Australia and Central Africa (Sambia). In some areas of Laos, for example, more than 40% of the human population are seropositive. *G. binucleatum* is probably the only zoonotic species in South America, cumulating in Mexico and Ecuador. Final hosts are fish-eating carnivores. G. *hispidum* and G. *doloresi* are found in pigs in Asia (*G. hispidum* also in Europe); *G. nipponicum* infests weasels in Japan.

Transmission. The life cycle of *Gnathostomum* spp. includes two intermediate hosts. Human infections occur by ingestion of third stage larvae in second intermediate hosts (freshwater fishes, frogs, and snails) or paratenic hosts (e.g., chicken). In addition, ingestion of stages in first intermediate hosts (*Cyclops* spp.) may cause infections in humans. Third stage larvae (from paratenic hosts) may also percutaneously invade the host. Intrauterine infections occur.

The adult parasites inhabit the stomach wall of their final hosts. Eggs are shed with the feces. Water fleas (*Cyclops* spp.) become infected by first-stage larvae in the egg and must be ingested by second intermediate hosts (fishes, frogs, and snails) where the parasite encysts in the musculature as third-stage larvae. They have to be ingested by the final host. In humans, the parasites do not reach sexual maturity but penetrate the stomach wall and migrate to various inner organs.

Clinical Manifestations. Epigastric pains may occur a few days after infection; 3 to 4 weeks p.i. (or sometimes later), the larvae reach a size of 5 mm and induce itching and/or painful erythematous, migrating swellings of the skin (subcutaneous gnathostomiasis) or mucosa. Larvae may break through the skin.

In visceral gnathostomiasis, inflammatory reactions develop in inner organs. They may persist over years, associated with intermittent complaints. Also, the eyes can be invaded by the parasites. Invasion of the CNS can be life threatening. Infection is usually accompanied with intense eosinophilia.

Diagnosis. Clinical diagnosis of subcutaneous gnathostomiasis is confirmed by excision and taxonomic determination of the larvae. In other forms of the disease, the trilogy eosinophilia, migrating skin reactions and disposing food habits are indicative. Imaging techniques (MRT) are helpful. Specific serological techniques are available.

Differential Diagnosis. Cutaneous larva migrans and sparganosis must be considered in cases of subcutaneous localization and invasions of other metazoa in the case of visceral forms.

Therapy. Treatment is done by surgery. For specific chemotherapy, albendazole, 400 mg once or twice a day orally for 21 days or ivermectin, 200 µg/kg/day orally for 2 days may be used. Relapses must be expected up to 7 months after treatment.

Prophylaxis. Raw or undercooked meat of fish, frogs, or poultry should be avoided in Asia. Drinking water from natural sources should be boiled before use.

REFERENCES

Alvarez-Guerrero C et al., *Gnathostoma binucleatum*: pathological and parasitological aspects in experimentally infected dogs. *Exp. Parasitol.* 127, 84–89, 2011.

Anataphruti MT, Nuamtanong S, Dekumyoy P, Diagnostic values of IgG4 in human gnathostomiasis. *Trop. Med. Int. Health* 10, 1013–1021, 2005.

Bhattacharjee H, Das J, Medhi J, Intraviteal gnathostomiasis and review of the literature. *Retina* 27, 67–73, 2007.

Bhende M, Biswas J, Gopal L, Ultrasound biomicroscopy in the diagnosis and management of intraocular gnathostomiasis. *Am. J. Ophthalmol.* 140, 140–142, 2005.

Diaz-Camacho SP et al., Acute outbrake of gnathostomiasis in a fishing community in Sinaloa, Mexico. *Parasit. Int.* 52, 133–140, 2003.

García-Márquez LJ et al., Morphological and molecular identification of *Gnathostoma binucleatum* (Nematoda: Gnathostomatidae) advanced third stage larvae (AdvL3) in the state of Colima, Mexico. *Rev. Mex. Biodiversidad* 80, 867–870, 2003.

Herman JS et al., Gnathostomiasis acquired by British tourists in Botswana. *Emerg. Infect. Dis.* 15, 594–597, 2009.

Magana M et al., Gnathostomiasis: clinicopathologic study. *Am. J. Dermatopathol.* 26, 91–95, 2004.

Nontasut P et al., Double-dose ivermectin vs albendazole for the treatment of gnathostomiasis. *Southeast Asian J. Trop. Med. Public Health* 36, 650–652, 2005.

Pillai GS et al., Intraocular gnathostomiasis: report of a case and review of literature. *Am. J. Trop. Med. Hyg.* 86, 620–623, 2012.

Sawanyawisuth K et al., MR imaging findings in cauda equine gnathostomiasis. *Am. J. Neuroradiol.* 26, 39–42, 2005.

Sieu TM et al., Comparison of Vietnamese cultured and wild swamp eels for infection with *Gnathostoma spinigerum*. *J. Parasitol.* 95, 246–248, 2009.

Strady C et al., Long-term follow-up of imported ganothostomiasis shows frequent treatment failure. *Am. J. Trop. Med. Hyg.* 80, 33–35, 2009.

Vargas TJ et al., Autochthonous gnathostomiasis, Brazil. *Emerg. Infect. Dis.* 18, 2087–2089, 2012.

Vonghachack Y et al., Sero-epidemiological survey of gnathostomiasis in Lao PDR. *Parasitol. Int.* 59, 599–605, 2010.

4.5.9 GONGYLONEMIASIS

Gongylonemiasis is a rare human disease of the oral cavity due to nematodes of the genus *Gongylonema*.

Etiology. *Gongylonema pulchrum* is the prevailing species in humans. Male and female worms reach lengths of 50 and 130 mm, respectively.

Occurrence. The genus, including the species *G. pulchrum*, is found worldwide in various animals (ruminants, pigs, and others). Approximately 60 human cases have been reported from all continents.

Transmission. Humans become infected by the accidental ingestion of intermediate hosts, for example, various coprophagous bugs, cockroaches, and others, which have taken up the eggs from feces of infected final hosts. Infection is also possible by the uptake (e.g., in water) of free larvae, released by intermediate hosts. Ingested larvae migrate from the stomach within the mucosa to the upper esophagus and into the oral cavity. In definite hosts, the parasite predominantly invades the esophageal mucosa and reaches sexual maturity 2 months p.i.

Clinical Manifestations. Parasites are found in mucosal lesions and migrating in the mucosa of the oral cavity after an incubation period of several weeks. The clinical picture is characterized by sensation of migrating foreign bodies in/on the oral mucosa, local inflammation, bleeding, and in general moderate pain.

Diagnosis. Exact diagnosis depends on the isolation and characterization of the worms.

Therapy. Treatment is extraction of the worms. A local antiphlogistic treatment may favor the egress of the parasite from the mucosa and supports extraction.

Prophylaxis. The only preventive measure is personal hygiene in food consumption.

REFERENCES

Allen JD, Esquela-Kerscher A, *Gongylonema pulchrum* infection in a resident of Williamsburg, Virginia, verified by genetic analysis. *Am. J. Trop. Med. Hyg.* 89, 755–757, 2013.

Molavi GH, Massoud J, Gutierrez Y, Human *Gongylonema* infection in Iran. *J. Helminthol.* 80, 425–428, 2006.

Pasuralertsakul R, Yaicharoen R, Sripochang S, Spurious human infection with *Gongylonema*: nine cases reported from Thailand. *Ann. Trop. Med. Parasitol.* 102, 455–457, 2008.

Pessan B et al., The first case of human gongylonemiasis in France. *Parasite* 20, 5, 2013.

Urch T et al., Humane Infektion mit *Gongylonema pulchrum*. *Dtsch. Med. Wochenschr.* 130, 2566–2568, 2005.

4.5.10 HOOKWORM INFECTION (INFECTION WITH *ANCYLOSTOMA CEYLANICUM*)

Hookworms are gut-dwelling nematodes, inhabiting the small intestine of their specific hosts. They may cause intestinal discomfort and anemia due to their continuous and excessive blood sucking. Two species represent specific parasites of humans: *Necator americanus* is found in the Americas and the eastern and southeastern parts of Asia, *Ancylostoma duodenale* predominates in Africa, the Middle East, and many Asian regions. A third species, *Ancylostoma ceylanicum*, a common parasite of dogs and cats in tropical Asia, was previously supposed to only occasionally infect humans. However, it became known that the infection is much more common in humans than suggested and the disease needs to be considered in more detail than previously thought. *A. ceylanicum* is the only animal hookworm species causing patent natural infections in humans.

For other hookworm related zoonoses see chapter 4.5.6 (Eosinophilic enteritis) and chapter 4.5.13 (Larva migrans cutanea).

Etiology. *Ancylostoma ceylanicum* is a nematode of 6 to 8 mm (males) and 8 to 10 mm (females) in length. Similar to other hookworms, the anterior end is bent dorsally, giving the worm a hook-like shape. The marked buccal capsule is armed by cutting plates with teeth. The worms are grey or reddish in color due to blood in their alimentary tract. Two haplotypes are known; one seems specific for humans, the other is found in humans, dogs, and cats.

Occurrence. *A. cheylanicum* occurs throughout South Asia, Southeast Asia and Australia. It is the second most common human hookworm species in Asia. In a rural area of Malaysia, *N. americanus* predominated but amongst hookworm egg positive persons, *A. ceylanicum* was found in 12.8% as single infection and in 10.6% of mixed infections. In other surveys, 6 to 23% of hookworm positive patients were infected with *A. ceylanicum*. Current estimates assume a number of 19 to 73 million infected people in regions of known endemicity.

Reservoir hosts are dogs and cats. A prevalence of up to >90% are found in the Asia-Pacific region, for example, in stray dogs in Malaysia. In rural villages in India, 93 to 98% of the dogs shed *A. ceylanicum* eggs. In areas where *A. ceylanicum* and *A. caninum* coincide, *A. ceylanicum* predominates or the incidence is similar for both species.

Transmission. Hookworms are transmitted in a direct cycle. Adult females release eggs with few blastomeres that are shed in the feces. First stage larvae develop in the environment, hatch and mature to ensheathed third stage larvae (L3; the sheath is a remnant of the second stage larva cuticle) within a few days. Larvae are highly motile and may survive under tropical conditions for several weeks. Humans become infected by percutaneously invading or orally ingested (e.g., adhering to vegetables) L3. As walking barefooted represents a distinct risk factor for human *A. ceylanicum* infections, the percutaneous route seems to be the mayor route of infection. The parasites pass a blood-heart-lung-migration, penetrate into the alveoli, and they are brought up by the ciliated epithelium or by coughing. They are swallowed back into the small intestine and then attach to the epithelium by their buccal capsule. In experimental human infections with 1200 L3, eggs were found beginning 5 weeks p.i. Egg excretion continued at relatively low levels until 30 weeks p.i., when the infection was terminated by treatment. It is noteworthy that the related parasite *A. duodenale* is lactogenously transmitted to neonates due to larval stages spread in the maternal organism.

Clinical Manifestations. Invading larvae may cause papular reactions (ground itch), particularly after repeated infections. The infection may be associated with considerable intestinal discomfort, such as abdominal distension, epigastric pain, and diarrhea. The parasites grasp plugs of mucosa into their toothed buccal capsule and open small blood vessels to get access to blood. Thus, anemia with iron deficiency and hypalbuminemia is a principle sequela of the feeding habit of hookworms and may develop particularly in malnourished patients. Estimates of the daily blood loss assume that approximately 0.01 to 0.02 ml will be lost per worm per day in infected dogs. Often occult blood is found in the feces because the parasites change their location at the intestinal wall. Children may be affected by long-term effects, that is, impaired physical and cognitive development.

Diagnosis. The oval, thin-shelled eggs measure approximately 70 by 45 µm and they may be detected in the feces. Freshly excreted eggs contain only 2 to 8 cells but embryonation proceeds rapidly. Differentiation from other hookworm species can be done by copro-molecular diagnostic tools. Eosinophilia is common in *A. ceylanicum* infections.

Differential Diagnosis. Infections with other intestinal nematodes (other hookworm species, trichostrongyles, *Oesophagostomum* spp.) and other causes for anemia must be considered.

Therapy. Effective drugs are benzimidazoles (e.g., albendazole, 400 mg, or mebendazole, 100 mg twice a day for 3 days orally) and pyrantel pamoate, 25 mg/kg for 2 days orally.

Prophylaxis. Barefoot walking should be avoided in known endemic areas. Pet dogs and cats should be dewormed. Vegetables and fruits with contact to the ground should be carefully washed before eating.

REFERENCES

Anten JF, Zudema PJ, Hookworm infection in Dutch servicemen returning from West New Guinea. *Trop. Geograph. Med.* 64, 216–224, 1964.

Brookers S Bethony J, Hortez PJ, Human hookworm infection in the 21. century. *Adv. Parasitol.* 58, 197–288, 2004.

Carroll SM, Grove DI, Experimental infections of humans with *Ancylostoma ceylanicum*: clinical, parasitological, haematological and immunological findings. *Trop. Geograph. Med.* 38, 38–45, 1986.

Hsu YC, Lin TJ, Images in clinical medicine. Intestinal infection with *Ancylostoma ceylanicum*. *N. Engl. J. Med.* 366: e20, 2012.

Jiraanakul V et al., Incidence and risk factors of human hookworm infections through high resolution melting (HRM) analysis. *PLoS One* 7, e41996, 2011.

Ngui R, Lim YA, Chua KH, Rapid detection and identification of human hookworm infections through high resolution melting (HRM) analysis. *PLoS One* 7, e41996, 2012.

Palmers, CS et al., The veterinary and public health significance of hookworms in dogs and cats in Australia and the status of *A.ceylanicum*. *Vet. Parasitol.* 145, 304–313, 2007.

Phosuk I et al., Molecular detection of *Ancylostoma duodenalis, Ancylostoma ceylanicum*, and *Necator americanus* in humans in northern and southern Thailand. *Korean J. Parasitol.* 51, 747–749, 2013.

Traub RJ, *Ancylostoma cheylanicum*, a re-emerging but neglected parasitic zoonosis. *Int. J. Parasitol.* 43, 1009–1015, 2013.

4.5.11 LAGOCHILASCARIASIS

Lagochilascariasis is a rare disease in humans. Patients are afflicted with worm-containing, fistular nodules, which are mostly found in the neck or head regions.

Etiology. The agent is *Lagochilascaris minor*, an ascarid nematode up to 20 mm long (females).

Occurrence. Human infections are only known from tropical regions in Central and South

America. All afflicted people (~80 cases have been recognized so far) were inhabitants of remote jungle forest areas. The final animal hosts are probably felids.

Transmission. The developmental cycle of *L. minor* is known in principle, but details are not clear. Humans are probably infected by ingestion of infected intermediate hosts (agoutis, mice, and other rodents). However, it can currently not be excluded that embryonated eggs are infectious for humans as well. In addition, patients seem to suffer often endogenous autoinfections, as nodules may contain all stages of the parasite, with eggs developing continuously into larvae.

When rodents are infected with embryonated eggs, larvae are found in inner organs and subcutaneous and fatty tissue and they become encapsulated. Feeding of infected rodents but not of embryonated eggs to cats results in the development of adult *L. minor* in their esophagus, pharynx, and cervical lymph nodes. However, endogenous autoinfections can also happen in cats.

Clinical Manifestations. *L. minor* causes usually chronic, up to hen's egg-sized, nodular swellings in the neck, but also in the throat, nasal sinuses, tonsils, brain, and lungs. The purulent discharge contains eggs and the various parasite stages (adult and larvae), which can sometimes be in large numbers. The general condition of the patient is severely disturbed. In two cases, the patients died. The occurrence of numerous different developmental stages of the parasite in one lesion suggests endogenous autoinfections by parasite eggs deposited in the nodules.

Diagnosis. Diagnosis is based on the clinical picture and the demonstration of parasites (eggs, larvae, adults) in the lesions. The eggs measure 50 by 65 µm, have a thick shell with granulated surface, and resemble the eggs of *Toxocara cati*. Dependent on the localization of the parasites, the eggs may be swallowed and can be found in the feces.

Differential Diagnosis. Furuncles, carbuncles, and abscesses of other etiology must be considered in the differential diagnosis. Eggs in the feces may be mistaken for eggs of *Ascaris lumbricoides*.

Therapy. Reports on the efficacy of chemotherapy are inconsistent. Treatment with levamisole, 150 mg/week orally for 3 months, and albendazole, 400 mg/day orally for several weeks, seem to be effective. Relapses may occur. Living worms were still found in nodules after treatment with ivermectin, 0.3 mg/kg/day orally for 8 weeks. Drug administration for 4 additional weeks seemed to be effective. In some cases, the nodules have been surgically removed.

Prophylaxis. The mode of transmission is not known. Strict personal hygiene is recommended.

REFERENCES

Aquino RTR et al., Lagochilascariasis leading to severe involvement of ocular globes, ears and meninges. *Rev. Inst. Med. Trop. Sao Paulo* 50, 355–358, 2008.

Barrera-Pérez M et al., *Lagochilascaris minor* Leiper, 1909 (Nematoda: Ascaridiae) in Mexico: three clinical cases from the Peninsula of Yucatan. *Rev. Inst. Med. Trop. Sao Paulo* 54, 315–317, 2012.

Campos DM et al., Experimental life cycle of *Lagochilascaris minor* Leiper, 1909. *Rev. Inst. Med. Trop. Sao Paulo* 34, 277–287, 1998.

De Freitas JG et al., *Lagochilascaris minor*: experimental infection of C57BL/6 and BALB7c isogenic mice reveals the presence of adult worms. *Exp. Parasitol.* 119, 325–331, 2008.

Roig JL et al., Otomastoiditis with right retroauricular fistula by *Lagochilascaris minor*. *Braz. J. Otorhinolaryngol.* 76, 407, 2010.

4.5.12 LARVA MIGRANS CUTANEA (CREEPING ERUPTION)

Larva migrans cutanea (also known as cutaneous larva migrans or creeping eruption) is a mostly acute syndrome of the skin that is caused by migrating larvae of parasitic nematodes. Humans are accidental hosts.

Etiology. The disease is caused by nematode larvae that invade the host percutaneously similar to hookworms (Ancylostomatidae) and *Strongyloides* spp. The most important parasites are *Ancylostoma braziliense* and *Uncinaria* *stenocephala*, which are hookworms of dogs. Other hookworms, such as *A. caninum* (from dogs), *A. tubaeforme* (from cats) and *Bunostomum phlebotomum* (from cattle), may occasionally be involved.

Occurrence. Hookworms and *Strongyloides* spp. occur in animals worldwide. *A. braziliense* is found predominantly in tropical and subtropical areas; *U. stenocephala* is a parasite of moderate climates. The other species are found preferentially under warmer climatic conditions. Human infections may occur in all areas of moderate or warm climates.

Transmission. Humans can be infected percutaneously when infective larvae can penetrate the bare skin. The moist and warm environmental conditions of beaches are highly suitable for the larval development from the eggs deposited in feces, for example, by dogs. This explains the high incidence of human infections on urban beaches of South America and South Africa, which are often polluted by dog feces. Contaminated playgrounds are also sources of infection (see "Larva Migrans Visceralis"; chapter 4.5.12).

In natural hosts, the parasites pass a blood-heart-lung-migration, penetrate the alveolar walls, are then brought up by the ciliated epithelia or by coughing, before being swallowed, settling in the small intestine and starting egg production, in the case of hookworms approximately 3 weeks p.i. In humans as a paratenic host, the development stops at the latest in the lungs (for exceptions see chapter 4.5.19).

Clinical Manifestations. Papules develop at the penetration site. Subsequently, in the classical form, which is mainly caused by *A. braziliense*, the larvae migrate a few mm to cm per day, between the corium and stratum granulosum in the skin. The burrows appear on the skin surface as elevated alterations, up to 2 mm wide, with surrounding erythema, edema, and crusts (Fig. 4.45). Patients feel tantalizing itching and pricking pain. Secondary infections may occur after scratching. Symptoms usually disappear after 2 to 8 weeks but may persist in untreated cases for up to 2 years.

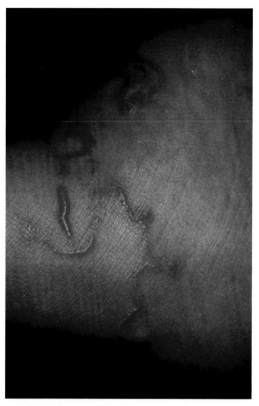

Figure 4.45 | Larva migrans cutanea (creeping eruption). Inflamed tracks of the dog hookworm *Ancylostoma braziliense* under the skin (picture: P. Janssen-Rosseck, Düsseldorf, Germany).

After infection with *A. caninum*, more follicular alterations and pustules develop. However, this species in general tends to invade in humans blood vessels and to spread in the organism. Eosinophilic infiltrations in the lung and pneumonia have been described as sequelae in these cases.

Diagnosis. The clinical picture is typical. Eosinophilia is not always present.

Differential Diagnosis. Similar symptoms may be found by larvae of *Ancylostoma duodenale*, *Necator americanus*, and *Strongyloides stercoralis*, which infest humans as adult parasites, and also by maggots of flies.

Gnathostoma spinigerum causes migrating, subcutaneous swellings but sometimes may also induce similar alterations (infections may occur after consuming raw fish, e.g., in

Southeast Asia). In addition, cercarial dermatitis and *Dracunculus* infections must be considered.

Therapy. Treatment is recommended with albendazole, 400 mg twice a day orally for 3 to 7 days or ivermectin, 200 µg/kg/day orally for 2 days. Attempts to kill migrating larvae by local freezing are usually unsuccessful and contraindicated because of tissue injury. Antipruritic agents may be applied to reduce itching.

Prophylaxis. Dogs and cats should be kept away from beaches and playgrounds. Shoes should be worn if the ground is polluted by animal feces. Beaches in humid regions populated by dogs and cats should not be visited. Dogs and cats should be examined for parasites and treated.

REFERENCES

Archer M, Late presentation of cutaneous larva migrans: a case report. *Cases J.* 12, 7553, 2009.

Bowman DD et al., Hookworms of dogs and cats as agents of cutaneous larva migrans. *Trends Parasitol.* 26, 162–167, 2010.

Heukelbach J, Feldmeier H, Epidemiological and clinical characteristics of hookworm-related cutaneous larva migrans. *Lancet Infect. Dis.* 8, 302–309, 2008.

Jensenius M, Maeland A, Brubakk O, Extensive hookworm-related cutaneous larva migrans in Norwegian travellers to the tropics. *Travel Med. Infect. Dis.* 6, 45–47, 2008.

Kannathasan S et al., A simple intervention to prevent cutaneous larva migrans among devotees of the Nallur Temple in Jaffna, Sri Lanka. *PloS One* 8, e61816, 2013.

Rivera-Roig V, Sánchez JL, Hillyer GV, Hookworm folliculitis. *Int. J. Dermatol.* 47, 246–248, 2008.

Senba Y et al., Case of creeping disease treated with ivermectin. *J. Dermatol.* 36, 86–89, 2009.

Shimogawara R et al., Hookworm-related cutaneous larva migrans in patients living in an endemic community in Brazil: immunological patterns before and after ivermectin treatment. *Eur. J. Microbiol. Immunol. (Bp)* 3, 258–266, 2013.

Siriez JY et al., Individual variability of the cutaneous larva migrans (CLM) incubation period. *Pediatr. Dermatol.* 27, 211–212, 2010.

Tamminga N, Bierman WF, de Vries PJ, Cutaneous larva migrans acquired in Brittany, France. *Emerg. Infect. Dis.* 15, 1856–1858, 2009.

Tan SK, Liu TT, Cutaneous larva migrans complicated by Löffler syndrome. *Arch. Dermatol.* 146, 210–212, 2010.

Te Booij M, de Jong E, Bovenschen HJ, Löffler syndrome caused by extensive cutaneous larva migrans: a case report and review of the literature. *Dermatol. Online J.* 16, 2, 2010.

Vanhaecke CA et al., Etiologies of creeping eruption: 78 cases. *Br. J. Dermatol.* 170, 1166–1169, 2013.

4.5.13 LARVA MIGRANS VISCERALIS

Larva migrans visceralis or visceral larva migrans (VLM) is a syndrome caused by the invasion of inner organs or the eye by nematode larvae. Humans are paratenic hosts.

Etiology. Potential agents are all nematodes that are able to invade visceral organs. The disease is mostly caused by larvae of *Toxocara canis* and *T. cati* (syn. *T. mystax*), ascarid worms of dogs and cats, respectively (toxocariasis). More rare, but important from a clinical point of view, are infections with *Baylisascaris procyonis*, an ascarid parasite of raccoons.

Occurrence. *Toxocara* infections are common worldwide in carnivorous animals. *T canis* is found predominantly in dogs. Eggs are usually shed by <6-month-old animals (prevalence up to 80%). Up to 80% of cats in Central Europe excrete *T. cati* eggs in the feces. Raccoons are often (>60%) infected with *B. procyonis*. An important parasite with respect to VLM is also *A. suum*, the ascarid of pigs. It is one of the most common nematodes in pigs worldwide.

Human infections occur worldwide. Antibodies to *T. canis* as an indicator of the infection are found worldwide in 2 to 14% of the human population with a higher prevalence in children than in adults. There is a higher prevalence in people living in the countryside than in inhabitants of urban areas. The relative rarity of clinically apparent cases suggests a clinically inapparent course in most infections. Approximately 20 human cases of infections with *B. procyonis* have been reported. Except two cases in Germany, they occurred in North America.

Transmission. Infection occurs by oral ingestion of embryonated (containing infective larva) eggs. Infective larvae develop within the eggs in the environment in the course of weeks (freshly excreted eggs are not infective). Embryonated eggs survive for months in the ground.

Important sources of eggs are playgrounds and sandboxes polluted with feces of definite hosts. The contamination rate of playgrounds is usually high. Seventy percent of playgrounds were found to be contaminated with infective eggs of *Toxocara*, for example, in large cities of Western Europe, whereby *T. cati* eggs predominated. Sandboxes in particular represent suitable environments for the maturation of *Toxocara* larvae, and are preferential defecation sites of cats. Further sources of infection are inner organs of paratenic hosts (livers) or, in case of *A. suum*, of the definite host, if they are ingested raw or undercooked. Raccoons use to defecate in so-called latrines, that is, defecation places, which are used together by groups of animals, and may represent places of dangerous accumulation of *B. procyonis* eggs.

After ingestion of embryonated eggs, larvae hatch in the small intestine of final or paratenic hosts, invade the intestinal wall and are spread hematogenously via the liver and the heart to the lung. In young dogs, they penetrate the alveolar wall and reach the small intestine via trachea and esophagus. In humans as a paratenic host, the migration ends on the way to the lung or in the lung, or the larvae enter the arterial system and they are disseminated throughout the body. They leave the blood vessels and enter the parenchyma, where they are generally encapsulated by connective tissue. Encapsulated larvae may survive for years and they may become reactivated.

Clinical Manifestations. The infective dose and the localization of the larvae in the patient determine the clinical picture. In many cases, the infection remains asymptomatic and it is not recognized. Clinical manifestations result in three symptom complexes: VLM, ocular larva migrans (OLM), and cerebral larva migrans (CLM).

VLM occurs mainly in children of <6 years of age. Pica is a significant diagnostic hint. Major symptoms are fever, abdominal pain, coughing, and asthmatic complaints. Eosinophilia and leukocytosis are common. The lungs show transient infiltrations with eosinophils (Löffler's syndrome). Without reinfection, patients recover

within weeks. In persistent reinfections, additional organs are involved, with lymphadenopathia, splenomegaly, urticaria, interstitional pneumonia, anorexia, and weight loss.

OLM is observed rather independent of the patient's age and is usually caused by a single larva in one eye (diffuse unilateral subacute neuroretinitis syndrome). Studies in Ireland showed an incidence of 10 per 100 000 in schoolchildren. In the United States, approximately 1% of all visual disturbances are caused by OLM. Visual acuity is reduced in OLM patients. The disease can manifest as endophthalmitis, uveitis, chorioretinitis or with intraretinal granulomas. A motile larva may be occasionally found ophthalmoscopically; OLM often lacks eosinophilia and leukocytosis.

CLM after *Toxocara* infections is relatively rare (~50 documented cases) although *T. canis* is shown to be neurotropic in rodent infections. CLM is associated with acute or subacute meningitis or meningoencephalitis. About 60% of the patients recovered completely. In contrast, *B. procyonis* is strongly neurotropic in humans. Thus, CNS (eosinophilic meningoencephalitis) and ocular symptoms prevail. Prognosis is often poor; 25% of known patients died, and except in a few cases, survivors showed severe central nervous and ocular sequelae.

Diagnosis. The clinical picture of VLM with eosinophilia, hepatomegaly, and swelling of the abdominal lymph nodes, occasionally elevated levels of hepatic aminotransferases and increased levels of serum IgE is suggestive. The diagnostic method of choice is an ELISA using metabolic larval antigens. Serology may fail in OLM. Ophthalmoscopy is required. Larvae of *Toxocara* spp. and *B. procyonis* may be differentiated by their lengths of 400 μm and 1500 μm, respectively. Differentiation is also possible by serologic investigation (immunoblotting).

In CLM, pleocytosis with a high participation of eosinophils (>10%) is often found in the CSF. Demonstration of humoral antibodies may fail. Reliable antibody concentrations are rather found in the CSF.

Differential Diagnosis. In case of involvement of the CNS, poliomyelitis and epilepsy must be excluded. In OLM, toxoplasmosis and retinoblastoma must be considered. Pulmonary symptoms require consideration of psittacosis and asthma bronchiale.

Therapy. There is no proven effective chemotherapy although clinical improvement has been reported after treatment with albendazole, 400 mg twice a day orally for 5 days or mebendazole, 100 to 200 mg twice a day orally for 5 days. In case of OLM and CLM, anthelmintic treatment is combined with corticosteroids (prednisolon, 40 to 60 mg/day for 4 weeks). Ocular larvae are eliminated by direct photocoagulation or surgery.

Prophylaxis. Children should be kept away from contaminated playgrounds. Pets (dogs, cats, raccoons) should be subjected to parasitological examination and antiparasitic treatment.

REFERENCES

Aydenizöz-Ozkayhan M, Yagci BB, Erat S, The investigation of *Toxocara canis* eggs in coats of different dog breeds as a potential transmission route in human toxocariasis. *Vet. Parasitol.* 152, 94–100, 2008.

Bauer C, Baylisascariosis – infections of animals and humans with 'unusual' round worms. *Vet. Parasitol.* 193, 404–412, 2013.

Dangoudoubiyam S, Kazacos KR, Differentiation of larva migrans caused by *Baylisascaris procyonis* and *Toxocara* species by Wesaestern blotting. *Clin. Vaccine Immunol.* 16, 1563–1568, 2009.

Fillaux J, Magnaval JF, Laboratory diagnosis of human toxocariasis. *Vet. Parasitol.* 193, 327–336, 2013.

Fisher M, *Toxocara cati*: an underestimated zoonotic agent. *Trends Parasitol.* 19, 167–170, 2003.

Gavignet B et al., Cutaneous manifestations of human toxocariasis. *J. Am. Acad. Dermatol.* 59, 1031–1042, 2008.

Good B et al., Ocular toxocariasis in schoolchildren. *Clin. Infect. Dis.* 39, 173–178, 2004.

Hoffmeister B et al., Cerebral toxocariasis after consumption of raw duck liver. *Am. J. Trop. Med. Hyg.* 76, 600–602, 2007.

Hotez PJ, Wilkins PP, Toxocariasis: America's most common neglected infection of poverty and a helminthiasis of global importance. *PLoS Negl. Trop. Dis.* 3, e400, 2009.

Kustimur S et al., *Toxocara* prevalence in adults with bronchial asthma. *Trans. R. Soc. Trop. Med. Hyg.* 101, 270–274, 2007.

Macpherson CN et al., The epidemiology and public health importance of toxocariasis: a zoonosis of global importance. *Int. J. Parasitol.* 43, 999–1008, 2013.

Nakamura-Uchiyama F et al., A case of *Ascaris suum* visceral larva migrans diagnosed by using *A. suum* larval excretory-secretory (ES) antigen. *Scand. J. Infect. Dis.* 38, 221–224, 2006.

Okada F et al., Pulmonary computed tomography findings of visceral larva migrans caused by *Ascaris suum*. *J. Comput. Assist. Tomogr.* 31, 402–408, 2007.

Page LK et al., Backyard raccoon latrines and risk for *Baylisascaris procyonis* transmission to humans. *Emerg. Infect. Dis.* 15, 1530–1531, 2009.

Pai PJ et al., Full recovery from *Baylisascaris procyonis* eosinophilic meningitis. *Emerg. Infect. Dis.* 13, 928–930, 2007.

Rodman J, Pizzimenti J, In vivo diagnostic imaging of ocular toxocariasis. *Clin. Exp. Optom.* 92, 146–149, 2009.

Rubinsky-Elefant G et al., Human toxocariasis: diagnosis, worldwide seroprevalences and clinical expression of the systemic and ocular forms. *Ann. Trop. Med. Parasitol.* 104, 3–23, 2010.

Schoenardie ER et al., Seroprevalence of *Toxocara* infection in children from southern Brazil. *J. Parasitol.* 99, 537–539, 2013.

Smiths H et al., How common is human toxocariasis? Towards standardizing our knowledge. *Trends Parasitol.* 25, 182–188, 2009.

Stensvold CR et al., Seroprevalence of human toxocariasis in Denmark. *Clin. Vaccine. Immunol.* 16, 1372–1373, 2009.

Uga S, Minami T, Nagata K, Defecation habits of cats and dogs and contamination by *Toxocara* eggs in public sandpits. *Am. J. Trop. Med. Hyg.* 54, 122–126, 1996.

4.5.14 OESOPHAGOSTOMIASIS

Oesophagostomiasis is a chronic disease of the colon with nodular alterations of the intestinal wall.

Etiology. The agent responsible for the disease is *Oesophagostumom bifurcum*, a common nematode of the large intestine of various primates in Africa. Occasionally, the species *O. aculeatum* and *O. stephanostomum*, common in African primates, are found in humans.

Occurrence. Human infections are found predominantly in Africa, south the Sahara, particularly in North Ghana and in the northern part of Togo. A local prevalence of >50% was reported in these areas.

Transmission. Infection occurs by oral ingestion of infective third-stage larvae adhering, for example, on vegetables. The female parasites release eggs that are shed with the feces. The ensheathed infective larva (the sheath is a remnant of the second-stage larval cuticle) develops under optimum conditions within 6 to 7 days and hatches from the egg. After ingestion, the infective larva invades the wall of the large intestine, induces the formation of small nodules, develops and molts to the fourth stage, which migrates back into the intestinal lumen. Sexual maturity is reached in the natural host after 30 to 40 days. The larval development in the colonic wall may be arrested after repeated infections. In these cases, the nodules not only persist, but they also become enlarged.

The importance of animal reservoirs for human *Oesophagostomum* spp. infections seem less than previously suggested. Genetic studies showed distinct differences between human- and ape-derived worm populations. In addition, the primate population is too small in the highly endemic areas to play an important role in the epidemiology of oesophagostomes. Furthermore, fertile worm populations have been found in humans in the highly concerned regions of Ghana and Togo, which is different from previous suppositions that worms remain in an infertile stage in humans. Therefore, transmission from person-to-person seems possible, at least in these areas.

Clinical Manifestations. Infections may be inapparent. Disease is associated with nodules in the intestinal wall, which may lead to severe obstructive changes of the large bowel and the formation of tumor-like, painful masses (*Tumeur de Dapaong*) or to multinodular reactions. In the last of these cases, the intestinal wall, predominantly in the ileocecal region, is interspearsed with pee-sized nodules that contain pus and an infertile worm.

Infections are mostly found in adolescents but rarely in children <5 years of age. Intraperitoneal adhesions are formed that can lead to abscesses and fistulas of the abdominal wall, which also may contain nematode larvae.

Diagnosis. The oval, thin-shelled eggs, 90 by 40 μm in size, with blastomeres are detected in patent infections. The nodular reactions of the intestinal wall can be demonstrated by sonography and laparoscopy. For serology, an ELISA that detects IgG4 antibodies is valuable.

Differential Diagnosis. The eggs can be mistaken for hookworm (*Ancylostoma dudenale*) eggs. For final differentiation, the third-stage larvae must be cultivated. Colorectal cancer must be excluded.

Therapy. Effective chemotherapy uses albendazole, 400 mg twice a day orally for 3 days, or mebendazole, 100 mg twice a day orally for 3 days. Albendazole also proved to be effective for the multinodular form of the disease. Patients with severe alterations of the intestine need surgical resection. In moderate cases, restitution is obtained within 6 to 12 months.

Prophylaxis. Personal hygiene (careful cleaning of the hands after contact with potentially contaminated material) reduces the risk of infection.

REFERENCES

Gasser RB, de Gruijter JD, Polderman AM, Insights into the epidemiology and genetic make-up of *Oesophagostomum bifurcum* from human, and non-human primates using molecular tools. *Parasitology* 132, 453–460, 2006.

Ghai RR et al., Nodule worm infection in humans and wild primates in Uganda: cryptic species in a newly identified region of human transmission. *PLoS Negl. Trop. Dis.* 8, e2641, 2014.

Krief S et al., Nodular worm infection in wild chimpanzees in western Uganda: a risk for human health? *PLoS Negl. Trop. Dis.* 4, e630, 2010.

Van Lieshout L et al., *Oesophagostomum bifurcum* in non-human primates is not a potential reservoir for human infection in Ghana. *Trop. Med. Int. Health* 10, 1315–1320, 2005.

Ziem JB et al., Impact of repeated mass treatment on human *Oesophagostomum* and hookworm infections in northern Ghana. *Trop. Med. Int. Health.* 11, 1764–1772, 2006.

Ziem JB et al., *Oesophagostomum bifurcum*-induced nodular pathology in a highly endemic area of northern Ghana. *Trans. R. Soc. Trop. Med. Hyg.* 99, 417–422, 2005.

4.5.15 STRONGYLOIDIASIS

Strongyloidiasis is an often asymptomatic, or sometimes (particularly in immunosuppressed patients) severe, occasionally fatal disease after infection with nematodes of the genus *Strongyloides*.

Etiology. Two species of the genus, *Strongyloides stercoralis* and *S. fuelleborni*, play a role. In addition, a parasite that is regarded as a subspecies of the latter species, *S. fuelleborni kellyi*, is reported from Papua New Guinea, predominantly in small children. Its zoonotic character, however, is doubted. All parasitic stages are parthenogenetic females. They are hair-thin, 2 to 3 mm in length, and parasitize the small intestine.

Occurrence. The parasites are found predominantly in humid, warm regions with minimum temperatures of 20 °C (prevalence of 10% and more), but less frequently in other geographical areas (Eastern and Southern Europe). Approximately 80 million people may be infected worldwide.

S. stercoralis is a cosmopolitan and occurs in dogs, cats, and monkeys, as well as in humans. For example, a study in Brazil showed a prevalence in dogs of 70%. *S. fuelleborni* is only found in the Old World in humans and primates.

Transmission. Infection occurs percutaneously by filariform third-stage larvae. In addition, galactogenous infections and autoinfections are important (see Fig. 4.46).

After percutaneous infection, the larvae migrate to the lung via lymph and blood vessels, penetrate the alveolar walls, and reach the small intestine via the trachea and esophagus. They invade the mucosa and pass two moltings to develop into adult, parthenogenetic females, which produce eggs after a prepatent period of at least 17 days. Galactogenous infections occur by women, immune to *Strongyloides* spp., where incoming larvae may settle in the breasts and in the surrounding tissue as hypobiotic larvae. They are activated during lactation and shed with the milk.

In the case of *S. stercoralis*, the first stage larvae hatch already in the intestine, whereas in the case of *S. fuelleborni*, eggs are shed that contain an embryo. In both cases, the infective larva develops in the environment. A particular characteristic of *S. stercoralis* is its ability to cause autoinfections when the first stage larvae molt to the infective stage already in the gut. Due to continuous autoinfections, *S. stercoralis* may persist for years in the host, controlled by an effective immune apparatus. Impairment of the immune system, however, may allow uncontrolled autoinfections, resulting in overwhelming worm populations.

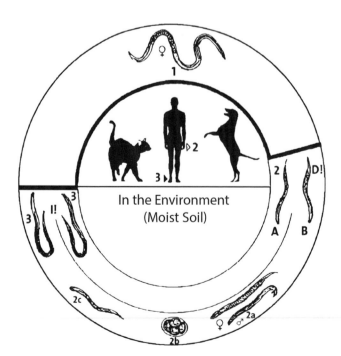

Figure 4.46 | Developmental cycle of *S. stercoralis*. (1) Adult parthenogenetic female *S. stercoralis* (2.2 to 2.5 mm) in the mucosa of the small intestine; (2) rhabditiform first-stage larva (0.20 to 0.25 mm) passed with feces (D, diagnostic stage); (2a) free-living male (0.7 to 0.9 mm) and female (ca. 1 mm) *S. stercoralis*; (2b) egg (0.07 mm) deposited by the free-living female; (2c) first-stage larva hatched from the egg; (3) filariform, infective third-stage larva (0.55 to 0.60 mm; I, infective stage) developed either via a free-living sexual worm generation or from a first-stage larva shed with the feces (2) invades percutaneously. The figure does not take into consideration endogenous autoinfections and possible repeated development of free-living generations.

Another peculiarity of the genus *Strongyloides* is its ability to switch from the parthenogenetic parasitic population to sexually propagating populations. When first stage larvae are released into the environment, besides the infective larvae, other larvae are formed that develop to free-living male or female worms, which multiply sexually. Subsequently, either further sexual cycles occur or new infective larvae develop. The molecular mechanisms of this change of generations are unclear but both exogenous factors, for example, dryness as an unsuitable condition for free-living stages and endogenous (host) factors (e.g., specific immunity) seem to play a role. In principle, this particular plasticity may represent a special survival strategy of the parasite.

Clinical Manifestations. Light infections are often asymptomatic. In chronic cases, patients suffer from abdominal pain, nausea, intermittent diarrhea, persisting for weeks, urticaria, and weight loss. Intermittently occurring urticaria may persist for 2 days and is accompanied by small cutaneous lesions resembling insect bites. Larva currens, that is, episodic meandering skin alterations that start from the anus and disappear after 2 days is pathognomonic. It is caused by autoinfections with third-stage larvae, which migrate in the skin. The high motile activity of the larvae (migration distances of 5 to 10 cm per h have been reported) allows a discrimination from cutaneous larva migrans. Dry cough is occasionally observed due to larvae invading the lung.

Severe, complicated forms of strongyloidiasis—hyperinfection syndrome, disseminated strongyloidiasis—with enterocolitis, malabsorption, sepsis due to extended damage of the mucosa, pulmonary hemorrhages, pneumonia, and meningitis are usually associated with the host's immunosuppression. Immunosuppression, either due to medication (e.g., application of systemic steroids) but also to intercurrent illness (HIV-1 and HIV infections, other diseases including parasitic infections with immunomodulating effects, e.g., kala azar) allows a dramatic increase of numbers of autoinfectious larvae, dissemination of the parasites, and involvement of multiple organs. Disseminated strongyloidiasis is associated with high mortality rates of more than 80%.

Diagnosis. The Baerman funnel and agar plate larva culture technique are used to detect *S. stercoralis* larvae in duodenal aspirates and in stools. The latter technique is more sensitive. The first-stage larvae, which can be isolated from fresh feces, measure 350 to 400 µm in length but are difficult to identify. The third-stage infective larva from culture techniques is more characteristic, that is, it is slender, 400 to 700 µm in length, and shows a long (40 to 45% of the body length) cylindric (filariform) esophagus. In the case of *S. fuelleborni* infections, eggs can be demonstrated by flotation or the SAF technique. Eggs measure 50 by 30 µm, have a thin shell, and contain an embryo. In both infections, examination of the duodenal juice gives more reliable results than fecal examination. If demonstration of larvae or eggs fails in suspected cases, serology or molecular probes can be employed. An ELISA using an extract of infective larvae is recommended. However, sensitivity and specificity of the assay are only partly satisfying.

Differential Diagnosis. A broad spectrum of abdominal diseases and cutaneous larva migrans must be considered.

Therapy. Because of the threat by hyperinfections, asymptomatic patients should be subjected to chemotherapy. Ivermectin, 200 µg/kg/day orally for 2 days is recommended. Albendazole, 400 mg twice a day orally for 7 days seems less effective. In case of hyperinfection, the anthelmintic treatment should be continued for 2 to 3 weeks and should be supported by symptomatic treatment and, if required, antibacterial therapy.

Prophylaxis. Barefoot walking should be avoided in areas of endemicity. In potentially endangered patients (e.g., patients returning from tropical areas) immunosuppressive treatment should not be done unless *Strongyloides* infections are excluded.

REFERENCES

Abrescia FF et al., Reemergence of strongyloidiasis, northern Italy. *Emerg. Infect. Dis.* 15, 1531–1533, 2009.

Agrawal V, Agarwal T, Goshal UC, Intestinal strongyloidiasis: a diagnosis frequently missed in the tropics. *Trans. R. Soc. Trop. Med. Hyg.* 103, 242–246, 2009.

Ashford RW, Barnish G, Viney ME, *Strongyloides fuelleborni kellyi*: infection and disease in Papua New Guinea. *Parasitol. Today* 6, 314–318, 1992.

Brügemann J et al., Two donor-related infections in a heart transplant recipient: one common, the other a tropical surprise. *J. Heart Lung Transplant.* 29, 1433–1437, 2010.

Buonfrate D et al., Severe strongyloidiasis: a systematic review of case reports. *BMC Infect. Dis.* 13, 78, 2013.

CDC, Notes from the field: strongyloidiasis in a rural setting in southeastern Kentucky, 2013. *MMWR Morb. Mortal. Wkly. Rep.* 62, 843, 2013.

Einsiedel L, Fernandes L, *Strongyloides stercoralis*: a cause of morbidity and mortality for indigenous people in Central Australia. *Intern. Med. J.* 38, 697–703, 2008.

Evans AC et al., Bushman children infected with the nematode *Strongyloides fülleborni*. *S. Afr. Med. J.* 80, 410–411, 1991.

Gill GV et al., Chronic *Strongyloides stercoralis* infection in former British Far East prisoners of war. *QJM* 97, 789–795, 2004.

Gonzaléz A et al., Clinical and epidemiological features of 33 imported *Strongyloides stercoralis* infections. *Trans. R. Soc. Trop. Med. Hyg.* 104, 613–616, 2010.

Hirata T et al., Increased detection rate of *Strongyloides stercoralis* by repeated stool examinations using the agar plate culture method. *Am. J. Trop. Med. Hyg.* 77, 683–684, 2007.

Koticha A et al., *Strongyloides stercoralis* hyperinfection syndrome in patients of prolonged steroid treatment : two case reports. *J. Indian Med. Ass.* 111, 272–274, 2013.

Lichtenberger P et al., Hyperinfection strongyloidiasis in liver transplant recipient treated with parenteral ivermectin. *Transpl. Infect. Dis.* 11, 137–142, 2009.

Marcos LA et al., *Strongyloides* hyperinfection syndrome: an emerging infectious disease. *Trans. R. Soc. Trop. Med. Hyg.* 102, 314–318, 2008.

Montes M, Shawhney C, Barros N, *Strongyloides stercoralis*: there but not seen. *Curr. Opin. Infect. Dis.* 23, 500–504, 2010.

Olsen A et al., Strongyloidiaisis – the most neglected of the tropical neglected diseases. *Trans. R.: Soc. Trop. Med. Hyg.* 103, 967–972, 2009.

Rets A, Gupta R, Haseeb MA, Determinants of reactivation of inapparent *Strongyloides stercoralis* infection in patients hospitalized for unrelated admitting diagnoses. *Eur. J. Gastroenterol. Hepatol.* 25, 1279–1285, 2013.

Roxby AC, Gottlieb GS, Limaye AP, Strongyloidiasis in transplant patients. *Clin. Infect. Dis.* 49, 1411–1423, 2009.

Schar F et al., *Strongyloides stercoralis*: global distribution and risk factors. *PloS Negl. Trop. Dis.* 7, e2288, 2013.

Vaiyavatjamai P et al., Immunocompromised group differences in the presentation of intestinal strongyliodiasis: *Jpn. J. Infect. Dis.* 61, 5–8, 2008.

Wang C et al., Strongyloidiasis: an emerging infectious disease in China. *Am. J. Trop. Med. Hyg.* 88, 420–425, 2013.

4.5.16 SYNGAMIASIS

Syngamiasis is a rare helminthiasis in which worms become established in the trachea and larynx.

Etiology. The agent, *Mammomonogamus laryngeus*, is a reddish-brown nematode measuring 6 mm (males) or up to 23 mm (females) in length. Worms live in the trachea attached to the mucosa, and are joined in copulo, presenting themselves in form of an upsilon (the male representing the short thigh).

Occurrence. The parasite occurs in Southeast Asia, India, Central and South America, and the Caribbean. Human infections (approximately 100 cases are so far known) are reported from the Caribbean, Brazil, and Southeast Asia. Natural hosts of *M. laryngeus* are cattle and other ruminants (buffaloes: prevalence of 30%), but the spectrum is rather broad, for example, it includes orangutans in Sumatra.

Transmission. Humans are infected by accidental oral ingestion of infective larvae either free or within the egg. The developmental cycle of *M. laryngeus* has not yet been completely elucidated; however, it may correspond with the cycle of other members of the family Syngamidae. Accordingly, the larvae invade the intestinal wall, are disseminated via the liver and heart to the lung, penetrate the alveolar wall and migrate upwards to their final destination. Eggs are first shed 3 weeks p.i. It is assumed that transport hosts (beetles, earthworms, and snails) may play a role in the infection of the natural hosts.

Clinical Manifestations. The major sign is a heavy, dry, chronic cough that develops approximately 1-week p.i. (incubation period). Hemoptysis may occur. Pulmonary symptoms are transient. Asthma-like symptoms have been observed.

Diagnosis. The worms can be demonstrated by endoscopy. Occasionally, they may be coughed up. Ellipsoid eggs (45 by 80 μm) can be observed in sputum and feces after the end of the prepatent period.

Differential Diagnosis. Provided no worms are found, all causes of a chronic, dry cough, for example, common cold and interstitional pneumonia must be considered.

Therapy. Recognized worms must be removed by endoscopy. Mebendazole, 200 mg/day orally for 10 days or 400 mg/day orally for 3 days is recommended.

Prophylaxis. Vegetables should be carefully washed. Blades of grass, etc., should not be put into the mouth.

REFERENCES

Castano JC et al., First report of *Mammomonogamus (Syngamus) lanryngeus* human infection in Colombia. *Biomedica* 26, 337–341, 2006.

Eamsobhana P et al., *Mammommonogamus* roundworm (Nematoda: Syngamidae) recovered from the duodenum of a Thai patient: a first and unusual case originating from Thailand. *Trans. R. Soc. Trop. Med. Hyg.* 100, 387–391, 2006.

Fiotová I et al., Presence and species identification of the gapeworm *Mammomnogamus laryngeus* (Raillet, 1899) (Syngamidae: Nematoda) in a semi-wild population of Sumatran orang utan (*Pongo abelii*) in Indonesia. *Res. Vet. Sci.* 84, 232–236, 2008.

Marques SM, Quadros RM, Pilati C, *Mammomonogamus laryngeus* (Railliet, 1899) infection in buffalos in Rio Grande do Sul, Brazil. *Vet. Parasitol.* 130, 241–243, 2005.

Turner P et al., A case of human syngamosis. *Travel Med. Infect. Dis.* 1, 231–233, 2003.

Van Aken D et al., *Mammomonogamus laryngeus* (Raillet, 1899) infections in cattle jn Mindanao, Philippines. *Vet. Parasitol.* 64, 329–332, 1996.

4.5.17 THELAZIASIS

Thelaziasis is an inflammatory disease of the conjunctiva caused by infestation with nematodes of the genus *Thelazia*.

Etiology. The major species infecting humans are *Thelazia callipaeda, T. californiensis, and*

T. rhodesi. They measure 9 mm (males) and 15 mm (females) in length.

Occurrence. *T. callipaeda* occurs in Southeast Asia and southern and Central Europe. The principle hosts are dogs and wild canids. *T. californiensis* is found in the western United States where it infects wild carnivores. *T. rhodesi* is a parasite of ruminants occurring throughout the Old World, particularly in southern Europe (Italy).

Transmission. The parasites are transmitted by insects with licking-sucking mouthparts, for example of the genus *Musca* and *Fannia*. The flies take up the first-stage larvae with conjunctival secretions. Third-stage larvae develop, which leave the insect through the mouthparts during licking, for example, of conjunctival fluid and establish in the conjunctival sack.

Clinical Manifestations. Thelaziasis is usually a mild disease and resembles a foreign-body conjunctivitis.

Diagnosis. The proof of thelaziasis is demonstration of the worms.

Therapy. Therapy consists of removal of the worms, eventually combined with irrigation.

Prophylaxis. Significant prophylactic measures are not known.

REFERENCES

Dutto M, Thelaziose oculaire chez l'homme en Italie du Nord. *Bull. Soc. Pathol. Exot.* 101, 9–10, 2008.

Kim HW et al., Intraocular infestation with *Thelazia callipaeda. Jpn. J. Ophthalmol.* 54 370–372, 2010.

Malacrida F et al., Emergence of canine ocular thelaziosis caused by *Thelazia callipaeda* in southern Switzerland. *Vet. Parasitol.* 157, 321–327, 2008.

Otranto D, Dutto M, Human thelaziasis, Europe. *Emerg. Infect. Dis.* 14, 647–649, 2008.

Shen J et al., Human thelaziosis – a neglected parasitic disease of the eye. *J. Parasitol.* 92, 872–875, 2006.

Sohn WM, Na BK, Yoo JM, Two cases of human thelaziasis and brief review of Korean cases. *Korean J. Parasitol.* 49, 265–271, 2011.

Viriyavejakul P et al., *Thelazia callipaeda*: a human case report. *SE Asian J. Trop. Med. Public Health* 43, 851–85, 2012.

Xue C, Tian N, Huang Z, *Thelazia callipaeda* in human vitreous. *Can. J. Ophthalmol.* 42, 884–885, 2007.

Yagi T et al., Removal of *Thelazia callipaeda* from the sub-conjunctival space. *Eur. J. Ophthalmol.* 17, 266–268, 2007.

4.5.18 TRICHINELLOSIS (TRICHINOSIS)

Trichinellosis (trichinosis) is a mild to fatal disease that occurs after infection with nematodes that settle in the intestine and release larvae, which invade the striated muscles.

Etiology. The agents belong to a complex of species with 12 currently known gene pools. Nine of these pools are identified with named species: *Trichinella spiralis, T. nativa, T. britovi, T. murrelli, T. nelsoni,* and *T. patagoniensis,* belonging to the so-called encapsulated clade, and *T. pseudospiralis, T. papuae,* and *T. zimbabwensis,* the members of the so-called nonencapsulated clade. Three additional genotypes, T 6, T 8, and T 9, are closely related to *T. nativa, T. britovi,* and *T. murrelli,* respectively. The species differ in inducing a collagen capsule, surrounding the infective larva in the muscle cell ("encapsulated") or not ("nonencapsulating"), and with regard to infectivity and pathogenicity to various host species, to ecology as well as to their geographic occurrence (Tab. 4.11).

Occurrence. The genus is almost globally distributed. Australia seems the only continent free of autochthonous infections. The parasites occur more frequently in temperate climates than in the tropics.

T. spiralis and *T. pseudospiralis* are cosmopolitans, while *T. nativa* and genotype T6 are found in the arctic and subarctic zones of the Holoarctis. *T. britovi* occurs in the temperate zone of the Palearctic region and *T. nelsoni* and genotype T8 are found in tropical Africa. *T. murrelli* occurs in the temperate zone of North America and genotype T 9 was reported from Japan. *T. patagoniensis* was recently found in a cougar in Argentina. *T. papuae* is present in New Guinea, and *T. zimbabwensis* is a parasite in Sub-Sahara Africa. Species found in Europe are *T. britovi, T. spiralis, T. nativa,* and, increasingly *T. pseudospiralis.*

The genus shows limited host specificity. All species parasitize in mammals, the three species that form nonencapsulated muscle stages, in addition, invade birds (*T, pseudospiralis*), reptiles including turtles (*T. papuae*), or predominantly reptiles (*T. zimbabwensis*). Although all species can infect mammals, host-parasite relationships vary. Reproductivity and persistence, for example, in pigs, are high in the case of *T. spiralis,* moderate or less in the cases of *T. britovi, T. nelsoni,* and *T. papuae,* and low in the other species.

Human infections are common in Eastern Europe, the former Soviet Union, Kenya, Alaska, and continental Asia. In Poland, three to 15 human infections became known per year in 1989 to 1993. Based on necropsies, a prevalence of 2% was estimated in Chile in 1992. More than 20 000 cases, including 230 deaths, were notified from 1964 to 1997 in China, and still 828 cases with 11 deaths in 2000 to 2003. The mean incidence of human trichinellosis in the European Union came to 0.1 per 100 000 inhabitants in 2008 (altogether 670 cases). Escalated rates exist in Lithuania, Bulgaria (0.9), and particularly Romania (2.3; regionally >80). In the United States, there were approximately 400 cases per year, in which 10 to 15 of them were fatal, were notified in the middle of the last century; altogether 230 cases with three deaths were reported for the years 1991 to 1996; 66 cases were observed from 2002 to 2007.

Eight of the 12 known *Trichinella* species/genotypes were found in humans (see Tab. 4.11). In the other cases, their partly limited occurrence and particular ecology may be the reasons for not having been found so far involved in human trichinellosis. However, it cannot be excluded that they are also able to cause illness in humans under suitable circumstances. For example, *T. zimbabwensis* is highly pathogenic at least to monkeys after experimental infections.

Transmission. Humans become infected after consumption of raw or undercooked meat. Infestation is almost limited to the striated musculature (Fig. 4.47). An important source of

Table 4.11 | *Trichinella* spp. and genotypes: geographic distribution and host spectrum

SPECIES/GENOTYPE	GEOGRAPHICAL DISTRIBUTION	MAIN NATURAL HOST SPECTRUM	INFECT. PIGS/ WILD BOARS	HUMAN INFECTION REPORTED	COMMENTS
Encapsulated clade					
T. spiralis	Cosmopolitan	Pigs, wild boars, carnivores, rodents	+++	Yes	Low cold resistance
T. nativa	Arctic/subarctic region	Carnivores (terrestrial and marine)	+/−	Yes	High cold resistance
Genotype T6[1]	Canada, USA	Carnivores	?	Yes	High cold resistance
T. britovi	Europe, Northwest Africa, Southwest Asia	Carnivores, wild boar	++	Yes	Moderate cold resistance
Genotype T8[2]	South Africa, Namibia	Carnivores	?	No[5]	
T. murrelli	North America	Carnivores	−	Yes	
Genotype T9[3]	Japan	Carnivores	?	No[5]	
T. nelsoni	East and South Africa	Wild animals, predominantly carnivores	+/−	Yes[6]	Not resistant to coldness, long survival in dead tissue
T. patagoniensis	South America (Argentina)	Wild carnivores	+/−	No[5]	
Nonencapsulated clade					
T. pseudospiralis[4]	Cosmopolitan	Carnivores, pigs, birds	+	Yes	Not resistant to coldness
T. papuae	Papua New Guinea	Domestic and wild pigs, reptiles	++	Yes	
T. zimbabwensis	*Sub*-saharan Africa	Reptiles, various mammals	+	No[7]	

[1] Closely related to *T. nativa*.
[2] Closely related to *T. britovi*.
[3] Closely related to *T. murrelli*.
[4] Three genotypes (Palearctic, Neoarctic, Australian type).
[5] Limited occurrence of the species/genotype must be considered.
[6] Not verified on a molecular level.
[7] Highly pathogenic in nonhuman primates after experimental infection.

infection is the pig; 58% of cases reported in the United States (1991 to 1996) could be related to this source. In Central Europe, infested pig meat had been the source of infection in more than 2000 cases since 1970. Meanwhile, infection rates in pigs decreased markedly, particularly in areas with industrial approaches to pig farming. In the European Union, current mean incidences in pigs might be 0.1 to 1.0 per 10^6 slaughtered pigs. In the United States, the prevalence in pigs varies, but might be, in general, a thousand times higher.

However, in Romania, which is a highly endemic area, still 0.1% of slaughtered pigs were found infected with *Trichinella* spp. in 2004. Linkages resulting in infections of pigs may occur through infected rodents that represent competitors of the pig at the tough, at least

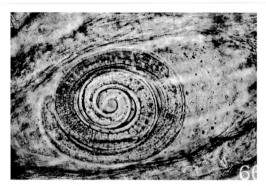

Figure 4.47 | *Trichinella spiralis* larvae in the musculature (squeezing preparation) (picture: Institute for Parasitology, Giessen, Germany).

under backyard farming conditions. Furthermore, it should not be overlooked that a certain amount of risk exists in particular types of organic pig production, when, for example, in Europe, sylvatic cycles with the fox as host of *T. britovi* merge with the domestic cycle that predominantly involves *T. spiralis*. Free-range pigs were definitely shown to be infected with *Trichinella* spp. to a larger extent than conventionally reared animals.

An important role is also played in Europe by wild boars (>1700 human cases since 1970). Prevalence rates in this species yield up to 0.5% and 0.9% in Poland and Romania, respectively. In particular countries, other special sources of infection may be important. Thus, considerable epidemics have been seen in France and Italy since 1975 (3000 cases) after consumption of infected horsemeat. The horses had mostly been imported from North and South America (the epidemiological details, leading to infection of horses are not known). In North Africa, humans became infected after eating the meat of camels. Bears or marine mammals (walruses) are important transmitters in other geographical regions. Epidemics were also reported after consumption of meat from a cougar or from dogs and—due to particular animal feeding conditions in China—from sheep and goats.

The larvae are released from the ingested musculature by digestion and they invade the mucosa of the upper small intestine. They develop within a few days between the lamina propria and the epithelium to adult worms and start producing larvae. The adult parasites survive for 4 to 6 weeks during which, in the case of *T. spiralis*, 1000 to 1500 larvae per female worm are produced and released in a suitable host. The larvae measure 80 μm in length, are lymphogenously spread, and invade the striated muscle cells, which are transformed by the parasite to nurse cells. The larvae grow to a length of 1 mm after 4 weeks and begin to coil. Subsequently, within 5 to 6 weeks, except for *T. pseudospiralis*, *T. papuae*, and *T. zimbabwensis*, they are encapsulated. The cycle closes without any phase in the environment when larvae (they must be at least 17 days old) are ingested by a new host. The developmental cycle of *T. spiralis* is shown in Fig. 4.48.

Encapsulated larvae survive and remain infectious even when the capsule is calcified. The survival time of *T. spiralis* in humans may be >30 years. Obviously, the larvae of *T. britovi* die earlier.

Clinical Manifestations. The severity of the disease depends on the number of ingested larvae and the *Trichinella* species. Approximately 70 larvae are suggested as the minimum dose to cause disease in humans in the case of *T. spiralis* [for example, larval counts in pigs yielded 7.4 and 188 larvae per g musculature in the hind leg, after moderate (1000 larvae) and heavy experimental infections (20 000 larvae), respectively].

The incubation period may vary (6 to 40 days). In the beginning (the intestinal phase) gastrointestinal symptoms prevail, that is, nausea, vomiting, epigastric pains, and diarrhea or constipation; fever is usually low. With the onset of the visceral phase during the second to eighth week p.i., additional symptoms are headache, arthralgias, increasing fever, cough, myalgias, conjunctivitis, and hemorrhages. Neurologic complications, for example, deafness, encephalitis, and convulsions, are observed. Facial edema, particularly periorbital edema, is an important sign. Maculopapular exanthems are observed rather often. The overall symptoms of fatigue, weakness, headache, arthralgias, and anorexia

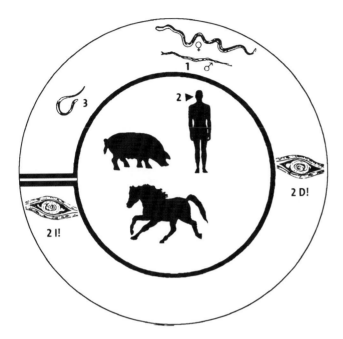

Figure 4.48 | Developmental cycle of *Trichinella spiralis*. (1) Adult male (1.0 to 1.6 mm) and female *T. spiralis* (3.0 to 4.0 mm) in the mucosa of the small intestine (e.g., of pigs, horses, humans); (2) encapsulated *T. spiralis* larva (capsule, 0.4 to 0.5 mm) in striated muscle (D, diagnostic stage; I. infective stage); (3) free larva of *T. spiralis* (0.8 to 1 mm) in the small intestine.

resemble those of influenza. Clinical symptoms may cease after a few days but may also persist for 5 to 6 weeks. In severe infections, patients are impaired by myalgia to such an extent that swallowing, speaking, breathing, and chewing become difficult. The most frequent cause of death in fatal cases is myocarditis due to invasion of the cardiac muscle and subsequent heart failure. The previously high death rate in *Trichinella* infections can be avoided by improved diagnostic techniques and treatment. After remission of acute signs, even untreated patients usually become asymptomatic in spite of persisting *Trichinella* larvae in the musculature. However, late sequelae with rheumatoid complaints, myalgia, and cardiac symptoms are possible (chronic trichinellosis). *T. spiralis* and *T. nativa* are generally more virulent in humans than the other species; in particular, the intestinal phase is more severe.

Diagnosis. The clinical picture and the fact that clusters of people are involved allow presumptive diagnosis. However, one must consider that incubation time and severity of the symptoms may vary depending on the number of larvae ingested.

Patients should be asked about consumption of raw or undercooked meat, for example, of pigs or wild boars, or in countries where official meat inspection includes the examination for *Trichinella*, whether inspection was performed properly. Leftover meat should be examined for *Trichinella* larvae.

Eosinophilia that occurs 1 week after infection and persists for 2 to 3 months and increased levels of muscle-specific enzymes (creatine phosphokinase, lactic dehydrogenase, and hydroxybutyrate dehydrogenase) are suggestive of the diagnosis. Involvement of the cardiac muscle suggests severe infection.

Serologic investigations are important. Assays indicative of the infection in the second to fifth week are the indirect immunofluorescence test employing encysted larvae as antigens and ELISAs using extracts or excretory-secretory products of muscle larvae. Excretory-secretory antigens of the so-called TSL-1 group respond to the several species. Appearance of antibodies may be delayed after *T. britovi* infections in comparison with antibody responses to *T. spiralis*; however, there is usually good correlation between antibody titers (first occurrence and levels) and the infectious dose. Maximum antibody levels are observed in the second and third month p.i.

Trichinella larvae can be directly demonstrated in muscle biopsy specimens (Fig. 4.47). The density of larvae in the muscle depends on the duration of the infection and the infectious dose, that is, attempts to demonstrate larvae may fail early after infection. Chronic forms of trichinellosis may be difficult to diagnose. Antibody levels decrease continuously in long-lasting infections, even in the presence of living larvae. Thus, only positive data are of diagnostic value.

Species determinations on a morphological basis are neither possible with adult parasites nor with larvae but may be performed at the molecular level. An International Trichinella Reference Centre (http://www.iss.it/site/Trichi nella/index.asp) provides assistance with diagnostic problems.

Differential Diagnosis. Influenza, myalgia, enteritis, and cardiac disorders of other etiology must be excluded. *Sarcocystis* infections, which can also develop after ingestion of raw or undercooked pork, must be considered because of similar intestinal disorders.

Therapy. Patients are treated with albendazole, 400 mg twice a day orally for 8 to 14 days or mebendazole, 200 to 400 mg three times a day orally for 3 days, subsequently 400 to 500 mg three times a day for 10 days. Corticosteroids, 1 mg/kg/day, are used for critically ill patients suffering from severe myositis and myocarditis.

Prophylaxis. Meat, particularly from carnivorous and omnivorous animals, should not be eaten raw or undercooked unless it is properly examined for *Trichinella* larvae. According to European Union law, pigs and solid-hoofed animals, but also wild boars, bears, badgers, nutrias, and some other animals, are to be subjected to official inspection for contamination with *Trichinella* if the meat is scheduled for consumption by humans (EG, Edict No. 2075/2005). Under certain circumstances, systemic *Trichinella* testing can be replaced by a risk-based surveillance system.

Freezing of meat is supposed to be equivalent to direct examination provided the meat is kept at a temperature of −25 °C for 10 to 20 days depending on the thickness of the cut. Reasonable doubts, however, are indicated, whether this regulation is sufficient in regard to the high resistance of *T. britova, T. nativa,* and *Trichinella* T6 to low temperatures. The efficacy of high pressure processing of the meat as an alternative technique can currently not be adequately judged. Pickling and smoking do not always kill the larvae. This must be particularly considered in the case of uncooked sausages, which in some areas may contain wild boar meat. *Trichinella* larvae are killed in food (uncooked sausages or ham) only if the proportion of salt exceeds 4% and the water content is <25%.

REFERENCES

Akar S et al., Frequency and severity of musculoskeletal symptoms in humans during an outbreak of trichinellosis caused by *Trichinella britovi. J. Parasitol.* 93, 341–344, 2007.

Alban L et al., Towards a standardised surveillance for *Trichinella* in the European Union. *Prev. Vet. Med.* 99, 148–160, 2011.

Balecu A et al., Identifying risk factors for symptoms of severe trichinellosis – a case study of 143 infected persons in Brasov, Romania, 2001–2008. *Vet. Parasitol.* 194, 106–109, 2013.

Blaga R et al., Animal *Trichinella* infection in Romania: geographical heterogeneity for the last 8 years. *Vet. Parasitol.* 159, 290–294, 2009.

Boutsini S et al., Emerging *Trichinella britovi* infections in free ranging pigs in Greece. *Vet. Parasitol.* 199, 278–282, 2014.

Cacagno M. A. et al., Description of an outbreak of human trichinellosis in an area of Argentina historically regarded as *Trichinella*-free: the importance of surveillance studies. *Vet. Parasitol.* 200, 251–256, 2014.

Cui J, Wang ZQ, Kennedy MW, The re-emergence of trichinellosis in China? *Trends Parasitol.* 22, 54–55, 2006.

European Community, Regulation (EC) no. 2075/2005 of the European Parliament and of the Council of 5 December 2005 laying down specific rules on official control for *Trichinella* in meat. *Off. J. Eur. Commun.* 338, 60–82, 2005.

Gajadhar AA et al., *Trichinella* diagnostics and control: mandatory and best practices for ensuring food safety. *Vet. Parasitol.* 159, 197–205, 2009.

Kennedy ED et al., Trichinellosis surveillance – United States, 2002–2007. *MMWR Surveill. Summ.* 58, 1–7, 2009.

Kusolsuk T et al., The second outbreak of trichinellosis caused by *Trichinella papuae* in Thailand. *Trans. R. Soc. Trop. Med. Hyg.* 104, 433–437, 2010.

Lo YC et al., Human trichinosis after consumption of soft-shelled turtles, Taiwan. *Emerg. Infect. Dis.* 15, 2056–2058, 2009.

Marucci G, Pezzotti P, Pozio E, Ring trial among National Reference Laboratories for parasites to detect *Trichinella spiralis* larvae in pork samples according to the EU directive 2075/2005. *Vet. Parasitol.* 159, 337–340, 2009.

Moller LN et al., *Trichinella* infection in a hunting community in East Greenland. *Epidemiol. Infect.* 138, 1252–1256, 2010.

Neghina R et al., Trichinellosis and poverty in a Romanian industrial area: an epidemiological study and brief review of literature. *Foodborne Pathog. Dis.* 7, 757–761, 2010.

Porto-Fett AC et al., Evaluation of fermentation, drying, and/or high pressure processing on viability of *Listeria monocytogenes*, *Escherichia coli* O157:H7, *Salmonella* spp., and *Trichinella spiralis* in raw pork and Genoa salami. *Int. J. Food Microbiol.* 140, 61–75, 2010.

Pozio E et al., Molecular taxonomy, phylogeny and biography of nematodes belonging to the *Trichinella* genus. *Infect. Genet. Evol.* 9, 606–616, 2009.

Ribicich M et al., Evaluation of the risk of transmission of *Trichinella* in pork production systems in Argentina. *Vet. Parasitol.* 159, 350–535, 2009.

Schuppers ME et al., A study to demonstrate freedom from *Trichinella* spp. in domestic pigs in Switzerland. *Zoonoses Public Health* 57, e 130-5.doi:10.1111/j.1863-2378.2009.01299.x, 2009.

Tint D et al., Cardiac involvement in trichinellosis: a case of left ventricular thrombosis. *Am. J. Trop. Med. Hyg.* 81, 313–316, 2009.

Zimmer IA et al., Detection and surveillance for animal trichinellosis in GB. *Vet. Parasitol.* 151, 233–241, 2008.

4.5.19 TRICHOSTRONGYLIDIASIS

Trichostrongylidiasis (Trichostrongylosis) is a usually mild gastrointestinal disease due to nematodes of ruminants.

Etiology. The trichostrongyles occurring in humans belong mainly to the genus *Trichostrongylus* or more rarely to the genera *Marshallagia* or *Mecistocyrrus*. In natural ruminant hosts, the parasites develop up to a length of 40 mm and inhabit the abomasum (the third compartment of the stomach of ruminants) and the small intestine.

Occurrence. Trichostrongyles are found worldwide, with varying geographical distribution of the different genera and species. All herbivorous animals kept on pastures are usually infected with various species. Young animals are usually more heavily infected than older animals. Human infections are known from all continents. The prevalence is often high; for example, in parts of the Middle East (Iran and Iraq), 25% of the inhabitants may be infected.

Transmission. Trichostrongyles are transmitted by oral ingestion of infective third-stage larvae contaminating plant material. They develop from eggs that are excreted by infected ruminants. The third stage is reached within one to several weeks dependent on the environmental temperature.

Infections are common in people living in close contact with animals, for example, under the same roof and burning animal feces in fires. Forming and drying for this purpose of older feces that already contain infective larvae, easily results in contamination of the hands. Infections can also occur via contaminated vegetables or drinking water. The larvae pass through a short tissue phase in the crypts or glands of the stomach/small intestine and develop to mature worms that start to produce eggs 3 weeks after infection.

Clinical Manifestations. In light infections, patients are asymptomatic or suffer from mild, gastrointestinal disorders. Severe infections cause persistent diarrhea and sometimes colicky abdominal pain. Anemia has been reported occasionally.

Diagnosis. The diagnosis is based on the demonstration of thin-shelled eggs of 90 by 50 μm. Shape, size, and blastomeres inside allow differentiation from eggs of other intestinal nematodes. The diagnosis can be confirmed by cultivation of third-stage larvae, which are characteristically shaped according to the genus.

Differential Diagnosis. Enteritis of other etiology must be ruled out.

Therapy. Pyrantel pamoate, 11 mg/kg (max. 1 g) orally, or albendazole, 400 mg orally, or mebendazole 100 mg twice a day for 3 days orally, are recommended.

Prophylaxis. Personal hygiene (cleaning the hands after contact with potentially contaminated material) reduces the risk of contracting trichostrongylidiasis. Adequate cleaning and cooking of all vegetables are important precautions.

REFERENCES

Becouet R et al., Contribution à l'étude de la trichostrongylose humaine (à propos de 71 observations). *Ann. Soc. Belg. Med. Trop.* 62, 139–155, 1982.

Boreham RE et al., Human trichostrongyliasis in Queensland. *Pathology* 27, 182–185, 1995.

El Shazly AM et al., Intestinal parasites in Dakahlia governate, with different techniques in diagnosing protozoa. *J. Egypt. Soc. Parasitol.* 36, 1023–1034, 2006.

Lattes S et al., *Trichostrongylus colubriformis* nematode infections in humans, *France. Emerg. Infect. Dis.* 17, 1301–1302, 2011.

Phosuk I et al., Molecular evidence of *Trichostrongylus colubriformis* and *Trichostrongylus axei* infections in humans from Thailand and Lao PDR. *Am. J. Trop. Med. Hyg.* 89, 376–379, 2013.

Ralph A et al., Abdominal pain and eosinophilia in suburban goat keepers –trichostrongylosis. *Med. J. Aust.* 184, 467–469, 2006.

Thibert JB, Guiguen C, Gangneux JP, Human trichostrongylidosis: case report and microscopic difficulties to indentify ancylostomidae eggs. *Ann. Biol. Clin.* 64, 281–285, 2006.

Watthanakulpanich D et al., Prevalence and clinical aspects of human *Trichostrongylus colubriformis* infection in Lao PDR. *Acta Trop.* 126, 37–42, 2013.

Yong TS et al., Differential diagnosis of *Trichostrongylus* and hookworm eggs via PCR using ITS-1 sequence. *Korean J. Parasitol.* 45, 69–74, 2007.

4.5.20 OTHER ZOONOTIC INFECTIONS BY NEMATODES

Physaloptera caucasica (order Spirurida) is found in the digestive tract (esophagus up to the small intestine) of monkeys of the suborder Simiae. It is the only species of the genus also found in humans. Human infection was common at least in the early 20th century in tropical Africa. The developmental cycle is not known. The infection probably occurs by ingestion of beetles, crickets, or cockroaches that contain infective larvae. The large parasites (up to 10 cm long) attach to the mucosa and cause inflammation and erosions. Due to the variable location of the worms from the esophagus to the small intestine, the clinical picture may vary from vomiting to bloody diarrhea and abdominal pain. The eggs, found in the feces, are 50 by 40 μm in size and contain an embryo. Treatment should use benzimidazoles, eventually administered for a longer period.

Ternidens deminutus occurs in the large intestine of various simian hosts in Africa and Asia. Infections of humans are known with a variable prevalence in southern Africa. The developmental cycle is not clear; however, it seems the parasite develops without intermediate hosts, and infection occurs by oral ingestion of a third-stage larva. *T. deminutus* sucks blood and microcytic, hypochromic anemia has been reported in severe infections. Occasionally, nodules have been found as in oesophagostomiasis (see "Oesophagostomiais"; chapter 4.5.13). Diagnosis is based on the demonstration of eggs, which are 80 by 50 μm in size and thin-shelled, with blastomeres, and resemble those of hookworms, oesophagostomes, and trichostrongyles. For treatment and prophylaxis, see "Oesophagostomiasis" above.

Roundworm infections with *Ascaris lumbricoides* belong to the most common helminthiases in humans. Globally >1200 million people may be infected. A high prevalence is particularly found in developing countries under inadequate hygienic conditions. In contrast, human *Ascaris* infections are observed only sporadicaly and with unclear epidemiology in areas with high hygienic standards, for example, in industrial countries in Central Europe. Genetic analyses showed that such cases in Denmark were caused by *A. suum*, a common pig parasite, which cannot be morphologically differentiated from *A. lumbricoides*, whereas the agent in human roundworm infections in tropical countries is exclusively the latter species. This means that ascariasis in Denmark is a zoonosis and it seems probable that the situation is similar in other industrial countries as well. There is, however, an open discussion on whether *A. lumbricoides* and *A. suum* represent, not two, but one single species.

A. suum behaves in humans in accordance with *A. lumbricoides*. The infection occurs by ingestion of embyonated eggs (see *Toxocara* spp.; chapter 4.5.12). The larvae hatch in the intestine, and after a heart-lung-migration they reach the pharynx via the trachea, are swallowed, and settle in the small intestine. After experimental infections of humans with *A. suum*, fewer and smaller worms developed than after infections with *A. lumbricoides*. The prepatent period lasted 8 to 10 weeks. In the course of the larval migration in humans, symptoms may develop that resemble "Larva Migrans Visceralis" (see chapter 4.5.12). The intestinal phase is often asymptomatic but may be associated with vomiting, abdominal pain, and diarrhea. Mebendazole, albendazole, and pyrantel pamoate are effective drugs against *A. suum*. Effective prophylaxis needs proper hygiene in handling pigs and pig manure.

Toxocara cati (see chapter 4.5.12) was also found at an adult stage in children (>20 cases). In these cases it is supposed that larval stages of the parasite (fourth stages?) were ingested, which are commonly shed by puppies with heavy infections.

REFERENCES

Eberhard ML, Alfano E, Adult *Toxocara cati* infection in US children: report of four cases. *Am. J. Trop. Med. Hyg.* 59, 404–406, 1998.

Anderson TJC, *Ascaris* infections in humans in North America: Molecular evidence for cross-infection. *Parasitology* 110, 215–219, 1995.

Fisher M, *Toxocara cati:* an underestimated zoonotic agent. *Trends Parasitol.* 19, 167–170, 2003.

Goldsmith JM, The African hookworm problem: an overview. In: *Parasitic helminths and zoonoses in Africa* (eds. MacPherson CNL, Craig PS), Unwin Hyman London, pp 101–137, 1991.

Hemsrichart V, *Ternidens deminutus* infection: first pathological report of a human case in Asia. *J. Med. Assoc. Thai.* 88, 1140–1143, 2005.

Liu GH et al., Comparative analyses of the complete mitochondrial genomes of *Ascaris lumbricoides* and *Ascaris suum* from humans and pigs. *Gene* 492, 110–116, 2012.

Nejsum P et al., Ascariasis is a zoonosis in Denmark. *J. Clin. Microbiol.* 43, 1142–1148, 2005.

Nejsum P et al., Assessing the zoonotic potential of *Ascaris suum* and *Trichuris suis*: looking to the future from an analysis of the past. *J. Helminthol.* 86, 148–155, 2012.

Schindler AR et al., Definition of genetic markers in nuclear ribosomal DNA for a neglected parasite of primates, *Ternidens deminutus* (Nematoda: Strongylida) – diagnostic and epidemiological implications. *Parasitology* 131, 539–546, 2005.

4.6 Zoonoses Caused by Acanthocephala

4.6.1 ACANTHOCEPHALIOSIS

Acanthocephaliosis is an uncommon human intestinal disease. Clinical symptoms are rare. It is caused by Acanthocephala ("thorny-headed worms"), a class of the phylum Nemathelmintha.

Etiology. The class Acanthocephala includes three orders with numerous species that infest mammals, birds, fish, and reptiles. Agents of human disease are predominantly *Macracanthorhynchus* (*M.*) *hirudinaceus, Moniliformis* (*Mo.*) *moniliformis*, and *M. ingens*. As the class is not very host specific, other species (*Acanthocephalus rauschi, A. buffoni, Bolbosoma* spp., and *Corynosoma strumosum*) may invade humans.

The body of acanthocephalans is cylindrical and bears an evaginable proboscis anteriorly, which is an armed structure with rows of hooks (Fig. 4.49), which is inserted into the intestinal mucosa of the host. Acanthocephala lack an intestine and absorb their nourishment through their tegument like cestodes. They are heterosexual with marked sex dimorphism. Some species are considerably large. *M. hirudinaceus* grows up to 5 to 9 cm (males) or 20 to 65 cm (females) in length. *Mo. moniliformis* in rats reach lengths of 3 to 5 cm (males) and 14 to 27 cm (females). In humans, these parasites

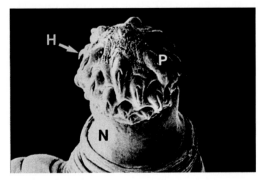

Figure 4.49 | *Macracanthorhynchus hirudinaceus* (Acanthocephala): front end with retractable proboscis (P) with hooks (H) and neck (H) (picture: H. Taraschewski, Karlsruhe, Germany).

are smaller. The length of worms of other genera occasionally detected in humans is approximately 1 cm.

Occurrence. The giant thorny-headed worm *M. hirudinaceus* is found almost worldwide in pigs and wild boars. It is common in southeastern Europe and in Asia but rare in Central and Western Europe. *M. ingens* is a parasite of pigs and raccoons. *Mo. moniliformis* is a cosmopolitan with a broad host spectrum. Rodents are the main final hosts. The genus *Acanthocephalus* is found in Asia in amphibia. *Bolbosoma* spp. and *C. strumosum* infest marine mammals.

Human acanthocephaliosis is generally a rare disease; however, it seems to be relatively common in some areas of China.

Transmission. Acanthocephalans develop through a two-host cycle. Intermediate hosts are Crustacea, Myriapoda and insects; *M. hirudinaceus* and *Mo. moniliformis* are transmitted by beetles and cockroaches. Humans are infected by ingestion of these intermediate hosts. Apart from accidental ingestion, special eating habits play a role. In some areas, for example, China, roasted beetles and cockroaches are used as traditional remedies. It is also epidemiologically important that some *Acanthocephalus, Bolbosoma*, and *Corynosoma* species use fish, amphibians, and reptiles as paratenic hosts. Thus, infections may be transmitted when these animals are eaten raw or undercooked.

The female parasites produce eggs with a thick, multilayered shell that carry a hooked embryo, the acanthor larva. Eggs are ingested by the arthropods, and the larvae encyst as a cystacanth in the intermediate host. In the case of *M. hirudinaceus*, beetle larvae (e.g., larvae of the cockchafer) become infested. The cystacanths develop within 10 to 12 weeks, persist throughout the pupal stage, and they are found in the mature beetle.

Clinical Manifestations. The usual symptoms, diarrhea and abdominal pain, are nonspecific. However, as the parasites insert their probiscis deeply in the mucosa, perforation of the intestine and subsequent peritonitis may occur.

Occasionally, the parasites are found in granulomas on the serosa in the peritoneal cavity.

Diagnosis. The ovoid, thick-shelled eggs in the feces are pathognomonic. In the case of *M. hirudinaceus*, they are 60 to 90 µm in size and dark brown with irregular surface. Eggs of *Mo. moniliformis* have a similar size, are semitransparent, and therefore, show the hooked larva.

Differential Diagnosis. Intestinal disorders of other etiology must be considered.

Therapy. Niclosamide (one 2 g dose) can be used as therapy. Ivermectin was effective in *M. hirudinaceus* infected pigs. Benzimidazoles are inefficient. Bowel perforation requires surgical intervention.

Prophylaxis. Care should be taken to avoid contamination of food with beetles and cockroaches. Raw or undercooked crustaceans and fish should not be eaten.

REFERENCES

Arizono N, Kuramochi T, Kagei N, Molecular and histological identification of the acanthocephalan *Bolbosoma cf. capitatum* from the human small intestine. *Parasitol. Int.* 61, 715–718, 2012.

Beaver PC et al., Acanthocephalan, probably *Bolsoma*, from the peritoneal cavity of a man in Japan. *Am. J. Trop. Med. Hyg.* 32, 1016–1018, 1983.

Berenji F, Fata A, Hosseininejad Z, A case of *Moniliformis moniliformis* (Acanthocephala) infection in Iran. *Korean J. Parasitol.* 45, 145–148, 2007.

Ikeh EI, Anosike JC, Okon E, Acanthocephalan infection in man in northern Nigeria. *J. Helminthol.* 66, 241–242, 1992.

Leng YJ, Huang WD, Liang PN, Human infection with *Macracanthorhynchus hirudinaceus* Travassos, 1916 in Guangdong Province, with notes on its prevalence in China. *Ann. Trop. Med. Parasitol.* 77, 107–109, 1983.

Messina AF et al., *Moniliformis moniliformis* infection in two Florida toddlers. *Pediatr. Infect. Dis.* 30, 726–727, 2011.

Prociv P et al., First record of human acanthocephalan infections in Australia. *Med. J. Aust.* 152, 215–216, 1990.

Radomyos P, Chobchuanchom A, Tungtrongchitr A, Intestinal perforation due to *Macracanthorhynchus hirudinaceus* infection in Thailand. *Trop. Med. Parasitol.* 40, 476–477, 1989.

Sahar MM et al., A child with an acanthocephalan infection. *Ann. Saudi Med.* 26, 321–324, 2006.

4.7 Zoonoses Caused by Arthropods

The phylum Arthropoda consists of more than a million described species. A small number of these invertebrates, including representatives of all arthropod classes (Arachnida, Diplopoda, Chilopoda, Insecta, Crustacea) affect the health of humans and animals directly or indirectly. The role of arthropods as vectors of pathogenic agents is described in the respective chapters. Of particular zoonotic importance are arachnids with ticks and mites as pathogens and some groups of insects, that is, bugs, dipterans, and fleas, which will be discussed in some detail. Lice are not included as zoonotic agents because they are highly host-specific as lice of animals do not infest humans.

REFERENCES

Aspöck H (ed.), *Krank durch Arthropoden.* Denisia, Oberösterreichisches Landesmuseum Linz, Austria, ISBN 1608–8700, 2010.

Kettle DS (ed.), *Medical and Veterinary Entomology. 2nd ed.: Wallingford: CAB International.* ISBN 0–85196-83, 1995.

Mullen G, Durden L (eds.),*Medical and Veterinary Entomology.* London: Academic Press. ISBN 0–12-510451–0, 2002.

4.7.1 ZOONOSES CAUSED BY TICKS

Ticks, like mites, belong to the class Arachnida and to the subclass Acari. Ticks are obligate, bloodsucking ectoparasites, with sometimes low host specificity and vectors of a variety of important pathogens of humans and animals (viruses, bacteria, rickettsiae, protozoa, and helminths) (Table 4.13). Pathogens are mostly transmitted via saliva during blood feeding but transmission may also occur through excrements of the ticks, for example, in the cases of *Coxiella burnetii*, which causes Q-fever, or, in case of argasid ticks, via the coxal fluid, as in the case of spirochetes, the agents of relapsing fever.

Bites of ticks may cause local skin irritations, hemorrhages and edemas due to toxic secretion of the salivary glands. Toxins of some tick species can cause fever, spasms, and paralysis (tick toxicosis, tick paralysis).

4.7.1.1 Tick Bites

Etiology. Two families of ticks exist, which differ in their morphology and biology: Ixodidae, "hard ticks," with about 670 species, and Argasidae, "soft ticks," with about 160 species. The most important genera and the diseases transmitted by them are listed in Tabs 4.12 and 4.13. About 85% of the tick species have developed a more or less strict host preference.

Ticks are unsegmentated arthropods. Merely the capitulum, carrying the mouthparts and the extremities are demarcated from the body (Figs 4.50 and 4.51). The capitulum of hard ticks projects forwards from the body and is visible from the dorsal aspect; in soft ticks, the capitulum and the mouthparts are situated anteriorly on the ventral surface and are not visible from the dorsal aspect. Hard ticks show a hard, chitinous dorsal shield (scutum) that covers the whole body of the males but only a small portion behind the capitulum in females and the developmental stages (Fig. 4.50). Soft ticks have a leather-like integument without a dorsal shield (Fig. 4.51). The mouthparts of ticks consist of one pair of chelicerae (cutting tools), one pair of pedipalps (sensing devices), and beneath them, that is, ventrally, the hypostome (piercing tool) (Fig. 4.52).

In general, all developmental stages of ticks (larvae with six legs, nymphs and adults with eight legs) suck the blood of vertebrates; blood feeding is essential prior to each developmental step (molting to the next stage) and egg deposition.

Hard ticks pass three developmental stages (larva, nymph, and adults) after hatching from the egg and all take blood at each stage for 2 to 7 days on a vertebrate host. The majority of ixodid ticks develop as three-host-ticks (see Tab. 4.10), whereby each developmental stage leaves its host after finishing the blood meal, molts on the ground to the next stage, and invades a new host (Fig. 4.53). Some species have adopted a cycle with two hosts or only one host. In the case of two-host-ticks, the larva and the nymph stay on the same host for feeding, and the nymph drops off and molts at the ground to an adult, which then invades a new host. One-host-ticks complete their development from larvae to adults on the same host. In all cases, the engorged, mated female deposits several thousands of eggs on one occasion on the ground and dies after egg deposition. Closing the cycle in three-host-ticks lasts at least 1.5 years, and under field conditions may require 2 to 3 years or even longer in cool climates. Each of the stages survives starving for about 1.5 years.

The life cycle of argasid ticks differs considerably from that of ixodids. They develop through one larval stage and several nymphal stages to adults. Larvae of the genus *Argas* feed for several days on one host; the other stages feed on their hosts usually at night for 20 to 30 min before each molting or egg laying (female argasid ticks repeatedly lay batches of 50 to 80 eggs). Argasid ticks concentrate the ingested blood rapidly in the course of feeding,

and thereafter, segregate surplus liquids and electrolytes as coxal fluid via the coxal apparatus, which opens just behind the coxae of the first pair of legs. In some species of the genus *Ornithodorus*, the larvae do not suck blood but develop to nymphs inside the egg; the further development is similar to that of *Argas* spp. Nymphal stages of *Otobius megnini* may stay for weeks to months on their hosts. The adults of this species do not feed.

Occurrence. The general geographic distribution of tick genera is summarized in Tab. 4.12 and 4.13. However, many species differ considerably in their demand on the biotope and the occurrence of a particular species may therefore vary regionally and locally.

The most frequent species of hard ticks in Western Europe is *Ixodes ricinus* (castor bean tick, capricorn beetle) representing about 95% of the total tick population. Typical biotopes are bushy areas, parks, heathland, moorland,

Table 4.12 | Important genera of ticks, geographical distribution and number of hosts during development

FAMILY AND GENUS	GEOGRAPHICAL DISTRIBUTION	NUMBER OF HOSTS DURING DEVELOPMENT
Ixodidae		
Hyalomma	Africa, South and Central Asia (relatively resistant against dryness)	One-, two-, three-host-ticks
Rhipicephalus	Africa and temperate zones (Mediterranean)	Mostly three-host-ticks, some species imported to Australia and South America are two-host-ticks
Boophilus	Savanna areas of Africa, Asia, Australia, and America (mainly on ungulates)	One-host-ticks
Amblyomma	Tropical and subtropical areas worldwide	Mostly three-host-ticks
Dermacentor	All continents; some species tolerate cold	Three-host-ticks
Ixodes	All continents, mostly temperate zones (only a few species in the tropics)	Three-host-ticks
Haemaphysalis	Mainly Old World (only three of 155 species in the New World)	Three-host-ticks
Argasidae		
Argas	Worldwide, mainly birds and bats	
Ornithodoros	Eastern and southern Africa (*O. moubata*) and arid areas in Africa, Near East, and India (*O. savigny*)	
Otobius	North and South America; imported to Africa and India	

Table 4.13 | Ticks as vectors of diseases (selection)

GENUS	DISEASE	CAUSATIVE AGENT	DISTRIBUTION	MAIN VECTOR
Family Ixodidae				
Ixodes	Tick borne encephalitis (TBE)	TBE group, Flaviviridae	Europe, North Asia	*I. ricinus, I. persulcatus*
	Powassan encephalitis	TBE group, Flaviviridae	North America	*I. cookei*
	Kemerovo virus disease	Orbivirus, Reoviridae	West Siberia	*I. persulcatus*
	Human granulocytic anaplasmosis	*Anaplasma phagocytophilum*	USA Europe	*I. scapularis I. pacificus, I. ricinus*
	Lyme Borreliosis	*Borrelia burgdorferi sensu lato*	Northern Hemisphere	*I. scapularis, I. pacificus, I. ricinus, I. persulcatus*
	Tularemia	*Francisella tularensis*	Northern Hemisphere	*Ixodes* spp., *I. ricinus* (*Dermacentor* sp. *Amblyomma americanum*)
	Babesiosis	*Babesia divergens, B. microti*	Europe North America	*I. ricinus, I. scapularis*
Dermacentor	Omsk hemorrhagic fever	TBE group, Flaviviridae	West Siberia	*D. reticulatus*
	Rocky Mountain spotted fever	*Rickettsia rickettsii*	North America	*D. andersoni D. variabilis*
	Colorado tick fever	Orbivirus, Reoviridae	Rocky Mountains	*D. andersoni*
	Tick-borne lymphadenopathy (TIBOLA)	*Rickettsia slovaca*	Eurasia	*D. marginatus*
	Q fever	*Coxiella burnetii*	Worldwide except New Zealand	*Dermacentor* spp.
Hyalomma	Crimean-Kongo hemorrhagic fever	Nairovirus, Bunyaviridae	Africa, Near East	*H. marginatum*
	Japanese spotted fever	*Rickettsia japonica*	Japan	*Hyalomma* spp.
Haemaphysalis	Kyasanur forest disease	TBE group, Flaviviridae	North India	*H. spinigera*
	Siberian tick typhus	*Rickettsia sibirica*	Russia, China	*Haemaphysalis* spp.
Rhipicephalus	Mediterranean spotted fever	*Rickettsia conorii*	Mediterranean area	*R. sanguineus*
	Rocky Mountain spotted fever	*Rickettsia rickettsii*	Mexico, USA	*R. sanguineus*
Amblyomma	African tick bite fever	*Rickettsia africae*	South Saharan Africa	*A. hebraeum, A, variegatum*
	Rocky Mountain spotted fever	*Rickettsia rickettsii*	South America	*A. cajennense*
	Human monocytic ehrlichiosis	*Ehrlichia chaffeensis, Ehrlichia ewingii*	North America	*A. americanum*
	American spotted fever	*Rickettsia parkeri*	USA, Atlantic coast, Gulf of Mexico	*A. maculatum*
Family Argasidae				
Argas	Avian spirochetosis; no infections in humans	*Borrelia anserina*	Worldwide, usually on birds and bats	*A. persicum*
Ornithodorus	Tick-borne relapsing fever	*Borrelia duttonii, B. hermsii, B. turicatae*	East Africa, North and Central America	*O. moubata, O. hermsii, O. turicata*

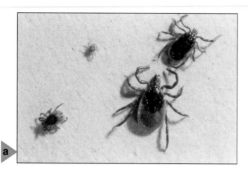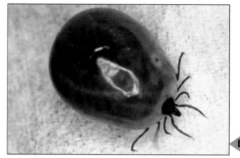

Figure 4.50 (a,b) | Developmental stages of ixodid ticks, for example, *Ixodes ricinus*. (**a**) Larva (six legs), nymph and adult stages. The chitinous shield covers the whole body in case of the male and part of the body in case of the other stages (picture: www.zecken.de). (**b**) Engorged female tick with massively enlarged body (picture: H. Mehlhorn, Düsseldorf, Germany).

and fern strips at the border of forests. *I. ricinus* starts activity at approximately 7 °C and accumulates in May and June. It depends on sufficient moisture. *I. ricinus* has no host preference and humans are often attacked. Rodents and often roe dear maintain the *I. ricinus* population. Among the other 11 *Ixodes* species occurring in Europe, some are only found in defined environments and infest defined hosts, for example, *I. trianguliceps*, in burrows of voles.

Other more rare hard tick species such as *Dermacentor marginatus*, *D. reticulatus*, and *Haemaphysalis punctata* only rarely attack humans; although *D. reticulatus* has expanded regionally in recent decades and is more often found on humans. *Rhipicephalus sanguineus*, the brown

dog tick, which is abundant in Southern Europe, infests buildings in Central Europe and becomes a pest.

In North America, the *Ixodes* species are represented by *I. scapularis* (*I. dammini*), the blacklegged tick or deer tick and *I. pacificus*, the western blacklegged tick. The former is widely distributed in the northeastern and upper midwestern US, the latter occurs along the Pacific coast. Both species are carriers of pathogens, for example, *Borrelia burgdorferi* (Tab. 4.13).

Dermacentor variabilis, the American dog tick, is the most common tick species in the United States and is widely distributed in the eastern part of the US and in limited areas of the Pacific coast. *D. andersoni*, the Rocky Mountain wood tick, is common in the Rocky Mountains states. *Dermacentor* spp. transmit *Rickettsia rickettsii* and other pathogens (Tab. 4.13). *Amblyomma americanum*, the lone star tick, is primarily found in the southeastern and eastern United States. The related species, *A. maculatum*, the gulf coast tick, is restricted to coastal areas along the Atlantic coast and the Gulf of Mexico. *A. americanum* feeds mainly on white tailed deer, the natural reservoir for *E. chaffeensis* (Tab. 4.13). *R. sanguineus*, the brown dog tick, is found throughout the United States. All stages feed mainly on dogs but can infest also other mammals and humans. As recently found, these ticks can transmit *R. rickettsii*.

Soft ticks of the genus *Argas* are common in warmer regions of America (southwest of the

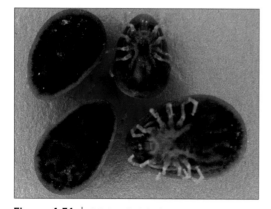

Figure 4.51 | Adult soft ticks (*Argas reflexus*); dorsal (left) and ventral aspects. Mouthpieces are only visible from the ventral aspect (picture: H. Mehlhorn, Düsseldorf, Germany).

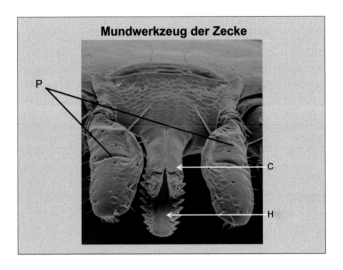

Figure 4.52 | Mouthparts of an ixodid tick (*Ixodes ricinus*); dorsal aspect with chelicerae (C), hypostome (H), and pedipalps (P) (picture: H. Mehlhorn, Düsseldorf, Germany).

United States, Central and South America), Europe, North Africa, and the Near East. In Europe, the thermophilic pigeon tick *Argas reflexus* occurs up to 55°N. It is common in pigeon houses and other buildings occupied by pigeons but attacks all species of domestic and wild birds. Occasionally humans become infested, for example, when pigeons have been expulsed from buildings and hungry ticks search for blood sources. *A. reflexus* is absent in the Americas; however, similar problems may arise there by the fowl tick *A. persicus*.

Otobius spp. are common in both Americas, India, and South Africa. Their habitats resemble those of *Argas* spp. The main hosts are dogs, ruminants, and pigs; *Otobius* spp. occasionally infest humans. Representatives of the genus *Ornithodoros* live outdoors in the Americas, Africa, and the Middle East. *Ornithodoros*

moubata and *O. savignyi* have adapted to domestic animals and humans. There seems to be even a "hut-dwelling" strain of *O. moubata* with rodents as reservoir hosts.

Transmission (Host finding). Ticks are temporary ectoparasites and find their hosts by mechanical (vibration), thermal, and chemical (CO_2) signals, and actively invade them. Humans are usually accidental hosts of predominantly nymphs and adults, while larvae often prefer small mammals such as rodents. Ticks preferentially infest soft parts of the skin and in humans attach to the neck, armpit, hollow of the knee, and wrinkles of the abdominal skin.

Clinical Manifestations. Ticks are pool feeders, that is, they induce a blood pool in front of their mouthparts in the host's skin on which they feed.

Figure 4.53 | Developmental cycle of a three-host tick (e.g., *I. ricinus*).

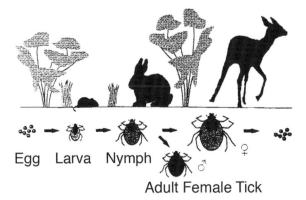

Egg Larva Nymph

Adult Female Tick

In principle, they pierce the skin with their chelicerae, insert the chelicerae together with the hypostome into the wound, and secrete saliva with lytic components, opening small blood vessels. The feeding canal is built dorsally by the chelicerae and ventrally by the hypostome. In case of ixodid ticks, which feed for several days, the mouthparts are fixed in the skin by a proteinaceous "cement" (which makes ticks so hard to remove).

Due to anesthetic and other components in the tick saliva, tick bites are usually painless and do not invoke much inflammation, unless pathogens (i.e., borreliae) are transmitted. Repeated infestations, however, may be accompanied by edema, erythema, inflammation, and subcutaneous hemorrhages. Sometimes, small abscesses may develop when the tick was not removed properly, that is, when mouthparts remain in the skin. Bites of *Argas* spp. are detectable as itching, erythematous lesions.

Larvae of *Otobius megnini* infest the ear and the auditory canal, often accompanied by secondary infections.

Diagnosis. Hard ticks are usually found *in situ* because of their sustained feeding. *Argas* spp. feed at night on humans, so that usually only itching sensations are found in the morning.

Differential Diagnosis. Bites of argasid ticks resemble those of bugs that should be considered.

Therapy. Ticks should be removed carefully and completely, and as early as possible to interrupt possible transmission of pathogens. If possible, ticks should not be annoyed *in situ*, for example, by application of oil or glue, as this may force them to release saliva, which can be associated with the release of pathogens. Removal is best done with pointed forceps (watchmaker forceps). Local reactions are treated topically.

Buildings infested with acarid ticks (or, in Central Europe, with *R. sanguineus*), must be cleared with acaricides, presumably with pyrethroids. These measures should be carried out by professionals.

Prophylaxis. Tick biotopes, for example, forest borders in Central Europe, should be avoided during the tick season. Repellents applied on the skin have only a temporary effect. Longer lasting effects are achieved by permethrin derivatives that can be used to impregnate clothing. Hiking boots and tightly fitting clothes may help to protect. Pigeons should not be allowed to settle in buildings (lofts) to prevent the establishment of *Argas* spp. Preventive treatment of dogs is recommended (tick collars) to avoid the introduction of ticks into buildings, for example, of *R. sanguineus*.

4.7.1.2 Tick Toxicoses (Tick Paralyses)

Tick toxicoses manifest in humans as paralysis.

Etiology, Occurrence, and Transmission. Worldwide, 55 ixodid and 14 argasid tick species out of 10 genera are suspected to cause paralysis, although convincing data do not exist in all cases. From the medical point of view, *Dermacentor andersoni* (the Rocky Mountain wood tick) in the western parts of North America, *D. variabilis* (the American dog tick) in the eastern parts of North America, and *Ixodes holocylus* (the Australian paralysis tick) in the eastern coastal areas of Australia are the most important species. In these cases, the disease is caused by adult female ticks. Approximately eight additional species have been incriminated, but only with one to three usually not well documented cases each.

Clinical Manifestations. Tick paralysis is a neurological syndrome characterized by ascending bilateral flaccid paralysis that progresses over hours and days. The patient becomes restless and sometimes shows nausea, dizziness, and vomiting. Headache, general muscle weakness, and numbness and tingling of the extremities are observed. An ascending flaccid paralysis follows, affecting legs, arms, and neck. Speech disorders, dysphagia, and dyspnea may appear rapidly. The disease may be fatal if paralysis of the respiratory muscles occurs. Mortality rates of 10 to 12% are reported. One female tick is able to induce the clinical signs. Different toxins seem to be produced by the various species.

Several tick species are economically important in tick paralysis of animals, for example, *Ixodes rubicundus* and *Rhipicephalus evertsi evertsi* in sheep in South Africa. Some *Argas* spp. affect all kinds of birds by paralysis, which is exclusively induced by the larvae. Other types of toxicoses in animals in East Africa result from *Hyalomma truncatum* infestations.

Diagnosis. Tick paralyses are diagnosed by the typical clinical picture and by demonstration of the ticks. They usually occur seasonally, that is, in spring and summer.

Differential Diagnosis. Other intoxications and CNS diseases, for example, poliomyelitis and peripheral neuropathy, must be considered.

Therapy. Patients should be hospitalized immediately and treated symptomatically. In the case of *Dermacentor* infestations, complete recovery follows quickly after removal of the tick, whereas symptoms often continue or progress for 1 to 2 days after removal of *I. holocyclus*. In the case of *I. holocyclus*, an effective hyperimmune serum is available for medical and veterinary use.

Prophylaxis. Measures for prophylaxis are the same as those mentioned in "Tick Bites" above.

REFERENCES

Campbell BS, Bowles DE, Human tick bite records in a United States Air Force population, 1989–1992: Implications for tick borne disease risk. *J. Wilderness Med.* 5, 405–412, p1994.

CDC, Ticks – geographical distribution. *CDC 24/7*, 2014.

Dworkin MS, Shoemaker PC, Anderson DE Jr, Tick paralysis: 33 human cases in Washington State, 1946–1996. *Clin. Infect. Dis.* 29, 1435–1439, 1999.

Guglielmon AA et al., The Argasidae, Ixodidae and Nuttallielidae (Acari: Ixodida) of the world: a list of species names. PDF (http://repository.up.ac.za/handle/2263/17278), 2012.

Fritsche TR, Arthropods of medical importance. In: Murray, P.R. (ed. in chief): *Manual of Clinical Microbiology*. 7th ed. ASM Press, Washington D.C. Parasitology cap. 114, ppp. 1449–1466, 1999.

Gothe R, Neitz AWH, Tickparalysis: pathogenesis and etiology. *Adv. Dis. Vector. Res.* 8, 177–204, 1991.

Horak JG et al., Ixodid ticks feeding on humans in South Africa: with notes on preferred hosts, geographical distribution, seasonal occurrence and transmission of pathogens. *Exp. Appl. Acarol.* 27, 113–136, 2002.

Kettle DS, Medical and veterinary entomology. C. A. B. International, Wallingford, U.K., en2nd edition, 1995.

Krant W, Walter DE, A manual of Acarology. Texas Tech University Press, Lubbock, Texas, 2009.

Medlock JM et al., Driving forces for changes in geographical distribution of *Ixodes ricinus* ticks in Europe. *Parasites Vect.* 6, p1, 2013.

Salafsky B et al., Short report: study on the efficacy of a new long-acting formulation of N, N-diethyl-m-toluamide (DEET) for the prevention of tick attachment. *Am. J. Trop. Med. Hyg.* 62, 169–172, 2000.

Sonenshine D E, Tick paralysis and other tickborne toxicoses. In: SonenshineDE: *Biology of ticks*. Oxford University Press, New York, Oxford. Vol. 2, 320–330, 1993.

Stromdahl EY, Prevalence of infection in ticks submitted to the human tick test kit program of the U.S. Army Center for Health Promotion and Preventive Medicine. *J.Med. Entomol.* 38, 67–74, 2001.

Uspensky I, Ioffe-Uspensky I, The dog factor in brown dog tick *Rhipicephalus sanguineus* (Acari: Ixodidae) infestations in and near human dwellings. *Int. J. Med. Microbiol.* 291 Suppl. 33, 156–163, 2002.

4.7.2 ZOONOSES CAUSED BY MITES

Mites are arachnids and related to ticks. About 30 000 species occur worldwide. Most of them are free-living but there are also numerous parasitic genera living as ectoparasites or endoparasites of medical and particularly of veterinary importance. Mites are relatively small animals of a body length of 0.2 to 4 mm, with six legs as larvae and eight legs as nymphs and adults (Fig. 4.54). Their mouthparts lack a hypostome.

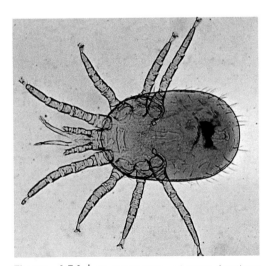

Figure 4.54 | *Ornithonyssus sylvarum* (northern poultry mite); 0.7 × 0.45 mm in size).

Etiology. Numerous mite species, predominantly of the families Trombiculidae (chigger mites), Cheyletiellidae (predatory mites), Dermanyssidae (bird mites), Halarachnidae (lung mites), and Sarcoptidae (scabies mites, mange mites) are at all stages, or at particular stages, parasites of humans and animals (Tab. 4.14). In addition, blood-sucking or lymph-sucking species may transmit other pathogens such as viruses, rickettsiae, or parasites.

Dust mites (Tyroglyphidae and Pyroglyphidae) that feed on food stocks and dust can induce severe allergies in humans (house dust allergy). These mites are not considered to be zoonotic agents.

Mites develop from eggs, laid by a female, to a larva, and molts to two or three nymphal stages (protonymph, sometimes deutonymph, tritonymph) and to fertile males and females. Feeding is necessary between the molts and for egg production

Occurrence. Trombiculid mites occur worldwide with >3000 species. They are free-living predators; however, the larvae of approximately 50 species infest humans and animals. Unfed larvae measure approximately 0.25 mm.

Eutrombicula alfreddugesi and *Trombidium irritans* (chigger mites; red chigger) occur in the United States and Mexico, predominantly on sheltered grasslands. Mites prefer warm temperatures (at maximum 38 °C) and a relative humidity of approximately 85%. In cooler regions, there is usually only one larval generation per year, resulting in a strict seasonality of the larval population. Larval activity lasts from May to October. They feed on mammals, birds, and reptiles.

Neotrombicula autumnalis (harvest bug) and related species (*N. inopinata*) play the same role in Central Europe. They are found up to an altitude of 3000 m but are often restricted to narrowly limited areas (gardens and parks). The ecological factors, favoring the abundance of *N. autumnalis* or interfering with it, are unknown. At least, excessive accumulations of the larvae also depend on the availability of enough suitable hosts, that is, rodents and birds, in the particular area. Larvae abound in summer and autumn and disappear with early frosts.

Trombicula akamushi and *Eutrombicula sarcina* occur in tropical and subtropical countries of Asia (India, Japan, China, and the Pacific Islands). *Leptotrombiculum* spp. (kedani mites) in East Asia are responsible for transmission of *Orientia tsutsugamushi*, the etiologic agent of scrub typhus (tsutsugamushi fever; see "Scrub Typhus"). These tropical species develop throughout the year.

A variety of other biting mites may occasionally infest humans and animals. The blood-sucking red bird mite, *Dermanyssus gallinae*, occurs worldwide in stables as an ectoparasite of chickens, pigeons, and other domestic poultry and may attack humans. *Ornithonyssus sylvarum* is common in domestic and wild birds in northern America and Europe, and *Ornithonyssus bursa* is found on the same spectrum of hosts in the tropics. *Ornithonyssus bacoti* is a cosmopolitan ectoparasite of rodents. *Pneumonyssus simicola* (family Halarachnidae) occurs in the lungs of rhesus monkeys (up to 100% may be

Table 4.14 | Important zoonotic mites and symptoms caused in humans

FAMILY	GENUS	MAJOR HOST	SYMPTOMS OR DISEASE IN HUMANS
Trombiculidae	*Neotrombicula* *Eutrombicula* *Leptotrombiculum*	Mammals, birds	Severe itching
Cheyletiellidae	*Cheyletiella*	Dogs, cats	Dermatitis
Dermanyssidae	*Dermanyssus*	Poultry, wild birds	Skin irritation, pruritus
Halarachnidae	*Pneumonyssus*	Monkeys	Alterations in the bronchi and bronchioli
Sarcoptidae	*Sarcoptes*	Canids, cattle, pigs	Pseudomange

infected) and more rarely of other primates. It may infest personnel of zoos and other animal husbandries.

The scabies (mange) mites of domestic and wild animals (genus *Sarcoptes*) are spread worldwide and may be transmitted to humans by contact. The validity of the various species is under discussion.

Transmission. Larvae (0.2 to 0.5 mm in length) of Trombiculidae hatch from eggs deposited in the soil. They ascend on plants to a height of 6 to 8 cm and cling to passing suitable hosts. The larvae are most active in sunny, dry weather and in late afternoon. The engorged larvae drop off the host after 5 to 7 days and molt on the ground to nonparasitic nymphs. The transmission of *Cheyletiella* spp. to humans occurs by close contact with infested animals (dogs, cats, and rabbits).

Dermanyssus spp. usually leave their hiding places in poultry stables at night and search hosts for blood sucking. They infest humans occasionally. More serious attacks by hungry mites occur—at daytime—when humans enter infested stables, which had not been used by poultry for a long time. Human infestations with *Ornithonyssus* spp. occur after fledglings have left their nest, for example, swallows' nests on buildings, and hungry mites migrate into these building, searching for hosts. *O. bacoti* may invade humans handling pet or laboratory reared rodents. Occasionally, humans are also infected when pests (mice, rats) have been exterminated in houses, that is, the mites lack their original hosts and humans are attacked substitutedly. *Pneumonyssus* spp. are spread by coughing or sneezing of infected animals and invade the bronchi and brochioli of humans.

Sarcoptes spp. (Fig. 4.55) are permanent, stationary parasites with all developmental stages infecting the host. Transmission occurs by close contact, and transmigration of young, inseminated female mites (larval or nympheal stages do not leave the burrows in the skin). Thus, for example, *S. scabiei var. bovis* may be transmitted from cattle to a milker (dairyman's itch), *S. scabiei var. canis* may transmigrate onto humans handling dogs, or butchers or hog growers may

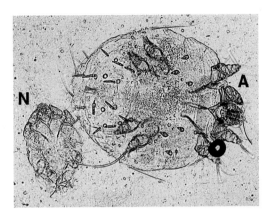

Figure 4.55 | *Sarcoptes* sp. (A) Adult (0.4 × 0.3 mm) and (N) nympheal stage out of the skin (picture: Institute for Parasitology, Giessen, Germany).

be infested by *S. scabiei var. suis*. *Sarcoptes* infections are common in domestic animals, particularly in pigs although mean prevalence may vary; for example, in Europe between 5% (Denmark) and >90% (Bulgaria) of pigs are infested. Indoor-housed cattle are more often infested with mange mites (during wintertime) than those on pasture. In horses, mange is extinguished in many countries. However, mange is a current problem in many wild-living animal populations, especially in foxes. Thus, mites may be transmitted to hounds, which then may be a source of human infections. It is also important that *Sarcoptes* mites are able to survive for up to several weeks apart from hosts, for instance on tools like brushes.

Clinical Manifestations. Trombiculosis (trombidiosis, chigger bites). Larvae of trombicule mites cause severe itching sensations, predominantly in thin-skin areas, for example, in the knee hollow, the groin and armpits, and areas where clothes can cling to (ankles above the shoe tops). The larvae scratch the skin with their chelicerae and form a proteinaceous feeding tube of a length of about 0.3 mm, the stylostome (histosiphon), through which the parasite sucks dissolved tissue. After approximately 10 h, inflammation and intense pruritus develop; they persist for 7 to 10 days, independent of whether the larvae persists or if it was stripped off.

Sarcoptic mange (animal scabies, pseudo-scabies, or fraud mange): The female mites burrow in the skin and deposit eggs. One to 2 days, or sometimes even hours after contact with *Sarcoptes*-infected animals, patients complain of intense pruritus. Small, hyperemic papular-vesicular eruptions are seen. Without reinfection, the disease is self-limiting because the animal-specific mites cannot complete their life cycle or the development stops after one or two cycles. Reinfections, however, may cause severe cutaneous alterations with inflammation on an immunopathological basis and para- and hyperkeratosis.

Other mite infestations: *Cheyletiella* infestation causes intensely itching dermatitis with papules and pustules. *Dermanyssus* spp. and *Ornithonyssus* spp. induce local skin irritations and strong pruritus. *Pneumonyssus simicola* accumulates in nodules in bronchi and bronchioli, which resemble tuberculosis granulomata. Pulmonary function is usually not impaired.

Straw itch mites or grain mites of the genus *Pyemotes* have gained increasing attention as pathogenic agents, and must therefore be mentioned here, although they are not zoonotic agents according to WHO definition (see page XV). *Pyemotes* spp. are predators of arthropods, especially of insects, and humans are attacked accidentally, even sometimes en masse. The genus comprises about 20 species with specific hosts in a wide array of insects, which are often pests of plants, stored products, or in wood. The mites exhibit a peculiar cycle: the hind body of fertilized females bulges enormously from their progeny that develops inside the females going through all molts within the female; the offspring is borne as adults of 0.2 mm in size, most of them females. Mated, they disperse to find new hosts. In humans, they cause a disease often termed dermatozoonosis. The bites cause skin lesions as red wheals with a central vesicle, or necrosis. The exanthemas often do not enlarge centrifugally but strip-like in one direction. Asthma, paralysis, and other symptoms may occur. Epidemics were reported in connection with stored grain, with swarms of periodical cicadas, or while resting under trees with massive infestation of oak gall mites.

In addition, furniture beetles (*Anobium punctatum*) were identified as hosts of the mites and source for *Pyemotes* attacks in humans.

Diagnosis. Trombiculosis is diagnosed clinically. Demonstration of the orange-red larvae (0.2 to 0.5 mm in size) on the human skin is only rarely possible as the parasites are usually removed by scratching or scrubbing of clothing.

Cheyletiella spp. can be demonstrated by applying transparent plastic adhesive tapes onto the altered skin, which may be subsequently applied to glass slides and examined microscopically.

Dermanyssus spp. and *Ornithonyssus* spp. are usually not found on the hosts because they leave the host rapidly after the blood meal and hide, for example, in cracks. If detected at all, the red bird mites may be sometimes found on light-protected regions of the body.

In *Pneumonyssus* infection, a brownish, pathognomonic pigment is detected at the site of infestation. Scabies mites are detected in deep skin swabs, which have to be treated and cleared by potassium hydroxide, which dissolves tissue remnants but does not affect the chitinous exoskeleton of the parasites. However, in case of pseudoscabies, usually only a few parasites occur. Therefore, history (professional exposure or contact with animals, particularly with those showing skin lesions) is often important.

Differential Diagnosis. Inflammatory dermatoses (pruric and papular skin diseases) for other etiology (chemical, physical, or microbiological) must be considered. Trombidiosis is often mistaken for flea bites.

Therapy. Trombidiosis, *Dermanyssus*, and *Ornithonyssus* infestations do not usually require causal treatment, as the parasites do not persist. Itching may be treated symptomatically by antipruritic drugs (antihistamines or corticosteroids or local application of 70% ethanol).

Pseudoscabies may need only symptomatic treatment if further contact with affected animals is discontinued. If required, drugs recommended for human scabies may be applied (e.g., permethrin, ivermectin, and lindane).

Except ivermectin, these drugs are also effective against *Cheyletiella*.

Prophylaxis. To avoid trombiculosis, infested areas (meadows and grassland) should not be visited during late summer and autumn. Repellents, based on diethyltoluamine (sprays, solutions, or pins) may be protective. To avoid *Dermanyssus* infestation, infested buildings must be sanitized by appropriate acaricides, for example, pyrethroids. To avoid *Pneumonyssus* and animal specific *Sarcoptes* infestations, contacts with infested animals must be avoided. Infested animals should be treated with acaricides. However, *Sarcoptes* mites are able to survive outsides their hosts for weeks. Therefore, stables, outer courtyards, kennels, and harnesses must be treated as well, most effectively with pyrethroids.

REFERENCES

Beck W, Occurence of a house-infesting tropical rat mite (*Ornithonyssus bacoti*) on murides and human beings. *Travel Med. Infect. Dis.* 6, 245–249. 2008.

Broce A et al., *Pyemotes herfsi* (Acari: Pyemotidae), a mite new to North America as a cause of bite outbreaks. *J. Med. Entomol.* 43, 610–613, 2006.

Burgess J, *Sarcoptes scabiei* and scabies. *Adv. Parasitol.* 33, 235–293, 1994.

Del Guidice P et al., *Pyemotes ventricosus* dermatitis, southeastern France. *Emerg. Infect. Dis.* 14, 1759–1761, 2008.

Frances SP et al., Seasonal occurrence of *Leptotrombidium deliense* (Acari: Trombiculidae) attached to sentinel rodents in an orchard near Bangkok, Thailand. *J. Med. Entomol.* 36, 869–874, 1999.

Houck MA, Qin H, Roberts HR, Hantavirus transmission: potential role of ectoparasites. *Vector Borne Zoonotic Dis.* 1, 75–79, 2001.

Keh B, Lane RS, Shachter SP, *Cheyletiella blakei*, an ectoparasite of cats, as cause of cryptic arthropod infestations affecting humans. *West. J. Med.* 146, 192–194, 1987.

Kettle DS, Medical and Veterinary Entomology, en2nd edition. CAB International, Wallingford, Oxon, UK, 1995.

Lathia B, *Eutrombicula alfreddugesi*. Animal diversity web, *U-M Museum of Zoology*, 2012.

Lucky AW et al., Avian mite bites acquired from a new source, pet gerbils: report of 2 cases and review of the literature. *Arch. Dermatol.* 137, p167–170, 2002.

Meinking TL et al., The treatment of scabies with ivermectin. *New Engl. J. Med.* 333, 26–30, 1995.

Moro CV et al., Diversity, geographic distribution and habitat-specific variations of microbiota in natural populations of the chicken mite, *Dermanyssus gallinae*. *J. Med. Entomol.* 48, 788–796, 2011.

Nordenfors H, Hoglund J, Long term dynamics of *Dermanyssus gallinae* in relation to mite control measures in aviary systems for layers. *Br. Poult. Sci.* 41, 533–540, 2000.

Sceppa JA et al., What's eating you? Oak leaf itch mite (*Pyemotes herfsi*). *Cutis* 88, 114–116, 2011.

Schöler A, Maier WA, Kampen H, Multiple environment factor analysis in habitats of the harvest mite *Neotrombicula autumnalis* (Acari: Trombiculidae) suggests extraordinarily high euryoecious biology. *Exp. Appl. Acarology* 39, 41–62, 2006.

Shatrov AB, Stylostome formation in trombiculid mites (Acariformes, Trombiculidae). *Exp. Appl. Acarology*, 49, 261–280, 2009.

Smith GA et al., The summer penile syndrome: Seasonal acute hypersensitivity reaction caused by chigger bites on the penis. *Pediatr. Emerg. Care* 14, 116–118, 1998.

Stekolnikov AA et al., *Neotrombicula inopinata* (Acari: Trombiculidae) - a possible agent of trombiculiasis in Europe. *Parasites Vectors* 7, p90, 2014.

Wagner R, Stallmeister N, *Cheyletiella* dermatitis in humans, dogs and cats. *Br. J. Dermatol.* 143, 1110–1112, 2000.

4.7.3 ZOONOSES CAUSED BY DIPTERA

Diptera are winged insects. The class Insecta includes approximately 70% of all known animal species. The body of an insect is organized into three distinct segments, that is, head, thorax, and abdomen. The head carries a pair of sensory antennae, usually large compound eyes, and three pairs of mouthparts that may be variably shaped according to the mode of feeding of the organism (e.g., chewing, licking, blood sucking). The thorax is composed of three segments and it bears the locomotion facilities, which are three pairs of legs and wings. The abdomen is usually segmented and it encloses the inner organs. Normally two pairs of membranous wings are found in insects. In Diptera, however, the posterior pair is reduced to a pair of knobbed, so-called halteres, ballancers that support the stability of the flight. Diptera pass a complete metamorphosis. Several larval stages (instars) develop. They are apodous and often show a reduced head. The type of the puppa varies with the various suborders of Diptera.

Two clinical features caused by Diptera are of medical importance, that is, diseases caused directly by blood-sucking species and a disease complex, summarized under the term "myiasis," which is caused by larvae of several genera of flies, invading living tissues.

4.7.3.1 Dipteran Bites

Etiology. A variety of dipteran families depend on blood sucking, either as a living source or for the production of eggs; others suck blood at least occasionally. Hematophagous Diptera include various families of the suborder Nematocera, that is, mosquitoes (Culicidae; Fig. 4.56), blackflies [buffalo gnats, turkey gnats (Simuliidae); Fig. 4.57], sand flies (Phlebotomidae; Fig. 4.58), and midges (Ceratopogonidae; Fig. 4.59), as well as flies with piercing-sucking mouthparts of the suborders Brachycera [horseflies (Tabanidae)], Cyclorapha ["true" flies, e.g., the stable fly (*Stomoxis calcitrans*)], and tsetse flies (Glossinidae). In the cases of the Nematocera and Brachycera, only the females suck blood; in the case of the Cyclorapha, both sexes are hematophagous.

Tab. 4.13 summarizes Diptera of medical importance (except of myiasis flies), and their involvement in the biological transmission of infectious diseases.

Occurrence. Mosquitoes (Culicidae) are slender insects with a small head and long extremities, the body resting with an angle to the surface (*Anopheles*) or parallel to the surface (*Aedes, Culex*, others; Fig. 4.56). Mosquitoes, including the main genera *Anopheles, Aedes, Culex*, are distributed worldwide. About 3200 species have been described. All species need stagnant or slowly flowing water as appropriate breeding sites. Depending on the genus, eggs are deposited on damp soil or vegetation, in moist tree holes, containers, pools, swamps, or directly into the water. Some mosquitoes, for instance *Anopheles* spp., need clean, natural waterbodies, but recently *A. stephensi* has also been found in artificial urban biotopes. Artificial facilities, such as tins or car tires, are typically used as breeding sites by *Aedes* species. Thus, species such as the yellow fever mosquito, *Ae. aegypti*, or the "tiger mosquito," *Ae. albopictus*, are easily spread in tanks by ships or in tires, and can colonize suitable biotopes in new areas.

In temperate regions, mosquitoes hibernate as eggs, larvae or adults, according to the species. Under suitable conditions, the whole cycle needs between 1 and 4 weeks, depending on weather conditions and species.

Sand flies (Phlebotominae) are hairy, small Nematocera of only 1.3 to 4 mm in size with long legs. The English name applies to their "sandy" color (Fig. 4.58). Phlebotominae are a subfamily of the moth flies (Psychodidae) and contain about 400 species. The various genera are mainly found in tropical and subtropical regions but important species still occur up to 55°N. Genera of medical importance are *Phlebotomus* in the Old World and *Lutzomyia* in the New World. They transmit leishmanises. Phlebotominae are mostly exophilic but some have become endophilic. Sand flies are inactive during daylight, when they seek dark, moist places. They show a "hopping" flight and fly more or less only under calm conditions and close to the ground. Larvae need breeding sites rich in organic matter.

Blackflies (Simuliidae) are small (1 to 5 mm), robust, dark-colored Diptera with a hunchbacked thorax (Fig. 4.57). Blackflies have a worldwide distribution. They need running water as breeding sites. The females lay their eggs in the water, attached to plants or rocks. Blackflies develop through 6 to 9 aquatic larval stages. They are especially abundant in the tropics and in the northern temperate and subarctic zones. In temperate climates, they may occur in enormous numbers in suitable areas during late spring and early summer (eggs or larvae hibernate in water and continue development with rising temperatures). Blackflies attack their hosts viciously in the open field during the day but do not enter buildings. They traverse distances of several km.

Midges (Ceratopogonidae) are small (1 to 3 mm), squat insects of worldwide distribution. Approximately 5400 species are known. The most important species belong to the genus *Culicoides* (Fig. 4.59). They lay their eggs in damp places, the margins of ponds, and swamps rich in organic matter. They are diurnal and usually have only a narrow range where they fly (a few 100 m). Midges hibernate in the egg stage.

Table 4.15 | Diptera of zoonotic importance and pathogens transmitted by them (selection)

GENUS	DISEASE	PATHOGEN	DISTRIBUTION
Suborder: Nematocera			
Family: Culicidae (mosquitoes)			
Anopheles	Malaria	*Plasmodium* spp.	Tropics, subtropics
	O'nyong-nyong fever	Alphavirus, Togaviridae	Africa
	Lymphatic filariasis	*Wuchereria bancrofti, Brugia malayi, Brugia timori*	Africa, Southeast Asia, Southeast Indonesia
Aedes	Chikungunya fever	Alphavirus, Togaviridae	Sub-Saharan Africa, Southeast Asia, Central America
	Epidemic Polyarthritis	Alphavirus, Togaviridae	Australia, Indonesia
	Dengue fever	Dengue virus Flaviviridae	Southeast Asia, India, Central/South America, Central Africa
	Yellow fever	Yellow fever virus, Flaviviridae	Central Africa, South America
	Rift-valley fever	Phlebovirus, Bunyaviridae	Africa
	Lymphatic filariasis	*Wuchereria bancrofti, Brugia malayi*	Indopacific region
Culex	Equine encephalomyelitis (WEE, EEE, VEE)	Alphavirus, Togaviridae	USA, Central America, South America
	Sindbis fever, Ockelbo disease	Alphavirus, Togaviridae	Old World
	Japanese encephalitis (JE)	JE virus, Flaviviridae	Southeast Asia, India, Japan
	West Nile fever	West Nile virus, Flaviviridae	Worldwide (except Australia)
	Murray Valley encephalitis (MVE)	MVE virus, Flaviviridae	Australia
	St. Louis encephalitis (SLE)	SLE virus, Flaviviridae	North and South America
	Rift Valley fever	Phlebovirus, Bunyaviridae	Africa
	Lymphatic filariasis	*Wuchereria bancrofti, Brugia malayi, Brugia timori*	Most tropical regions of Southeast Asia, Indopacific region
Family: Psychodidae (moth flies)			
Phlebotomus	Old World Leishmanioses	*Leishmania* spp.	Mediterranean region, Central Asia, North Africa
	Sand fly fever, Pappataci fever	Phlebovirus, Bunyaviridae	Mediterranean region
Lutzomyia	New World Leishmanioses	*Leishmania* spp, *Viannia* spp.	South America
Family: Ceratopogonidae (midges)			
Culicoides	Oropouche fever	Oropouche virus, Bunyaviridae	South America
	Filariasis	*Mansonella perstans, M. ozzardi, M. streptocerca*	Africa, South America, South America West and Central Africa
Family: Simuliidae (black flies)			
Simulium	Onchocerciasis	*Onchocerca volvulus*	Africa, South America

continued

Table 4.15 *continued*

GENUS	DISEASE	PATHOGEN	DISTRIBUTION
Suborder Brachycera			
Family: Tabanidae (horse flies)			
Chrysops	Loiasis	*Loa loa*	Sub-Saharan Africa
Tabanus, Haematopota	Tularemia	*Francisella tularense*	Northern Hemisphere
Family: Glossinidae (tsetse flies)			
Glossina	Sleeping sickness	*Trypanosoma brucei gambiense, T. b. rhodesiense*	Sub-Saharan Africa

Horseflies (Tabanidae) are large (10 to 30 mm), blood-sucking insects, distributed worldwide with 4000 species. The most important genera are *Tabanus, Haematopota*, and *Chrysops*. A characteristic feature is the big bean-shaped head with well-developed eyes (Fig. 4.60). Females bite and feed on warm-blooded animals, they are notorious pests of animals and some species readily attack humans. Tabanids are strong fliers and live most frequently near water. They breed in moist earth or leaf mold.

Flies (Cyclorapha) are the advanced Diptera. All families are found worldwide except tsetse flies (Glossinidae), which occur exclusively in Africa, south of the Sahara. Many species are blood sucking ectoparasites but only a few, for example, *Stomoxys* spp. and tsetse flies, attack humans. They are different from other Cyclorapha that lay eggs, as tsetse flies give birth to fully developed third instar larvae. Also belonging to the group of the so-called Pupipara are the louse flies (Hippoboscidae) that occasionally suck blood on humans. The larvae of many cycloraphan flies are causative agents of myiasis (see chapter 4.7.3.2).

Transmission (Host finding). Diptera are active during the day and/or night, depending on the genus. Many mosquito species are nocturnal or crepuscular. Most mosquitoes have a well-defined activity cycle, for example, some attack at dusk, others at midnight. Mosquitoes of the rainforest, blackflies, horseflies, tsetse flies, and others are active during the daytime. Diptera find their hosts by chemical signals (e.g., CO_2, butyric acid, or valerianic acid in body perspiration) and optic signals.

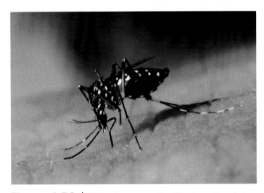

Figure 4.56 | Female mosquito (*Aedes albopictus:* tiger mosquitoe) during blood feeding (picture: R. Pospichil, Bergheim, Germany).

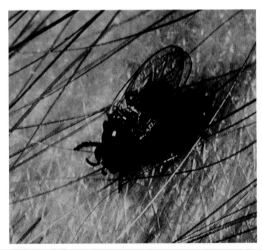

Figure 4.57 | Blackfly (*Simulium* sp.) causing painful lesions (picture: H. Mehlhorn, Düsseldorf, Germany).

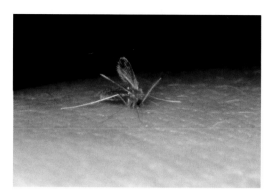

Figure 4.58 | Female sand fly (*Phlebotomus mascittii*) during blood feeding (picture: T. Naucke, Bonn, Germany).

Clinical Manifestations. Bites of Diptera cause local symptoms, such as erythema, swelling, urticaria, pruritus, and pain. Bites of phlebotomes, Simuliidae, Ceratopogonidae (*Culicoides* spp.), and Tabanidae are particularly painful and may induce severe urticarial reactions. Occasionally, skin lesions persist for a week or longer, for example, after phlebotome and blackfly bites. Some people exposed to repeated blackfly bites show severe facial swellings, edematous eyelids, and often bloodshot conjunctivae, as well as circulation problems. Indeed, serious, sometimes lethal disease, caused by salivary toxins of Simuliidae, as it is known for grazing animals after mass infestation, does not usually occur in humans, although a hemorrhagic, sometimes lethal syndrome in humans in Brazil has been related to attacks by blackflies.

Culicoides species are known as plagues for humans and animals because of their painful bites and their abundance. The bites cause severe reactions accompanied with wheals and pustule formation. *Culicoides* bites may cause allergic skin reactions in horses.

Tabanids (horse flies) injure the hosts by relatively large, painful bite wounds and secondary hemorrhages. In humans, usually locally circumscribed, erythematous wheals develop that decline in most cases after some hours. The bites of the stable fly (*Stomoxys calcitrans*) cause only temporary itching papules.

The effects of tsetse fly bites on humans may vary individually and depend on the *Glossina* species. Bites are often not immediately recognized, but small hemorrhages invariably develop, which may be followed by tender, hard swellings. Serious generalized reactions to the bites of tsetse flies are reported. Severe skin reaction to tsetse fly bites may suggest an infection with trypanosomes, representing a trypanosome chancre (see chapter 4.2.11).

Diagnosis. Diagnosis is based on clinical signs.

Differential Diagnosis. In cases of uncomplicated skin reactions, trombiculosis and bites of fleas and bugs must be considered. Systemic reactions may resemble anaphylactic reactions.

Therapy. In general, cutaneous reactions to insect bites disappear within a few hours or days. In particular cases, local disinfection to

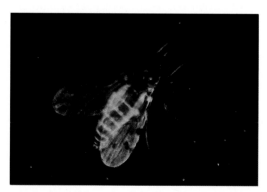

Figure 4.59 | Midge (*Culicoides* sp.), transmitter of various pathogens and cause of painful and itching biting lesions (picture: R. Pospischil, Bergheim, Germany).

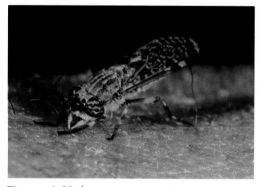

Figure 4.60 | Common horse fly (*Haematopota pluvialis*), an abundant species in Europe, the Near East and the Palearctic zone (picture: R. Pospischil, Bergheim, Germany)

prevent secondary infections may be performed. Cooling compresses are used to reduce pain and itching. Persistent reactions in humans are treated locally with corticoids. In systemic reactions, treatment with antihistamines or corticoids is recommended.

Prophylaxis. Repellents, for instance diethyltoluamid solution, provide temporary protection. To avoid the infestation by adult dipterans, long trousers or shirts and long sleeves are advisable, particularly in the evening. In tropical areas, mosquito nets should be used at night (preferably with a mesh size of 0.2 mm to also protect against sand flies).

Infested buildings can be cleaned by insecticides (e.g., pyrethroids). Pools, water pipes, etc., infested with larvae of Nematocera can be treated by the application of *Bacillus thuringiensis*, or one of its recombinant proteins, that selectively kills dipteran larvae. Areas infested with simuliids and tabanids should be avoided during the daytime.

REFERENCES

Adler PH, McCreadie JW, Black flies (Simuliidae) In: Mullen, G. and L. Durden (eds.) *Medical and Veterinary Entomology*, Academic Press, Amsterdam, 183–200, 2009.

Anderson GS, Belton B, Kleider N, Hypersensitivity of horses in British Columbia to extracts of native and exotic species of *Culicoides* (Diptera: Ceratopogonidae). *J. Med. Entomol.* 30, 657–663, 1993.

Becker N et al., *Mosquitoes and their control*. Kluwer Academic/Plenum Publisher NY., 2003.

Borkent A, Biting midges (Ceratopogonidae). In: Marquard, W.C. (ed.) *Biology of Disease Vectors*. Elsevier Academic Press, Amsterdam, 113–126, 2005.

Kettle DS, *Medical and Veterinary Entomology*, 2nd ed C.A.B. International, Wallingford, UK, 1995.

Killick-Kendrick M, Killick-Kendrick R, Biology of sandfly vectors of Mediterranean canine leishmaniasis. *Proc. Int. Canine Leishmaniasis Forum, Barcelona, Spain* 26–31, 1999.

Molloy DP 1990. Progress in the biological control of black flies with *Bacillus thuringiensis israelensis* with emphasis on temperate climates. In: De Bariac H, Sutherland DJ (eds.), Bacterial control of mosquitoes and black flies: Biochemistry, Genetics and Applications of *Bacillus thuringiensis israelensis* and *Bacillus sphaericus*. Rutgers Univ. Press, New Brunswick, N.J., 161–186, 1990.

4.7.3.2 Myiasis

Myiasis is the infestation of living vertebrate tissues by first-stage dipteran larvae and the development to third-stage larvae. After the last molt, the third stage larvae leave the host and undergo a pupal stage to develop to mature flies (metamorphosis). Myiasis can be obligatory or facultative (optional). Larvae of obligatory myiasis flies depend on living tissue for their development. Optional myiasis flies deposit their eggs or larvae only occasionally into skin lesions or onto mucosal surfaces but they can also develop in organic debris.

Etiology and Occurrence. Various genera and species of the order Diptera are known as causative agents for the various types of human myiasis. The major species, their geographical distribution, and animal reservoirs are listed in Tab. 4.16.

Transmission. Transmission of eggs or larvae to the host is not uniform. Some genera deposit eggs or larvae onto the skin and the larvae penetrate the skin actively (so-called primary myiasis: *Lucilia, Calliphora, Dermatobia, Hypoderma,* and *Gasterophilus* species). In most cases of cutaneous or subdermal myiasis, the female flies deposit the eggs into wounds (often minute lesions) or at the margin of dermal lesions. Eggs may be also deposited onto used underwear, from where, if worn again, hatched larvae can invade, for example, in the case of urogenital myiasis.

Exceptions are *Cordylobia* spp. and *Auchmeromyia luteola* that deposit their eggs onto the floor of houses or in soil. *Dermatobia hominis* developed a particular transmission strategy by depositing the eggs onto other flies or mosquitoes, which may serve as transporters (phoresis).

Clinical Manifestations. Wound myiasis: Species that cause wound myiasis usually deposit their eggs into wounds and under surgical bandages. The larvae stay for about 5 days. They feed on necrotic tissue and secrete bactericidal moieties that can prevent secondary infections. Under controlled conditions, *L. sericata* (Fig. 4.61) larvae are used for cleaning and

Table 4.16 | Major forms of myiasis and their etiologic agents in humans

MYIASIS TYPE	AGENT	GEOGRAPHICAL DISTRIBUTION	MAJOR RESERVOIR HOST
Dermals/ subdermal myiasis	*Cordylobia anthropophaga* (Tumbu or mango fly)	Africa, south of the Sahara	Dogs, other animal species
	Cordylobia rodhaini	Tropical Africa	Mainly rodents
	Cochliomya hominivorax (New World screwworm)	Central and South America	Cattle, many other species
	Chrysomya bezziana (Old World screwworm)	Africa, Asia, Middle East	Cattle and other mammals
	Dermatobia hominis (human bot fly or tropical warble fly)	Central and South America	Cattle and other mammals
Wound myiasis	*Lucilia sericata*	Worldwide	Sheep
	Lucilia cuprina	Worldwide	Sheep
	Calliphora spp. (blowflies)	Worldwide	Facultative myiasis[1]
	Sarcophaga spp. (flesh flies)	Worldwide	Facultative myiasis[1]
"Creeping" myiasis	*Hypoderma* spp.	Worldwide	Cattle
	Gasterophilus spp.	Worldwide	Equids
Ophthalmomyiasis (nasopharyngeal)	*Oestrus ovis* (botflies)	Worldwide	Sheep
	Wohlfahrtia magnifica (Old World fleshfly)	Mediterranean	Rodents (rats), lagomorphs
	Wohlfahrtia nuba	West Africa to Pakistan	Ruminants (camels)
	Rhinoestrus purpurea	Europe, Africa, Asia	Equids
Auricular myiasis	*Wohlfahrtia* spp.	Worldwide	Rodents
	Cochliomya hominivorax	Central and South America	Cattle, numerous other species
	Musca domestica	Worldwide	Facultative myiasis[1]
Sanguinivorous myiasis	*Auchmeromya luteola* (Congo floor maggot)	Africa, south of the Sahara	Pigs
Urogenital myiasis	*Calliphora* spp. (bluebottle flies)	Worldwide	Sheep, other mammals (facultative myiasis)
	Musca domestica	Worldwide	Facultative myiasis[1]
	Fannia spp.	Worldwide	Facultative myiasis[1]
Rectal myiasis	*Fannia* spp.	Worldwide	Facultative myiasis[1]
	Musca domestica	Worldwide	Facultative myiasis[1]
	Calliphora spp.	Worldwide	Numerous species
Intestinal (pseudo) myiasis	*Calliphora* spp.	Worldwide	Numerous species
	Fannia spp.	Worldwide	Facultative myiasis[1]
	Musca domestica	Worldwide	Facultative myiasis[1]
	Sarcophaga spp.	Worldwide	Facultative myiasis[1]

[1] No definable reservoir.

sanitizing poorly healing wounds (so-called maggot therapy).

Dermal/subdermal myiasis: Larvae of *Cordylobia* spp., *Cochliomya* spp. (New World screwworms in Central and South America), and *Chrysomia* spp. (Old World screwworm) burrow several centimeters deep, causing subdermal lesions, located on various parts of the body, in which the larvae feed and develop to stage 3 within 5 to 8 days.

D. hominis (tropical warble fly or macaw worm) causes painful lesions in the skin of the head, arms, back, abdomen, thigh, axilla, or orbit (Fig. 4.62), which are accompanied with swellings of the local lymph nodes. If undisturbed, larvae feed for an extraordinary long

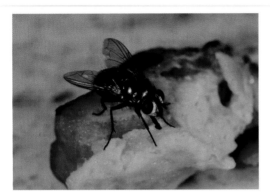

Figure 4.61 | *Lucilia sericata* (common green bottle fly or sheep blow fly): its larvae cause wound myiasis worldwide.

period of 4 to 12 weeks on the host. *D. hominis* is a common cause of ocular myiasis in Colombia.

Creeping myiasis: This complex of symptoms is caused by larvae that penetrate into the subcutaneous tissues where they migrate, sometimes for considerable distances. In definitive hosts, the larvae develop after extensive migrations in subdermal outwardly opened boils (*Hypoderma* spp.; cattle botflies) or in the gastrointestinal tract of equids (*Gasterophilus* spp.). In humans, the larvae penetrate the skin and cause itching swellings, as well as extended circuitous tunnels in the lower epidermis, where they may persist for long periods. However, in general they do not develop further.

Ophthalmomyiasis: The disease develops when ova or the actual larvae are deposited on the eyelids or adjacent skin, and in the

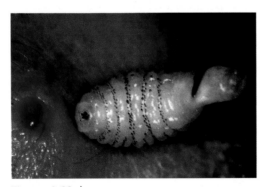

Figure 4.62 | Myiasis. Shown is a maggot (second-instar larva) of *Dermatobia hominis* removed from the subcutis. Note the opening at the migration channel (picture: P. Janssen-Rosseck, Düsseldorf, Germany).

conjunctival sac. Occasionally, they may burrow under the conjunctiva and rarely through the sclera into the eyeball. The symptoms arise quickly with painful irritating effects and range from catarrhal conjunctivitis to severe anterior uveitis. Ophthalmomyiasis is frequently caused by *Oestrus ovis* (Sheep Bot Fly) in the Mediterranean area and in the Near East, but also in Central Europe. In their natural hosts (see Tab. 4.16), the larvae invade the nasopharynx, a site that is rarely infested in humans. Invasion of the inner eye with severe damages was observed by *Hypoderma*, *Sarcophaga*, and *Wohlfahrtia* larvae.

Auricular myiasis: The symptoms of auricular myiasis, caused by *Cochliomya* spp. and *Wohlfahrtia* spp. (sarcophagid flies in Europe, Asia, North Africa, and North America) are similar to those of dermal myiasis: deep discharging and disfiguring lesions in the auditory canal and nasal cavity may extend to cartilage and bone, sometimes reaching the brain.

Sanguinivorous myiasis: The larvae of the agent *A. luteola* are usually deposited on the floor of houses. They cause skin lesions and feed on blood, mainly at night. They attack repeatedly; 5 to 20 blood meals are required for development during a period of approximately 10 weeks.

Urogenital and rectal myiasis is caused by invasion of the vagina, ureter, or rectum by larvae of Calliphoridae (blow flies). The major reason is poor personal hygiene. Occasionally, eggs or larvae are deposited onto worn underwear, from where, if it is worn again, they may invade the host.

Intestinal myiasis or pseudomyiasis is caused by accidental ingestion of eggs or larvae, for example, of the house fly, *Musca domestica*, with contaminated food. The larvae may survive the transport down the gastrointestinal tract and may cause severe irritations, intestinal pain, vomiting, and diarrhea, sometimes ulcerations. They may be found in feces or sometimes in vomit.

Diagnosis. Myiasis is diagnosed clinically and by demonstration of larvae. Depending on the type of myiasis, the larvae are found in lesions, wounds, in feces, urine, or vomit. Species differentiation considers the shape of the posterior spiracles of the larvae and structures of the cephalopharyngeal skeleton.

Differential Diagnosis. Skin alterations and diseases of other etiology (parasites, bacteria, or fungi) should be taken into consideration. In cases of creeping myiasis, the lesions resemble those of larva migrans cutanea (creeping eruption; see chapter 4.5.11).

Therapy. The first aim of myiasis therapy is the removal of the maggots (e.g., with forceps). Larvae of *C. anthropophaga* can be expressed from their boils by pressure. Occasionally, surgical measures may be necessary. Secondary infections need antibiotic treatment. Intestinal (pseudo)myiasis can be treated with laxatives.

Prophylaxis. There are no prophylactic measures except personal hygiene. Economically important myiasis flies in animals (e.g., *Cordylobia hominivorax* and *Chrysomya bezziana*) are controlled by extensive measures, particularly by "sterile male technique." Female flies mate only once; therefore, fertile males are displaced by sterilized males (e.g., by radiation). Decimation of the fly population by insecticides before the release of sterile males is supportive.

REFERENCES

Bailey MS, Tropical skin diseases in British military personnel. *J. R. Army Med. Corps* 159, 224–228, 2013.

Boggild AK, Keystone JS, Kain KC, Furuncular myiasis: a simple and rapid method for extraction of intact *Dermatobia hominis* larvae. *Clin. Infect. Dis.* 35, 336–338, 2002.

Carillo I et al., External ophthalmomyiasis: a case series. *Int. Ophthalmol.* 33, 167–169, 2013.

Delhaes L et al., Case report: recovery of *Calliphora vicina* first instar larvae from a human traumatic wound associated with a progressive necrotizing bacterial infection. *Am. J. Trop. Med. Hyg.* 64, 159–161, 2001.

FAO. 1991. The World Screwworm Eradication Programme. FAO, Rome.

Hall MR, Wall R, Myiasis of humans and domestic animals. *Adv. Parasitol.* 35, 257–334, 1995.

Jelinek T et al., Cutaneous myiasis: review of 13 cases in travelers returning from tropical countries. *Int. J. Dermatol.* 34, 624–626, 1995.

Kan B et al., Reindeer warble fly-associated human myiasis, Scandinavia. *Emerg. Infect. Dis.* 19, 830–832, 2013.

Kearney MS et al., Ophthalmomyiasis caused by the reindeer warble fly larva. *J. Clin. Pathol.* 44, 276–284, 1991.

Macdonald PJ et al., Ophthalmomyiasis and nasal myiasis in New Zealand: a case series. *N. Z. Med. J.* 112, 445–447, 1999.

Rotte M, Fields M, That's not an abscess! Furuncular myiasis. *Ann. Emerg. Med.* 62, p98, 2013.

Sampson CE, Maguire J, Eriksson E, Botfly myiasis: case report and brief review. *Ann. Plast. Surg.* 46, 150–152, 2001.

Shakeel M et al., Unusual pseudomyiasis with *Musca domestica* (housefly) larvae in a tracheotomy wound: a case report and literature review. *Ear Nose Throat J.* 92, E38–41, 2013.

Sherman RA, Wound myiasis in urban and suburban United States. *Arch. Intern. Med.* 160, 2004–2014, y2000.

Tamir J et al., *Dermatobia hominis* myiasis among travelers returning from South America. *J. Am. Acad. Dermatol.* 48, 630–632, 2003.

Victoria J, Trujillo R, Barreto M, Myiasis: a successful treatment with topical ivermectin. *Int. J. Dermatol.* 38, 142–144, 1999.

4.7.4 ZOONOSES CAUSED BY FLEAS (SIPHONAPTERA)

4.7.4.1 *Flea bites*

Fleas, except the genus *Tunga*, are irritating, temporary ectoparasites of humans and animals and transmitters of pathogens.

Etiology. More than 2500 species of fleas of >200 genera have been classified. They are wingless, laterally flattened insects, 1 to 6 mm in length and characterized by an enlarged third pair of legs. Both sexes regularly feed on blood. In general, fleas infest a broad range of hosts, although some species are host specific. About 95% of the known species feed on mammals and around 5% prefer birds.

Humans are frequently infested by fleas of domestic or wild animals, for instance, the dog flea *Ctenocephalides canis*, the cat flea (*C. felis*) (Fig. 4.63), the oriental rat flea, *Xenopsylla cheopis*, and the northern rat flea, *Nosopsyllus fasciatus*. In addition, there is the sticktight (bird) flea *Echidnophaga gallinacea*, or the so-called human flea, *Pulex irritans* (originally a parasite of wild carnivores; meanwhile rather rare in Central Europe).

Tab. 4.17 lists the medically important flea species, their preferred hosts, and the pathogens transmitted by them.

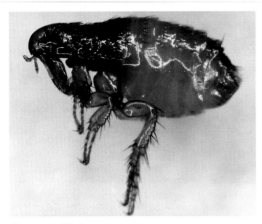

Figure 4.63 | *Ctenocephalides felis* (cat flea) (picture: H. Mehlhorn, Düsseldorf, Germany).

Occurrence. Fleas occur worldwide. They live outdoors and indoors, infest dwellings, barns, but also public facilities, such as schools, cinemas, and transportation.

Transmission. They are activated and attracted by mechanical (vibrations), visual, olfactory (CO$_2$), and thermic signals. In general, humans are not attacked as long as hosts that are more appropriate are available. Fleas move by jumping, using their enlarged third pair of legs. Some species can jump over distances up to 150 times their body length. If possible, they suck blood daily for 2 to 25 min but they may starve for months.

About 1 day after copulation, the female fleas deposit eggs wherever they can, for example, onto the host from where they drop in nests or directly on the ground. Eggs are laid repeatedly (up to 10 times 20 to 50 eggs) after a blood meal. In general, three maggot-like larval stages develop and feed on organic debris or undigested blood, excreted by adult fleas. Fleas pass a pupal stage in a cocoon, spun by the third stage larva. The development depends on environmental conditions. At optimum temperatures and under moist conditions, the cycle may be closed within approximately 14 days. Hatching of the adult fleas from the cocoon is provoked by mechanical (vibrations), thermic, and chemical (CO$_2$) signals.

Clinical Manifestations. Fleas are capillary feeders. Their bites are usually arranged in groups or lines because a flea bites repeatedly before it actually sucks blood (a failure in hitting capillaries?). Within minutes, an itching

Table 4.17 | Fleas of zoonotic importance, their preferential hosts and agents transmitted by them

SPECIES	HOSTS	AGENTS TRANSMITTED
Pulex irritans	Humans, pigs, dogs, cats	*Yersinia pestis*, cysticercoids of *Hymenolepis* spp., and *Dipilidium caninum*
Ctenocephalides canis	Dogs, cats humans, foxes, other mammals	Cysticercoids of *Hymenolepis* spp. and *Dipylidium caninum*
Ctenocephalides felis	Cats, dogs, humans	*Bartonella henselae*, *Rickettsia felis*, cytocercoids of *Hymenolepis* spp., and *Dipylidium caninum*
Nosopsyllus fasciatus	Rats, other rodents, humans	*Yersinia pestis*
Xenospilla cheopis[1]	Rats, mice, humans, domestic animals	*Yersinia pestis*, *Rickettsia typhi*
Spilopsyllus cuniculi	Rabbits, humans	*Francisella tularensis*
Archeopsilla erinacei	Hedgehogs, humans, other mammals	
Ceratophyllus gallinae	Poultry, other birds, humans, cats	
Echidnophaga gallinacea[1]	Fowl-like birds, dogs, humans	
Tunga penetrans[1]	Humans, dogs, other mammals	Soil bacteria, e.g., *Clostridium tetani*

[1] In tropical areas.

erythema develops with or without a wheal. Hypersensitivity, in humans predominantly of the delayed type, may emerge after repeated exposure, resulting in severely itching, indurated papules within 12 to 24 h. Secondary infections may occur after scratching.

Diagnosis. Multiple eruptions, often in a line, are typical.

Differential Diagnosis. Trombidiosis (in temperate regions depending on the season), and other infestations with hematophagous arthropods, especially of bed bugs, must be considered. Mosquito bites may sometimes evoke similar symptoms.

Therapy. Flea bites are treated symptomatically, particularly to mitigate pruritus. Superinfected bites may need antibiotic treatment. However, continuous reinfestations may occur without effective control measures (prophylaxis).

Prophylaxis. Infested areas, for example, the deserted resting places of cats, should be avoided or treated. Nest boxes for free-living birds should be cleaned during the winter (fleas are immotile at low temperatures). Repellents, for example, *N,N*-diethyl-*m*-toluamide, have some deterrent effect.

Flea infestations of pets should be controlled effectively. Insecticide collars protect for several months. Highly active, killing (knock-down) substances with long-lasting activity are available, for instance, imidoclopride, fipronil, and some synthetic pyrethroids. Insect growth regulators (IGRs: methopren and pyriproxifen, lufenurone) can be administered orally and are taken up by the fleas with the blood meal. Passing into the eggs, they disrupt the development of the flea larvae or act as chitin synthesis inhibitors. IGRs and knock-down compounds are often administered in combination in order to prevent infective flea populations in the environment.

Flea control should include measures to clean the environment, for instance resting places of pets (only 1% of the total flea population resides on the host). Rigorous vacuum cleaning (also of undersides of carpets, upholstery) can eliminate a large proportion of developing stages. In addition, spraying with insecticides and IGRs can be performed. Effects of outdoor measures are more questionable, if not targeted at particular (e.g., resting) places of the animals. Finally, mineral materials can be applied, for instance, diatomaceous earth (silica) for treatment of outdoor areas or boric acid for indoor rooms. They are supposed to act by dehydration and are nontoxic alternatives.

Most insecticides (organophosphates, pyrethroids, and carbamates) do not kill the eggs of the fleas. Thus, the treatment of the environment must be repeated in 1-week intervals.

REFERENCES

Beck W, Clark HH, Differential diagnosis of medically relevant flea species and their significance in dermatology. *Hautarzt* 48, 714–719, 1997.

Craven RB et al., Reported cases of human plague infections in the United States, 1970–1991. *J. Med. Entomol.* 30, 758–761, 1993.

Halos L et al., Flea control failure? Myths and realities. *Trends Parasitol* 30, 228–235, 2014.

Kern WH Jr **et al.**, Outdoor survival and development of immature cat fleas (Siphonaptera: Pulicidae) in Florida. *J. Med Entomol* 36, 207–211, 1999.

Mackey SL, Wagner KF, Dermatologic manifestations of parasitic diseases. *Infect Dis Clin North Am* 8, 713–743, 1994.

Rhodich N, Roepke RK, Zschiesche E, A randomized, blinded, controlled and multicentered study comparing the efficacy and safety of Bravecto (fluralaner) against Frontline (fipronil) in flea- and tick-infested dogs. *Parasit Vectors* 7, 83. doi 10.1186/1786/1756-3305-7-83, 2014.

Robinson WH, Distribution of cat flea larvae in the carpeted household. *Vet Dermatol* 6, 145–150, 1995.

4.7.4.2 Tungiasis (Chigoe Flea infestation)
Tungiasis is a painful, tropical dermal disease due to the invasion of the skin by female sand fleas or chigoe fleas (not to be confused with "chigger"; see chapter 4.7.2).

Etiology. The disease is caused by females of the chigoe flea, *Tunga penetrans* (jigger). The very small males are free-living. The fertilized females (initially only 1 mm in length) burrow into the skin of their hosts. They may finally reach a size of 1 cm in diameter.

Occurrence. *Tunga penetrans* originates from Latin America and the Caribbean but it was spread to Africa where it is now found in the entire Sub-Saharan region. It occurs sporadically in tropical Asia (i.e., China) and Oceania, and according to recent reports in western Europe. *T. penetrans* prefers dry, dusty environments that may be also found in unclean houses and huts. Often seasonal pattern are observed with high abundances of the disease during the hot and dry seasons.

Humans and many species of domestic and wild animals, including birds, may be infested. A crude prevalence of up to 50% is not uncommon during the dry season in humans in endemic areas.

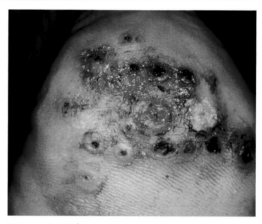

Figure 4.64 | Tungiasis. Multiple lesions on the heel caused by *Tunga penetrans* (picture: H. Feldmeier, Hamburg, Germany).

Transmission. Fertilized females burrow into the exposed skin, for example, of barefooted walking people and start to produce eggs after 8 to 12 days. During this time, its abdomen enlarges considerably, finally reaching the size and shape of a pea (jigger). The flea produces about 200 eggs that are passed continuously into the environment over a period of several weeks. Subsequently, the parasite dies. Larvae hatch from the eggs, pass three stages, and pupate after 2 weeks.

Clinical Manifestations. The penetration site becomes painful after 2 to 3 days. The growing, maturing female causes extreme pruritus, purulent inflammation, and lymphangitis (Fig. 4.64). After the death of the flea, it may be rejected and the lesion may desiccate; however, due to the main location of the parasite in the feet and scratching, secondary infections are common, and in worse cases, the infection may result in gangrene and sepsis. Tetanus is common in unvaccinated patients.

Any part of the body may be affected, although it mostly occurs in the soles of the feet, the skin between the toes and around the toenails, and the hands, arms and genitals, particularly when people sleep on the floor. Usually only one or two fleas are present but hundreds can be found. There is no protective immunity, even after repeated infestations.

Diagnosis. Chigoe infestation is diagnosed clinically.

Differential Diagnosis. Myiasis must be considered.

Therapy. Fleas should be removed as early as possible by aseptic surgery, avoiding burst of the parasite. Otherwise, severe inflammatory reactions are inevitable. Secondary infections need topical antibiotic treatment. Topical application of phenol-containing solutions is reported to kill the parasite and facilitate its extraction. Various other recommendations are found in the literature, for example, an oral treatment with ivermectin, 0.2 mg/kg. However, data obtainable are not representative so far.

Prophylaxis. Shoes should be worn to prevent flea attacks. Simple hygienic measures, for example, sweeping and cleaning houses and floors, are effective. Spraying insecticides onto infested soil is used successfully to eliminate the larvae of the parasite. According to recent studies, a plant-derived repellent (Zanzarin, based on coconut oil) spread on the skin of the feet protects better than wearing shoes. Domestic animals have to be treated with suitable insecticides in order to reduce the reservoir.

REFERENCES

Arranz J et al., Four imported cases of tungiasis in Mallorca. *Travel Med Infect Dis* 9, 161–164, 2011.

Cooper JE, An outbreak of *Tunga penetrans* in a pig herd. *Vet Rec* 80, 365–366, 1967.

Feldmeier H, Sentongo E, Krantz I, Tungiasis (sand flea disease): a parasitic disease with particular challenges for public health. *Eur J Clin Microbiol Infect Dis* 32, 19–26, 2013.

Heukelbach J, Revision on tungiasis: treatment options and prevention. *Expert Rev Anti Infect Ther* 4, 151–157, 2006.

Heukelbach J et al., Topical treatment of tungiasis, a randomized, controlled trial. *Am J Trop Med Parasitol* 97, 743–749, 2003.

Kehr JD et al., Morbidity assessment in sand flea disease (tungiasis). *Parasitol Res* 100, 413–421, 2007.

Kimani B, Nyagero J, Ikamari L, Knowledge, attitude and practices on jigger infestation among household members aged 18 to 80 years: a case study of a rural location in Kenyia. *Pan Afr Med J* 13, Suppl. 2012.

Mazigo HD et al., Tungiasis infestation in Tanzania. *J Infect Dev Ctries* 29, 187–189, 2010.

Pampiglione S et al., Sand flea (*Tunga* spp.) infections in humans and domestic animals: state of the art. *Med Vet Entomol* 23, 172–186, 2009.

Thielecke M et al., Prevention of tungiasis and tungiasis-associated morbidity using the plant-based repellent Zanzarin: a randomized, controlled field study in rural Madagascar. *PLoS Negl Trop Dis* 9, pe2426, 2013.

Veraldi S, Carrera C, Schianchi R, Tungiasis has reached Europe. *Dermatology* 201, p382, 2000.

Winter B et al., Tungiasis-related knowledge and treatment practices in two endemic communities in northeast Brazil. *J Infect Dev Ctries* 3, 458–466, 2009.

4.7.5 INFESTATIONS BY HETEROPTERA (BED BUGS AND TRIATOMINE BUGS)

Heteroptera represent a species-rich order of insects (about 30 000 species). Two families, Cimicidae and Reduviidae, include blood-sucking species and are of medical importance as pests and transmitters of diseases, respectively.

Etiology. All members of the 22 genera of the family Cimicidae are blood-sucking parasites. Only two species are common ectoparasites of humans, the bed bug *Cimex lectularius* (Fig. 4.65), and the closely related tropical bed bug, *C. hemipterus*. In addition, there are several almost animal-specific species that only attack humans occasionally; typical examples for this in Europe are the pigeon bug, *Cimex columbarius*, and the swallow bug, *C. hirundinis*, that may invade buildings after the birds have left their nests. Cimicidae are red-brown in color, flattened, oval in shape, and 5 to 7 mm long (females are larger than males). They are secondarily wingless as the forewings are reduced to very small structures (pads) and the hind wings are entirely lacking.

Within the Reduviidae, members of the subfamily Triatominae are of particular importance as vectors of *Trypanosoma cruzi*, the agent of Chagas' disease (see chapter 4.2.4). They are large insects (up to 3 cm in length) with a leaf-like abdomen and a cone-shaped head. The adults possess four well-developed wings. They are known as conenose, kissing, or assassin bugs. In South America, they have local names such as chipo in Venezuela, barbiero in Brazil,

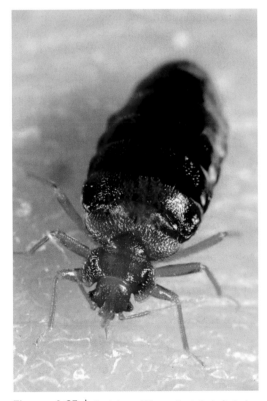

Figure 4.65 | Bed bug (*Cimex lectularius*) during the blood meal (picture: R. Pospischil, Bergheim, Germany).

and vinchuca in Argentina. Approximately 140 species in 18 genera are described. The most important genera are *Triatoma, Rhodnius, Panstrongylus* and *Dipetalogaster*; 12 species are known to transmit *T. cruzi*.

Occurrence. Bed bugs live in close association with humans. *Cimex lectularius* occurs worldwide and *C. hemipterus* in the tropics and subtropics. They infest humans, bats, other mammals, and birds. Bed bugs are nocturnal insects and hide during daytime near the resting places of their hosts in crevices and cracks, bedsteads, mattresses, behind pictures, under loose wallpapers, etc. They may also pass to a neighboring building.

One hundred of the 140 known species of triatomines occur in the New World, mostly in tropical and subtropical areas of South and Central America. Some species are found in India and Southeast Asia. In addition, the only species occurring in Africa, *Triatoma rubrofasciata*, is widespread in the tropics. Some triatomine species (sylvatic types) feed at daytime, but most are nocturnal. They often colonize the artificial habitats built by humans, simple and primitive homes (crevices in mud walls, palm roofs, furniture), stables, chicken houses, and pig sties in rural areas. The primary habitats of triatomines are nests or resting sites of wild animals (marsupials, rodents, carnivores, bats, and birds). They may also occur under rocks and loose barks and in stone walls.

Transmission (Host Finding). Blood-sucking bugs are attracted by warm temperature and CO_2. All stages suck blood that is required for molting and egg production. A blood meal may last 10 to 25 min. The females lay eggs in batches (altogether 200 eggs) in the course of 1 to 2 months in their hiding places. The time until hatching depends on the environmental temperature. In the case of *Cimex* spp., development does not proceed at temperatures below 13 °C. The larvae resemble adults and, like the other stages, feed on blood. There are five larval stages (also called nympheal stages). The life cycle of bed bugs lasts from 4 weeks up to 4 to 7 months, whereas it lasts up to 1 year in

Triatominae. Heteroptera are long-living insects and survive long periods (months) of starvation.

Clinical Manifestations. Bed bug bites are preferably found on unclothed parts of the body (face, neck, breast, forearms, and lower legs). The actual bite is usually painless and often not recognized by the resting host. However, severely itching, hemorrhagic sensations and urticarial wheals may develop within hours. The lesions often occur in linear groups and can be very annoying. Repeated exposure may result in delayed-type hypersensitivity to bug saliva. Scratching may lead to secondary infections.

In bed bugs, up to 40 pathogens of humans were found, but transmission was never confirmed. In the case of hepatitis B, the virus undergoes a transstadial transmission and it may be mechanically transmitted in feces of the bugs.

Diagnosis. Diagnosis is made according to the clinical picture. Bed bugs (also dead ones) have a typical unpleasant smell due to stink glands. Black traces of feces of the bugs are often found surrounding the bugs' hiding places.

Differential Diagnosis. Flea bites and bites of other haematophagous insects have to be considered.

Therapy. Skin sensations may need symptomatic treatment to reduce pruritus and anti-inflammatory treatment by topical application of corticosteroids.

Prophylaxis. Buildings with bed bug infestation must be sanitized with sprays or foggers containing pyrethroids as residual insecticides. Organophosphates or carbamates may be used as well, but treatment has to be repeated several times in weekly intervals because the eggs can survive it. Special attention should focus on the hiding places of the bugs.

Triatomines may be affected in a similar way. In areas where Chagas' disease is endemic, control is performed on a large scale by house spraying of residual insecticides (pyrethroids). In addition, slow-release formulations are used successfully. Important measures are improving houses to eliminate the hiding places of the bugs (cracks, holes, and crevices), and replacement of palm-thatched roofs by solid, durable constructions.

REFERENCES

Blow JA et al., Stercorarial shedding and transstadial transmission of hepatitis B virus by common bed bugs (Hemiptera: Cimicidae). *J Med Entomol* 38, 694–700, 2001.

Cecere MC et al., Improved chemical control of Chagas disease vectors in the dry Chaco region. *J Med Entomol* 50, 394–403, 2013.

Delaunay P, Human travelling and travelling bed bugs. *J Travel Med* 19, 373–379, 2012.

Delaunay P et al., Bedbugs and infectious diseases. *Clin Infect Dis* 52, 200–210, 2011.

Goddard J, De Shazo R, Bed bugs (*Cimex lectularius*) and clinical consequences of their bites. *J Am Med Ass* 301, 1358–1366, 2009.

Gurtler R et al., Detecting domestic vectors of Chagas' disease: a comparative trial of six methods in north-west Argentina. *Bull WHO* 73, 487–494, 1995.

Marbud TS et al., Spatial, and temporal patterns of *Cimex lectularius* (Hemiptera: Cimicidae) reporting in Philadelphia. *J Med Entomol* 51, 50–54, 2014.

Pinto RJ, Cooper R, Kraft SK, Bed Bug Handbook: The complete guide to bed bugs and their control. Pinto&Associates Inc. Mechanicsville MD (USA), 2007.

Salvatella R et al., Ecology of *Triatoma rubrovaria* (Hemiptera, Triatominae) in wild and peridomestic environments of Uruguay. *Mem Inst Oswaldo Cruz* 90, 325–328, 1995.

Sansom JE, Reynolds NJ, Peachey RD, Delayed reaction to bed bug bites. *Arch Dermatol* 128, 272–273, 1992.

Tharakaram S, Bullous eruption due to *Cimex lectularius*. *Clin Exp Dermatol* 24, 241–242, 1999.

Vallve SL, Rojo H, Wisnivesky-Colli C, Urban ecology of *Triatoma infestans* in San Juan, Argentina. *Mem Inst Oswaldo Cruz* 91, 405–408, 1996.

Whang C, Zhang A, Liu C, Repellency of selected chemicals against the bedbug (Hemiptera: Cimicidae). *J Econom Entomol* 106, 373–379, 2013.

Zeledon R, Montenegro VM, Zeledon O, Evidence of colonization of man-made ecotropes by *Triatoma dimidiata* (Latreille, 1811) in Costa Rica. *Mem Inst Oswaldo Cruz* 96, 659–660, 2001.

4.8 Zoonoses Caused by Pentastomids

Pentastomids (tongue worms) were not clearly classified for a long time; however, they now belong to their own phylum Pentastomida. They are heterosexual. Adult stages (1 to 16

cm in length) usually settle in the respiratory tract. The parasites are elongated, the cuticle is transversely striated, and the body is cylindrical or flattened. The flattened ventral surface of the anterior end shows the oral aperture and four additional slit-like openings (Greek: pente: five; stoma: mouth).

4.8.1 PENTASTOMIDOSIS, LINGUATULOSIS (HALZOUN, MARRARA SYNDROME)

Etiology. Pentastomids are common in reptiles with most of the known >60 species. Four species occur in carnivorous mammals and one species in birds (gulls). Visceral human pentastomidosis is caused in >90% of the cases by intermediate stages of *Linguatula serrata* (final hosts: carnivors) and *Armillifer armillatus* (final hosts: snakes). In addition, at least seven other species are known as agents of visceral pentastomiasis (Tab. 4.18). In rare cases of infections with adult *L. serrata*, humans are final hosts.

Occurrence. *L. serrata* is a cosmopolitan parasite in the nasal passages of dogs and other canids. Natural intermediate hosts are herbivorous animals. In areas where it is highly endemic, such as the Middle East, North Africa, and India, up to 50% of the dogs and 15 to 40% of the goats and sheep are infected. Human infections with intermediate stages are known worldwide. Infections with adult stages are rarely found in North Africa and the Middle East.

Armillifer armillatus occurs in the respiratory tract of snakes (pythons and vipers) in Central and West Africa. The prevalence in humans in these areas varies from 0.01% to 7.5%. Other species, such as *A. agkistrodontis*, are found in humans in China as intermediate stages. *A. grandis* occurs in the Congo basin and *A. moniliformis* is found in pythons in Southeast Asia. Human infections may be very common; for example, >40% of aborigines in Malaysia were found to be infected.

Transmission. When humans act as intermediate hosts, infection occurs by ingestion of vegetables or water, contaminated with eggs, usually from dog feces (*L. serrata*) or snake feces

Table 4.18 | Pentastomids infecting humans

SPECIES	GEOGRAPHICAL DISTRIBUTION	COMMON FINAL HOSTS	COMMON INTERMEDIATE HOSTS
*Linguatula serrata**	Cosmopolitan	Canids	Herbivorous animals
Armillifer armilatus	Central, West Africa	Snakes (pythons, vipers)	Rodents, other mammals
A. grandis	Congo basin	Snakes	Rodents, other mammals
A. moniliformis	Southeast Asia	Pythons	Various mammals
A. agkistrodontis	Asia (China)	Snakes	Rodents
Porocephalus crotali	America	Crotalid snakes	Small mammals
P. taiwana	East Asia (China)	Snakes	Rodents
Leiperia cincinnalis	South Africa	Crocodiles	Fishes
Railletiella hemidactyli	Asia	Lizards	Insects (cockroaches)

* In case of *L. serrata*: Humans may be both intermediate and final hosts, in all other cases only intermediate hosts.

(*Armillifer* spp.). Handling of living or dead snakes (e.g., in ritual acts) and consumption of undercooked snake meat are risk factors. Infections with adult *L. serrata* develop after ingestion of infectious stages (nymphs) with raw or undercooked viscera of animals (e.g., goats, sheep, or cattle).

Adult parasites live in the nasal and respiratory passages (*L. serrata*) or the lungs of the final hosts. Eggs of pentastomids are discharged by coughing or sneezing and shed with feces. They contain a larva that hatches in the intestine of intermediate hosts, invades the intestinal wall, and is spread with the blood stream to

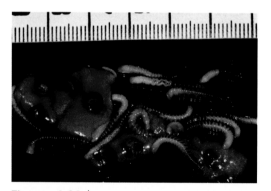

Figure 4.66 | Adult pentastomids and visceral (encysted) larval stages (nymphs) in a dog (picture: N. Pantchev, IDEXX Laboratories, Ludwigsburg, Germany).

various organs. After a series of moltings, a nymphal stage (4 to 5 mm in size) develops, which is found in a small cyst. The larva may leave the cyst and migrate through the visceral cavities of the intermediate host. Infections in final hosts occur after ingestion of nymphs (see Fig. 4.65).

Clinical Manifestations. Visceral infestation with larval pentastomids is often asymptomatic. Parasites may be found incidentally during surgery or at autopsy in the liver (superficially under the liver capsule), mesenteric lymph nodes, spleen, and lung. Invasion of uncommon sites (eyes and brain) may cause respective symptoms.

Nasopharyngeal linguatulosis after ingestion of nymphs in viscera of animals is rarely found but it may cause severe irritations in the nasal and respiratory passages. Nymphs may reach the final site and attach, probably within hours, causing pain and inflammation accompanied by edema of the surrounding mucosa, the larynx, and the Eustachian tubes, followed by sneezing and paroxysmal cough, which sometimes expels the worm. Hoarseness, dyspnea, dysphagia, and vomiting are common. The disease is known as *halzoun* in Lebanon or *Marrara* syndrome in the Sudan. A rarely occurring early temporary acute phase is explained as a hypersensitivity reaction due to previous visceral infection.

Diagnosis. Diagnosis is based on the clinical symptoms and demonstration of parasites. Imaging techniques may support diagnosis of visceral infections. Serologic techniques are used but are not validated.

Differential Diagnosis. In visceral linguatulosis, sparganosis and fasciolosis should be considered. In cases of nasopharyngeal infestations, other causes of irritation and pain sensation in the nasal and respiratory passages should be considered.

Therapy. Chemotherapy is not known. Surgery may be indicated. In nasopharyngeal linguatulosis, developing parasites are often expelled early after infection, although the adults may survive in dogs for more than 1 year.

Prophylaxis. Cleaning of vegetables, boiling and/or filtering of drinking water, and avoiding contact with snakes should protect from visceral pentastomidosis. Consumption of undercooked snake meat has been found to be a risk factor. To prevent nasopharyngeal linguatulosis, viscera of slaughtered animals should not be eaten raw.

REFERENCES

Chen SH et al., Multi-host model-based identification of *Armillifer agkistrodontis* (Pentastomida), a new zoonotic parasite from China. *PLoS Negl Trop Dis* 4, pe647, 2010.

Dakubo J, Naaeder S, Komodji S, Totemism and the transmission of human pentastomiasis. *Ghana Med J* 42, 165–168, 2008.

Lai C et al., Imaging features of pediatric pentostomiasis infection: a case report. *Korean J Radiol* 11, 480–484, 2010.

Latif B et al., Human pentostomiasis caused by *Armillifer moniliformis* in Malaysian Borneo. *Am J Trop Med Hyg* 85, 878–881, 2011.

Machado MA et al., Unusual case of pentastomosis mimicking liver tumor. *J Gastroenterol Hepatol* 21, 1218–1220, 2006.

Ma KC, Qiu MH, Rong YL, Pathological differentiation of suspected cases of pentastomiasis in China. *Trop Med Int Health* 7, 166–177, 2002.

Morsy TA, El-Sharkawy IM, Lashin AH, Human nasopharyngeal linguatuliasis (Pentasomida) caused by *Linguatula serrata*. *J Egypt Soc Parasitol* 29, 787–790, 1999.

Nourollahi Fard SR et al., The prevalence of *Linguatula serrata* nymphs in goats slaughtered in Kerman slaughterhouse, Kerman, Iran. *Vet Parasitol* 171, 176–178, 2010.

Pan C et al., Heavy infection with *Armillifer moniliformis*. *Chin Med J* 118, 262–264, 2005.

Tappe D, Büttner DW, Diagnosis of human visceral pentastomiasis. *PLoS Negl Trop Dis* 3, pe320, 2009.

Tappe D, Winzer R, Büttner DW, Linguatuliasis in Germany. *Emerg Infect Dis* 12, 1334–1336, 2006.

Yagi H et al., The Marrara syndrome: a hypersensitivity reaction of the upper respiratory tract and buccopharyngeal mucosa to nymphs of *Linguatula serrata*. *Acta Trop* 62, 127–134, 1996.

Yao MH, Wu F, Tang LT, Human pentastomiasis in China: case report and literature review. *J Parasitol* 94, 1295–1298, 2008.

Ye F et al., Severe pentastomiasis in children: a report of 2 cases. *SE Asian J TropMed Public Health* 44, 25–30, 2013.

Appendix A

A.1 Animal Bite Infections

In the United States, approximately 4 to 5 million episodes of animal bites occur every year, resulting in approximately 300 000 visits to emergency departments, 10 000 hospitalizations, and 20 deaths, mostly among young children. In England and Wales, 200 000 people per year seek medical help in hospitals after dog bites; in France, the number is 500 000. In Germany, 35 000 people per year are bitten by dogs; 1 to 2% of them are treated in ambulatory care units.

Ninety percent of animal bites are from dogs and cats. Three to 18% of dog bites and 28 to 80% of cat bites become infected, with occasional sequelae of purulent arthritis, septic shock, endocarditis, and meningitis. However, bites from several other, sometimes exotic, animal species should not be overlooked even though they occur rarely.

Animal bites may be due to accidental exposure (in children or dog owners), occupational exposure (in farmers, laboratory personnel, veterinarians, or animal trainers), or recreational exposure (in tourists, hunters, trappers, wilderness campers, or owners of exotic pets). Even licking by pet dogs or cats may transmit potentially pathogenic bacteria that may induce severe, occasionally lethal disease, particularly in patients with immune deficiencies.

A broad spectrum of etiological agents has been found in bite wounds, particularly in those inflicted by dogs and cats. There are only a few case reports of bites from more exotic animals and their number must be considered incomplete. About 85% of bites harbor bacteria originating from teeth and oral cavities of the animal or from the cutaneous flora of the victim. Fungi have rarely been reported, possibly due to insufficient media and/or incubation time.

A.1.1 DOG BITES AND BITES BY FOXES, SKUNKS, AND RACCOONS

Wounds from dog contact can be tears, evulsions, punctures, or scratches. The risk of infection is greatest for crush injuries, punctures, and hand wounds (rate, approximately 40% for each). About 90% of clinically infected wounds and 80% of wounds in patients presenting <8 h after injury yield potentially pathogenic bacteria. Most wounds contain aerobically growing bacteria, and anaerobes are only found in 30 to 40%. Transmission of rabies would be the most serious consequence of a bite, it may also occur as a consequence of bites by foxes, skunks, and raccoons.

Most infections resulting from dog bite injuries are localized to the area of injury. However, many of the microorganisms involved are capable of causing systemic infections, particularly in victims suffering from edema or compromised lymphatic drainage in the involved extremity, or from a weakened immune system.

In 20 to 50% of cases, *Pasteurella* spp. are detected, mainly *P. canis* (50% of all canine pasteurellae), *P.multocida* subsp. *multocida*, and *P. stomatis* (12% each*), *P. multocida* subsp. *septica* (10%), *P. dagmatis* (4%), and *P. multocida* subsp. *gallicida* (2%). Other frequently detected bacteria include *Staphylococcus* spp., that is, *S. aureus* (20%), *S. epidermidis* (18%), *S. warneri* (6%), *S. intermedius* (2%), and others; *Streptococcus* spp. such as *S. mitis* (22%), *S. mutans* and *S. pyogenes* (12% each), *S. sanguinis* (8%), *S. intermedius* (6%), and *S. constellatus* (4%); *Neisseria* spp. such as *N. weaveri* (14%), *N. zoodegmatis* (10%), and *N. animaloris* (6%); *Corynebacterium* spp. (Centers for Disease Control and Prevention group *G*, 6%; *C. minutissimum*, 4%); *Moraxella* spp. and *Enterococcus faecalis* (10% each); *Bacillus* spp. (8%); *Pseudomonas* spp., *Brevibacterium* spp., *Actinomyces* spp., *Gemella morbillorum*, *Escherichia coli* (6% each); *Proteus mirabilis*, *Klebsiella* spp., *Citrobacter* spp., *Stenotrophomonas maltophilia*, *Flavobacterium* spp., *Bergeyella zoohelcum*, *Micrococcus* spp., *Lactobacillus* spp. (4% each). Particularly dangerous are bite wounds infected with *Capnocytophaga canimorsus* (see chapter 2.26.5). Other aerobically growing bacteria have been found in <2% of all dog bite wounds.

Pure anaerobic cultures are rare. The most frequent anaerobes isolated from dog bite wounds are *Fusobacterium nucleatum* (16%); *Bacteroides tectus*, *Prevotella heparinolytica*, and *Propionibacterium acnes* (14% each); *Prevotella intermedia* and *Peptostreptococcus anaerobius* (8% each); *Porphyromonas macacae* and *P. cansulci* (6% each). They, as well as other more rarely isolated species (e.g., *C. tetani*) occur most often together with aerobically growing bacteria.

---

*Percentages listed according to Abrahamian and Goldstein (2011). Bacteria found in <2% have not been mentioned for any bites.

A.1.2 CAT BITES

Both cat bites and scratches may become infected with components of the feline oral flora. The teeth of cats are slender but extremely sharp.

Bacteria isolated from bites by exotic and wild felines, for example, tigers, cougars, and lions, are similar to those introduced by domestic cat bites. In 75 to 90%, cat bite wounds are infected with *Pasteurella* spp., mainly with *P. multocida* subsp. *multocida* (ci. 50% of all feline pasteurellae isolated), *P. multocida* subsp. *septica* (28%), *P. dagmatis* (7%), and *P. stomatis* (4%). Next in frequency are staphylococci (*S. epidermidis*, 18%; *S. warneri*, 11%; *S. aureus* and *S. lentus*, 4% each). Among the neisseriae, *N. weaveri* (14%) and *N. zoodegmatis* (9%) prevail. Among the moraxellae, *M. catarrhalis* (11%), among the coryneforms, *Leifsonia aquatica* (14%), *C. minutissimum* (7%), and *Corynebacterium group G* (5%) are the most frequent species. Other isolates have been *Bergeyella zoohelcum*, *Capnocytophaga* spp. (see chapter 2.26.5), and *Acinetobacter* spp. (7% each). Other nonfermentative Gram-negative rods such as *Pseudomonas* spp. and *Alcaligenes* spp., Grampositive rods such as *Brevibacterium* spp., *Erysipelothrix rhusiopathiae*, *Rothia dentocariosa* and *Actinomyces* spp., fastidious Gram-negative rods such as *Riemerella anatipestifer* and *Actinobacillus* spp., as well as *Gemella morbillorum* have been found more rarely. The most frequent anaerobes isolated were *Fusobacterium nucleatum* (25%), *Propionibacterium acnes* (16%), *F. russii* (14%), *Porphyromonas gulae* (11%), *Prevotella heparinolytica* and *P. canoris* (9% each), *P. macacae* (7%), and *Peptostreptococcus anaerobius* (5%).

Furthermore, cat bites can transmit *Bartonella henselae* (see chapter 2.3) and, in endemic areas, *Francisella tularensis* (see chapter 2.23), *Yersinia pestis* (see chapter 2.16), and *Sporothrix schenckii* (see chapter 3.5) and rabies virus.

A.1.3 SIMIAN BITES

Simian bites are said to be some of the worst animal bites, causing more edema and infections than many other bites. From wound specimens, streptococci (*S. anginosus, S. mitis, S. agalactiae, S. sanguinis*), neisseriae (*N. subflava, N. sicca*), staphylococci (*S. epidermidis, S. intermedius*), enterococci (*E. faecalis, E. durans*), *Klebsiella pneumoniae, Escherichia coli, Haemophilus parainfluenzae, Eikenella corrodens, Candida albicans, Clostridium* spp., *Bacteroides* spp., and *Fusobacterium* spp. have been isolated.

Bites of old world monkeys (*Macaca* spp. and *Cynomolgus* spp.) may pose a risk of infection with herpesvirus simiae (cercopithecine herpesvirus). The seroprevalence of this virus in adult animals may be >70%, and 2 to 3% of those excrete the virus. It may also be transmitted to other captive simian species if they are kept in contact with *Macaca* spp. or successively housed in the same cage.

A.1.4 ALLIGATOR BITES

Alligator/crocodile bites are rare and data on infections are few. Among the bacteria isolated were enterobacteriaceae (*Pantoea agglomerans, Citrobacter diversus, Serratia fonticola, Proteus vulgaris*), nonfermenters (*Pseudomonas aeruginosa*), *Enterococcus* spp., *Vibrio vulnificus, Aeromonas hydrophila, Clostridium* spp., *Bacteroides* spp., *Fusobacterium* spp., and, rarely, fungi.

A.1.5 SQUIRREL BITES

Squirrel bites have caused infections due to viridans streptococci, *Staphylococcus epidermidis, Veillonella parvula, Propionibacterium granulosum, Sporothrix schenckii*, and, in endemic regions, *Francisella tularensis*.

A.1.6 LIZARD BITES

Captive iguanas may react aggressively. *Serratia marcescens* and *Staphylococcus aureus* have been isolated from bite wounds.

A.1.7 FISH BITES

Marine bacteria are known to cause wound infections in humans that arise from swimming or walking in salt water with unprotected breaks in the skin. Halotolerant or halophilic bacteria, such as *Vibrio* spp., *Shewanella* spp.,

Staphylococcus and *Micrococcus* spp., have been isolated from such wounds. Fish bites by themselves have rarely caused wound infections. In some of them, *Vibrio vulnificus, V. parahaemolyticus, Halomonas venusta, Photobacterium damsela, Erysipelothrix rhusiopathiae, Aeromonas hydrophila*, and *V. carchariae* were found. The latter two and *Clostridium* spp. were also isolated from wounds caused by piranha bites.

A.1.8 BAT BITES

Rabies virus, mainly serotype 1 and 4 (in Africa) may be transmitted by bats, particularly by hematophagous vampire bats. In Finland and Scotland, lethal cases of rabies were observed following bites of a broad-winged bat (*Eptesicus serotinus*).

A.1.9 SHARK BITES

Nowadays, about 75% of victims of shark attacks survive. Frequently, there is no significant loss of tissue; instead, laceration patterns indicate that bites are most likely caused by open-mouth raking, resulting in severe cuts and slashes. *Vibrio alginolyticus, V. carchariae, V. fluvialis, V. vulnificus* and *V. parahaemolyticus, Pseudomonas* spp., *Shewanella* spp., *Aeromonas* spp., *Citrobacter* spp., *Klebsiella* spp., *Staphylococcus* spp., and *Micrococcus* spp. have been isolated from such wounds.

A.1.10 HAMSTER/GUINEA PIG/FERRET BITES

Acinetobacter spp., *Leptospira* spp., *Francisella tularensis*, and the lymphocytic choriomeningitis virus may be transmitted by hamster bites. *Haemophilus influenzae* and pasteurellae have been isolated from guinea pig bites, and *Pasteurella* spp., *Corynebacterium* spp., and *Rothia* spp. from ferret bites.

A.1.11 CAMEL BITES

Camels do not bite if kept in adequate quarters but can bite, if irritated, which can give rise to severe, even fatal lacerations. These wounds have yielded growth of *Staphylococcus aureus*,

Streptococcus pyogenes, Pseudomonas aeruginosa, and *Bacillus* spp. From the oral flora of camels, *Moraxella catarrhalis, Klebsiella pneumoniae,* and *Escherichia coli* have also been isolated. Camels and dromedaries may be infected with MERS coronavirus.

A.1.12 OPOSSUM BITES

Very few reports are extant. The oral flora of opossums contain *Staphylococcus* spp., *Streptococcus* spp., *Pasteurella multocida, Aeromonas* spp., *Citrobacter* spp., *Eikenella corrodens,* and *Escherichia coli.*

A.1.13 HORSE BITES

Most horse bites contain a mixed aerobic-anaerobic flora with *Pasteurella* spp. (*P. multocida,* occasionally *P. caballi*), *Actinobacillus* spp. (*A. lignieresii, A. suis, A. equuli*), *Streptococcus* spp. (*S. mutans, S. anginosus, S. equi*), *Staphylococcus aureus, Neisseria* spp., *Escherichia coli,* and anaerobes (*Prevotella melaninogenica, Bacteroides spp, Clostridium* spp.)

A.1.14 RAT AND MOUSE BITES

Bacteria can be isolated from 30% of all rat bite wounds but the infection rate is only 2%. *Staphylococcus epidermidis* (43%), *Bacillus subtilis, Corynebacterium* spp., viridans streptococci, *Leptospira* spp., and, rarely, *Streptobacillus moniliformis* and *Spirillum minus,* (the former more frequently in the Americas, the latter in Asia), have been reported. Lymphocytic choriomeningitis virus can also be transmitted by mouse or rat bites.

A.1.15 SHEEP BITES

Actinobacillus lignieresii and *Pasteurella multocida* have been isolated.

A.1.16 SNAKE BITES

Every year, approximately 8000 people in the US are bitten by snakes, mostly by rattlesnakes, cobras, and vipers. Extensive tissue necrosis predisposes the victim to infections from the snake's normal oral flora in addition to members of the fecal flora of its prey. The normal oral flora of the snake consists of a mixture of aerobically and anaerobically growing bacteria, such as enterobacteriaceae, staphylococci, streptococci, as well as *Aeromonas, Enterococcus, Clostridium,* and *Bacteroides* spp. Infected wounds following snake bites generally reflect this flora.

A.1.17 PIG BITES

Pigs are aggressive animals but there are few reports of pig bites in the literature. Again, mixtures have been isolated consisting of *Pasteurella* spp. (notably, *P. aerogenes*), *Actinobacillus suis, Streptococcus* spp. (*S. agalactiae, S. dysgalactiae, S. suis*), *Staphylococcus* spp., enterobacteriaceae, and *Bacteroides* spp.

A.1.18 SEAL BITES

Seal finger is a well-known infection in sealers occurring either after seal bites or by skinning/handling seals. *Erysipelothrix rhusiopathiae, Corynebacterium* spp., *Mycoplasma phocicerebrale,* and some as yet unidentified coccobacilli have been isolated.

A.1.19 BIRD BITES

Rooster pecks, swan bites, and bites resulting from an owl attack have rarely caused infections (*Streptococcus bovis, Clostridium tertium, Aspergillus niger, Pseudomonas aeruginosa,* and *Bacteroides* spp.).

A.1.20 BEAR BITES

Since 1900, approximately two bear attacks per year have been reported for the US and Canadian national parks. There are a few reports dealing with bacteria isolated from bear bite wounds. These were enterobacteriaceae (notably, *Serratia* spp.), *Aeromonas* spp., *Bacillus* spp., *Staphylococcus* spp., *Streptococcus sanguinis,* and *Neisseria sicca.*

Clinical Manifestations. Wounds caused by animal bites are of four main types: lacerations, crush injuries, punctures, and abrasions. Depending on the animal, the wound typically involves a combination of two or more of these types. Wounds resulting from dog bites consist of tears or evulsions, punctures, or scratches (see above). Bites from rodents and domestic cats usually produce puncture wounds that may be deep and then penetrate bones and joints, causing purulent arthritis, osteomyelitis, or local abscesses. Bites from horses or other ungulates typically do not break the skin but can cause severe crush injuries.

Patients who present within 8 h after injury usually present with crush injuries, disfiguring wounds, and/or the need for rabies or tetanus prophylaxis. Patients presenting later usually have established infections manifested by local cellulitis, pain at the site of injury, and purulent, often grey and malodorous discharge. Fever, lymphangitis, and regional lymphadenopathy may occur. If the microorganism disseminates, septicemia, meningitis, and endocarditis may develop, though rarely.

Immunosuppression, malignant tumors, splenectomy, diabetes mellitus, liver disease, and local edema of the affected area predispose the patient to more rapidly spreading and/or more severe diseases.

Diagnosis. An exact history should ascertain the animal species involved and risk factors of the victim. Physical examination should include a diagram of location and extent of all injuries, range of motion, nerve and tendon functions, joint penetration, and presence of edema or crush injury. Specimens for Gram stain and aerobic, as well as anaerobic, culture should be obtained from the wound. X-ray is indicated if there is the possibility of a fracture or if bones or joints have been penetrated.

Therapy. Copious quantities of normal saline should be used for irrigation in order to reduce the bacterial load in the wound. Puncture wounds may be irrigated with a 20 ml syringe (18 gauge needle) inserted into the wound in the direction of the puncture. Devitalized tissue should be carefully debrided and any foreign material removed. Infected wounds and those seen >24 h after the bite should be left open.

Antimicrobial therapy should cover most potential pathogens, that is, aerobes and anaerobes. Amoxicillin-clavulanic acid 875/125 mg, (p.o.) 2×/day is the drug of choice. It is given as a 3 to 5 day course to patients with moderate to severe wounds that are seen <8 h after the bite with crush injury, edema, or wounds involving bones or joints. The same treatment is recommended for hand wounds, cat bites, punctures (particularly if close to a joint), and for wounds in patients with an underlying disease that could predispose them to a more serious infection. Patients with an overtly infected bite wound should be treated for 10 to 14 days; purulent arthritis and osteomyelitis require longer courses of treatment.

Tetanus toxoid should be administered if a booster injection has not been given during the past 5 years. Patients who have never been fully immunized may require a primary immunization series as well as a simultaneous tetanus immunoglobulin administration.

Rabies vaccination should be considered, especially in cases of bites from wild animals. Rabies in rodents, including squirrels, hamsters, rats, and mice, is uncommon but does exist; raccoons, skunks, bats, foxes, coyotes, bobcats, and other carnivores are often afflicted and should be considered rabid unless proven otherwise by laboratory tests. The postexposure rabies immunization schedule for unvaccinated persons includes (i) human rabies immunoglobulin, 20 IU/kg infiltrated around the wound(s), with the remainder injected intragluteally; and (ii) intramuscular injected human diploid cell vaccine on days 0, 3, 7, 14, and 28.

Elevation of the injured area is essential and should be continued for several days until the edema has resolved. Hands with bite wounds should be immobilized with a splint for several days.

For outpatients, follow-ups should occur at 24 and 48 h. Simian bite wounds should be irrigated immediately and scrubbed thoroughly, and cultures for herpesvirus simiae and determination of antibody performed. Asymptomatic people with an initially positive viral wound culture should be treated with acyclovir (5×800 mg p.o./day), and every effort should be made to confirm or rule out evidence for an active infection. The absence of continuous viral shedding or of clear-cut seroconversion after 14 days indicates that therapy can be discontinued but the patient should remain under medical supervision. In cases of encephalitis, patients should be treated with acyclovir 3×15 mg/kg/day intravenously.

REFERENCES

Abrahamian FM, Goldstein EJ, Microbiology of animal bite wound infections. *Clin. Microbiol. Rev.* 24, 231–246, 2011.

Akahane T et al., A case of wound dual infection with Pasteurella dagmatis and Pasteurella canis resulting from a dog bite – limitation of Vitek-2 system in exact identification of Pasteurella species. *Eur. J. Med. Res.* 16, 531–536, 2011.

Badejo OA, Komolafe OO, Obinwogwu DL, Bacteriology and clinical course of camelbite wound infections. *Eur. J. Clin. Microbiol. Infect. Dis.* 18, 918–921, 1999.

Baker AS, Ruoff KL, Madoff S, Isolation of Mycoplasma species from a patient with seal finger. *Clin. Infect. Dis.* 27, 1168–1170, 1998.

Barnham M, Pig bite injuries and infection: report of seven human cases. *Epidemiol. Infect.* 101, 641–645, 1988.

Benaoudia F, Escande F, Simonet M, Infection due to Actinobacillus lignieresii after a horse bite. *Eur. J. Clin. Microbiol. Infect. Dis.* 13, 439–440, 1994.

Berkowitz FE, Jacobs DWC, Fatal case of brain abscess caused by rooster pecking. *Pediatr. Infect. Dis. J.* 6, 941–942, 1987.

Brenner DJ et al., Capnocytophaga canimorsus sp. nov. (formerly CDC group DF-2), a cause of septicemia following dog bite, and C. cynodegmi sp. nov., a cause of localized wound infection following dog bite. *J. Clin. Microbiol.* 27, 231–235, 1989.

Buck JD et al., Bacteriology of the teeth from a great white shark: potential medical implications for shark bite victims. *J. Clin. Microbiol.* 20, 849–851, 1984.

Escande F, Vallee E, Aubart F, Pasteurella caballi infection following a horse bite. *Zbl. Bakt.* 285, 440–444, 1997.

Flandry F et al., Initial antibiotic therapy for alligator bites: Characterization of the oral flora of Alligator mississippiensis. *Southern Med. J.* 82, 262–266, 1989.

Fraser SL et al., Rapidly fatal infection due to Photobacterium (Vibrio) damsela. *Clin. Infect. Dis.* 25, 935–936, 1997.

Gaver-Wainwright MM et al., Misdiagnosis of spider bites: bacterial associates, mechanical pathogen transfer, and hemolytic potential of venom from the hobo spider, Tegenaria agrestis (Araneae: Agelenidae). *J. Med. Entomol.* 48, 382–388, 2011.

Goldstein EJC et al., Bacteriology of rattlesnake venom and implications for therapy. *J. Infect. Dis.* 140, 818–821, 1979.

Goldstein EJC, Citron DM, Finegold SM, Role of anaerobic bacteria in bite-wound infections. *Rev. Infect. Dis.* 6, S177–S183, 1984.

Goldstein EJC et al., Recovery of an unusual Flavobacterium group IIb-like isolate from a hand infection following pig bite. *J. Clin. Microbiol.* 28, 1079–1081, 1990.

Goldstein EJC, Pryo EPIII, Citron DM, Simian bites and bacterial infection. *Clin. Infect. Dis.* 20, 1551–1552, 1995.

Goldstein EJC, Current concepts on animal bites: bacteriology and therapy. *Curr. Clin. Topics Infect. Dis.* 19, 99–111, 1999.

Haddad V et al., Localized lymphatic sporotrichosis after fishinduced injury (Tilapia sp.). *Med. Mycol.* 40, 425–427, 2002.

Haenen OLM, Evans JJ, Berthe F, Bacterial infections from aquatic species: potential for and prevention of contact zoonoses. *Rev. Sci. Tech.* 32, 497–507, 2013.

Hsieh S, Babl FE, Serratia marcescens cellulitis following an iguana bite. *Clin. Infect. Dis.* 28, 1181–1182, 1999.

Kaiser RM et al., Clinical significance and epidemiology of NO-1, an unusual bacterium associated with dog and cat bites. *Emerg. Infect. Dis.* 8, 171–174, 2002.

Lam KK et al., A cross sectional survey of snake oral bacterial flora from Hong Kong, SAR, China. *Emerg. Med. J.* 28, 107–114, 2011.

Montejo MK et al., Bergeyella zoohelcum bacteremia after a dog bite. *Clin. Infect. Dis.* 33, 1608–1609, 2001.

Murphy E, Microbiology of animal bites. *Clin. Microbiol. Newslett.* 30, 47–49, 2008.

Oehler RL et al., Bite-related and septic syndromes caused by cats and dogs. *Lancet Infect. Dis.* 9, 439–447, 2009.

Pavia AT et al., Vibrio carchariae infection after a shark bite. *Ann. Intern. Med.* 111, 85–86, 1989.

Pers C, Gahrn–Hansen B, Frederiksen W, Capnocytophaga canimorsus septicemia in Denmark, 1982–1995: review of 39 cases. *Clin. Infect. Dis.* 23, 71–75, 1996.

Talan DA et al., Bacteriologic analysis of infected dog and cat bites. *N. Engl. J. Med.* 340, 85–92, 1999.

von Graevenitz A et al., Human infection with Halomonas venusta following fish bite. *J. Clin. Microbiol.* 38, 3123–3124, 2000.

Appendix: Infections and Intoxications Transmissible by Foodstuffs of Animal Origin

B.1 Viruses

In a recent survey of foodborne illnesses requiring hospitalization, viruses were found as causative agents three times more frequently than bacteria. The death toll of foodborne viral infections, however, is less than one-fifth of the death toll of foodborne bacterial illnesses. Norwalk-like agents are the most important causes of foodborne illness with 23 million cases per year worldwide, followed by rotaviruses, astroviruses, and hepatitis A virus (Tab. B1).

Outbreaks of Norwalk-like agents and hepatitis A have been traced to eating oysters or mussels that were captured in seawater that was contaminated by human feces. The hepatitis A virus has also been transmitted via fruits and salads that were contaminated with the virus from human excretions. Nine hepatitis E epidemics have been documented in the People's Republic of China since 1982. Five of them were waterborne and four were foodborne, and they occurred in six of 30 provinces or autonomous regions. Hepatitis E most frequently affects young adults, with fewer cases in children and the elderly. In Europe, family infections with hepatitis E virus may occur in households of hunters.

Enteroviruses, and probably hepatitis A virus, can be transmitted passively by flies and other arthropods when they have access to contaminated excrement and to food. Strictly speaking, none of these foodborne viruses can be considered zoonotic. They are human viruses and their spread is facilitated by poor hygiene. Strategies for their control must be directed toward improvement of hygienic measures among humans rather than for animals. However, truly zoonotic viruses may be transmitted by foodstuffs of animal origin as well.

Tickborne flaviviruses (tickborne encephalitis and Kyasanur Forest viruses) have been transmitted to humans by way of raw milk from viremic goats and cattle. These animals are inapparently infected with the tickborne encephalitis virus. There is no definite proof that rabies virus can be transmitted by way of milk from infected cows, sheep, or goats. The foot-and-mouth disease virus was transmitted to humans via milk in an early experiment conducted during the 19th century; however, clinical manifestation of human infection with foot-and-mouth disease is rare, and this route of infection is not a major cause of human disease. It may, however, contribute to the spread of the virus in livestock. Human infections with avian influenza A viruses (chicken), or swine influenza A virus,

Table B1 | Important foodborne virus infections

VIRUS	CLINICAL SIGNS	INCUBATION TIME	FOOD STUFFS
Norovirus	Abdominal pain, vomiting, diarrhea	1–2 days	Oysters, shellfish
Rotavirus	Vomiting, diarrhea	1–3 days	Contaminated food, beverages
Astrovirus	Vomiting, anorexia, fever, watery diarrhea	3–4 days	Contaminated food and water, oysters
Hepatitis A virus	Hepatitis without jaundice	2–6 weeks	Contaminated food and water, oysters, shellfish, crabs, crayfish
Hepatitis E virus	Hepatitis, mostly anicteric	30 days	Contaminated food and water, game, wild boar, domestic pigs
Adenoviruses	Enteritis, respiratory diseases	5–10 days	Contaminated water
Enteroviruses	Fever, myositis, carditis, meningitis, encephalitis	7 days	Contaminated water

Ebola virus (chimpanzees and bats), Marburg virus (green monkeys and bats), Crimean Congo hemorrhagic fever virus (camels, cattle, and ostriches), Rift Valley fever virus (cattle and sheep), Nipah virus (pigs), Lassa virus [*Mastomys natalensis* (the multimammate rat)], rabies virus (cattle and deer), and foot-and-mouth disease virus may be associated with slaughter and use of animals for human food. Type 3 of hepatitis E virus may be present in domestic and wild pigs and in other wild animals. Hantaviruses and arenaviruses are excreted in the urine and feces of their rodent hosts; wherever the rodents or their excrements come into contact with human food, infections may result. These are important examples of foodborne zoonotic diseases of viral origin. Imported monkeys have transmitted human viruses such as hepatitis B, measles, and herpes.

The urgent need to control the microbiological quality of animal feed has only become evident recently. Human infections with prions (bovine spongiform encephalopathy and new variant Creutzfeldt-Jakob disease) may also be regarded as a foodborne zoonotic infection. The viruses causing foot-and-mouth disease and Newcastle disease may be spread via discarded human food, which is sometimes fed to pigs despite legal restrictions.

B.2 Bacteria

There are many reasons for the recent increase in foodborne zoonotic diseases. The reasons could be global trade and travel including immigration, worldwide food distribution, mass feedings, changing consumption habits, and an increase in immunosuppressed people.

In truly zoonotic foodborne infections, the primary reservoir of bacteria are animals from which they can be transmitted through food to humans (e.g., *Brucella, Campylobacter,* enterohemorrhagic *Escherichia coli, Listeria, Salmonella,* and occasionally, *Staphylococcus aureus, Streptococcus* spp., and *Vibrio*). In other infections, the causative bacterium resides primarily in soil that may contaminate foodstuffs (e.g., *Bacillus cereus, Clostridium botulinum, C. perfringens*). In a third group, the bacteria are primarily aquatic, infections are waterborne and animals do not seem, at least for now, to have a role in transmission even though they may carry the bacteria [e.g., *Aeromonas* (see chapter 2.26.2), *Edwardsiella, Plesiomonas, Vibrio*]. A last group contains certain bacteria that are transmitted from human-to-human only and through water or foodstuffs (e.g., *Shigella,* and occasionally, *Staphylococcus aureus*).

Tab. B.2 lists, in alphabetical order, bacterial agents that could be transmitted by food.

Table B2 | Important Bacteria Transmitted by Food[1]

BACTERIA	CONSPICUOUS SYMPTOMS	INCUBATION PERIOD	MOST IMPORTANT FOOD
Aeromonas spp.	Diarrhea (causative?) see Chap. 2.26.2	1–6 h	Seafood? Water sources
Bacillus cereus	Vomiting	1–6 h	Boiled rice kept unrefrigerated
Brucella spp.	see Chapter 2.5		
Campylobacter jejuni, C. coli	see Chapter 2.6		
Clostridium botulinum	Muscle weakness, fatigue, blurred vision, diplopia, dry mouth, hoarseness, difficulty swallowing, occasional diarrhea, terminal respiratory failure and cardiac arrest	12–72 h	Insufficiently sterilized food (home-canned vegetables, alkaline/low-acid foodstuffs in oil or airtight packaging, ungutted salted fish
Clostridium perfringens	Diarrhea, nausea, cramps	8–16 h	Insufficiently heated/reheated meat, poultry exposed to slow cooling
***Escherichia coli*[2]**			
EHEC	see Chap. 2.9		
EPEC	severe diarrhea, fever rare	?	Contaminated infant formula
EIEC	diarrhea (frequently bloody)	1–7 d	Potato/egg salad, lettuce, contaminated unrefrigerated food
ETEC	watery diarrhea, resembles light cases of cholera, abdominal pain	6–48 h	ditto
EAEC	watery diarrhea	8–18 h	Contaminated unrefrigerated food
Listeria monocytogenes	see Chapter 2.13		
Plesiomonas shigelloides	Diarrhea (causative?)	?	Seafood
Salmonella spp.	see Chapter 2.20		
Shigella spp.	Diarrhea (often bloody)	1–7 d	Potato/egg salad, lettuce
Staphylococcus aureus	Nausea, vomiting, hypotension	1–6 h	Eggs, meat, fish, milk
Streptococcus pyogenes	Pharyngitis, upper respiratory infection	1–4 d	Milk, potato and egg salad
Vibrio cholerae	see Chapter 2.24.1		
V. parahaemolyticus	Diarrhea, vomiting, often fever see Chap. 2.24.2	4–30 h	Insufficiently cooked seafood (shellfish)
V. vulnificus	Septicemia in patients with liver disease/immune defects/alcoholism/hemochromatosis see Chap. 2.24.2	12 h–30 d	Raw seafood (oysters)
Yersinia enterocolitica	see Chapter 2.25		

[1] Including some non-zoonotic bacteria (e.g., *C. botulinum*)
[2] EAEC, enteroaggregative E. coli; EHEC, enterohemorrhagic E. coli; EIEC, enteroinvasive E. coli, EPEC, enteropathogenic E. coli; ETEC, enterotoxigenic E. coli

Table B3 | Mycotoxins transmitted by animal foodstuffs

TOXIN	EFFECT	IMPORTANT SOURCE
Aflatoxin M	toxic, cancerogenic	Milk, milk products
Ochratoxin A	(nephro) toxic, cancerogenic, teratogenic, immunosuppressive	Blood and kidney from pigs, blood and liver from poultry, occasionally milk and milk and milk products

For a discussion of pathogenic mechanisms, means of transmission, critical number of organisms, prophylaxis and treatment, the reader is referred to the references because a thorough coverage of all (not only zoonotic) foodborne infections and intoxications is beyond the framework of this volume.

B.3 Fungi (Mycotoxins)

Mycotoxins, that is, metabolic products of certain molds, such as *Aspergillus*, *Fusarium*, and *Penicillium* spp., may be transmitted by foodstuffs of animal origin (Tab. B.3). As a rule, the chain involves farm animals that have taken up these fungi in moldy feedlots.

B.4 Parasites

Food can become a source of human infection with parasites. This can either be after accidental contamination, for example, by vegetables with infective stages of parasites that are sufficiently resistant to environmental influences (cysts, oocysts, larval stages) or when animals used for human food serve as intermediate or paratenic (transport) hosts of parasites.

A variety of protozoa (Tab. B.4.1) develops resistant cysts that are shed in the feces of their definite hosts and they persist for weeks or up to years in surface water or soil. This holds for *Entamoeba histolytica* and other amoeba, *Balantidium coli* and *Giardia duodenalis*. Oocysts that are particularly resistant are generated

Table B4.1 | Important protozoan infections transmitted by food

PARASITIC AGENT	MOST CONSPICUOUS SYMPTOMS	INCUBATION PERIOD	MOST IMPORTANT FOODSTUFFS
Balantidium coli	Diarrhea, enteritis	?	Any contaminated food
Cryptosporidium spp.	Diarrhea	5–28 days	Drinking water
Entamoeba histolytica	Diarrhea	1–7 days	Any contaminated food
	Abscesses in parenchymatous organs (see chapter 4)	Months to years	
Giardia lamblia	Diarrhea, gastrointestinal discomfort	6–15 days	Drinking water
Sarcocystis spp.	Diarrhea	1–2 days	Raw or undercooked pork or beef
Toxoplasma gondii	See chapter 4	See chapter 4	Raw or undercooked meat (pork, from sheep, goats, poultry?)
Trypanosoma cruzi	Generalized disease (see chapter 4)	10–30 days	Fruits, fruit juices contaminated with feces of infected reduviid bugs

after sexual multiplication by members of the class Coccidea. In the case of *Cryptosporidium* spp., *Toxoplasma gondii*, and *Sarcocystis* spp., they are released in feces into the environment where they rapidly mature and have to be ingested by suitable hosts for further development. In the case of *T. gondii*, oocysts excreted by cats represent only one type of infective stages for humans. In addition, in the cases of *T. gondii* and *Sarcocystis* spp., humans may be also infected by the ingestion of tissue cysts in raw or insufficiently cooked tissues of intermediate hosts. *T. gondii* cysts can be found in

all warm-blooded animals; cysts of *Sarcocystis* spp., infective for humans, develop in cattle and pigs.

Within the metazoa, trematodes and cestodes show generally complex heterogenous life cycles with one or more intermediate hosts. In the case of trematodes (flukes), the cycles are mostly water-bound. Concerning the major zoonotic trematodes (Tab. B.4.2), *Fasciola hepatica* and *Fasciolopsis buski* encyst to infectious metacercariae on plants, whereas *Opisthorchis* spp., *Clonorchis sinensis*, dwarf flukes, and lung flukes develop through two intermediate hosts and

Table B4.2 | Important helminth infections transmitted by food

PARASITIC AGENT	MOST CONSPICUOUS SYMPTOMS	INCUBATION PERIOD	MOST IMPORTANT FOODSTUFFS
Angiostrongylus cantonensis	Cerebral symptoms	1 to several weeks	Raw or undercooked crabs, crayfish, snails
Angiostrongylus costaricensis	Acute abdomen	>10 days	Raw or undercooked crabs, crayfish, snails
Anisakis spp., *Pseudoterranova* spp.	Epigastric pains, vomiting	Hours to several days	Raw or undercooked saltwater fish, squid
Capillaria philippinensis	Gastrointestinal symptoms (variable, see chapter 4)	?	Raw or undercooked freshwater or brackishwater fish
Clonorchis sinensis	Variable (cholangitis, see chapter 4)	Weeks	Raw or undercooked freshwater fish
Diphyllobothrium latum	Usually asymptomatic; 2% develop megaloblastic anaemia	Months	Raw or undercooked freshwater fish
Dracunculus medinensis	Painful blister or ulcer on the leg, impaired general condition	10–12 months	Drinking water
Echinostoma revolutum and many other dwarf fluke spp.	Diarrhea, abdominal pain	Weeks	Freshwater snails and mussels
Fasciola hepatica	Variable (see chapter 4)	2 weeks to months	Plants from natural sites contaminated with metacercariae
Fasciolopsis buski	Epi- and hypogastric pain, diarrhea	1–2 months	Water chestnuts contaminated with metacercariae
Opisthorchios felineus	See *Clonorchis sinensis*	Weeks	Raw or undercooked freshwater fish
Paragonimus spp.	Chest pain, cough, fever	5–10 weeks	Freshwater crabs, crayfish
Taenia saginata	Usually asymptomatic		Raw or undercooked beef
Taenia solium	See chapter 4	See chapter 4	Raw or undercooked pork
Trichinella spp.	See chapter 4	6–40 days	Raw or undercooked meat from various animals (pigs, wild boars, horses, and others)

encyst to infectious metacercariae in fish, frogs, or crustaceans, which are commonly used for human nutrition. In the first case, humans become infected by accidental ingestion of contaminated water plants, for example, watercress or of floating metacercariae. In the latter cases, infections occur by consumption of the raw or undercooked second intermediate hosts. Due to local eating habits, incidences in the human population are often high and diseases are common. Uncontrolled fish production by aqua culture techniques may be hazardous (see chapters 4.3.1 and 4.3.6 for carcinogenic effects of liver flukes).

Concerning cestodes, *Taenia* infections and diphyllobothriasis represent typical foodborne zoonoses due to the uptake of larval stages by consumption of raw or undercooked beef or pork and freshwater fish, respectively. *T. saginata* is found in cattle worldwide. Although great efforts have been made and are still ongoing in industrial countries to fight this zoonosis, success is still insufficient. *T. solium* and *Diphyllobothrium* infections are of more local importance. Cysticercosis due to *T. solium* and echinococcoses develop after accidental ingestion of tapeworm eggs by smear infections, or in the case of *Echinococcus multilocularis*, for example, by eating raw or undercooked berries or mushrooms contaminated by feces of infected foxes.

Diverse food-derived zoonotic nematode infections may occur after ingestion of raw or undercooked intermediate or paratenic hosts such as snails, crabs, frogs, reptiles, or partly, freshwater fishes. They can cause cerebral or intestinal angiostrongyliasis, gnathostomiasis, gongylonemiasis, and lagochilascariasis. The spectra of complementary hosts are complex; in some cases, meat of birds and rodents must be considered as a source of infection. Anisakiasis (herring worm disease) is caused by larvae of anisakids that are transmitted to humans in raw or undercooked saltwater fish. Ingestion of such larvae results in severe tissue responses in the bowel and hypersensitivity reactions due to larval allergens. Lasting problems are observed in many areas of the world due to *Trichinella* spp. The host spectrum of the genus is extremely broad, and together with local eating habits

(eating raw or undercooked meat), it is responsible for perseverative infections. Dracunculiasis is an example for infection via drinking water. It is transmitted to humans by infected copepods in contaminated drinking water and it was a scourge of humanity in many tropical areas. Indeed, it seemed almost to be defeated by eliminating the vectors and supplying the population in endemic areas with clean water; however, ongoing wars in the regions concerned rise doubts on the real success.

Arthropods are generally not transmitted by food. An exception may be represented by larvae of various flies (*Musca* spp., *Calliphora* spp., *Sarcophaga* spp.), deposited on unprotected meat. In cases where they are ingested by humans, they may cause intestinal (pseudo) myiasis.

Acanthocephalan parasites are transmitted to humans by intermediate hosts such as various beetles and by cockroaches. These animals are eaten in some areas, for example, in China, as traditional remedies. However, it is also epidemiologically important that some species use fish, amphibians, and reptiles as paratenic hosts. Pentastomids infecting humans are mostly parasites of dogs and snakes. Human infections may occur after consumption of vegetables contaminated with feces of infected animals, but also by undercooked snake meat, or, in case of linguatulosis, of viscera of animals (sheep, goats), which serve as paratenic hosts.

B.5 Fish Poisoning

Poisonings from the consumption of fish have increased worldwide, particularly due to increased tourism (Tab. B5). Fish may also transmit some of the agents listed in Tab. B2 and Tab. B4.

B.6 Shellfish Poisoning

Consumption of shellfish or other crustaceans may lead to food intoxication (Tab. B6). Shellfish may also transmit bacteria, viruses, and parasites to humans.

Table B5 | Zoonoses Transmitted to Man by Various Animal Species (Selection)

DISEASE	DOG	CAT	EQUINES	CATTLE	SHEEP, GOAT	PIG	MONKEY	RODENTS	BAT	WILD ANIM.	AMPHIBIANS	FISH	BIRDS
Acanthocephalosis						+						+	
Actinobacillosis			+		+								
Amebiasis		+											
Ancylostomiasis		+											
Angiostrongyliasis										+		+	
Anisakiasis												+	
Anthrax			+	+	+					+			
Argentine h.f.								+					
Balantidiasis						+	+						
Baylisascaris inf.										+			
Bolivian h.f.								+					
Bovine spongif. enc.				+									
Brucellosis	+			+	+	+				+			
Buffalo pox[1]			+[1]										
Californian enc.								+					
Camel pox			+[1]					+					
Campylobacteriosis	+			+		+		+		+			+
Capillariasis										+		+	
Capnocytophaga inf.	+	+											
Cat scratch disease		+											
Central Europ. enc.	+		+	+	+			+	+	+	+		+
Chagas disease	+	+											
Chikungunya f.							+						
Chlamydiosis		+			+	+		+					+
Clonorchiasis	+	+				+				+		+	
Coenuriasis	+									+			

Table B5 *continued*

DISEASE	DOG	CAT	EQUINES	CATTLE	SHEEP, GOAT	PIG	MONKEY	RODENTS	BAT	WILD ANIM.	AMPHIBIANS	FISH	BIRDS
Colorado tick f.								+					
Cow pox				+									
Crimean–Congo h.f.				+	+			+					
Cryptosporidiosis	+			+	+	+				+			
Dengue f.							+						
Dicrocoeliasis				+	+								
Dioctophymiasis	+	+								+	+	+	
Diphyllobotriasis	+	+				+						+	
Dipylidiasis	+	+											
Dirofilariasis	+												
Ebola v.inf.									+				
Echinococcosis	+	+								+			
Echinostomiasis	+	+										+	
EEE	+	+											+
EHEC inf.				+									
Ehrlichiosis	+												
Elephantpox										+			
Encephalomyocarditis						+		+		+			
Epid. polyarthritis	+			+	+			+					+
Erysipeloid					+	+				+		+	
Fascioliasis				+	+					+			
Fasciolopsiasis						+							
Filariasis (Brugia)	+	+											
Flea-bite induced dermatosis	+	+											
Food & Mouth dis.				+	+	+				+			
Gastrodiscoides inf.						+							
Giardiasis	+			+	+			+					
Glanders			+										

	C1	C2	C3	C4	C5	C6	C7	C8	C9	C10	C11	C12	C13
Gnathostomiasis						+					+	+	+
Gongylonemiasis				+		+						+	
Hantavirus inf.								+					
Hendravirus inf.			+							+			
Hepatitis E, Type 3						+						+	
Heterophysiasis				+						+		+	
Hymenolepsiasis			+					+					
Influenza A inf.													+
Japanese enc.	+	+	+										+
Kyasanur forest d.	+						+			+			+
Larva migrans	+	+											
Lassa fever								+					
Leishmaniasis	+												
Leptospirosis	+		+	+		+		+		+			
Listeriosis				+	+	+				+	+		
Louping ill					+	+		+		+			+
Lyme borreliosis	+		+	+	+	+		+		+			
LCM							+	+		+			
Marburg virus inf.							+		+	+			
Mayaro f.							+						+
Mediterranean s.f.	+												
Melioidosis	+		+		+	+		+					
MERS[2]									+				
Mesocestoides inf.	+		+										
Metagonimiasis													+
Microsporiasis	+		+				+	+		+			
Microsporidiosis	+		+					+					
Milker's nodules				+									
Mite infestation	+		+				+	+					

Table B5 continued

DISEASE	DOG	CAT	EQUINES	CATTLE	SHEEP, GOAT	PIG	MONKEY	RODENTS	BAT	WILD ANIM.	AMPHIBIANS	FISH	BIRDS
Monkeypox							+	+					
Murine typhus		+						+					
Murray valley enc.													+
Mycobacterium sp. (fish, aquarium)												+	
Nanophyetus salm.inf.	+	+								+		+	
Newcastle dis.													+
Nipah virus enc.									+				
Oesophagostomiasis							+						
Omsk h.f.								+					
Opisthorchiasis		+										+	
Oropouche f.							+						
Pappataci f.								+					
Paragonimiasis	+	+				+				+		+	
Pasteurellosis	+	+			+	+		+		+	+		
Pentastomidosis											+		
Plague		+						+		+			
Pneumocystosis	+												
Powassan v.	+							+	+[3]	+			
Pustular dermatitis					+								
Q fever	+			+	+			+		+			+
Rabies	+	+		+	+	+			+	+			
Rat bite f.								+		+			
Recurrent f.		+						+		+			
Rickettsialpox								+		+			
Rift valley fever				+	+								
Rocio enc.													+
RMSF	+									+			

Disease	1	2	3	4	5	6	7	8	9	10	11	12	13	14	15	16	17	18
Russ.spring-summer enc.	+							+					+		+		+	+
Salmonellosis	+							+				+	+		+		+	+
Sandfly fever			+			+		+						+				
Sarcoptes inf.	+		+		+			+					+				+	
Sarcosporidiosis								+				+	+		+	+		
SARS	+[4]																	+
Schistosomiasis			+			+												
Semliki forest f.		+																
Simian herpes v.d.												+		+				
Simian imm.-def. v.d.										+								
Simian malaria										+								
Sindbis f.																		+
Sparganosis															+		+	
Sporotrichosis	+													+		+		
Spotted f.ricketts.												+		+				
Staphylococcal inf	+		+					+				+	+	+			+	
SLE																		+
Stomatitis papulosa									+									
Streptococcal inf.	+		+					+				+	+	+		+	+	
Strongyloidiasis	+							+				+		+	+			
Swine vesic.d.								+										
Syngamosis	+		+						+									
Taeniasis asiatica/saginata								+				+		+				
Taeniasis solium												+		+				
Tanapox v.inf.										+					+			
Thelaziasis	+								+									
Tick dermatosis	+	+																
Toxoplasmosis	+											+		+		+		

Table B5 *continued*

DISEASE	DOG	CAT	EQUINES	CATTLE	SHEEP, GOAT	PIG	MONKEY	RODENTS	BAT	WILD ANIM.	AMPHIBIANS	FISH	BIRDS
Trichinellosis			+			+				+			
Trichophytosis	+	+	+	+	+	+	+	+		+			
Tricho-strongyloidiasis				+	+					+			
Trypanosomiasis				+									
Tsutsugamushi f.								+					
Tuberculosis	+	+	+	+	+		+			+			
Tularemia	+	+		+	+			+		+			
VEE			+						+				+
Vesicular stomatitis			+	+	+								
VHF								+					
Vibriosis incl.Cholera												+	
Wesselsbron d.	+		+	+	+					+			+
WEE			+									+	
West Nile f.	+		+										
Whitewater-Arroyo f.								+					
Yabapox v.d.							+						
Yellow fever							+						
Yersiniosis	+	+	+	+	+	+		+		+			+

Abbreviations: d, disease; enc, encephalitis ; EEE, eastern equine encephalitis ; EHEC, enterohemorrhagic Escherichia coli; f, fever; h, hemorrhagic; imm.-def, immunodeficiency; inf, infection; LCM, lymphocytic choriomeningitis; ricketts, ricketts., rickettsioses; RMSF, Rocky Mountain spotted fever; salm, salmincola; SLE, St Louis encephalitis; spong, spongiform;t, tick; v, virus; VEE; Venezuelan equine encephalitis; vesic, vesicular; VHF, Venezuelan hemorrhagic fever; WEE, western equine encephalitis.

Dogs includes all Canines, Cats includes all felines, Wild animals excludes monkeys and birds; Amphibians includes monkeys and birds; Amphibians includes snakes and tortoises; Fish includes shellfish.
[1] Buffalo
[2] Dromedary, camel
[3] Aardvark, Skunk, Fox
[4] Civet cat

Table B6 | Food poisoning from fish consumption

TOXIN	MOST CONSPICUOUS SYMPTOMS	INCUBATION PERIOD	MOST IMPORTANT SOURCES
Ciguatera toxins (ciguatoxin, gambierol, maitotoxin, scaritoxin)	Nausea; vomiting; watery diarrhea; abdominal pain; metallic taste; paresthesias onlips and oral mucosa are followed by numbness extending to the limbs; reversal of cold-hot sensation; pruritus on palms and soles; arthralgia; myalgia: in severe cases, heart arrhythmias, hypotension, dizziness; ataxia, seizures, lethargy, even coma. Acute symptoms last for 8–10 h; neurological symptoms last for weeks and even months. Mortality is <1%.	From minutes to approx 6 h, occasionally up to 30 h	Tropical or semitropical marine coral reef fish, mainly in the Caribbean Sea and Indian and Pacific Oceans; less often in Florida, Hawaii. Ciguatera toxins are produced by dinoflagellates (*Gambierdiscus toxicus* and *Ostreopsis lenticularis*) that are eaten by herbivorous fish which finally fall victim to predatory fish.
Palytoxin	Muscle spasms that intensify to uncontrollable tonic contractions of all muscle groups; tremor; nausea; vomiting; abdominal cramps; diarrhea; paresthesias; reversal of cold-hot sensation; acute respiratory distress; cardiac failure. Palytoxin is a potent tumor promoter.	Several hours	Palytoxin is synthesized by marine zoanthids (corals), e.g., *Palythoa* spp. and *Zoanthus* spp. It has been hypothesized but not proven that symbiotic algae and/or bacteria might be involved in palytoxin synthesis. The toxin has been detected in a wide range of marine animals, e.g., in sponges, corals, shellfish, polychaetes, crustaceans, and fish that feed on crustaceans and zoanthids as well. Marine animals are resistant to palytoxin, which exhibits extreme toxicity in mammals. Intoxications have been reported due to in-gestion of triggerfish (*Melichthys vidua*), filefish (*Alutera scripta*), parrot-fish (*Ypsicarus ovifrons*), mackerel (*Decapterus macrosoma*), and crabs (*Lophozozymus pictor* and *Demania reynaudii*).
Clupeotoxin	Metallic and bitter taste of the fish, nausea, abdominal cramps, vomiting, diarrhea, hypotension, headache, paresthesias, myalgia, paralysis, seizures	Minutes to a few hours	Herring, sardines, anchovies
Tetrodotoxin	Paresthesias first on lips and oral mucosa extending to the limbs and followed by numbness; nausea; ataxia; muscle cramps. In severe cases, general weakness, somnolence, ataxia, slurred speech, muscle cramps, dysphagia, difficulty breathing, hypotension, flaccid respiratory musculature. Mortality is up to 60%.	10–20 min, up to 3 h	Puffer fish (*Fugu rubripes, Fugu vermicularis, Fugu pardalis, Sphaeroides* spp.). Tetrodotoxin is produced by marine bacteria, e.g., *Pseudomonas* spp., *Micrococcus* spp., *Acinetobacter* spp., *Alteromonas* spp., and *Vibrio* spp., and bioaccumulates in the puffer fish. Tetrodotoxin has also been detected in marine snails, crabs, octopuses, newts and toads.
Histamine (scombroid toxin)	Urticaria, pruritus, perspiration, burning sensations of mouth and throat, hypotension, abdominal pain, nausea, vomiting, diarrhea. Symptoms last for 12–24 h.	15 min–1 h	Mahi-mahi, tuna, sardines, mackerel. Histamine in fish is produced by postmortem contamination with *Enterobacteriaceae*.
Botulinum toxin type E	See Table B1	12–24 h	Salted, smoked, or canned fish

Table B7 | Intoxications caused by consumption of crustaceans

TOXIN	MOST CONSPICUOUS SYMPTOMS	INCUBATION PERIOD	MOST IMPORTANT SOURCES
Saxitoxin, gonyautoxins (paralytic shellfish poisoning)	Tingling sensations on lips and oral mucosa extending to the face and limbs are followed by numbness, general weakness, somnolence, ataxia, and dizziness. Symptoms last for 12–48 h. In severe cases, dysphagia, difficulty in breathing, and flaccid paralysis of respiratory musculature occur. The mortality rate is approximately 10–15%.	5 min–4 h	Mussels, clams, scallops. Toxin is produced by dinoflagellates, e.g., *Gonyaulax* spp., *Alexandrium* spp., and *Gymnodinium catenatum*, presumably in connection with endosymbiotic bacteria. (Gene exchange? Gene transfer by phages?)
Domoic acid (amnesic shellfish poisoning)	Diarrhea, vomiting, abdominal cramps, headache, ataxia, amnesia, confusion; in severe cases, coma. Permanent memory defects can occur.	15 min–6 h	Mussels. Toxin is produced by dinoflagellates, e.g., *Pseudonitzschia pungens forma multiseries, Pseudonitzschia australis,* and *Pseudonitzschia pungens forma pungens.*
Brevetoxins (neurotoxic shellfish poisoning)	Facial paresthesias, which extend to the limbs, are followed by numbness, ataxia, reversal of cold-hot sensation. Symptoms last for <36 h.	5 min–4 h	Mussels. Toxin is produced by dinoflagellates, e.g., *Ptychodiscus brevis* and *Gymnodinium breve.*
Pectenotoxins, yessotoxin, dinophysistoxins, okadaic acid (diarrheic shellfish poisoning)	Nausea, vomiting, abdominal pain, severe diarrhea (up to 20 evacuations per day). Symptoms last for <3 days.	5–6 h	Mussels. Toxin is produced by dinoflagellates, e.g., *Dinophysis acuminata, Dinophysis fortii,* and *Prorocentrum lima.*

B.7 Phytotoxins Transmitted by Bats

In Guam, flying foxes (*Pteropus tokudae* and *P. marianus*) have been eaten by the indigenous people on ceremonial occasions and at social gatherings. Flying foxes, which sometimes consume up to two and a half times their body weight per night in fruit and nectar, find the seeds of *Cycas rumphii* to be highly palatable. However, the seeds contain neurotoxins, that is, beta-methyl-amino-L-alanine and cycasin and its aglycone, methylazoxymethanole, which are accumulated in the adipose tissue of the cycad-eating flying foxes. Due to consumption of flying foxes containing neurotoxins, people contract neurodegenerative diseases known as amyotrophic lateral sclerosis/parkinsonism-dementia complex with a high fatality rate.

REFERENCES

Anderson AD et al., Multistate outbreak of Norwalk-like virus gastroenteritis associated with a common caterer. *Am. J. Epidemiol.* 154, 1013–1019, 2001.

Archer DL, Young FE, Contemporary issues: diseases with a food vector. *Clin. Microbiol. Rev.* 1, 377–398, 1988.

Arcuri EF et al., Toxigenic status of Staphylococcus aureus isolated from bovine raw milk and Minas frescal cheese in Brazil. *J. Food Protect.* 73, 2225–2231, 2010.

Brenden RA, Millewr MA, Janda JM, Clinical disease spectrum and pathogenic factors associated with Plesiomonas shigelloides infections in humans. *Rev Infect Dis* 10, 303–316, 1988.

Callis JJ, Evaluation of the presence and risk of foot and mouth disease virus by commodity in international trade. *Rev. Sci. Tech.* 15, 1075–1085, 1996.

Chan TY, Chiu SW, Wild mushroom poisonings in Hong Kong. *Southeast Asian J. Trop. Med. Public Health* 42, 468–469, 2011.

Centers for Disease Control (CDC), Community outbreaks of shigellosis – United States. *MMWR Morb. Mort Wkly. Rep.* 39, 509–519, 1990.

Centers for Disease Control and Prevention (CDC), Neurologic illness associated with eating Florida pufferfish, 2002. *MMRW Morb. Mortal. Wkly. Rep.* 51, 321–323, 2002.

Centers for Disease Control and Prevention (CDC), Surveillance of food-borne disease outbreaks- United States, 2008. *MMWR Morb. Mortal. Wkly. Rep.* 60, 1197–1202, 2011.

Cliver DO, Viral foodborne disease agents of concern. *J. Food Prot.* 57, 176–178, 1994a.

Cliver DO, Epidemiology of viral foodborne disease. *J. Food Prot.* 57, 263–266, 1994b.

Cox PA, Sacks OW, Cycad neurotoxins, consumption of flying foxes, and ALS-PDC disease in Guam. *Neurology* 58, 956–959, 2002.

Donaldson AI, Risks of spreading foot and mouth disease through milk and diary products. *Rev. Sci. Tech.* 16, 117–124, 1997.

Doores S, Food safety – current status and future needs. *American Academy of Microbiology*, Washington, D.C., 1999.

Dorny P et al., Emerging food-borne parasites. *Vet. Parasitol.* 163, 196–206, 2009.

Eurosurveillance Editorial Team: The European Union summary report on trends and sources of zoonoses, zoonotic agents and food-borne outbreaks in 2011. *EuroSurveillance* 18, 20449.

Fosse J et al., On farm contamination of pigs by food-borne bacterial zoonotic hazards – an exploratory study. *Vet. Microbiol.* 147, 209–213, 2011.

Feried A, Abruzzi A, Food-borne trematode infections of humans in the United States of America. *Parasitol. Res.* 106, 1263–1280, 2010.

Fried B, Graczyk TK, Tamang L, Food-borne intestinal trematodiasis in humans. *Parasitol. Res.* 93, 159–170, 2004.

Fürst T, Keiser J, Utzinger J, Global burden of human food-borne trematodiasis. A systemic review and meta-analysis. *Lancet Infect. Dis.* 12, 210–221, 2012.

Gajadhar AA et al., Trichinella diagnostics and control: mandatory and best practices for ensuring food safety. *Vet. Parasitol.* 159, 197–205, 2009.

Gleibs S, Mebs B, Studies on the origin and distribution of palytoxin in a caribbean coral reef. *Toxicon* 33, 1531–1537, 1995.

Hall AH, Spoerke BH, Mushroom poisoning: identification, diagnosis, and treatment. *Pediatr. Rev.* 8, 291–298, 1987.

Hermans D et al., Poultry as host for the zoonotic pathogen Campylobacter jejuni. *Vector Borne Zoonotic Dis.* 12, 89–98, 2012.

Isonhood JH, Drake M, Aeromonas species in foods. *J. Food Prot.* 65, 575–582, 2002.

Iwamoto M et al., Epidemiology of seafood-associated infecftions in nthe United States. *Clin. Microbiol. Rev.* 23, 399–411, 2010.

Janda JM, Abbott SL, Infections associated with the genus Edwardsiella: the role of Edwardsiella tarda in human disease. *Clin. Infect. Dis.* 17, 742–748, 1993.

Jenkins EJ et al., Tradition and transition: parasitic zoonoses of people in Alaska, northern Canada, and Greenland. *Adv. Parasitol.* 82, 33–204, 2013.

Johansson A et al., Genetic diversity of Clostridium perfringens type A isolates from animals, food poisoning outbreaks and sludge. *BMC Microbiol.* 6, 47, 2006.

Kapperud G et al., Outbreak of Shigella sonnei infection traced to imported iceberg lettuce. *J. Clin. Microbiol.* 33, 609–614, 1995.

Kodama AM et al., Clinical and laboratory findings implicating palytoxin as cause of ciguatera poisoning due to Decapterus macrosoma (mackerel). *Toxicon* 27, 1051–1053, 1989.

Kurdova-Mintcheva R, Jordanova D, Ivanova M, Human trichinellosis in Bulgaria – epidemiological situation and trends. *Vet. Parasitol.* 159, 316–319, 2009.

Lund BM, Foodborne disease due to Bacillus and Clostridium species. *Lancet* 336, 982–986, 1990.

Mamminna C et al., A food-borne outbreak of Salmonella enteritica serotype Brandenburg as a hint to compare human, animal and food isolates identified in the years 2005–2009 in Italy. *J. Prev. Med. Hyg.* 52, 9–11, 2011.

Mead PS et al., Food-related illness and death in the United States. *Emerg. Inf. Dis.* 5, 607–625, 1999.

Mebs D, Occurrence and sequestration of toxins in food chains. *Toxicon* 36, 1519–1522, 1998.

Medus CJB et al., Salmonella infections in food workers identified through routine Public Health Surveillance in Minnesota: impact on outbrake recognition. *J. Food. Prot.* 73, 2053–2058, 2010.

Mullendore JL et al., Improved method for the recovery of hepatitis A virus from oysters. *J. Virol. Methods* 94, 25–35, 2001.

Nataro JP, Kaper JB, Diarrheagenic Escherichia coli. *Clin. Microbiol. Rev.* 11, 142–201, 1998.

Ravel A et al., Epidemiologicaland clinical description of the top three reportable parasitic diseases in a Canadian community. *Epidemiol. Infect.* 141, 431–442, 2013.

Rippey SR, Infectious diseases associated with molluscan shellfish consumption. *Clin. Microbiol. Rev.* 7, 419–425, 1994.

Scallan E et al., Foodborne illness acquired in the United States – major pathogens. *Emerg Infect. Dis.* 17, 7–15, 2011.

Shao D et al., A brief review of foodborne zoonoses in China. *Epidemiol. Infect.* 139, 1497–1504, 2011.

Sixl W et al., Rare transmission mode of FSME (tickborne encephalitis) by goat´s milk. *Geogr. Med. Suppl.* 2, 11–14, 1989.

Songer JG, Clostridia as agents of zoonotic disease. *Vet. Microbiol.* 140, 399–404, 2012.

Stafford R et al., An outbreak of Norwalk virus gastroenteritis following consumption of oysters. *Commun. Dis. Intell.* 21, 317–320, 1997.

Stolle A, Sperner B, Viral infections transmitted by food of animal origin: the present situation in the European Union. *Arch. Virol., Suppl.*, 13, 219–228, 1997.

Svensson L, Diagnosis of foodborne viral infections in patients. *Int. J. Food. Microbiol.* 59, 117–126, 2000.

Tauxe RV, Emerging foodborne diseases: an evolving public health challenge. *Emerg. Infect. Dis.* 3, 425–434, 1997.

Toledo R, Esteban JG, Fried B, Current status of foodborne trematode infections. *Eur. J. Clin. Microbiol. Infect. Dis.* 31, 1705–1718, 2012.

van Damme LR, Vandepitte J, Isolation of Edwardsiella tarda and Plesiomonas shigelloides from mammals and birds in Zaire. *Rev. Elev. Med. Vet. Pays Trop.* 37, 145–151, 1984.

Yolken RH, et al., Antibody to human rotavirus in cow's milk. *New Engl. J. Med.* 312, 605–610, 1985.

Yoshida N, Tyler KM, Llewellyn MS, Invasion mechanisms among food-borne portozoan parasites. *Trends Parasitol.* 27, 459–466, 2011.

Zhou P et al., Food-borne parasitic zoonoses in China: perspective for control. *Trends Parasitol.* 24, 190–196, 2008.

Appendix: Iatrogenic Transmission of Zoonotic Agents

Iatrogenic transmission of pathogens is generally possible for agents that circulate in the blood or infect tissues to be transplanted. Severe complications may arise, particularly if the agent is able to subsequently proliferate in the recipient. Apart from using contaminated tools, for instance, needles and syringes, iatrogenic transmission occurs mainly in the course of transfusion of blood or blood products and in organ transplantation. Major problems arise by the fact that usually relatively large amounts of agents are transmitted and the recipient is, in general, a sick person, impaired by an eventually reduced resistance or immunocompetence. Transmissions of the following zoonotic agents by transfusion of blood and blood products have been reported:

- Viruses: Colorado tick fever virus, dengue fever virus, West Nile fever virus, Ross River fever virus, herpes B virus, lymphocytic choriomeningitis virus, rabies virus, yellow fever 17D vaccine. HIVs originating from monkeys have been established as human infectious agents;
- Bacteria: *Anaplasma phagocytophilum, Brucella* spp. *Campylobacter jejuni, Ehrlichia ewingii, Listeria monocytogenes, Rickettsia rickettsii, Salmonella, Yersinia enterocolitica*;

- Parasites: *Babesia* spp., *Leishmania* spp., *Plasmodium* spp., *Toxoplasma gondii, Trypanosoma cruzi, Trypanosoma gambiense, Trypanosoma rhodesiense*.

Transmission by solid organ transplantation occurred with the West Nile fever virus, rabies virus (by cornea transplantation), prions (by cornea and dura mater transplantation), *Brucella, Mycobacterium tuberculosis, Toxoplasma gondii*, and *Strongyloides stercoralis*.

Iatrogenic transmission of zoonotic viruses is a special issue in the context of zoonotic diseases. Viruses and other agents from calves or sheep have probably been transmitted to humans by the smallpox vaccine, which is now out of use. Similarly, it is now acknowledged that simian virus 40 has been transmitted to humans in poliomyelitis vaccines. SV40, an oncogenic virus, was present in poliomyelitis virus vaccine produced before 1961. It was also found in some human meningiomas. It has, however, been argued that a virus closely related to the simian virus might have been present in the human population before the start of poliomyelitis vaccination. Other viruses, for example, simian retroviruses, were also present in vaccines of simian origin for human use in the early years before it was known that this problem existed. In contrast, a possible contamination with herpes B virus was recognized early enough to avoid contamination when monkey kidneys were used for production of poliomyelitis vaccines. The Marburg virus has been isolated from kidney cell cultures prepared from kidney cells of infected monkeys. The use of live poliomyelitis vaccines grown on chimpanzee-derived kidney cells in early vaccination studies has been implicated by some in the transmission of simian immunodeficiency virus to the human population, a political claim never corroborated scientifically. Vaccines grown in embryonated chicken or duck eggs are known to contain avian retroviruses, requiring the use of eggs from certified virus-free flocks for vaccine production.

The use of a recombinant virus based on the vaccinia virus as a vaccine "shuttle," which is in use for the vaccination of foxes against rabies, may be dangerous for people suffering from immunosuppression if it were transmitted.

Scrapie, a prion disease of sheep, has been transmitted experimentally via blood transfusion from sheep-to-sheep. Transmission of prions from person-to-person via blood transfusion remains a potential problem. Prions have been transmitted in human corneal transplants and dura mater, as has the rabies virus.

The technique of xenotransplantation may create an important additional risk for transmission of zoonotic infections. Transgenic pigs, the organs of which may be tolerated by human recipients, have already been developed. It has been shown that mice can be infected with hepatitis B virus when their livers are colonized by human hepatocytes. In the same way, porcine organs or cells transplanted to humans might render the recipient susceptible to infection with porcine viruses that may cross the species barrier rapidly. The problem is aggravated by the fact that organ recipients may have to be treated with immunosuppressants.

The use of feeder cells of murine origin for isolation and cultivation of human embryonic stem cells may be associated with the transmission of murine viruses, for example, lymphocytic choriomeningitis virus, which is highly pathogenic for humans. The risk of virus transmission is also associated with the use of murine monoclonal antibodies for human therapy.

Zoonotic bacteria (see above) have rarely been transmitted or caused symptoms by blood transfusion in the recipient. An exception is *Yersinia enterocolitica*, which has been transmitted via transfusion, but even this has been an exceptional event occurring with a frequency of only 1 in 10^5 to 10^7 in blood transfusions. It has generally been due to prolonged storage of blood from an asymptomatic donor with *Y. enterocolitica* bacteremia, with subsequent multiplication by the psychotropic bacterium and release of endotoxin that can be fatal. Even rarer has been transmission of infected donor organs by zoonotic bacteria; single cases have been recorded for *Brucella* and *Mycobacterium tuberculosis*.

Iatrogenic transmission of zoonotic parasites to humans concerns predominantly protozoa. Thus, in areas of the USA endemic for *Babesia microti*, babesiosis is considered one of the most frequent transfusion-transmitted human infections. According to estimates, up to 3.7% of blood and blood products collected in these areas may contain the parasite. At its intraerythrocytic stage, it survives >35 days storage of blood at 4 °C, as well as cryopreservation of blood cells. *Plasmodium* spp., for instance, are clearly less resistant to storage at such temperatures.

Iatrogenic transmission of *Leishmania* spp. and trypanosomes is a common problem in endemic areas. Particularly in the case of leishmaniasis, the selection of suitable uninfected donors is difficult because the relatively high rate of latent cases who do not respond in antibody assays. Reliable results, at the most, may be obtained by molecular techniques. There exist various current attempts to overcome the problems by pathogen inactivation in blood samples, although the methods are not yet applicable in practice.

In the case of *T. cruzi*, iatrogenic transmission plays an important role. Years ago, in some countries, 5 to 20% of all infections were supposed to be caused by blood transfusion. The situation has improved due to compulsatory antibody screening of blood donors, blood, and blood product by reliable assays.

Iatrogenic *Toxoplasma gondii* infections may be life threatening, particularly in recipients of solid organ transplants, whereas hemopoietic stem cell recipients seem to suffer more often from activation of their own persistent latent infections. Transmission by blood transfusion seems to be relatively rare due to the limited occurrence of the parasite in the peripheral blood.

The risk of transmission varies with the transplanted organ and seems to be particularly high after heart transplantation. Clinical symptoms develop within approximately 3 months, whereby myocardititis, encephalitis, and pneumonitis prevail. Dissemination occurs frequently. Chorioretinitis was reported as a common first sign. Serological investigations of donors and recipients are recommended to estimate particular risks. For chemoprophylactic treatment of recipients (see Constanzo et al., 2010).

Among metazoan parasites, iatrogenic infections with *Strongyloides stercoralis* may be a cause of serious disease. The usual developmental cycle includes a percutaneous invasion by third-stage larvae, a tissue migration to the lungs where they break through the alveoles, are then swallowed, and finally settle in the small intestine where the parthenogenetic females produce eggs (see chapter 4). The parasite tends to autoinfections when infective larvae already develop in the intestine and start tissue migration immediately or after skin penetration in the perianal region. This type of larvae may be transplanted together with hemopoietic stem cells or in solid organs to recipients where it completes its development. The complications arise by a tendency of the parasite to cause "hyperinfections" by continuous autoinfections in immunosuppressed people such as transplant recipients.

Chronic *S. stercoralis* infections are common in many tropical and subtropical areas and are asymptomatic in about 50% of the cases. In-depth diagnostic analysis of potential transplant donors is recommended, in particular, if there is a history of travelling to endemic areas. Drugs of choice are benzimidazoles and ivermectin (see chapter 4).

There are some other reports on iatrogenic transmission of metazoan stages, for example, of microfilariae, but they are irrelevant because such stages do not cause damage nor do they proliferate in the recipients. At the most, sparganum infections by measures of traditional medicine in Asia are to be mentioned. These infection occur when chopped meat of frogs accidentally infected with larval stages of pseudophyllid cestodes is applied, for example, to wounds from where the larvae invade the patient

REFERENCES

Alves da Silva A et al., The risk factors for and effects of visceral leishmaniasis in graft and renal transplant recipients. *Transplantation* 95, 721–727, 2013.

Blusch JH, Patience U, Martin: pig endogenous retroviruses and xenotransplantation. *Xenotransplantation* 9, 242–251, 2002.

Boneva RS, Folks TM, Chapman LE, Infectious disease issues in xenotransplantation. *Clin. Microbiol. Rev.* 14, 1–14, 2001.

Centers for: Disease Control and Prevention (CDC), Update: detection of West Nile virus in blood donations – United States, 2003. *MMWR Morb. Mortal. Wkly. Rep.* 52, 916–919, 2003.

Centers for: Disease Control and Prevention (CDC), Anaplasma phagocytophilum transmitted through blood transfusion – Minnesota 2007. *MMWR Morb. Mortal. Wkly. Rep.* 57, 1145–1148, 2008.

Centers for Disease Control and Prevention (CDC), Transplantation-transmitted tuberculosis – Oklahoma and Texas, 2007. *MMWR Morb. Mortal. Wkly. Rep.* 57, 333–336, 2008.

Chapman L, Xenotransplantation: benefits and risks. *Emerg. Infect. Dis.* 7 (Suppl. 3), 545, 2001.

Chattopadhyay R, Majam VF, Kumar S, Survival of Plasmodium falciparum in human blood during refrigeration. *Transfusion* 51, 630–635, 2011.

Chokkalingam Mani B et al., Strongyloides stercoralis and organ transplantation. *Case Rep. Transplant.* 549038, 2013.

Constanzo MR et al., The International Society for Heart and Lung Transplantation guidelines for the care of heart transplant recipients. *J. Heart. Lung. Transplant.* 29, 914–956, 2010.

Derrouin F et al., Prevention of toxopülasmosis in transplant patients. *Clin. Microbiol. Infect.* 14, 1089–1101, 2008.

Economidou J et al., Brucellosis in two thalassemic patients infected by blood transfusions from the same donor. *Acta Haematol* 55, 244–249, 1976.

Ertem M et al., Brucellosis transmitted by bone marrow transplantation. *Bone Marrow Transplant.* 26, 225–226, 2000.

Ferber D, Virology. Monkey virus link to cancer grows stronger. *Science* 296, 1012–1015, 2002.

Filloy A, Garcia-Garcia O, Fernandez-Lorente L, Chorioretinitis as the first sign of acquired toxoplasmosis transmitted from donor following kidney transplantation: a case report and review of the literature. *Ocul. Immunol. Inflamm.* 21, 34–35, 2013.

Fishman JA, Infection in xenotransplantation. *J. Card. Surg.* 16, 363–373, 2001.

Gerber MA et al., The risk of acquiring Lyme disease or babesiosis from a blood transfusion. *J. Infect. Dis.* 170, 231–234, 1994.

Guinet F, Carniel E, Leclercq A, Transfusion-transmitted Yersinia enterocolitica sepsis. *Clin. Infect. Dis* 53, 583–591, 2011.

Harrington T et al., West Nile virus infection transmitted by blood transfusion. *Transfusion* 43, 1018–1022, 2003.

Iwamoto M et al., Transmission of West Nile virus from an organ donor to four transplant recipients. *New Engl. J. Med.* 348, 2196–2203, 2003.

Izquierdo I et al., Fatal Strongyloides hyperinfection complicating a Gram-negative sepsis after allogeneic stem cell transplantation: case report and review of the literature. *Case Rep. Hematol.* 860976, 2013.

Jafari M et al., Salmonella sepsis caused by a platelet transfusion from a donor with a pet snake. *N. Engl. J. Med.* 347, 1075–1078, 2002.

Jimenez-Marco T et al., Pathogen inactivation technology applied to a blood component collected from an asymptomatic carrier of Leishmania infection: a case report. *Vox. Sang.* 103, 356–358, 2012.

Leiby DA, Gill JE, Transfusion-transmitted tick-borne infections: a cornucopia of threats. *Transfus. Med. Rev.* 18, 293–306, 2004.

Leiby DA, Transfusion-transmitted Babesia spp.: bull's eye on Babesia microti. *Clin. Microbiol. Rev.* 24, 14–28, 2011.

Menon M et al., Listeria monocytogenes in donated platelets: a potential transfusion-transmitted pathogen intercepted through screening. *Transfusion* 53, 1974–1978, 2013.

Mesta L et al., Transfusion-transmitted visceral leishmaniasis caused by Leishmania mexicana in an immunocompromised patient: a case report. *Transfusion* 51, 1919–1923, 2011.

Morris MI, Fischer SA, Ison MG, Infections transmitted by transplantation. *Infect. Dis. Clin. North Am.* 24, 497–514, 2010.

Osthoff M et al., Disseminated toxoplasmosis after allogeneic stem cell transplantation in a seronegative recipient. *Transpl. Infect. Dis.* 15, e14–e19, 2013.

Pealer LN et al., Transmission of West Nile virus through blood transfusion in the United States in 2002. *N. Engl. J. Med.* 349, 1236–1245, 2003.

Pepersack F et al., Campylobacter jejuni post-transfusional septicemia. *Lancet 2*, 911, 1979.

Procopio AR et al., SV40 expression in human neoplastic and non-neoplastic tissues: perspectives on diagnosis, prognosis and therapy of human malignant mesothelioma. *Dev. Biol. Stand.* 94, 361–367, 1998.

Reading FC, Brecher ME, Transfusion related sepsis. *Curr. Opin. Hematol.* 8, 380–386, 2001.

Regan J et al., A confirmed: Ehrlichia ewingii infection likely acquired through platelet transfusion. *Clin. Infect. Dis.* 56, e105–107, 2013.

Reynolds L, McKee M, Possible risks of transmission of bloodborne infection via accupuncture needles in Guizhou province, southwest China. *J. Altern. Complement. Med.* 14, 1281–1285, 2008.

Sandler SG, Risks of blood transfusion. *Curr. Opin. Hematol.* 9, 509–510, 2002.

Sazama K, Bacteria in blood for transfusion. *A review. Arch. Pathol. Lab. Med.* 118, 350–365, 1994.

Scarlata F et al., Asymptomatic Leishmania infantum/chagasi infection in blood donors of western Sicily. *Trans. R. Soc. Trop. Med. Hyg.* 102, 394–396, 2008.

Strabelli TM et al., Toxoplasma gondii myocarditis after adult heart transplantation: successful prophylaxis with pyrimethamine. *J. Trop. Med.* 853562, 2012.

Strickler HD, Goedert JJ, Exposure to SV40-contaminated poliovirus vaccine and the risk of cancer – a review of the epidemiological evidence. *Dev. Biol. Stand.* 94, 235–244, 1998.

Strickler HD et al., Contamination of poliovirus vaccines with simian virus 40 (1955–1963) and subsequent cancer rates. *JAMA* 279, 292–295, 1998.

Weile J et al., First case of Mycobacterium tuberculosis transmission by heart transplantation from donor to recipient. *Int. J. Microbiol.* 303, 449–451, 2013.

Wylie BR, Transfusion transmitted infection: viral and exotic diseases. *Anaesth. Intensive Care* 21, 24–30, 1993.

Appendix: Zoonotic Diseases Notifiable at the National Level

Appendix D | *Zoonotic* Diseases Notifiable at the National Level, United States (2012) and Canada (2014)[1]

DISEASE	UNITED STATES	CANADA
Anthrax	+	+
Arboviral diseases	+[2]	+[3]
Babesiosis	+	
Brucellosis	+	+
Campylobacteriosis		+
Cholera	+[4]	+
Cryptosporidiosis	+	+
Ehrlichiosis/Anaplasmosis	+	
Giardiasis	+	+
Hantavirus pulmonary syndrome	+	+
Influenza A virus	+[5]	+[6]
Leptospirosis	+	
Listeriosis	+	+[7]
Lyme disease	+	+
Malaria	+	+
Paralytic shellfish poisoning		+
Plague	+	+
Psittacosis/Ornithosis	+	+
Q fever	+	
Rabies	+	+
Salmonellosis	+	+
SARS-CoV disease	+	+
Spotted fever rickettsioses	+	+

continued

Appendix D *continued*

DISEASE	UNITED STATES	CANADA
Trichinellosis	+	
Tuberculosis (incl. bovine)	+	+
Tularemia	+	+
Verotoxigenic *E. coli* (EHEC)	+[8]	+
Vibriosis other than Cholera	+[9]	
Viral hemorrhagic fevers	+[10]	+
Yellow fever	+	+

[1] +, Notifiable; blank, no mention in reference.
United States: www.cdc.gov/mmwr/mmwr_nd
Canada: dsol-smed.phac-aspc.gc.ca
[2] incl. disease due to California serogroup viruses, EEE virus, Powassan virus, SLE virus, West Nile virus, WEE virus, Dengue virus
[3] West Nile virus listed only
[4] toxigenic serotypes 01 and 0139
[5] novel viruses, associated pediatric mortality
[6] if laboratory confirmed
[7] invasive forms only
[8] incl. hemolytic-uremic syndrome
[9] any species of the family Vibrionaceae
[10] Diseases due to Crimean-Congo hemorrhagic fever virus, Ebola virus, Lassa virus, Lujo virus, Marburg virus, and New World Arenaviruses

REFERENCES

Centers for Disease Control and Prevention (CDC), Summary of Notifiable Diseases – United States, 2012; Adams DA, Coordinator. MMWR Morb. Mort. Wkly. Rep. 61, 1–121, 2014.

Final Report and Recommendations from the National Notifiable Diseases Working Group. Canada Communicable Disease Report 32, 1–16, 2006 (modified 2014).

Index

A

Acanthamoeba spp., 307, 309
Acanthocephala, 447–448
Acanthocephalan parasites, 488
Acanthocephaliosis, 447–448
Acinetobacter spp., 478, 479
Actin-assembly inducing protein (ActA), 219
Actinobacilloses, 280
Actinobacillus infections, 280
Actinobacillus spp., 232, 280, 478, 480
Actinomyces spp., 478
Active immunization, 36, 56
Acute respiratory distress syndrome (ARDS), 204, 312
Acute schistosomiasis, 380
Adult *Schistosoma* flukes, 380
Adult soft ticks, 452
Adult T-cell leukemia (ATL), 147, 148
Aedes (*Stegomyia*) *abnormalis*, 16
Aedes (*Stegomyia*) *triseriatus*, 6
Aedes aegypti (*A. aegypti*), 7, 8, 21
Aedes albopictus (*A. albopictus*), 462
Aedes caspius (*A. caspius*), 74
Aedes sollicitans (*A. sollicitans*), 11
Aedes triseriatus (*A. triseriatus*), 67
Aedes vexans (*A. vexans*), 11
A/E lesions. *See* Attachment and effacement lesions (A/E lesions)
Aeromonads, 280
Aeromonas spp. /infections, 260, 280–281, 479, 480, 485
Afipia spp., 181
African horse sickness. *See* Semliki Forest fever
African tick bite fever, 251–252
African *Trypanosoma* spp., 319
African trypanosomiasis, 351
  clinical manifestations, 352–353
  diagnosis, 354
  differential diagnosis, 354
  etiology, 351
  occurrence, 351–352
  prophylaxis, 355
  therapy, 354–355
  transmission, 352
AHF. *See* Argentinian hemorrhagic fever (AHF)
AIDS. *See* Acquired human immunedeficiency syndrome (AIDS)
Alabama rot, 209
Alaria alata (*A. alata*), 383, 384
Alaria americana (*A. americana*), 383, 384
Alaria genus, 383
Albuminuria, 55
Alcaligenes spp., 478
Aleppo boil, 337
Alkhurma virus hemorrhagic fever, 39–40
Alligator bites, 479
Allodermanyssus sanguineus (*A. sanguineus*), 252
Alphaviral zoonoses, 8
  clinical manifestations, 9–10
  occurrence, 9
  prophylaxis, 10
  transmission, 8–9
Alphaviruses. *See also* Bunyaviruses; Flaviviruses; Mosquito-borne flaviviruses
  agents, 8
  alphaviral zoonoses, 8–10
  Chikungunya fever, 21–23

Alphaviruses (*Continued*)
  EEE, 10–12
  epidemic polyarthritis, 18–20
  Mayaro fever, 25–26
  O'nyong-nyong fever, 24–25
  Semliki Forest fever, 16–17
  Sindbis fever, 17–18
  VEE, 14–15
  WEE, 12–14
Alveolar echinococcosis, 390, 393. *See also*
    Cystic echinococcosis
  clinical manifestations, 392–393
  diagnosis, 393
  differential diagnoses, 393
  etiology, 390
  in liver, 392
  occurrence, 390–392
  prophylaxis, 394
  therapy, 393–394
  transmission, 392
Alveolar echinococcus, 385
Ambisense technique, 88
Amblyomma, 180, 190, 203, 204, 248, 251, 450
Amebiasis, 307. *See also* Babesiosis
  clinical manifestations, 309
  diagnosis, 309–310
  differential diagnosis, 310
  etiology, 307
  occurrence, 308
  prophylaxis, 311
  therapy, 310–311
  transmission, 308–309
Amebic abscess, 310–311
Amebic dysentery, 310–311
Amebic keratitis, 308, 311
Ameboma, 309
American cutaneous and mucocutaneous
    leishmaniases, 339. *See also* Old World cutaneous
    leishmaniasis
  clinical manifestations, 339–341
  cutaneous leishmaniasis, 340
  diagnosis, 341
  differential diagnosis, 341
  etiology, 339
  occurrence, 339
  prophylaxis, 341
  therapy, 341
  transmission, 339
American Prospect Hill virus, 78
American trypanosomiasis. *See* Chagas' disease
Amerithrax, 176
Amphotericin B lipid complex, 336
Amyotrophic lateral sclerosis, 496

Anadromous species, 388
Anaplasma spp., 202, 499
  A. phagocytophilum, 203
  pathogenic for humans, 203
Anaplasmata, 202, 205
Anaplasmoses, 202, 204, 503
Ancylostoma spp.
  A. braziliense, 430
  A. braziliense, 430, 431
  A. caninum, 420
  A. ceylanicum, 428
  A. duodenale, 428, 429, 431, 435
Angiomatosis, 182, 183
Angiostrongyliasis, 410
  cerebral, 410–411
  intestinal, 411–412
Angiostrongylus cantonensis (*A. cantonensis*), 410
Angiostrongylus costaricensis (*A. costaricensis*), 411
Animal bite infections, 477
  Alligator bites, 479
  bat bites, 479
  bear bites, 480–482
  bird bites, 480
  bites by foxes, 477–478
  camel bites, 479–480
  cat bites, 478
  dog bites, 477–478
  ferret bites bites, 479
  fish bites, 479
  guinea pig bites, 479
  hamster bites, 479
  horse bites, 480
  lizard bites, 479
  mouse bites, 480
  opossum bites, 480
  pig bites, 480
  raccoons, 477–478
  rat bites, 480
  seal bites, 480
  shark bites, 479
  sheep bites, 480
  Simian bites, 478–479
  skunks, 477–478
  snake bites, 480
  squirrel bites, 479
Animal scabies. *See* Sarcoptic mange
Anisakiasis, 412
  clinical manifestations, 414
  diagnosis, 414
  differential diagnosis, 414
  etiology, 412–413
  occurrence, 413
  prophylaxis, 414–415

therapy, 414
transmission, 413–414
Anisakis spp., 412, 413
Anopheles spp., 17, 28, 346, 423, 460
  A. funestus, 24
  A. gambiae, 7, 24
Anthrax, 175
  clinical manifestations, 176, 177
  diagnosis, 177–178
  differential diagnosis, 178
  etiology, 175
  occurrence, 175, 176
  prophylaxis, 178
  reporting, 178
  therapy, 178
  transmission, 176
Anthrax carbuncle, 177
Anthrax vaccine adsorbed vaccine (AVA vaccine), 178
Anthrax vaccine precipitated vaccine, 178
Anthropophilic dermatophytes, 293
Anti-*Giardia*-IgG antibodies, 329
Anti-TBE hyperimmunoglobulin, 36
Antibiotics, 260
Antimicrobial therapy, 481
Anuria, 55
Apathogenic arboviruses, 17
Aphthovirus, 134
Apolipoprotein L1 (ApoL1), 363
Arboviruses, 3, 5, 47
Arbovirus infections, cycles of, 5–8
Arcanobacterium pyogenes (*A. pyogenes*), 291
Arcobacter infections, 281–282
ARDS. *See* Acute respiratory distress syndrome (ARDS)
Arenaviridae, 88
Arenaviruses, 88, 89
  Lassa fever, 92–94
  LCM virus, 88, 89–91
  zoonotic arenaviruses, 89
Argasidae/*Argas* spp., 189, 449
Argasid ticks, 450
Argentinian hemorrhagic fever (AHF), 95–97
Armillifer armillatus (*A. armillatus*), 473
Arthralgias, 21, 25
Arthroderma spp., 296
Arthropod-borne viruses. *See* Arboviruses
Arthropod-transmitted bunyaviruses, 65
Arthropoda, 449
Arthropods, 449, 488. *See also* Parasitic zoonoses
  diptera, 459–467
  fleas, 467–470
  heteroptera infestations, 471–473

mites, 455–459
ticks, 449–455
Ascaris lumbricoides (*A. lumbricoides*), 446, 447
Asian "tiger mosquito" (*Stegomyia albopicta*), 5
Aspergillus spp., 205, 480, 486
Assassin bugs, 471
Asymptomatic intestinal carriers, 310
ATL. *See* Adult T-cell leukemia (ATL)
Attachment and effacement lesions (A/E lesions), 206
Atypical fowl plague. *See* Newcastle disease
Auchmeromya luteola (*A. luteola*), 464
Auricular myiasis, 466
Austrobilharzia variglandis (*A. variglandis*), 364
AVA vaccine. *See* Anthrax vaccine adsorbed vaccine (AVA vaccine)
Avian influenza viruses, 131. *See also* Swine influenza virus
  clinical manifestations, 132
  diagnosis, 132
  differential diagnosis, 132–133
  etiology, 131
  occurrence, 131
  prophylaxis, 133
  therapy, 133
  transmission, 131–132

B
B-weapons, zoonotic viruses as, 4
Babesia divergens (*B. divergens*), 314
Babesia microti (*B. microti*), 500
Babesia spp., 312
  developmental cycle, 313
  in humans, 312
Babesiosis, 312. *See also* Amebiasis
  clinical manifestations, 314
  diagnosis, 314
  differential diagnosis, 314–315
  etiology, 312
  occurrence, 312–313
  prophylaxis, 315
  therapy, 315
  transmission, 313–314
Baby hamster kidney cells (BHK21), 9
Bacillary angiomatosis, 182
Bacille Calmette-Guérin vaccine (BCG vaccine), 226, 227
Bacillus spp., 478, 480
  B. anthracis, 175, 176
  B. cereus, 485
  B. thuringiensis, 464
Bacteremia, 177

Bacteria, 484–486, 499
Bacterial zoonoses, 175. *See also* Parasitic zoonoses;
  Viral zoonoses
  actinobacillus infections, 280
  aeromonas infections, 280–281
  anthrax, 175–178
  arcobacter infections, 281–282
  bartonelloses, 179–183
  bordetella infections, 282–283
  borrelioses, 183–191
  brucelloses, 191–194
  campylobacterioses, 195–198
  capnocytophaga infections, 283–284
  chlamydioses, 198–201
  C. pseudotuberculosis infections, 284–285
  D. congolensis, 286–287
  EHEC infections, 206–210
  ehrlichioses/anaplasmosis, 202–206
  erysipeloid, 211–213
  glanders, 214–215
  helicobacter infections, 287
  leptospiroses, 216–218
  listeriosis, 219–222
  melioidosis, 288–290
  mycobacterioses, 223–232
  pasteurelloses, 232–234
  plague, 234–237
  Q fever, 238–242
  rare and potential agents, 280
  rat bite fever, 242–244
  R. equi, 290
  rickettsioses, 244–257
  salmonelloses, 257–261
  staphylococcal infections, 262–263
  streptococcal infections, 264–268
  T. pyogenes, 291
  tularemia, 269–272
  vibrioses, 272–275
  yersinioses, 276–279
Bacteroide spp., 478, 479, 480
Balamuthia spp., 307
Balantidiasis, 315. *See also* Cryptosporidiosis;
  Giardiasis
  clinical manifestations, 316–317
  diagnosis, 317
  differential diagnosis, 317
  etiology, 315–316
  occurrence, 316
  prophylaxis, 317
  therapy, 317
  transmission, 316
Balantidium coli (*B. coli*), 315, 486
  developmental cycle, 316

Bang's disease, 192
Barmah forest fever, 18, 18, 19–20
Bartonellaceae, 202, 245
Bartonella spp., 179–180, 181
  endocarditis due to, 182
  medical and veterinarian significance,
    184–185, 190
Bartonelloses, 179
  Bartonella infections in immunocompromised
    patients, 182–183
  CSD, 180–182
  endocarditis, 182
  etiology, 179–180
  occurrence, 180
  transmission, 180
Bat-borne viruses, 3–4
Bat bites, 479
Bat rabies, 111, 112
Baylisascaris procyonis (*B. procyonis*), 432, 433
Bayou virus, 78
BCG vaccine. *See* Bacille Calmette-Guérin vaccine
    (BCG vaccine)
Bear bites, 480
  clinical manifestations, 480–481
  diagnosis, 481
  therapy, 481–482
Bed bug (*Cimex lectularius*), 471, 472
Benznidazole, 322
Bergeyella zoohelcum (*B. zoohelcum*), 233, 478
Bertiella spp., 408
Beta-retroviruses, 147
BHF. *See* Bolivian hemorrhagic fever (BHF)
BHK21. *See* Baby hamster kidney cells (BHK21)
Bilharziosis. *See* Schistosomiasis
Biosafety level 3 (BSL-3), 48, 178
Bioweapons, 176, 192, 214, 235, 239, 246,
    270, 288
Bird bites, 480
Bird migration, 8
Bites, 477
BIV. *See* Bovine immunodeficiency virus (BIV)
Black Creek Canal virus, 78
Blackflies (Simuliidae), 460, 462
Bolbosoma spp., 447, 448
Bolivian hemorrhagic fever (BHF), 95–97
Bordetella bronchiseptica (*B. bronchiseptica*), 282
Bordetella infections, 282–283
Borrelia spp., 85, 183
  B. burgdorferi, 7, 32, 204, 279, 452
  B. garinii, 36
  B. recurrentis, 189, 191
  medical and veterinarian significance,
    184–185, 190

Borrelioses, 183
  lyme borreliosis, 183–188
  relapsing fever, 189–191
Bovine immunodeficiency virus (BIV), 149
Bovine spongiform encephalopathy (BSE), 169–170
  clinical manifestations, 172
  diagnosis, 172
  differential diagnosis, 172
  etiology, 170
  genetic disposition, 172
  occurrence, 170–171
  prophylaxis, 172, 173, 174
  transmission, 171
Bradyzoites, 356
Brevibacterium spp., 478
Broad tapeworm, 386
Brucella spp., 179, 192, 194, 271, 279, 484, 499
  transmission chains, 193
Brucelloses, 191. *See also* Lyme borreliosis;
    Relapsing fever
  clinical manifestations, 192, 193
  diagnosis, 193–194
  differential diagnosis, 194
  etiology, 191–192
  occurrence, 192
  prophylaxis, 194
  reporting, 194
  therapy, 194
  transmission, 192, 193
Brucellosis, 103, 192, 193
Brugia filariasis, 422
  clinical manifestations, 423
  diagnosis, 423–424
  differential diagnosis, 424
  etiology, 422
  occurrence, 422–423
  prophylaxis, 424
  therapy, 424
  transmission, 423
Brugia spp., 421
  B. malayi, 421, 422, 423
  B. timori, 422, 423
BSE. *See* Bovine spongiform encephalopathy (BSE)
BSL-3. *See* Biosafety level 3 (BSL-3)
Bubo, 236
Buffalopox, 163
Bugs, 318, 319, 449, 471–473
Bunostomum, 431
Bunyaviruses, 65, 67. *See also* Alphaviruses;
    Flaviviruses; Mosquito-borne flaviviruses
  CCHF, 71–73
  La Crosse encephalitis, 68–69
  Oropouche fever, 70–71

RVF, 73–75
SFF, 76–77
Snowshoe hare virus, 68–69
Tahynavirus, 68–69
zoonotic bunyaviruses, 66–67
Burkholderia mallei (*B. mallei*), 214
Burkholderia pseudomallei (*B. pseudomallei*), 288
  infections, 288–290

C
CAA. *See* Circulating anodic antigen (CAA)
C. abortus, 199, 201
CAE. *See* Caprine arthritis encephalitis virus (CAE)
cAECT. *See* mini anion exchange centrifugation
    technique (cAECT)
California encephalitis. *See* La Crosse encephalitis
Calliphora spp., 464, 488
Camel bites, 479–480
Camelpox, 163–164
Campylobacterioses, 195
  clinical manifestations, 196, 197
  diagnosis, 197
  differential diagnosis, 197
  etiology, 195–196
  occurrence, 196
  prophylaxis, 198
  reporting, 198
  therapy, 197
  transmission, 196, 197
Campylobacter spp., 195, 197, 279
Candida spp., 229, 479
Capillaria aerophila (*C. aerophila*), 417
Capillaria hepatica (*C. hepatica*), 415
Capillaria philippinensis (*C. philippinensis*), 416
Capillariases, 415
  hepatic, 415–416
  intestinal, 416–417
  pulmonary, 417–418
Capnocytophaga canimorsus (*C. canimorsus*), 283
Capnocytophaga infections, 283–284
Caprine arthritis encephalitis virus (CAE), 149
5′cap snatching, 67
Cardiovirus, 134
Cat bites, 478
Cat flea (*Ctenocephalides felis*), 199, 201, 467, 468
Cat scratch disease (CSD), 180
  clinical manifestations, 180, 181
  clinical presentation, 182
  diagnosis, 181, 182
  differential diagnosis, 182
  etiology, 180
  occurrence, 180
  prophylaxis, 182

Cat scratch disease (CSD) (*Continued*)
  transmission, 180
  treatment, 182
Caulimoviridae, 147
Causative agents, 364
Caveolin phosphorylates FYN, 168
CCA. *See* Circulating cathodic antigen (CCA)
CCHF. *See* Crimean-Congo hemorrhagic fever (CCHF)
CDC. *See* Centers for Disease Control (CDC)
CEE. *See* Central European encephalitis (CEE)
Cefsulodin-irgasannovobiocin (CIN), 278
Centers for Disease Control (CDC), 187
Central European encephalitis (CEE), 27, 32
  clinical manifestations, 34–35
  diagnosis, 35–36
  differential diagnosis, 36
  etiology, 32
  occurrence, 32, 34
  prophylaxis, 36–37
  therapy, 36
  transmission, 34
Central European tick encephalitis (CEE). *See*
    Central European encephalitis (CEE)
Central nervous system (CNS), 300, 307
  Borreliae, 187
Ceratopogonidae, 460, 463
Cercariae, 364
Cercarial dermatitis, 363, 364, 365
  clinical manifestations, 364–365
  diagnosis, 365
  differential diagnosis, 365
  etiology, 364
  occurrence, 364
  prophylaxis, 365
  therapy, 365
  transmission, 364
Cerebral angiostrongyliasis, 410–411
Cerebral cysticercosis, 406
Cerebral larva migrans (CLM), 433
Cerebrospinal fluid (CSF), 9, 188
Cestodes, 384. *See also* Nematodes; Parasitic
    zoonoses; Trematodes
  coenurosis, 385–386
  cysticercoids, 384
  diphyllobothriasis, 386–388
  dipylidiosis, 389
  echinococcosis, 390–399
  hymenolepiasis, 399–401
  sparganosis, 401–402
  T. saginata, 402–404
  T. solium, 405–407
  zoonotic cestode infections, 408–409
CF. *See* Complement fixation (CF)

C. fetus subsp. *fetus*, 196
C. fetus subsp. *venerealis*, 195
Chagas' disease, 317
  clinical manifestations, 320–322
  congenital infections, 321
  diagnosis, 322
  differential diagnosis, 322
  edema of eyelids in child, 321
  etiology, 317–318
  occurrence, 318–319
  prophylaxis, 323
  therapy, 322–323
  transmission, 319–320
  triatomine bugs, 319
Chagoma, 321
Chemoprophylaxis, 315
Cheyletiella infestation, 458
Cheyletiella spp., 457
Chick embryo fibroblasts, 16
Chiclero's ulcer, 331, 340
Chigger bites, 457
Chiggerborne rickettsiosis. *See* Tsutsugamushi fever
Chigoe flea infestation, 469–470
Chikungunya fever, 8, 21
  clinical manifestations, 21–22
  diagnosis, 22
  differential diagnosis, 22
  etiology, 21
  occurrence, 21
  prophylaxis, 23
  therapy, 22–23
  transmission, 21
Chlamydiaceae, 199
Chlamydiae, 198
  possible danger in transmitting, 200
Chlamydiales, 199
Chlamydia spp./Chlamydioses, 199, 201, 279
Chlamydioses
  chlamydioses transmitted from mammals, 201
  etiology, 198–199
  psittacosis/ornithosis, 199–201
Chlamydophila, 199
Cholera, 273–274
Cholera toxin (CTX), 273
Chordopoxvirinae, 156, 157
Chronic kala-azar, 334
Chronic Lyme borreliosis, 187
Chronic progressive Lyme encephalomyelitis, 187
Chronic schistosomiasis, 380
Chronic wasting disease (CWD), 169
Chrysomia spp., 465
Chrysops spp., 422
Ciclero's ulcer, 340

Cimex spp., 472

CIN. *See* Cefsulodin-irgasannovobiocin (CIN)

Circulating anodic antigen (CAA), 381

Circulating cathodic antigen (CCA), 381

Citrobacter spp., 478, 479, 480

CJD. *See* Creutzfeldt-Jakob disease (CJD)

C. jejuni subsp. *jejuni*, 196

Clams, 3

Classical Lyme arthritis, 187

CLM. *See* Cerebral larva migrans (CLM)

Clonorchiasis, 366–367. *See also* Dicrocoeliais

Clonorchis sinensis (*C. sinensis*), 366

   developmental cycle of, 367

Clostridium spp., 479, 480, 484

CMV. *See* Cytomegalovirus (CMV)

CNS. *See* Central nervous system (CNS)

Cochliomya spp., 465, 466

Cockroaches, 308

Coenurosis, 385–386

Coli enterotoxemia, 209

Colorado fever. *See* Colorado tick fever

Colorado tick fever, 83–85

Coltivirus, 83

   Colorado tick fever, 83–85

   Eyach virus, 83

Common horse fly (*Haematopota pluvialis*), 463

Complement fixation (CF), 194

Complexes of *Flaviviridae*, 27

   agents causing yellow fever and dengue, 27–31

   mosquitoes, virus complex transmitted by, 27

   ticks, virus complex transmitted by, 27

Computed tomography (CT), 310

Conenose, 471

Conjunctivitis, 101

Contagious ecthyma of sheep, 165–166

Convalescence, 90

Cordylobia spp., 464

Coronaviruses, 139–140, 142

   MERS-COV, 144–146

   SARS, 141–144

Corynebacterium pseudotuberculosis infections, 284

Corynebacterium ulcerans infections, 285

Corynosoma spp., 447

Cotton rats (*Sigmodon hispidus*), 411

Cowpox, 164

Coxiella burnetii (*C. burnetii*), 238–240, 449

Coxiellae, 238

C. psittaci, 199

Creeping eruption. *See* Larva migrans cutanea

Creeping myiasis, 466

Creutzfeldt-Jakob disease (CJD), 169, 170

   differential diagnosis, 173

Crimean-Congo hemorrhagic fever (CCHF), 71

   clinical manifestations, 72

   diagnosis, 72

   differential diagnosis, 72

   etiology, 71

   occurrence, 71–72

   prophylaxis, 73

   therapy, 72–73

   transmission, 72

   virus, 67

Crimean Congo virus, 4

Crocodile bites. *See* Alligator bites

Crohn-like terminal ileitis, 196

Crosse virus, 67

Crustaceans, 488

CRVG. *See* Cutaneous and renal glomerular vasculopathy (CRVG)

Cryptosporidiosis, 324. *See also* Balantidiasis

   clinical manifestations, 325–326

   diagnosis, 326

   differential diagnosis, 326

   etiology, 324–325

   occurrence, 325

   prophylaxis, 327

   therapy, 326–327

   transmission, 325

Cryptosporidium spp., 324

   C. muris, 324

   developmental cycle of, 326

   in humans, 324

   oocysts, 325

CSD. *See* Cat scratch disease (CSD)

CSF. *See* Cerebrospinal fluid (CSF)

CT. *See* Computed tomography (CT)

Ctenocephalides canis (*C. canis*), 467

Ctenocephalides felis. *See* Cat flea (*Ctenocephalides felis*)

Ctenocephalides felis (*C. felis*), 180, 255, 468

CTX. *See* Cholera toxin (CTX)

Cuevavirus, 98

Culex annulirostris (*C. annulirostris*), 7

Culex mosquitoes, 42

Culex pipiens (*C. pipiens*), 46

Culex quinquefasciatus (*C. quinquefasciatus*), 46

Culex tarsalis (*C. tarsalis*), 7, 13, 46

Culex tritaeniorhynchus (*C. tritaeniorhynchus*), 28, 74

Culex univittatus (*C. univittatus*), 17

Culex univittatus (*C. univittatus*), 7

Culicoides species, 463

   C. paraensis, 70

Culicoides spp.. *See* Gnats (*Culicoides* spp.)

Culiseta melanura (*C. melanura*), 11

Cutaneous amebiasis, 309

Cutaneous and renal glomerular vasculopathy (CRVG), 209
Cutaneous anthrax, 176, 178
Cutaneous larva migrans. *See* Larva migrans cutanea
Cutaneous leishmaniases, 339, 340
CWD. *See* Chronic wasting disease (CWD)
Cyclophillida, 384, 387
Cyclops spp., 419
Cynomolgus spp., 479
Cystic echinococcosis, 395. *See also* Alveolar echinococcosis
   clinical manifestations, 397
   clinical picture, 398
   diagnosis, 397–398
   differential diagnoses, 398
   etiology, 395
   occurrence, 395–396
   prophylaxis, 398–399
   therapy, 398
   transmission, 396–397
Cysticerci, 403, 405, 406
Cysticercoids, 384
Cysticercosis, 405
Cysticercus cellulosae, 405
Cysticercus racemosus (*C. racemosus*), 406
Cytomegalovirus (CMV), 322

D

Dandy fever. *See* Dengue fever
DCL. *See* Diffuse cutaneous leishmaniasis (DCL)
DDT. *See* Dichlorodiphenyltrichloroethane (DDT)
DEC. *See* Diethylcarbamazine (DEC)
Deep trichophytosis. *See* Tinea barbae
Delayed-type hypersensitivity reactions, 43–44
Dengue fever (DEN fever), 27, 58
   animal infections with flaviviruses, 29
   clinical manifestations, 29, 62–63
   diagnosis, 29–30, 63
   differential diagnosis, 63
   distribution of dengue virus infection, 59–61
   etiology, 58
   infections, 22
   occurrence, 27–28, 58, 62
   prophylaxis, 30, 63–64
   therapy, 30, 63
   transmission, 28–29, 62
   vaccination and problem of immune enhancement, 30–31
   virus, 27
Dengue hemorrhagic fever (DHF), 58, 62–64
Dengue shock syndrome (DSS), 29, 58, 62–64
DEN hemorrhagic fever (DHF), 27
Dermacentor andersoni (*D. andersoni*), 454

Dermacentor apronophorus (*D, apronophorus*), 40
Dermacentor marginatus (*D. marginatus*), 7
Dermacentor reticulatus (*D. reticulatus*), 40
Dermacentor variabilis (*D. variabilis*), 452
Dermal/subdermal myiasis, 465–466
Dermanyssus gallinae (*D. gallinae*), 456
Dermanyssus spp., 457, 458
Dermatobia hominis (*D. hominis*), 464, 465, 466
Dermatophilosis, 286
Dermatophilus congolensis/infections, 286–287
Dermatophyte indicator medium (DIM), 295
Dermatophyte test medium (DTM), 295
Dermatophytoses, 293
   caused by *Microsporum* spp., 293–296
   caused by *Trichophyton* spp., 296–298
   zoophilic zoonotic species, 294
DHF. *See* DEN hemorrhagic fever (DHF); Dengue hemorrhagic fever (DHF)
Diarrheagenic *Escherichia coli*, 207
Dichlorodiphenyltrichloroethane (DDT), 3, 28
Dicrocoeliais, 368–369
Dicrocoelium spp., 367, 368
Dientamoeba fragilis (*D. fragilis*), 304
Diethylcarbamazine (DEC), 424
Diffuse cutaneous leishmaniasis (DCL), 331–332
DIM. *See* Dermatophyte indicator medium (DIM)
Dioctophyma renale (*D. renale*), 418
Dioctophymiasis, 418
Dipetalogaster spp., 472
Dipetalonema perstans (*D. perstans*), 422
Dipetalonema streptocerca (*D. streptocerca*), 422
Diphyllobothriasis, 386–388, 488
Diplogonoporus balaenoptera (*D. balaenoptera*), 386
Diplogonoporus balaenopterae (*D. balaenopterae*), 388
Diplogonoporus dalliae (*D. dalliae*), 388
Diplogonoporus dendriticum (*D. dendriticum*), 386, 388
Diplogonoporus grandis (*D. grandis*), 408
Diplogonoporus latum (*D. latum*), 386, 388
   developmental cycle, 387
Diplogonoporus nihonkaiense (*D. nihonkaiense*), 388
Diplogonoporus pacificum (*D. pacificum*), 388
Diplogonoporus stemmacephalum (*D. stemmacephalum*), 386, 388
Diplornaviruses. *See* Reoviruses
Diptera, 459. *See also* Heteroptera infestations
   dipteran bites, 460–464
   myiasis, 464–467
   zoonoses caused by, 459
Dipylidiosis, 389
Dipylidium caninum (*D. caninum*), 384, 389
Dirofilaria immitis (*D. immitis*), 425
Dirofilaria repens (*D. repens*), 425

Dirofilariasis, 425–426
Dirofilaria spp., 425
Dirofilaria striata (*D. striata*), 425
Dirofilaria tenuis (*D. tenuis*), 425
Dirofilaria ursi (*D. ursi*), 425
Discrete typing units (DTUs), 317
Distomatosis, 368–369, 376–378, 383
DNA viruses, 1
Dobrava virus, 78–79
Dog bites, 477–478
Dog flea (*Ctenocephalides canis*), 467
Dracunculiasis, 418, 488
   clinical manifestations, 419
   diagnosis, 419
   differential diagnosis, 419
   etiology, 419
   occurrence, 419
   prophylaxis, 420
   therapy, 419–420
   transmission, 419
DSS. *See* Dengue shock syndrome (DSS)
DTM. *See* Dermatophyte test medium (DTM)
DTUs. *See* Discrete typing units" (DTUs)
Duhring's disease, 158
Dust mites, 456
Dwarf fluke infections, 369–370
Dwarf tapeworm infection. *See* Hymenolepiasis

E
eae gene. *See* Intimin (*eae* gene)
Eastern equine encephalitis (EEE), 10
   clinical manifestations, 11
   diagnosis, 11
   differential diagnosis, 11–12
   etiology, 10
   occurrence, 10–11
   prophylaxis, 12
   therapy, 12
   transmission, 11
Eastern subtype of TBE. *See* Russian spring-summer meningoencephalitis (RSSE)
Ebola virus, 3, 4, 97, 98
Ebola virus hemorrhagic fever, 104. *See also* Marburg virus hemorrhagic fever
   clinical manifestations, 106–107
   diagnosis, 107
   differential diagnosis, 107
   etiology, 104
   occurrence, 104–105
   prophylaxis, 108
   therapy, 107–108
   transmission, 105–106
Echidnophaga gallinacea (*E. gallinacea*), 467

Echinococcosis, 390
   agents of alveolar and polycystic, 390
   alveolar, 390–394
   cystic, 395–399
Echinococcus granulosus (*E. granulosus*), 390, 395, 397
   developmental cycle, 397
   geographic distribution, 396
   strains/species of, 395
Echinococcus multilocularis (*E. multilocularis*), 390, 391, 392, 393, 396, 397
   eggs, 394
   geographic distribution, 391
Echinococcus shiquicus (*E. shiquicus*), 390
Echinostomatidae, 369
Edwardsiella, 484
EEE. *See* Eastern equine encephalitis (EEE)
EHEC adherence factor 1 (Efa1), 207
EHEC infections. *See* Enterohemorrhagic *Escherichia coli* infections (EHEC infections)
Ehrlichiae, 202, 205
Ehrlichia spp., 202
   E. ewingii, 205
   pathogenic for humans, 203
Ehrlichioses/Anaplasmosis, 202
   clinical manifestations, 204–205
   diagnosis, 205
   differential diagnosis, 205
   etiology, 202, 203
   occurrence, 203, 204
   prophylaxis, 205–206
   reporting, 206
   therapy, 205
EIA. *See* Enzyme immunoassay (EIA)
EIAV. *See* Equine infectious anemia virus (EIAV)
Eikenella corrodens (*E. corrodens*), 479, 480
Elementary bodies, 198–199, 200, 202
Elephantpox, 164–165
ELISA. *See* Enzyme linked immunosorbent assay (ELISA)
Ellinghausen-McCullough-Johnson-Harris (EMJH), 216
El Niño, 4, 79
Elocharis tuberosa (*E. tuberosa*), 374
EMC virus. *See* Encephalomyocarditis virus (EMC virus)
Emerging infections, 2
EMJH. *See* Ellinghausen-McCullough-Johnson-Harris (EMJH)
Encapsulated clade, 440
Encephalitis, 8, 11, 15
Encephalitozoon spp., 343
Encephalomyocarditis virus (EMC virus), 134, 138

Encepur® CEE vaccine, 36
Endemic typhus. *See* Murine typhus
Endocarditis, 182
Endogenous retroviruses, 152–153
5′-end scavenging, 6
Entamebae, 307
Entamoeba histolytica (*E. histolytica*), 307
 developmental cycle, 307, 308
 trophozoites with phagocytized erythrocytes, 307
Entamoeba spp., 308
 surface antigens, 310
Ent. bieneusi, 343
Ent. cuniculi, 344
Enteritis, 144, 196, 370, 374, 400
Enterobacteriaceae, 234, 238, 276, 479, 480
Enterococcus spp., 478, 479
Enterocytes, gamonts/gametes in, 356
Enterocytozoon spp., 342
Enterohemolysin, 207
Enterohemorrhagic *Escherichia coli* infections
 (EHEC infections), 206
 clinical manifestations, 208–209
 diagnosis, 209–210
 differential diagnosis, 210
 etiology, 206–208
 occurrence, 208
 prophylaxis, 210
 reporting, 210
 therapy, 210
 transmission, 208
Enteropathogenic *Escherichia coli*, 207
Enteroviruses, 134, 483
Ent. hellem, 344
Ent. intestinalis, 343
Entomopoxvirinae, 156, 157
Enzyme immunoassay (EIA), 209
Enzyme linked immunosorbent assay (ELISA),
 10, 40, 56, 67, 178, 310
Eosinophilic enteritis, 420–421
Eosinophilic meningitis.
 See Cerebral angiostrongyliasis
Eosinophilic meningoencephalitis.
 See Cerebral angiostrongyliasis
Epidemic polyarthritis, 18–20
Epidemic typhus, 253–254
Epimastigote stage, 319
Equine infectious anemia virus (EIAV), 149
Equine morbillivirus, 3
Erysipelas, 188, 213
Erysipeloid, 211–213
Erysipelothrix rhusiopathiae (*E. rhusiopathiae*), 211
Erythema infectiosum (*E. infectiosum*), 18, 20
Erythema migrans, 184, 186, 187

Escherichia coli (*E. coli*), 206, 207, 260, 306, 366, 478,
 479, 480, 484
Espundia, 339, 340
Ethambutol (ETB), 227
Ethylenimine (*aziridine*)-inactivated virus
 vaccines, 137
European or western subtype of TBE. *See* Central
 European tick encephalitis (CEE)
Eurytrema pancreaticum (*E. pancreaticum*), 383
Eutrombicula alfreddugesi (*E. alfreddugesi*), 456
Eutrombicula sarcina (*E. sarcina*), 456
Exanthemas, 8
Extensive resistance (XDR), 227
Extraintestinal amebiais, 310
Extraintestinal infestation, 409
Extrapulmonary tuberculosis, 225
Eyach virus, 83

F
Facial poxvirus lesion, 164
Farcy. *See* Glanders
Far Eastern Encephalitis. *See* Russian spring-summer
 meningoencephalitis (RSSE)
Fasciola gigantica (*F. gigantica*), 370
Fasciola hepatica (*F. hepatica*), 370, 371
 developmental cycle of, 373
 encysted metacercariae, 372
Fasciola hepatica (*F. hepatica*), 370, 371, 372, 487
Fascioliasis, 370–373
Fasciolopsiasis, 374–375
Fasciolopsis buski (*F. buski*), 374, 487
Favus, 296, 297, 298
febre de Mojui. *See* Oropouche fever
Feline immunodeficiency virus (FIV), 149
Female sand fly (*Phlebotomus mascittii*), 463
Ferret bites, 479
Fièvre boutonneuse. *See* Mediterranean
 spotted fever
Filariases, 421
 brugia filariasis, 422–424
 dirofilariasis, 425–426
Filoviridae, 97, 104
Filoviruses, 97, 99
 causing outbreaks, 98
 Ebola virus hemorrhagic fever, 104–108
 extended necroses, 98
 hemorrhagic diathesis, 98–99
 human infections, 97–98
 Marburg virus hemorrhagic fever, 99–103
 mononegavirales, 98
Fish bites, 479
Fish poisoning, 488–494
FIV. *See* Feline immunodeficiency virus (FIV)

Flaviviruses, 26. *See also* Alphaviruses; Bunyaviruses; Mosquito-borne flaviviruses
  agents, 26–27
  complexes of *Flaviviridae*, 27–31
  zoonoses caused by tick-borne flaviviruses, 32–41
Flavobacterium spp., 478
Fleas (Siphonaptera), 467
  flea bites, 467–469
  Tungiasis, 469–470
  zoonoses caused by, 467
Flies (Cyclorapha), 308, 462
Floodwater *Aedes*, 7
Florid plaques, 169
Flying fox. *See Roussettus aegyptiacus* (Flying fox)
Flying foxes, 4, 496
FMD. *See* Foot-and-mouth disease (FMD)
FMD virus. *See* Foot-and-mouth disease virus (FMD virus)
Foodborne virus infections, 484
Food industry, 261
Foodstuffs, transmission by, 483
  bacteria, 484–486
  bacteria transmitting by food, 485
  fish poisoning, 488–494
  foodborne virus infections, 484
  fungi, 486
  mycotoxins, 486
  parasites, 486–488
  phytotoxins transmitting by bats, 496
  shellfish poisoning, 488, 495
  viruses, 483–484
Foot-and-mouth disease (FMD), 4, 118, 119
  virus, 134, 135–137
Forest yaws. *See* Pian bois
Four Corners disease. *See* Hantavirus pulmonary syndrome (HPS)
Foxes, bites by, 477–478
Francisella philomiragia (*F. philomiragia*), 269
Francisella tularensis (*F. tularensis*), 269
Fraud mange. *See* Sarcoptic mange
Freshwater types, 388
Fruit-eating bats, 112–113
Fungal zoonoses
  dermatophytoses, 293–298
  pneumocystosis, 300–302
  sporotrichosis, 298–300
Fungi, 486
Fusarium spp., 486
Fusobacterium spp., 478, 479

G
GAE. *See* Granulomatous encephalitis (GAE)
Gasterophilus spp., 464, 466

Gastrodiscoides hominis (*G. hominis*), 383
Gemella spp., 478
Geonoses/sapronoses, 293
Giant liver fluke. *See Fasciola gigantica* (*F. gigantica*)
Giardia duodenalis (*G. duodenalis*), 328
Giardia intestinalis (*G. intestinalis*), 328
Giardiasis, 328–329. *See also* Balantidiasis
Gid, 385
Glanders, 214–215
Glossina fusca (*G. fusca*), 352
Glossina fuscipes (*G. fuscipes*), 352
Glossina morsitans (*G. morsitans*), 352
Glossina pallidipes (*G. pallidipes*), 352
Glossina palpalis (*G. palpalis*), 352
Glossina spp., 352, 463
Glossina swynnertoni (*G. swynnertoni*), 352
Glossina tachynoides (*G. tachynoides*), 352
Gnathostoma binucleatum (*G. binucleatum*), 426
Gnathostoma doloresi (*G. doloresi*), 426
Gnathostoma hispidum (*G. hispidum*), 426
Gnathostoma nipponicum (*G. nipponicum*), 426
Gnathostoma spinigerum (*G. spinigerum*), 426, 431
Gnathostomiasis, 426–427
Gnats (*Culicoides* spp.), 5
Gongylonema pulchrum (*G. pulchrum*), 427
Gongylonemiasis, 427–428
Grain mites. *See* Straw itch mites
Granulocytic anaplasmosis, 201
Granulocytopenia, 62
Granulomatous encephalitis (GAE), 309
Group-specific reactivity of flaviviruses, 26
Group B arboviruses. *See* Flaviviruses
Guinea pig bites, 479
Guineaworm infection. *See* Dracunculiasis
Gymnophalloides seoi (*G. seoi*), 370

H
H1N1 virus. *See* Swine influenza virus
H5N1. *See* Influenza A virus
HAART. *See* Highly active retroviral treatment (HAART)
HACCP. *See* Hazard analysis critical control point (HACCP)
Haemaphysalis, 27, 34, 40, 452
Haematopota, 462, 463
Haemophilus influenzae (*H. influenzae*), 128, 222, 266, 283, 479
Halomonas venusta (*H. venusta*), 479
Halophilic bacteria. *See* Halotolerant bacteria
Halotolerant bacteria, 479
Halteres, 459
Halzoun, 473, 474
Hamster bites, 479

Hantaviruses, 65, 78–82
Hantavirus pulmonary syndrome (HPS), 78, 132
  clinical manifestations, 80
  diagnosis, 80–81
  differential diagnosis, 81
  etiology, 78
  occurrence, 78–79
  prophylaxis, 82
  therapy, 81–82
  transmission, 79
Hard ticks, 449
HAT. *See* Humans, African trypanosomiasis (HAT)
Haverhill fever, 242, 243
Hazard analysis critical control point (HACCP), 367
HDC. *See* Human diploid cell culture (HDC)
Helicobacter spp. /infections, 287
Hemagglutinin inhibition (HI), 10
Hemolytic-uremic syndrome (HUS), 206, 209
Hemophagocytic lymphohistiocytosis (HLH), 132
Hemorrhagic conjunctivitis, 121
Hemorrhagic diathesis, 80, 98–99, 101
Hemorrhagic disease, 21
Hemorrhagic fever with renal syndrome (HFRS), 78
  clinical manifestations, 80
  diagnosis, 80–81
  differential diagnosis, 81
  etiology, 78
  occurrence, 78–79
  prophylaxis, 82
  therapy, 81–82
  transmission, 79
Hendra virus, 122–125
Hepatic capillariasis, 415–416
Hepatitis A virus, 483
Hepatitis E (Hep E), 138–139
Hepatovirus, 134
Hep E. *See* Hepatitis E (Hep E)
Herpes B virus, 153
  clinical manifestations, 154
  diagnosis, 154–155
  differential diagnosis, 155
  etiology, 153–154
  occurrence, 154
  prophylaxis, 155–156
  therapy, 155
  transmission, 154
Herpes simplex virus type 1 (HSV-1).
    See Herpesvirus hominis type 1 (HVH-1)
Herpesviridae, 153
Herpesviruses, 153
  herpes B virus, 153–156
Herpesvirus hominis type 1 (HVH-1), 153
Herpesvirus simiae, 153, 479

Herring worm disease. *See* Anisakiasis
HERV. *See* Human endogenous retroviruses (HERV)
Heterophyidae, 369
Heteroptera infestations, 471–473
HFRS. *See* Hemorrhagic fever with renal syndrome (HFRS)
HGA. *See* Human granulocytic anaplasmosis (HGA)
HGE. *See* Human granulocytic ehrlichiosis (HGE)
HI. *See* Hemagglutinin inhibition (HI)
Highly active retroviral treatment (HAART), 229, 327
HIV 1 and HIV 2, 2
  clinical manifestations, 150–151
  diagnosis, 151
  etiology, 149–150
  occurrence, 150
  prognosis, 152
  prophylaxis, 151–152
  therapy, 151
  transmission, 150
HI viruses. *See* Immunodeficiency viruses (HI viruses)
HLA. *See* Human Leukocyte Antigen (HLA)
HLH. *See* Hemophagocytic lymphohistiocytosis (HLH)
HME. *See* Human monocytic ehrlichiosis (HME)
Holarctica, 269
Hookworm infection, 428–429
Horse bites, 480
Horseflies (Tabanidae), 462
HPMPC. *See* (S)-1-(3-hydroxy-2-phosphonylmethoxypropyl)cytosine) (HPMPC)
HPS. *See* Hantavirus pulmonary syndrome (HPS)
HTLVs. *See* Human T-cell lymphotropic viruses (HTLVs)
Human-to-human transmission, 31
Human babesiosis, 312
Human diploid cell culture (HDC), 115
Human endogenous retroviruses (HERV), 152, 153
Human flea (*Pulex irritans*), 467
Human granulocytic anaplasmosis (HGA), 204
Human granulocytic ehrlichiosis (HGE), 204
Human Leukocyte Antigen (HLA), 187
Human monocytic ehrlichiosis (HME), 204
Humans, African trypanosomiasis (HAT), 351
Human T-cell lymphotropic viruses (HTLVs), 147–148
HUS. *See* Hemolytic-uremic syndrome (HUS)
HVH-1. *See* Herpesvirus hominis type 1 (HVH-1)
HVH-8 virus, 153
Hyalomma, 71–72
Hydatidosis, 395
Hydatid sand, 396

(S)-1-(3-hydroxy-2-phosphonylmethoxypropyl) cytosine) (HPMPC), 159
Hymenolepiasis, 399–401
Hymenolepis diminuta (H. diminuta), 400
Hymenolepis nana (H. nana), 399
  developmental cycle, 400
Hypalbuminemia, 429
Hypoderma spp., 464, 466

I

IARC. *See* International Agency for Research on Cancer (IARC)
Iatrogenic *Toxoplasma gondii* infections, 501
Iatrogenic transmission of zoonotic agents, 499
  blood transfusion and blood products, 499
  iatrogenic *Toxoplasma gondii* infections, 501
  Marburg virus, 500
Iatrogenic zoonosis, 3
IFA. *See* Immunofluorescence assay (IFA)
IgM. *See* Immunoglobulin M (IgM)
IGR. *See* Insect growth regulators (IGR)
IHA. *See* Indirect hemagglutination assay (IHA)
Immune serum, 103
Immunization of amplification hosts of flaviviruses, 31
Immunodeficiency viruses (HI viruses), 2
Immunofluorescence assay (IFA), 200, 314
Immunoglobulin M (IgM), 10
Immunohistology, 9
Immunoprophylaxis, 36
Inactivated phase vaccine, 242
Indian Civet (*Viverra zibetha*), 143
Indirect hemagglutination assay (IHA), 178, 310
Indirect immunofluorescence, 40
Individual orthopoxvirus infections
  buffalopox, 163
  camelpox, 163–164
  cowpox, 164
  elephantpox, 164–165
  monkeypox virus, 159–160
  vaccinia virus, 160–163
Inermic madagascariensis (I. cubensis), 408
Influenza-viruses, 127
  availability of "fitting" receptors, 129
  avian influenza viruses, 131–133
  binary code for influenza A viruses, 128
  gene exchange, 128
  pathogenicity, 128–129
  surveillance, 129
  swine influenza virus, 129–131
  viral RNA polymerases, 129
Influenza A virus, 4, 131
INH. *See* Isoniacid (INH)

Insect growth regulators (IGR), 469
Interferon gamma release assay, 226
Internalin, 219
International Agency for Research on Cancer (IARC), 366
Intestinal amebiasis, 309–310
Intestinal angiostrongyliasis, 411–412
Intestinal anthrax, 176, 178
Intestinal capillariasis, 416–417
Intestinal dwarf fluke infections. *See* Dwarf fluke infections
Intestinal infestation, 408–409
Intestinal myiasis, 466
Intimin (*eae* gene), 207
intraperitoneal injection (i.p. injection), 322
In vitro cultivation of amebae, 310
i.p. injection. *See* intraperitoneal injection (i.p. injection)
Isoniacid (INH), 227
Ivory Coast, 104
Ixodes persulcatus (I. persulcatus), 7
Ixodes ricinus (I. ricinus), 450, 452, 453
Ixodes rubicundus (I. rubicundus), 455
Ixodid ticks, 32, 39
  developmental stages, 452
  mouthparts, 453

J

Japanese encephalitis (JE), 27, 28, 41
  clinical manifestations, 42–43
  diagnosis, 43
  differential diagnosis, 43
  etiology, 41
  occurrence, 41–42
  prophylaxis, 43–44
  therapy, 43
  transmission, 42

K

Kagama fever, 205
Kala-azar, 7, 194, 332–337, 339
Kaposi sarcoma virus. *See* HVH-8 virus
Katayama syndrome, 380
Kedani disease. *See* Tsutsugamushi fever
Kemerovo complex. *See* Orbivirus
Kemerovo virus, 7
Keratopathia, 200
KFD. *See* Kyasanur Forest disease (KFD)
KHF. *See* Korean hemorrhagic fever (KHF)
Kissing bugs, 471
Klebsiella spp., 128, 478, 479, 480
Korean hemorrhagic fever (KHF), 78, 79, 80

Kunjin virus disease, 44–45
Kyasanur Forest disease (KFD), 3, 27, 39–40

L
La Crosse virus, 6
Lactobacillus spp., 478
Lagochilascariasis, 429–430
Lagochilascaris minor (*L. minor*), 429, 430
Lambliasis. *See* Giardiasis
Large babesia, 312
Large cell variant (LCV), 238
Large liver fluke. *See Fasciola hepatica* (*F. hepatica*)
Larva migrans cutanea, 430–432
Larva migrans visceralis, 432–434
Lassa fever, 92–94
Lassa virus, 2, 3
Latrines, 433
LCM virus. *See* Lymphocytic choriomeningitis virus (LCM virus)
LCV. *See* Large cell variant (LCV)
Lecithodendriidae, 370
LEE. *See* Locus of enterocyte effacement (LEE)
Leeches, 281
Legionellales, 245
Leifsonia aquatica (*L. aquatica*), 478
Leishmania donovani (*L. donovani*), 330, 335
   developmental cycle of, 332
Leishmaniasis, 330
   American cutaneous and mucocutaneous leishmaniases, 339–341
   Old World cutaneous leishmaniasis, 337–339
   species/species complexes, 330
   variants, 331–332
   visceral leishmaniasis, 332–337
Leishmaniasis recidivans (RL), 331
Leishmaniasis tegumentaria diffusa, 340–341
Leishmania spp./Leishmaniasisses, 330, 500
   human diseases, 331
   New World Cutaneous, 339–341
   Old World Cutaneous, 337–339
   Panamanian, 339–341
   visceral, 332
Leptobromidium scutellare (*L. scutellare*), 79
Leptopsylla segnis (*L. segnis*), 255
Leptospira spp., 216, 479, 480
Leptospiroses, 216
   agents, 216
   clinical manifestations, 217–218
   diagnosis, 218
   differential diagnosis, 218
   etiology, 216
   occurrence, 216, 217
   prophylaxis, 218

reporting, 218
   therapy, 218
   transmission, 217
Leptospirosis, 222
Leptotrombiculum spp., 456
Leptotrombidium spp., 245
LI. *See* Louping ill (LI)
Linguatula serrata (*L. serrata*), 473, 474
Linguatulosis, 473
   nasopharyngeal, 474
   visceral, 475
Liponyssoides sanguineus (*L. sanguineus*), 252
Lipopolysaccharide (LPS), 209
Liposomal amphotericin B, 336
Lipovnik virus, 7, 85
Listeria monocytogenes (*L. monocytogenes*), 219
Listeriolysin O (LLO), 219
Listeriosis, 219
   clinical manifestations, 221
   diagnosis, 221–222
   differential diagnosis, 222
   etiology, 219
   occurrence, 219, 220
   prophylaxis, 222
   reporting, 222
   therapy, 222
   transmission, 220–221
Lithium chloride-phenylethanol-moxalactam agar (LPM agar), 221
Lizard bites, 479
LLO. *See* Listeriolysin O (LLO)
Loa Loa, 422
Locus of enterocyte effacement (LEE), 207
Long polar fimbriae (Lpf), 207
Louping ill (LI), 27, 37–38
Louse flies (Hippoboscidae), 462
Lpf. *See* Long polar fimbriae (Lpf)
LPM agar. *See* Lithium chloride-phenylethanol-moxalactam agar (LPM agar)
LPS. *See* Lipopolysaccharide (LPS)
Lucilia sericata (*L. sericata*), 466
Lumbar CSF tap, 91
Lutzomyia spp., 180, 330, 333–334
Lyme arthritis, 187
   disease, 187, 503
   encephalomyelitis, 187
Lyme borreliosis, 183. *See also* Brucelloses; Relapsing fever
   clinical manifestations, 186–187
   diagnosis, 187–188
   differential diagnosis, 188
   etiology, 183–184
   occurrence, 184, 185

prophylaxis, 188
reporting, 188
therapy, 188
transmission, 185, 186
Lymphadenopathy, 353
Lymphatic filariasis, 423
Lymphocutaneous sporotrichosis, 299–300
Lymphocytic choriomeningitis virus (LCM virus), 88, 89, 500
   clinical manifestations, 90–91
   diagnosis, 91
   differential diagnosis, 91
   etiology, 89–90
   occurrence, 90
   prophylaxis, 91
   therapy, 91
   transmission, 90
Lymphocytoma, 186
Lyssavirus, 109, 111

M

MAA infections. *See Mycobacterium avium* subsp. *avium* infections (MAA infections)
Macaca fascicularis (*M. fascicularis*), 347
Macracanthorhynchus hirudinaceus (*M. hirudinaceus*), 447, 448
Macracanthorhynchus ingens (*M. ingens*), 447, 448
Maculopapular rash, 25, 101
Mad cow disease, 169
Maggot therapy, 465
Magnetic resonance imaging (MRI), 310
Magnetic resonance tomography (MRT), 360
MAH infections. *See Mycobacterium avium* subsp. *hominissuis* infections (MAH infections)
MAI complex. *See M. avium-intracellulare* complex (MAI complex)
Major histocompatibility complex (MHC), 321
Maladie du sommeil. See African trypanosomiasis
Malaria, 345
Malaria quartana, 345
Malaria rapid diagnostic tests, 347
Malaria tertian, 345
Malaria tropica, 345
Malignant pustule, 176
Malleus. *See* Glanders
MALT. *See* Mucosa-associated lymph tissue (MALT)
Mammomonogamus laryngeus (*M. laryngeus*), 438
Mansonella ozzardi (*M. ozzardi*), 422
MAP infections. *See Mycobacterium avium* subsp. *paratuberculosis* infections (MAP infections)
Marburg virus, 2, 98, 99, 100, 500

Marburg virus hemorrhagic fever, 99. *See also* Ebola virus hemorrhagic fever
   clinical manifestations, 101–102
   diagnosis, 102
   differential diagnosis, 102–103
   etiology, 99, 100
   occurrence, 100
   prophylaxis, 103
   therapy, 103
   transmission, 100–101
Maridi virus, 104
Marine anisakids, developmental cycle of, 413
Marine bacteria, 479
Marine types, 388
Marrara syndrome, 473–475
Marshallagia, 445
Mature spores, 343
M. avium-intracellulare complex (MAI complex), 229
Mayaro fever, 25–26
MDR. *See* Multiple resistance (MDR)
Mecistocyrrus, 445
Mediasiatica, 269
Mediterranean spotted fever, 249–251
Megachiroptera, 105
Megaparamyxovirus, 122
Melioidosis, 288–290
Menangle virus, 122
Mendel-Mantoux test (MMT), 226
Meningitis, 90
Meningonema peruzzii (*M. peruzzii*), 422
Meningoradiculitis Bannwarth, 186
Merozoites, 356
MERS-CoV. *See* Middle East respiratory syndrome Coronavirus (MERS-CoV)
Merthiolate-iodine formaldehyde techniques. *See* Sodium acetate-acetic acid formaldehyde techniques (SAF techniques)
Mesocercariae, 383
Mesocestoides, 408
Metacercariae, 363, 372
Metastrongylus apri (*M. apri*), 304
Methicillin-resistant *S. aureus* (MRSA), 262
Metorchis albidus (*M. albidus*), 375
MHC. *See* Major histocompatibility complex (MHC)
Micrococcus spp., 478, 479
Microsporida, 341, 343
   developmental cycle, 343
   infecting humans, 342
Microsporoses, 341
   clinical manifestations, 344
   diagnosis, 344
   differential diagnosis, 344
   etiology, 341–343

Microsporoses (*Continued*)
  occurrence, 343
  prophylaxis, 344
  therapy, 344
  transmission, 343
Microsporum spp., 293
  clinical manifestations, 294–295
  diagnosis, 295
  etiology, 293–294
  prophylaxis, 296
  therapy, 295–296
  tinea capitis, 294, 295
  transmission, 294
MID. *See* Minimum infective dose (MID)
Middle East respiratory syndrome Coronavirus
    (MERS-CoV), 4, 141, 144
  clinical manifestations, 145
  diagnosis, 145–146
  differential diagnosis, 146
  etiology, 144
  occurrence, 144–145
  prophylaxis, 146
  therapy, 146
  transmission, 145
Midges, 460, 463
Miliary tuberculosis, 225
Milker's nodules. *See* Pseudocowpox
Miltefosin, 336
mini anion exchange centrifugation technique
    (cAECT), 354
Minimum infective dose (MID), 258
Mites, 455
  clinical manifestations, 457
  diagnosis, 458
  differential diagnosis, 458
  etiology, 456
  infestations, 458
  occurrence, 456–457
  prophylaxis, 459
  sarcoptic mange, 458
  straw itch mites, 458
  therapy, 458–459
  transmission, 457
  zoonoses caused by, 455
  zoonotic mites and symptoms in humans, 456
MLEE. *See* Multilocus enzyme electrophoresis (MLEE)
MLTS. *See* Multilocus sequence typing (MLTS)
MMT. *See* Mendel-Mantoux test (MMT)
Modified virus Ankara (MVA), 159
Molina spp., 422
Moniliformis moniliformis (*M. moniliformis*), 447, 448
Moniliformis spp., 447
Monkey malaria, 345

clinical manifestations, 347
  diagnosis, 347
  etiology, 345
  occurrence, 345–346
  prophylaxis, 348
  therapy, 347–348
  transmission, 346–347
Monkeypox virus, 159–160
Mononegavirales, 98
Mononuclear phagocytic system (MPS), 330
Moraxella spp., 478, 480
Mosquito-borne flaviviruses. *See also* Alphaviruses;
    Bunyaviruses; Flaviviruses
  DEN fever, 58–64
  JE, 41–44
  MVE and Kunjin virus disease, 44–45
  RE, 48–49
  SLE, 46–47
  Wesselsbron fever, 52–53
  WNF, 49–51
  YF, 53–57
Mosquitoes, 5, 460
  cells, 9
  virus complex transmitted by, 27
Mouse bites, 480
MPS. *See* Mononuclear phagocytic system (MPS)
MRI. *See* Magnetic resonance imaging (MRI)
MRSA. *See* Methicillin-resistant *S. aureus* (MRSA)
MRT. *See* Magnetic resonance tomography (MRT)
Mucosa-associated lymph tissue (MALT), 287
Muerto Canyon virus disease. *See* Hantavirus
    pulmonary syndrome (HPS)
Multilocus enzyme electrophoresis (MLEE), 263
Multilocus sequence typing (MLTS), 263
Multiple eschars, 215
Multiple hydatid cysts, 397
Multiple resistance (MDR), 227
Murine typhus, 254–255
Murray Valley encephalitis (MVE), 27, 44–45
Musca, 465, 488
Musca domestica (*M. domestica*), 466
Muskrats (*Ondatra zibethica*), 40
MVA. *See* Modified virus Ankara (MVA)
MVE. *See* Murray Valley encephalitis (MVE)
Myalgia, 29
Mycobacteria, 223, 226
Mycobacterioses
  infections with *Mycobacterium tuberculosis*
    complex, 223–227
  Mycobacterium marinum infections, 228–229
  zoonotic mycobacterioses, 229
Mycobacterium abscessus (*M. abscessus*), 229
  avium subspecies, 230

chelonae, 228, 229
fortuitum, 228, 229
genavense, 229
marinum, 228
tuberculosis complex, 223
Mycobacterium avium subsp. *avium* infections (MAA infections), 230
Mycobacterium avium subsp. *hominissuis* infections (MAH infections), 230–231
Mycobacterium avium subsp. *paratuberculosis* infections (MAP infections), 231
Mycobacterium bovis (*M. bovis*), 227
Mycobacterium genavense infections, 232
Mycobacterium marinum infections, 228–229
Mycobacterium tuberculosis infections, 223–227
Mycoplasma phocicerebrale (*M. phocicerebrale*), 480
Mycoses, 293
Mycotoxins, 486
Myelitis, 90
Myiasis, 459–460, 464, 466
   clinical manifestations, 464–466
   diagnosis, 466–467
   differential diagnosis, 467
   etiology and occurrence, 464
   forms and etiologic agents in humans, 465
   prophylaxis, 467
   therapy, 467
   transmission, 464

N

Naegleria spp., 307, 308, 309
Nagana, 363
Nairovirus, 71
Nanophyetus salmincola (*N. salmincola*), 383
Nasopharyngeal linguatulosis, 474
NDV. *See* Newcastle disease virus (NDV)
NE. *See* Nephropathia epidemica (NE)
Necator americanus (*N. americanus*), 428, 431
Necroses, 98
Neisseria spp., 478, 480
Nematodes, 409. *See also* Parasitic zoonoses; Trematodes
   adult female, 409
   angiostrongyliasis, 410–412
   anisakiasis, 412–415
   capillariases, 415–418
   dioctophymiasis, 418
   dracunculiasis, 418–420
   eosinophilic enteritis, 420–421
   filariases, 421–426
   gnathostomiasis, 426–427
   gongylonemiasis, 427–428
   hookworm infection, 428–429

lagochilascariasis, 429–430
larva migrans cutanea, 430–432
larva migrans visceralis, 432–434
oesophagostomiasis, 434–435
other zoonotic infections, 446–447
strongyloidiasis, 435–437
syngamiasis, 438–439
thelaziasis, 439
trichinellosis, 440–444
trichostrongylidiasis, 445–446
Neorickettsia, 202
Neorickettsia helminthoeca (*N. helminthoeca*), 205, 383
Neorickettsia sunnetsu (*N. sunnetsu*), 204, 205
Neospora caninum (*N. caninum*), 304
Neotrombicula autumnalis (*N. autumnalis*), 456
Neotrombicula spp., 456
Nephropathia epidemica (NE), 78, 79, 80
Newcastle disease, 120–122
Newcastle disease virus (NDV), 121
new variant of CJD (nvCJD), 169–170
   clinical manifestations, 172
   criteria for diagnosis, 173
   diagnosis, 172
   differential diagnosis, 172
   etiology, 170
   genetic disposition, 172
   occurrence, 170–171
   prophylaxis, 172, 173, 174
   transmission, 171
New world Arenaviruses, 95–97
New World Hantaviruses. *See* Hantavirus pulmonary syndrome (HPS)
Nifurtimox, 322
Nipah virus, 122, 124–125
Nipah virus encephalitis, 124–126
NNN medium. *See* Novy-McNeal-Nicolle medium (NNN medium)
Non-neutralizing circulating immune complexes, 62
Nonencapsulated clade, 440
None zoonotic RNA virus species, 2
Nonstructural protein (NS protein), 65
Nontuberculous mycobacteria (NTM), 229
Nontyphoidal salmonellae, 258
Northern rat flea (*Nosopsyllus fasciatus*), 467
Norwalk-like agents, 483
Nosopsyllus spp., 467
Novartis vaccines, 36
Novicida, 269
Novy-McNeal-Nicolle medium (NNN medium), 322
NS protein. *See* Nonstructural protein (NS protein)
NTM. *See* Nontuberculous mycobacteria (NTM)

nvCJD. *See* new variant of CJD (nvCJD)
Nympheal stages, 472

O

Ocular larva migrans (OLM), 433
Ocular toxoplasmosis, 359
Oesophagostomiasis, 434–435
Oesophagostomum spp., 435
Oesophagostomum aculeatum (*O. aculeatum*), 434
Oesophagostomum bifurcum (*O. bifurcum*), 434
Oesophagostomum stephanostomum (*O. stephanostomum*), 434
Oestrus ovis (Sheep Bot Fly), 466
OHF. *See* Omsk hemorrhagic fever (OHF)
Old World cutaneous leishmaniasis, 337. *See also* Visceral leishmaniasis
  clinical manifestations, 338
  diagnosis, 338
  differential diagnosis, 338
  etiology, 337
  occurrence, 337–338
  prophylaxis, 339
  therapy, 338–339
  transmission, 338
Old World hantaviruses. *See* Hemorrhagic fever with renal syndrome (HFRS)
Oliguria, 55
OLM. *See* Ocular larva migrans (OLM)
Omsk hemorrhagic fever (OHF), 27, 40–41
Onchocerca spp., 304, 421
Onchocerca volvulus (*O. volvulus*), 422
Oncosphere, 396
O'nyong-nyong fever, 24–25
O'nyong-nyong virus, 24
Ophthalmomyiasis, 466
Opisthorchiasis, 375–376, 487
Opisthorchis, 367
Opisthorchis felineus (*O. felineus*), 375, 383
Opisthorchis viverrini (*O. viverrini*), 375
Opossum bites, 480
Orbiviruses, 83, 85
Orchopeas, 254
Orf virus, 165–166
  human infection with, 166
Oriental rat flea (*Xenopsylla cheopis*), 467
Orienta Tsutsugamishi (*O. Tsutsugamishi*), 79
Orientia tsutsugamushi (*O. tsutsugamushi*), 256
Orinetal sore, 337
Ornithodorus spp., 189, 450
Ornithonyssus spp., 457, 458
  O. bacoti, 456
  O. bursa, 456
  O. sylvarum, 455, 456

Ornithophilic mosquito species, 17
Ornithosis, 199–201
Oropharyngeal anthrax, 176
Oropouche fever, 70–71
Oroya fever, 179
Orthomyxoviruses, 128
  influenza-viruses, 127–133
  thogotoviruses, 133–134
Orthopoxviruses, 158–159
Orthoretrovirinae, 147
OspA. *See* Outer surface protein A (OspA)
Otobius megnini (*O. megnini*), 450, 454
Otobius spp., 450
Outer surface protein A (OspA), 185

P

Pacific oyster (*Crassostrea gigas*), 370
PALCAM agar. *See* Polymyxin B-acriflavin-lithium chloride-ceftazidime-esculin-mannitol agar (PALCAM agar)
PAM. *See* Primary meningoencephalitis (PAM)
Panaman leishmaniasis, 340
Panstrongylus spp., 318, 472
Pantoea agglomerans (*P. agglomerans*), 479
Pappataci fever. *See* Sandfly fever (SFF)
Papular stomatitis, 166, 167
Parachlamydia acanthamoebae (*P. acanthamoebae*), 201
Parachlamydiaceae, 199
Paragonimiasis, 376–378. *See also* Schistosomiasis
Paragonimus africanus (*P. africanus*), 376
Paragonimus heterotremus (*P. heterotremus*), 376
Paragonimus kellicotti (*P. kellicotti*), 376
Paragonimus mexicana (*P. mexicana*), 376
Paragonimus myazakii (*P. myazakii*), 376
Paragonimus skrjabini (*P. skrjabini*), 376
Paragonimus uterobilateralis (*P. uterobilateralis*), 377
Paragonimus westermani (*P. westermani*), 376
Paramyxoviridae, 119, 120, 122
Paramyxovirinae, 120
Paramyxoviruses, 119–120
  Newcastle disease, 120–122
  Nipah virus encephalitis, 124–126
  zoonoses caused by Hendra virus, 122–124
  zoonotic paramyxoviruses, 120
Parapoxvirus infections, 165
  contagious ecthyma of sheep, 165–166
  papular stomatitis, 166, 167
  pseudocowpox, 166, 167
Parasites, 486, 499
  acanthocephalan, 488
  helminth infections, 487
  metazoa, trematodes and cestodes, 487

protozoa, 486
protozoan infections transmitting by food, 486
Parasitic amebae, 307
Parasitic antigens, 310
Parasitic protozoa, 303
Parasitic zoonoses, 303. *See also* Viral zoonoses
  Acanthocephala, 447–448
  diagnostic methods in parasitology, 304
  intermediate hosts, 303
  parasitic protozoa, 303
  parasitological terms, 305–306
  pentastomids, 473–475
Parasitology, diagnostic methods in, 304
Parechovirus, 134
Parinaud's conjunctivitis, 270, 278
Parkinsonism-dementia complex. *See* Amyotrophic
  lateral sclerosis
Parvovirus, 2
Pasteurella spp., 232, 478, 479, 480
Pasteurelloses, 232–234
Pathogenicity islands, 257
PE. *See* Powassan encephalitis (PE)
Pediculus, 180, 190, 254
Pelecitus spp., 422
Pelican itch, 364
Peliosis, 182, 183
Penicillium spp., 486
Pentastomidosis, 473–475
Pentastomids, 474, 488
  infecting humans, 474
  pentastomidosis, 473–475
  zoonoses caused by, 473
Peptostreptococcus spp., 478
Peromyscus maniculatus (*P. maniculatus*), 84
PERV. *See* Porcine endogenous retroviruses (PERV)
PFGE. *See* Pulsed field gel electrophoresis (PFGE)
Pharyngitis, 101
Phlebotomus fever. *See* Sandfly fever (SFF)
Phlebotomus/Phlebotominae, 333, 460
Phlebotomus spp.. See sand flies (*Phlebotomus* spp.)
Photobacterium damsela (*P. damsela*), 479
Physaloptera caucasica (*P. caucasica*), 446
Phytotoxins transmitting by bats, 496
Pian bois, 339, 340
Picornaviridae, 134
Picornaviruses, 134
  EMC virus, 138
  FMD virus, 135–137
  SVD, 134–135
Pig bites, 480
Pigeon bug (*Cimex columbarius*), 471
Pipe head cercariae, 375
PKDL. *See* Post-kala-azar dermal leishmaniasis (PKDL)

Plague, 234, 503
  clinical manifestations, 236
  diagnosis, 236–237
  differential diagnosis, 237
  etiology, 234–235
  occurrence, 235
  prophylaxis, 237
  reporting, 237
  therapy, 237
  transmission, 235–236
Planorbis, 374
Plasmodium brasilianum (*P. brasilianum*), 346, 347
Plasmodium coatneyi (*P. coatneyi*), 346
Plasmodium cynomolgi (*P. cynomolgi*), 346, 347
Plasmodium eylesi (*P. eylesi*), 346
Plasmodium falciparum (*P. falciparum*), 347
Plasmodium inui (*P. inui*), 346
Plasmodium knowlesi (*P. knowlesi*), 345, 347
Plasmodium malariae (*P. malariae*), 345, 346
Plasmodium ovale (*P. ovale*), 345
Plasmodium schwetzi (*P. schwetzi*), 347
Plasmodium spp., 345–348, 500
Plasmodium vivax (*P. vivax*), 345
Plerocercoids, 388
Plesiomonas shigelloides (*P. shigelloides*), 484, 485
Pleuropulmonary amebiasis, 309
Pneumocystis carinii (*P. carinii*), 300, 301
Pneumocystis pneumonia (PCP). See Pneumocystosis
Pneumocystis spp. /Pneumocystosis, 300–302
Pneumonyssus infection, 458
Pneumonyssus simicola (*P. simicola*), 456, 458
Pneumonyssus spp., 456, 457, 458
Pneumovirinae, 120
Polymyxin B-acriflavin-lithium chloride-ceftazidime-
  esculin-mannitol agar (PALCAM agar), 221
Porcine disease, 125
Porcine endogenous retroviruses (PERV), 152
Porphyromonas spp., 478
Post-kala-azar dermal leishmaniasis (PKDL), 331
Postexposure vaccination, 37
Powassan encephalitis (PE), 27
Powassan virus encephalitis, 38–39
Pox-like disease, 159
Poxviridae, 155
Poxviruses, 1, 156
  individual orthopoxvirus infections, 159–165
  lesion transmission, 164
  Orthopoxvirus, 157
  Parapoxvirus, 157–158
  parapoxvirus infections, 165–167
  subfamilies, 156, 157
  zoonoses caused by orthopoxviruses, 158–159
  zoonoses caused by yabapoxviruses, 167

PPD. *See* Purified protein derivative (PPD)
PPI. *See* Proton pump inhibitor (PPI)
Praziquantel, 382
Pre-cyst, 301
Prevotella spp., 478, 480
Primary complex, 225, 270
Primary meningoencephalitis (PAM), 309
Primary myiasis, 464
Primate T-cell-lymphotropic viruses (PTLV), 147–148
Prion protein gene (PrP gene), 168
Prions, 168
  BSE and nvCJD, 169–174
  florid plaques, 169
  reproduction in lymphatic organs, 169
  transmissible spongiform encephalopathies, 167–169
Proglottids, 384
Propionibacterium spp., 478, 479
Proteinaceous infectious particles. *See* Prions
Proteus spp., 478, 479
Proton pump inhibitor (PPI), 287
Protozoa, 306. *See also* Parasitic zoonoses; Trematodes
  African trypanosomiasis, 351–355
  amebiasis, 307–311
  babesiosis, 312–315
  balantidiasis, 315–317
  Chagas' disease, 317–323
  cryptosporidiosis, 324–327
  giardiasis, 328–329
  leishmaniasis, 330–341
  microsporoses, 341–344
  monkey malaria, 345–348
  sarcosporidiosis, 348–351
  toxoplasmosis, 355–362
  zoonotic protozoal infections, 362–363
Provirus, 147
PrP gene. *See* Prion protein gene (PrP gene)
Pseudoamphistomum truncatum (*P. truncatum*), 375
Pseudoappendicitis, 278
Pseudocowpox, 166, 167
Pseudocysts, 356
Pseudomonas spp., 478–480
Pseudomyiasis. *See* Intestinal myiasis
Pseudophyllida, 384
Pseudophyllidea, 387
Pseudoscabies. *See* Sarcoptic mange
Pseudoterranova decipiens (codworm), 412
Pseudoterranova spp., 414
Pseudotuberculosis, 278
Psittacosis, 199, 201, 503
  clinical manifestations, 199–200
  diagnosis, 200
  differential diagnosis, 200
  occurrence, 199
  prophylaxis, 201
  reporting, 201
  therapy, 201
  transmission, 199
PTLV. *See* Primate T-cell-lymphotropic viruses (PTLV)
Pulex irritans (*P. irritans*), 467
Pulmonary anthrax, 176, 178
Pulmonary capillariasis, 417–418
Pulmonary distomatosis, 376–378
Pulsed field gel electrophoresis (PFGE), 263
Pupipara, 462
Purified protein derivative (PPD), 226
Purified rabies cell culture vaccines, 115
Pustule, malignant, 176
Puumala-like virus, 79
Puumala virus, 78
Pyemotes, 458
Pyrazinamide (PZA), 227

Q

Q-vax. *See* Inactivated phase vaccine
Q fever, 238, 503
  clinical manifestations, 240–241
  diagnosis, 241
  differential diagnosis, 241
  etiology, 238
  occurrence, 238, 239
  prophylaxis, 241–242
  reporting, 242
  therapy, 241
  transmission, 239–240
Quasispecies, 1–2

R

Rabies, 110, 477, 479
  clinical manifestations, 113–114
  diagnosis, 114–115
  differential diagnosis, 115
  etiology, 110
  infection chain, 111
  occurrence, 110, 111–112
  prophylaxis, 116–117
  recommendations for postexposure rabies prophylaxis, 111
  therapy, 115–116
  transmission, 112–113
  vaccination, 481
  virus, 479
Raccoons, 477–478
Raillietina spp., 408

Rat bite fever, 242
  clinical manifestations, 243
  diagnosis, 243–244
  differential diagnosis, 244
  etiology, 242–243
  occurrence, 243
  prophylaxis, 244
  therapy, 244
  transmission, 243
Rat bites, 480
16S rDNA analysis, 245
Rectal myiasis, 466
Relapsing fever, 189. *See also* Brucelloses; Lyme
    borreliosis
  Borrelia spp. of medical and veterinary significance,
      190
  clinical manifestations, 190–191
  diagnosis, 191
  differential diagnosis, 191
  etiology, 189
  occurrence, 189
  prophylaxis, 191
  therapy, 191
  transmission, 189
Reoviruses, 83
  Coltivirus, 83–85
  Orbivirus, 85
  rotavirus, 85–87
RES. *See* Reticuloendothelial system (RES)
Reston virus, 104
Reticulate bodies, 198, 199
Reticuloendothelial system (RES), 317
Retroviruses, 147
  endogenous retroviruses, 152–153
  lentiviruses, 149–152
  PTLV, 147–148
Reverse transcription polymerase chain reaction
    (RT-PCR), 15, 67, 69
  group-specific, 22, 24
RE virus. *See* Rocio encephalitis virus (RE virus)
Rhabdoviridae, 109
Rhabdoviruses, 109
  genetic program, 109, 110
  Lyssavirus, 109
  rabies, 110, 111–117
  recommendations for treatment of animal bites,
      110
  Vesiculovirus, 110
Rheumatic arthritis, 24
Rhinovirus, 134
Rhipicephalus conorii (*R. conorii*), 249–250
Rhipicephalus evertsi evertsi (*R. evertsi evertsi*), 455
Rhipicephalus spp., 190, 204, 248, 250, 450–452

Rhodnius prolixus (*R. prolixus*), 318, 472
Rhodococcus equi (*R. equi*), 290
  infections, 290
Rickettsia akari (*R. akari*), 252
  africae, 251
  conorii, 249–250
  mooseri, 254
  other spp., 251, 252
  prowazekii, 253, 254
  rickettsii, 248, 499
  typhi, 254, 255
Rickettsiaceae, 245
Rickettsiales, 202–203
Rickettsialpox, 252–253
Rickettsia spp., 244
Rickettsioses, 244, 502
  African tick bite fever, 251–252
  in Central Europe, 252
  epidemic typhus, 253–254
  features, 244–246
  human pathogenic *Rickettsia* spp., 245–246
  Mediterranean spotted fever, 249–251
  murine typhus, 254–255
  Rickettsialpox, 252–253
  RMSF, 248–249
  tsutsugamushi fever, 256–257
Riemerella anatipestifer (*R. anatipestifer*), 478
Rifampicin (RMP), 227
Rift Valley fever (RVF), 73
  clinical manifestations, 74–75
  diagnosis, 75
  differential diagnosis, 75
  etiology, 73
  occurrence, 73–74
  prophylaxis, 75
  therapy, 75
  transmission, 74
  virus, 4, 7, 65
RL. *See* Leishmaniasis recidivans (RL)
RMP. *See* Rifampicin (RMP)
RMSF. *See* Rocky mountain spotted fever (RMSF)
RNA viruses, 1
Roboviruses, 78
Rochalimaea, 245
Rocio encephalitis virus (RE virus), 3, 27, 28,
    48–49
Rocky mountain spotted fever (RMSF),
    248–249
Rodent-borne viruses. *See* Roboviruses
Rodentiosis, 278
Romana sign, 321
Ross river fever. *See* Epidemic polyarthritis
Ross River virus (RRV), 7, 18, 19

Rotavirus, 85
  clinical picture, 86–87
  diagnosis, 87
  differential diagnosis, 87
  etiology, 85–86
  occurrence, 86
  prophylaxis, 87
  therapy, 87
  transmission, 86
Rothia spp., 478, 479
Roussettus aegyptiacus (Flying fox), 97, 100,
    105, 112
RRV. *See* Ross River virus (RRV)
RSSE. *See* Russian spring summer encephalitis (RSSE)
RT-PCR. *See* Reverse transcription polymerase chain
    reaction (RT-PCR)
Rubella, 18, 20
Russian spring-summer meningoencephalitis (RSSE).
    See Russian spring summer encephalitis (RSSE)
Russian spring summer encephalitis (RSSE), 3, 27, 32
  clinical manifestations, 34–35
  diagnosis, 35–36
  differential diagnosis, 36
  etiology, 32
  occurrence, 32, 34
  prophylaxis, 36–37
  therapy, 36
  transmission, 34
RVF. *See* Rift Valley fever (RVF)

S
SAF techniques. *See* Sodium acetate-acetic acid
    formaldehyde techniques (SAF techniques)
Salivary trypanosomes, developmental cycle of, 352
Salmonella-Shigella (SS), 260
Salmonella spp./serovars, 257–261, 484, 499
Salmonelloses/Salmonellosis, 257, 503
  clinical manifestations, 259–260
  diagnosis, 260
  differential diagnosis, 260
  etiology, 257
  occurrence, 258
  prophylaxis, 260–261
  therapy, 260
  transmission, 258–259
Sand fly
  Phlebotominae, 460
  Phlebotomus species, 118
  species, 7
Sandfly fever (SFF), 76–77
Sandfly Naples (SFN), 76
Sandfly Sicilia (SFS), 76
Sandfly Toscana (SFT), 76

Sanguinivorous myiasis, 466
Sappinia spp., 309
Sarcocystis bovihominis (*S. bovihominis*), 349
Sarcocystis spp., 348–349, 487
  developmental cycle, 350
Sarcocystis suihominis (*S. suihominis*), 349
Sarcocystosis. *See* Sarcosporidiosis
Sarcophaga, 466, 488
Sarcoptes mites, 457
Sarcoptes spp., 457, 458, 459
Sarcoptic mange, 458
Sarcosporidiosis, 348
  clinical manifestations, 349–350
  diagnosis, 350
  differential diagnosis, 350
  etiology, 348–349
  occurrence, 349
  prophylaxis, 350–351
  therapy, 350
  transmission, 349
SARS-CoV. *See* Severe acute respiratory syndrome
    associated coronavirus (SARS-CoV)
SARS. *See* Severe acute respiratory syndrome (SARS)
Schistosoma mansoni (*S. mansoni*), 378, 379, 381
  cercariae, 379
  developmental cycle, 381
Schistosoma spp., 378, 379
  eggs, 379
  S. bovis, 378
  S. haematobium, 378, 379, 380, 382
  S. intercalatum, 378
  S. japonicum, 378, 379, 381, 382
  S. magrebowiei, 378
  S. malayensis, 378
  S. matheei, 378
  S. mekongi, 378
  S. rodhaini, 378
Schistosomiasis, 378
  chronic, 380
  clinical manifestations, 380
  diagnosis, 381–382
  differential diagnosis, 382
  etiology, 378
  of intestinal tract, 380
  occurrence, 378–379
  prophylaxis, 382
  sequelae of schistosomal infections, 380–381
  therapy, 382
  transmission, 379–380
Scrapie, 500
  in sheep, 170
Scrub typhus. *See* Tsutsugamushi fever
Scutula, 297

SCV. *See* Small cell variants (SCV)
SEA. *See* Soluble egg antigens (SEA)
Seal bites, 480
Seal finger, 480
Segmentina, 374
Semliki Forest fever, 16–17
Semliki Forest virus (SFV), 16
Seoul virus, 79
Septicemia, 212
Serodiagnosis, 22
Serodiagnostic methods, 329
Serogroup A. *See Streptococcus pyogenes* (*S. pyogenes*)
Serogroup B. *See Streptococcus agalactiae*
    (*S. agalactiae*)
Serologic techniques, 322
Serology, 193, 271
Serratia marcescens (*S. marcescens*), 479
Serratia spp., 479, 480
Severe acute respiratory syndrome (SARS), 141
    clinical manifestations, 143–144
    diagnosis, 144
    differential diagnosis, 144
    etiology, 141, 142
    occurrence, 142
    prophylaxis, 144
    therapy, 144
    transmission, 142–143
Severe acute respiratory syndrome associated
    coronavirus (SARS-CoV), 4, 141, 143
SFF. *See* Sandfly fever (SFF)
SFN. *See* Sandfly Naples (SFN)
SFS. *See* Sandfly Sicilia (SFS)
SFT. *See* Sandfly Toscana (SFT)
SFV. *See* Semliki Forest virus (SFV)
sGP. *See* soluble glycoprotein (sGP)
Shark bites, 479
Sheep bites, 480
Shellfish poisoning, 488, 495
Shewanella spp., 479
Shiga toxin *Escherichia coli* (STEC), 206
Shiga toxins (Stx), 206, 207
Simian bites, 478–479
Simian herpes infection, 153–156
Simian immunodeficiency virus (SIV), 149
Simian malaria. *See* Monkey malaria
Simian T-cell leukemia virus (STLV), 147
Simian virus 40 (SV40), 3
Simkaniaceae, 199
Sindbis fever, 17–18
Single point mutation, 1
Sin Nombre disease. *See* Hantavirus pulmonary
    syndrome (HPS)
Sin Nombre virus, 78

Siphonaptera, 467–469
SIV. *See* Simian immunodeficiency virus (SIV)
Skunks, 477–478
Sleeping sickness. *See* African trypanosomiasis
SLE virus. *See* St. Louis encephalitis virus (SLE virus)
SMAC. *See* Sorbitol-MacConkey agar (SMAC)
Small babesia, 312
Small cell variants (SCV), 238
Smears, 344
Snake bites, 480
Snowshoe hare virus, 68–69
Sodium acetate-acetic acid formaldehyde techniques
    (SAF techniques), 310
Sodium stibogluconate (SSG), 336
Soft ticks, 449
Soluble egg antigens (SEA), 381
soluble glycoprotein (sGP), 98
Sorbitol-MacConkey agar (SMAC), 209
Spargana, 401
Sparganosis, 401–402
Sparganum, 401
Sparganum proliferum (*S. proliferum*), 401
Spirillum minus (*S. minus*), 242, 480
Spirometra erinaceieuropaei (*S. erinaceieuropaei*), 401
Spirometra mansoni (*S. mansoni*), 401
Spirometra mansonoides (*S. mansonoides*), 401
Spirometra spp., 401
Spores, 343
Sporocyst, 301
Sporothrixschenckii/Sporotrichosis, 298, 478, 479
    clinical manifestations, 299
    diagnosis, 299
    etiology, 298
    prophylaxis, 300
    therapy, 299–300
Sporozoites, 356
Spotted fever diseases, 251–252
Spotted fever rickettsioses, 245, 246, 503
Squirrel bites, 479
SS. *See* Salmonella-Shigella (SS)
S. scabiei var. bovis, 457
S. scabiei var. canis, 457
SSG. *See* Sodium stibogluconate (SSG)
Staggers. *See* Gid
Staphylococcal infections, 262–263
Staphylococcus aureus (*S. aureus*), 479
Staphylococcus spp., 262, 478–480, 484
    infections, 262
STEC. *See* Shiga toxin *Escherichia coli* (STEC)
Stegomyia albopicta. *See* Asian "tiger mosquito"
    (*Stegomyia albopicta*)
Stegomyia albopicta (*S. albopicta*), 53, 58, 68
Stegomyia nivea (*S. nivea*), 62

Stegomyia triseriata (*S. triseriata*), 68
Stellantchasmus falcatus, 203
Stenotrophomonas maltophilia, 478
Sticktight (bird) flea (*Echidnophaga gallinacean*), 467
St. Louis encephalitis virus (SLE virus), 7, 27, 28, 46–47
STLV. *See* Simian T-cell leukemia virus (STLV)
Stomoxys spp., 185, 462, 463
Straw itch mites, 458
Streptobacillus moniliformis (*S. moniliformis*), 242–243, 480
Streptococcal infections, 264
  features, 264
  infections with other *streptococcus* spp., 267–268
  S. agalactiae, 267
  S. equi infections, 264–265
  S. pyogenes, 267
  S. suis infections, 266
Streptococcus agalactiae (*S. agalactiae*), 267, 480
  equi (groups C and G), 264, 480
  groups E, G, L, P, U, V, 267, 268
  iniae, 268
  other spp, 478, 479, 480, 484
  pyogenes (group A), 267, 480
  suis (group R, S, T), 266, 480
Streptococcus equi (*S. equi*), 264
  infections, 264–265
Streptococcus pyogenes (*S. pyogenes*), 267
Streptococcus suis (*S. suis*), 266
Strobila, 384
Strongyloides fuelleborni (*S. fuelleborni*), 436
Strongyloides fuelleborni kellyi (*S. fuelleborni kellyi*), 436
Strongyloides spp., 430, 431, 435
Strongyloides stercoralis (*S. stercoralis*), 431, 436
  developmental cycle, 436
Strongyloides stercoralis (*S. stercoralis*), 501
Strongyloidiasis, 435–437, 499, 501
Stx. *See* Shiga toxins (Stx)
Subgenomic polycistronic mRNA (26S RNA), 8
Subtype-specific reactivity of flaviviruses, 26
Surra, 363
SV40. *See* Simian virus 40 (SV40)
SVD. *See* Swine vesicular disease (SVD)
SVDV. *See* Swine vesicular disease virus (SVDV)
Swallow bug (*Cimex. hirundinis*), 471
Swine influenza virus, 129–131. *See also* Avian influenza viruses
Swine vesicular disease (SVD), 134–135
Swine vesicular disease virus (SVDV), 134
Syncytin I, 152
Syncytin II, 152
Syngamiasis, 438–439

T
Tabanids, 463
Tabanus spp. /Tabanidae, 185, 460
Tabardillo, 254–255
Tache noire, 250
Tachyzoites, 358
Taenia
  genus, 384
  infections, 488
Taenia brauni (*T. brauni*), 385
Taenia crassiceps (*T. crassiceps*), 409
Taenia glomerata (*T. glomerata*), 385
Taenia multiceps (*T. multiceps*), 385
Taenia serialis (*T. serialis*), 385
Taeniasis asiatica (*T. asiatica*), 402, 488
Taeniasis saginata (*T. saginata*), 402–404, 409, 488
Taenia solium (*T. solium*), 405–407, 409, 488
Tahynavirus, 68–69
Tanapox virus, 167
Tapeworms, 384
TBE. *See* Tick-borne encephalitis (TBE)
TCP. *See* Toxin-coregulated pilus (TCP)
Ternidens deminutus (*T. deminutus*), 446
Tetanus prophylaxis, 156
Tetanus toxoid, 481
Tetraparesis, 90
Tetrathyridia, 408
Thelazia californiensis (*T. californiensis*), 439
Thelazia callipaeda (*T. callipaeda*), 439
Thelazia rhodesi (*T. rhodesi*), 439
Thelaziasis, 439
Thelazia spp./Thelaziasis, 439
Thermophilic agents, 195
Thogoto virus, 127, 133–134
Thrombocytopenia, 62
Thrombotic-thrombocytopenic purpura (TTP), 206
TIBOLA. *See* Tick-borne lymphadenopathy (TIBOLA)
Tick-borne Dhori virus, 127
Tick-borne encephalitis (TBE), 27, 32
  areas in Eurasia, 33
  clinical manifestations, 34–35
  diagnosis, 35–36
  differential diagnosis, 36
  etiology, 32
  infectious cycle, 35
  occurrence, 32, 34
  prophylaxis, 36–37
  therapy, 36
  transmission, 34
  virus infection, 33–34
Tick-borne flaviviruses, 32, 483
  KFD and Alkhurma virus hemorrhagic fever, 39–40
  LI, 37–38

OHF, 40–41
Powassan virus encephalitis, 38–39
TBE, 32–37
Tick-borne lymphadenopathy (TIBOLA), 252
Tick bites, 449. *See also* Flea bites
   clinical manifestations, 453–454
   diagnosis, 454
   differential diagnosis, 454
   etiology, 449–450
   occurrence, 450–453
   prophylaxis, 454
   therapy, 454
   transmission, 453
Tick paralysis. *See* Tick toxicoses
Ticks, 449
   genera of ticks, geographical distribution and number of hosts, 450
   paralyses/toxicoses, 454–455
   sand flies, 5
   tick bites, 449–454
   tick toxicoses, 454–455
   as vectors of diseases, 451
   virus complex transmitted by, 27
   zoonoses caused by, 449
Tick toxicoses, 454–455
Tinea barbae, 296, 297
   capitis, 293
   corporis, 293
Tioman virus, 122
Tir. *See* Translocated intimin receptor (Tir)
Tongue worms. *See* Pentastomids
Toulon typhus, 254–255
Toxin-coregulated pilus (TCP), 273
Toxocara, 303, 432, 446
Toxocara canis (*T. canis*), 432
Toxocara cati (*T. cati*), 432, 433, 447
Toxoplasma gondii (*T. gondii*), 304, 355, 358
   developmental cycle and transmission, 356
   oocyst in feces of cat, 357
   tissue cyst in brain, 357
Toxoplasmosis, 304, 355, 487, 499
   acute *T. gondii* infection, 359
   clinical manifestations, 359
   diagnosis, 360
   differential diagnosis, 360
   etiology, 355–356
   in immunocompromised adults, 359
   occurrence, 356–357
   ocular, 359
   in pregnancy and congenital toxoplasmosis, 359–360

   prophylaxis, 361–362
   therapy, 360–361
   transmission, 357–359
Transfusion, transmission by, 500
Translocated intimin receptor (Tir), 207
Transmissible spongiform encephalopathies, 167–169, 170
Transmissible subacute dementia. *See* Bovine spongiform encephalopathy (BSE)
Transmission, iatrogenic, 499
Trapa bicornis (*T. bicornis*), 374
Trapa natans (*T. natans*), 374
Trematodes, 363. *See also* Parasitic zoonoses; Protozoa
   Cercarial dermatitis, 363–365
   clonorchiasis, 366–367
   dicrocoeliais, 368–369
   dwarf fluke infections, 369–370
   fascioliasis, 370–373
   fasciolopsiasis, 374–375
   opisthorchiasis, 375–376
   paragonimiasis, 376–378
   schistosomiasis, 378–382
   zoonotic trematode infections, 383–384
Trench fever, 182
Triatoma, 318, 472
Triatoma rubrofasciata (*T. rubrofasciata*), 472
Triatomine(s), 472
   bugs, 319
Trichinella larvae, 444
Trichinella papuae (*T. papuae*), 442
Trichinella pseudospiralis (*T. pseudospiralis*), 440, 442
Trichinella spiralis (*T. spiralis*), 440, 442
   developmental cycle, 443
Trichinella spp./Trichin (ell) osis, 440, 488
Trichinella zimbabwensis (*T. zimbabwensis*), 440, 442
Trichinellosis, 440
   clinical manifestations, 442–443
   diagnosis, 443–444
   differential diagnosis, 444
   etiology, 440
   occurrence, 440
   prophylaxis, 444
   therapy, 444
   transmission, 440–442
Trichinosis. *See* Trichinellosis
Trichobilharzia, 364
Trichobilharzia franki (*T. franki*), 364
Trichobilharzia ocellata (*T. ocellata*), 364
Trichobilharzia spp., 364

Trichophyton spp., 296
  clinical manifestations, 296–297
  diagnosis, 297–298
  etiology, 296
  superficial trichophytosis, 297
  therapy, 298
Trichophytosis, 296, 297
Trichostrongyles, 445
Trichostrongylidiasis, 445–446
Trichostrongylosis. *See* Trichostrongylidiasis
Trichostrongylus spp., 445
Trichuris, 304
Trombicula akamushi (*T. akamushi*), 456
Trombicula spp./Trombiculosis, 180, 256, 457
Trombiculid mites, 456
Trombiculosis, 457
Trombidiosis, 458
Trombidium irritans (*T. irritans*), 456
Trombidium spp., 456
Trophozoites, 307
Tropical bed bug (*Cimex hemipterus*), 471, 472
Tropical eosinophilia, 422
Tropical liver abscess, 309
Trueperella pyogenes (*T. pyogenes*), 291
Trypanosoma brucei evansi (*T. brucei evansi*), 363
Trypanosoma brucei gambiense (*T. brucei gambiense*),
  351, 352, 353, 354
Trypanosoma brucei rhodesiense (*T. brucei*
  rhodesiense), 351, 352, 353, 354
Trypanosoma congolense (*T. congolense*), 363
Trypanosoma cruzi (*T. cruzi*), 317, 471
  developmental cycle, 319
  infection of humans with, 320
Trypanosoma lewisi (*T. lewisi*), 362
Trypanosoma spp., 317, 330, 362, 471, 499
Trypanosomatidae, 351
Trypanosomes, 354, 500
Trypanosomiasis, 317
Tsetse-belt, 352
Tsetse flies (Glossinidae), 462
TSL-1 group, 443
Tsutsugamushi fever, 256–257
TTP. *See* Thrombotic-thrombocytopenic purpura
  (TTP)
Tuberculosis, 223
  clinical manifestations, 224, 225
  diagnosis, 225–226
  differential diagnosis, 226–227
  etiology, 223
  occurrence, 223–224
  prophylaxis, 227
  reporting, 227
  therapy, 227
  transmission, 224
Tularemia, 269–271
Tularensis, 269
Tunga penetrans (*T. penetrans*), 469, 470
Tungiasis, 469–470
26S RNA. *See* Subgenomic polycistronic mRNA
  (26S RNA)

U

Uncinaria spp., 430
  U. stenocephala, 430–431
Urban transmission cycles, 7–8
Urogenital myiasis, 466
Uta, 339, 340

V

Vaccination, 315
  campaigns, 37
  poliomyelitis, 3
  postexposure, 115
  prophylactic, 116
Vaccinia-rabies glycoprotein vaccines, 163
Vaccinia virus, 160
  clinical manifestations, 161
  confluent generalized vaccinia, 161
  diagnosis, 161, 162
  etiology, 160
  local pox after vaccination with, 161
  occurrence, 160
  prophylaxis, 162–163
  therapy, 162
  transmission, 160–161
Variable major protein (Vmp), 189
Variola virus, 156
VD. *See* Vesicular disease (VD)
VEE. *See* Venezuelan equine encephalitis (VEE)
Veillonella parvula (*V. parvula*), 479
Venezuelan equine encephalitis (VEE),
  14–15
Venezuelan hemorrhagic fever (VHF),
  95–97
Venezuelan horse encephalitis virus, 2
Verotoxigenic Escherichia coli, 206, 504
Verruca peruana, 179
Vesicular disease (VD), 119
Vesicular stomatitis (VS), 117–119
Vesicular stomatitis viruses (VSV), 118
Vesiculovirus, 110
VHF. *See* Venezuelan hemorrhagic fever (VHF)
Viannia, 330
Vibrio cholerae (*V. cholerae*), 273
  El Tor, 273
  spp., 275, 479, 484

Vibrioses, 272, 504
  cholera, 273–274
  disease due to other *vibrio* spp., 275
Vibrio spp., 272, 275
Viral glycoproteins, 8
Viral receptors, 86
Viral zoonoses, 1. *See also* Bacterial zoonoses;
    Parasitic zoonoses
  associated with prions, 167–174
  caused by alphaviruses, 8–26
  caused by arenaviruses, 88–94
  caused by bunyaviruses, 65–77
  caused by filoviruses, 97–108
  caused by flaviviruses, 26–41
  caused by hantaviruses, 78–82
  caused by herpesviruses, 153–156
  caused by mosquito-borne flaviviruses,
      41–64
  caused by new world arenaviruses, 95–97
  caused by orthomyxoviruses, 127–134
  caused by paramyxoviruses, 119–126
  caused by picornaviruses, 134–138
  caused by poxviruses, 156–167
  caused by reoviruses, 83–87
  caused by rhabdoviruses, 109–117
  classification principles, 1
  coronaviruses, 139–146
  cycles of arbovirus infections, 5–8
  hepatitis E, 138–139
  retroviruses, 147–153
  vesicular stomatitis, 117–119
  zoonotic viruses, 1–5
Virulence factors, 175
Virus(es), 1, 483–484, 499
  replication, 86
  vaccine, 43
Visceral larva migrans (VLM). See Larva migrans
    visceralis
Visceral leishmaniasis, 332
  child with kala-azar, 335
  clinical manifestations, 334–335
  diagnosis, 335–336
  differential diagnosis, 336
  etiology, 332–333
  excessive growth of eyelashes, 334
  occurrence, 333–334
  prophylaxis, 336–337
  therapy, 336
  transmission, 334
Visceral linguatulosis, 475
Visna virus (VV), 149
Viverra zibetha. *See* Indian Civet
    (*Viverra zibetha*)

Vmp. *See* Variable major protein (Vmp)
VS. *See* Vesicular stomatitis (VS)
VSV. *See* Vesicular stomatitis viruses (VSV)
VV. *See* Visna virus (VV)

W
Waddliaceae, 199
Washed sheep erythrocytes, antibiotics, and calcium
    ions (WSBA-Ca), 210
WEE. *See* Western equine encephalitis (WEE)
Weil-Felix reaction, 246
Wesselsbron fever, 52–53
Western equine encephalitis (WEE), 12–14, 46
West Nile fever (WNF), 27, 49–51
West Nile virus (WNV), 5, 7, 28
WHO. *See* World Health Organization (WHO)
WNF. *See* West Nile fever (WNF)
WNV. *See* West Nile virus (WNV)
Wolbachia, 421
World Health Organization (WHO),
    194, 308
Wound myiasis, 464, 465
WSBA-Ca. *See* Washed sheep erythrocytes,
    antibiotics, and calcium ions (WSBA-Ca)
Wuchereria bancrofti (*W. bancrofti*), 422
Wuchereria spp., 422, 424

X
XDR. *See* Extensive resistance (XDR)
Xenopsyllacheopis, 235, 255, 467
Xenotransplantation, 152, 500
XMRV, 2–3

Y
Yaba monkey tumor virus, 167
Yabapoxviruses, 167
YELAND. *See* Yellow fever vaccine associated
    neurologic disease (YELAND)
Yellow fever (YF), 27, 53
  animal infections with flaviviruses, 29
  areas with transmission risk, 54
  clinical manifestations, 29, 55
  diagnosis, 29–30, 55–56
  differential diagnosis, 56
  etiology, 53
  occurrence, 27–28, 53, 55
  prophylaxis, 30, 56–57
  therapy, 30, 56
  transmission, 28–29, 55
  vaccination and problem of immune enhancement,
      30–31
Yellow fever vaccine associated neurologic disease
    (YELAND), 57

Yersinia, 276
Yersinia enterocolitica (*Y. enterocolitica*),
    276–280, 500
  pestis 234
  pseudotuberculosis 276–280
Yersinia pestis (*Y. pestis*), 234
Yersinioses, 276
  clinical manifestations,
    277–278
  diagnosis, 278–279
  differential diagnosis, 279
  etiology, 276
  frequent manifestations of enteral, 278
  occurrence, 276–277
  prophylaxis, 279
  therapy, 279
  transmission, 277
Yersinioses, enteral, 278, 412
YF. *See* Yellow fever (YF)

Z
Zaire subtype of Ebola virus, 104
ZMapp, 108
Zoonotic bacteria, 500
Zoonotic cestode infections, 408
Zoonotic diseases notifiable at National level,
    503–504
Zoonotic mycobacterioses, 229
  MAA infections, 230
  MAH infections, 230–231
  MAP infections, 231
  Mycobacterium genavense infections, 232
Zoonotic protozoal infections, 362–363
Zoonotic trematode infections, 383–384
Zoonotic viruses, 1–3
  as B-weapons, 4
  Bat-borne viruses, 3–4
  diagnostic procedures, 5
  global distribution of zoonotic agents, 4–5